D0743274

CONTEMPORARY ORAL AND MAXILLOFACIAL PATHOLOGY

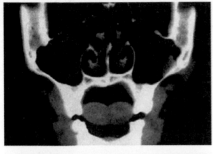

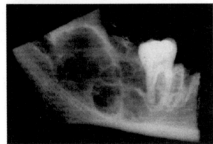

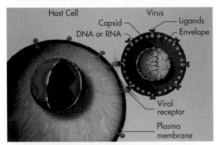

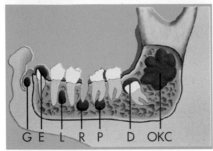

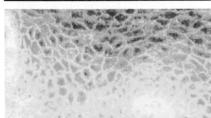

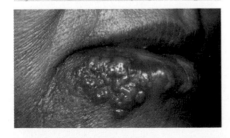

CONTEMPORARY ORAL AND MAXILLOFACIAL PATHOLOGY

J. PHILIP SAPP, D.D.S., M.S.

Diplomate,
American Board of Oral and Maxillofacial Pathology;
Professor,
Section of Diagnostic Sciences,
School of Dentistry,
University of California,
Los Angeles, California

LEWIS R. EVERSOLE, D.D.S., M.S.D., M.A.

Diplomate,
American Board of Oral and Maxillofacial Pathology;
Professor,
Section of Diagnostic Sciences,
School of Dentistry,
University of California,
Los Angeles, California

GEORGE P. WYSOCKI, D.D.S., Ph.D.

Diplomate,
American Board of Oral and Maxillofacial Pathology;
Professor and Chair,
Division of Oral Pathology,
Department of Pathology,
School of Medicine and Dentistry,
University of Western Ontario,
London, Ontario

with 839 illustrations

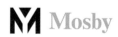 Mosby

St. Louis Baltimore Boston Carlsbad Chicago Naples New York Philadelphia Portland
London Madrid Mexico City Singapore Sydney Tokyo Toronto Wiesbaden

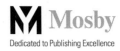

Mosby
Dedicated to Publishing Excellence

A Times Mirror
Company

PUBLISHER: Alison Harrison
EDITOR: Linda L. Duncan
DEVELOPMENTAL EDITOR: Jo Salway
PROJECT MANAGER: John Rogers
PRODUCTION EDITOR: Cheryl Abbott Bozzay
DESIGNER: Lee Goldstein
DESIGN MANAGER: Yael Kats

COVER

Clockwise from upper right:

· Diagram of the basic structure of a virus.
· Antral mucocele. CT scan of polypoid lesion on lateral wall of maxillary sinus.
· Pemphigus vulgaris. Characteristic "fishnet" pattern of antigen-antibody complexes surrounding cells at site of destruction of the epithelial intercellular cohesive system.
· Early stages of recurrent herpes labialis.
· Diagram of odontogenic cysts.
· Odontogenic myxoma. Multicellular lesion in resected mandible.

Printed in the United States of America
Composition by The Clarinda Company
Printing/Binding by Von Hoffmann Press, Inc.

Mosby–Year Book, Inc.
11830 Westline Industrial Drive
St. Louis, Missouri 63146

International Standard Book Number 0-8016-6918-9

96 97 98 99 00 / 9 8 7 6 5 4 3 2 1

To
present and future students and clinicians
who possess an ardent desire
to be truly knowledgeable of
the oral and maxillofacial diseases
that afflict humankind.

PREFACE

Contemporary Oral and Maxillofacial Pathology will help students acquire a sound basic knowledge of oral and maxillofacial diseases; it is a concise, organized source of current information in a visually pleasing format with ample color illustrations. It is not meant to be all inclusive in its coverage of the diseases that affect the oral and maxillofacial region but rather an aid for students who wish to acquire a working knowledge of the more common and important conditions found in patients. The less common entities and lesser known variants of common lesions have been either omitted or discussed very briefly. The breadth and depth of the subjects covered in the book should provide sufficient information for candidates preparing for certification in many specialities. The practicing clinician will find the book to be a useful chairside resource and a means to rapidly find and differentiate similarly named or closely associated conditions and to quickly become familiar with their pertinent features and management.

The book is formatted and designed to be user friendly for both students and clinicians. The concise style should obviate the need for instructors to provide substantial supplemental course handouts and the ample number of color illustrations, the need to purchase an accompanying color atlas. Color-screened definitions provide an overview of the distinguishing features of each disease and succinctly differentiate it from others that appear similar. The definitions also provide a means for the reader to scan through the book and quickly review pertinent information. The authors have made an effort to use either the most updated terminology or the most common usage.

The textbook has been specifically designed to encourage and facilitate a *basic understanding* of groups of disease processes rather than just memorization of factual information regarding individual entities. This approach is based on the premise that the higher the student's level of understanding of basic disease processes the higher the student's level of retention. To this end, the text utilizes short reviews of foundational information and an extensive amount of diagrams and other visual material. The reduced size of illustrations not only allows for a greater number of illustrations for each individual disease, it also allows for closer placement to the corresponding text so that the clinical and laboratory features of a disease will be more clearly understood when variations are encountered in a future clinical setting. Another important aid to learning and understanding is the addition of line tracings of the salient microscopic features of the more complex photomicrographs.

Additional Reading found at the end of each chapter is a selection of resources categorized according to disease. The citations selected represent recent publications and/or contain updated information and are not intended to be an exhaustive list. The occasional older citations were included because of their contribution to the development of an understanding of the condition. In some chapters *Additional Reading* contains a *General* category, which provides recent sources such as proceedings of workshops, monographs, and invited reviews covering broad categories of diseases, most of which contain thorough and in-depth bibliographies.

The chapters are organized in a manner that has been found to be convenient for most course instructors of oral and maxillofacial pathology, and one that allows some of the subject material to be taught at an earlier stage of a predoctoral curriculum. The order in which the conditions are presented will most likely dovetail with the sequencing of prerequisite and closely allied courses of the curriculum of most dental schools.

Chapter 1, *Developmental Disturbances of the Oral Region*, deals with common developmental conditions of the teeth, soft tissue, and bone. These conditions are usually covered early in most curriculums.

Chapter 2, *Cysts of the Oral Region*, is also easily comprehended early in the curriculum because the prerequisite is only a basic knowledge of odontogenesis and the embryology of the head and neck.

Chapter 3, *Infections of Teeth and Bone*, requires fundamental knowledge of bacteriology and the mechanisms of inflammation and repair. This chapter is presented from a pathologist's perspective and emphasizes those aspects of dental caries, pulpitis, and periapical lesions that are frequently not emphasized in other courses. The conditions are presented as part of a continuum of a single disease process.

Chapter 4, *Bone Lesions*, discusses the concept of nonneoplastic and noninflammatory alterations in bone formation within the jaws. The chapter also discusses the difficult concepts inherent in those entities categorized as benign bone lesions but that are in reality a collection of hyperplastic, hamartomatous, reactive conditions and few actual benign bone neoplasms.

Chapter 5, *Odontogenic Tumors*, begins with a review of the fundamental aspects of odontogenesis. The authors have found such a review necessary for students and clinicians to gain a complete understanding of the nomenclature, classification, and biologic nature of odontogenic lesions. To facilitate the learning process, the authors have presented a classification for the separation of these relatively rare malignant odontogenic lesions.

Chapter 6, *Epithelial Disorders*, is restricted to the preneoplastic, benign, and malignant conditions that affect the intraoral and perioral epithelial layers. This chapter also includes the pigmented lesions and those that metastasize to the soft tissues and bones.

Chapter 7, *Oral Infections*, is organized differently from the other chapters. The diseases are organized and presented under the genus and species of the infectious agents, which is the same format used in prerequisite microbiology courses. This format will facilitate the learning process because the student can more easily build upon the clinical information regarding oral diseases using the previously established framework. Because of the recent epidemic of the human immunodeficiency virus (HIV) and its impact on health care workers, a significant portion of the chapter is devoted to understanding the basic principles regarding a retroviral infection and its systemic and oral manifestations.

Chapter 8, *Immune-Mediated Disorders*, is unique in that it places all the conditions that are due to or suspected of being due to dysfunctions of the immune system together in one chapter, except for Sjögren syndrome and benign lymphoepithelial lesions, which are included in Chapter 10. The chapter emphasizes recent information on the basic mechanisms contributing to the pathogenesis of each of the desquamative diseases and their specific target antigens.

Chapter 9, *Connective Tissue Lesions*, contains the largest number of individual disease entities, which are categorized according to their tissue of origin. Within each category the lesions are further grouped as hyperplasias, hamartomas, and benign and malignant neoplasms. Because of the extensive amount of continuous minor trauma ("wear and tear") to the oral tissues due to mastication, abusive oral hygiene practices, and the presence of oral appliances, the reactive hyperplastic lesions of the fibrous connective tissue predominate the overall incidence of oral lesions.

Chapter 10, *Salivary Gland Disorders*, includes a review of the basic morphologic component of this tissue, the glandular secretory unit. The unit is diagrammed and reproduced in miniature throughout the chapter to help illustrate the basic alteration from normal that leads to the development of the disease process. It is included as an inset adjacent to each tracing of the pertinent histologic features of a salivary gland neoplasms, where it is used to correlate the basic neoplastic tumor cell with the theoretical cell of origin.

Chapter 11, *Physical and Chemical Injuries*, contains some entities discussed in Chapter 9. Those repeated consist of some of the reactive fibrous hyperplasias due to chronic mechanical irritation and those that result from taking selected medications. The tissue changes and other complications associated with treatments utilizing therapeutic doses of radiation are also included.

Chapter 12, *Diseases of Blood*, is a compilation of the conditions that would most likely be encountered in patients seen during a general or speciality practice. Since a large number of the conditions are dysfunctions of cells or of the clotting mechanism and are apparent only through laboratory results, there is generally a lack of illustrations of the clinical features associated with these conditions. This necessitated a greater dependence on diagrams and an additional heading for laboratory procedures and results for most entities.

ACKNOWLEDGMENTS

The production of a textbook in a specialized field is the culmination of many years of contemplating fundamental principles conveyed by early mentors; continually scrutinizing the literature to remain abreast of advances; and ardently collecting, developing, and refining illustrative material. Many of these activities can only be achieved with the help of professional colleagues. To those colleagues with whom the authors have interacted and benefited professionally, a heartfelt thanks is extended.

Particular acknowledgment is extended to Dr. William G. Shafer and the late Dr. Donald A. Kerr for their guidance and direction during the introductory and formative years of our careers. A special thanks is extended to Dr. David G. Gardner who provided collegial advice during the early academic years of one of the authors (JPS) and who willingly shared in the compilation of visual teaching materials, some of which appear in this textbook without specific acknowledgment.

The book would not have been possible without the help and cooperation of past and present colleagues with whom the authors have worked closely. Many of the illustrations are teaching materials procured collectively and shared with those colleagues. Special thanks and appreciation are extended to Dr. Tom Daley, University of Western Ontario; Dr. Russell Christensen and Dr. Frank Lucatorto, University of California, Los Angeles; Dr. Alan Leider, University of the Pacific; Dr. Ron Baughman, University of Florida; and Dr. William Sabes. For any images that may have been published that were inadvertently not acknowledged, we apologize. Every effort was made to follow up on any available information that would identify the actual source of the material that was in the teaching collections of the authors and used in this text. Since the origin of some of the material extends beyond a 20-year period, this was occasionally difficult.

We wish to acknowledge the exquisite computer-generated graphic illustrations produced by Mr. Patrick Masson of the UCLA School of Dentistry Illustration and Media Center and the help he provided during the preparation of the book.

We would also like to thank the editorial and production staff of Mosby–Year Book, Inc., especially Ms. Linda Duncan, the editor of the project, for her guidance, vision, and support in bringing the concept of the book to reality; Ms. Jo Salway, Developmental Editor; and Ms. Cheryl Abbott Bozzay, a very competent and highly professional production editor, for keeping the project under control at all times and for her patience, help, and understanding throughout the most difficult periods.

And finally, a special thanks is extended to our families, friends, and colleagues who were neglected in various ways during the arduous hours required to see the project to fruition.

J. PHILIP SAPP
LEWIS R. EVERSOLE
GEORGE P. WYSOCKI

C ONTENTS

DEVELOPMENTAL DISTURBANCES OF THE ORAL REGION

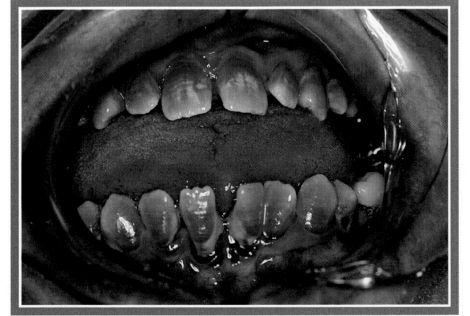

evelopmental disturbances of the oral region are discussed under three broad categories: (1) developmental disturbances affecting teeth, (2) developmental disturbances limited to soft tissue, and (3) developmental disturbances affecting bone.

TEETH

DISTURBANCES IN SIZE

Microdontia

■ MICRODONTIA: one or more teeth that are smaller than normal.

When all teeth in both arches are smaller than normal, the condition is termed *generalized microdontia*. If all the teeth are uniformly smaller than normal, which occurs in uncommon conditions such as pituitary dwarfism, the condition is termed *true generalized microdontia*. The term *relative generalized microdontia* is used when the mandible and maxilla are somewhat larger than normal but the teeth are of normal size, giving the illusion of generalized microdontia. In the latter, the teeth are spaced.

Microdontia involving one or two teeth is far more common than the generalized types. Individual teeth most frequently affected by microdontia are the maxillary lateral incisors ("peg laterals") and the maxillary third molars. In addition to being miniature teeth, they are often conically shaped (Figure 1-1) and congenitally absent. However, maxillary and mandibular second premolars, which are often congenitally absent, rarely exhibit microdontia. Supernumerary teeth are also smaller than normal and conically shaped.

FIGURE 1-1

Microdontia. Most common single tooth involvement of maxillary lateral incisor ("peg lateral").

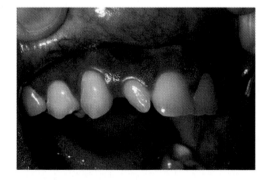

Macrodontia

■ MACRODONTIA: one or more teeth that are larger than normal.

When all teeth in both arches are measurably larger than normal, the condition is termed *true generalized macrodontia* and seen in rare conditions such as pituitary gigantism. The term *relative generalized macrodontia* is used to describe a condition in which the mandible and/or the maxilla are somewhat smaller than normal but the teeth are normal in size. In this condition, the arches exhibit crowding of teeth. Regional or localized macrodontia is occasionally seen on the affected side of the mouth in patients with hemifacial hypertrophy. Macrodontia of an individual tooth is occasionally seen but is rare and should not be confused with the fusion of two adjacent teeth.

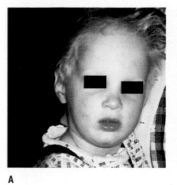
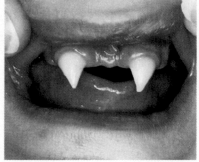
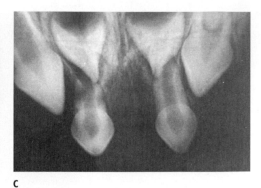

A

B

C

FIGURE 1-2

Anodontia. Young patient with ectodermal dysplasia. **A,** Lanugo hair. **B,** Two conical cuspids. **C,** Radiograph revealing several additional abnormally shaped unerupted permanent teeth. (Courtesy Dr. David G. Gardner.)

DISTURBANCES IN NUMBER

Total and Partial Anodontia

■ TOTAL ANODONTIA: congenital absence of all teeth.

■ PARTIAL ANODONTIA (HYPODONTIA): congenital absence of one or more teeth.

Total anodontia is a rare condition in which there are no deciduous and permanent teeth. It usually occurs in association with a generalized disorder such as hereditary ectodermal dysplasia. Ectodermal dysplasia is usually inherited as an X-linked recessive trait primarily in males, but an autosomal dominant form also occurs in females. All features are basic to defects in the development of the ectodermally derived structures, such as hair, sweat glands, and teeth. The hair may be absent or of the lanugo type (Figure 1-2, *A*) and the reduction or absence of sweat glands results in the inability to regulate body temperature. Although total anodontia may occur, most cases of ectodermal dysplasia exhibit some teeth that are anomalous in shape and are commonly cuspids and molars (Figure 1-2, *B* and *C*).

The more common form of anodontia is *partial anodontia*, also termed *hypodontia* or *oligodontia*, and involves one or more teeth (Figure 1-3). Although any tooth can be congenitally absent, certain teeth tend to be absent more often than others. The most common congenitally absent teeth are the third molars, followed by the maxillary lateral incisors and the second premolars. Although the percentage of congenitally absent teeth varies, as much as 35% of the general population have at least one congenitally absent third molar. Congenital absence of all third molars is common, but congenital absence of deciduous teeth is uncommon. When a deciduous tooth is congenitally absent, it is most often the maxillary lateral incisor. A close correlation exists between congenital absence of a deciduous tooth and congenital absence of the permanent successor, suggesting some genetic influence. Familial tendency for congenitally absent teeth is well recognized.

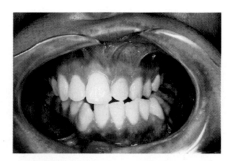

FIGURE 1-3

Hypodontia. Congenitially absent left maxillary central incisor resulting in underdevelopment of the maxilla and severe malocclusion.

FIGURE 1-4
Supernumerary teeth. A, An erupted miniature conically shaped extra tooth is present in the midline of the anterior palate ("mesiodens"). **B,** A similarly located extra tooth that is impacted and unable to erupt.

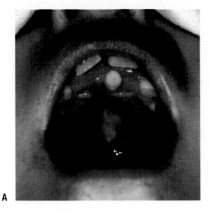
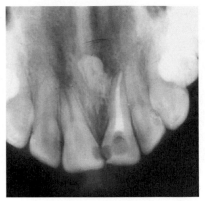

A   B

Supernumerary Teeth

■ SUPERNUMERARY TEETH: teeth in excess of the normal number.

Although these teeth can occur in any location, they have a predilection for certain sites. They are far more common in the maxilla (90%) than in the mandible (10%). A supernumerary tooth located between the maxillary central incisors, usually referred to as a **"mesiodens"** (Figure 1-4), is the most common, followed by fourth molars (paramolars) and lateral incisors. In the mandible the most common supernumerary teeth are premolars, although fourth molars and incisors are also occasionally seen. A supernumerary tooth may resemble the corresponding normal tooth (Figure 1-5), or it may be rudimentarily and conically shaped, bearing little or no resemblance to its normal counterpart. The mesiodens and the paramolars often exhibit conical crowns; the latter is located on the buccal or palatal aspect of the normal maxillary molars. Supernumerary deciduous teeth are uncommon; however, when they do occur, the most common is a maxillary lateral incisor. Supernumerary teeth may be single or multiple and erupted or impacted. Multiple supernumerary teeth, which are generally impacted, are characteristically seen in cleidocranial dysplasia.

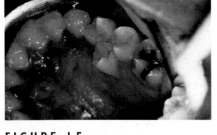

FIGURE 1-5
Supernumerary teeth. A fully developed normal extra premolar that has erupted lingually to the arch.

DISTURBANCES IN ERUPTION

The eruption time varies for deciduous and permanent teeth in humans. It is therefore difficult to assess the eruption times for any given individual. Only when the eruption time or sequence is obviously outside of the normal range can one consider that an eruption abnormality exists.

Premature Eruption
Erupted deciduous teeth present at birth are termed **natal teeth** (Figure 1-6). Deciduous teeth that erupt during the first 30 days of life are termed **neonatal teeth.** Premature eruption usually involves only one or two teeth, most commonly the deciduous mandibular central incisors. Although the etiology of this phenomenon is unknown, a familial pattern is sometimes observed. Natal teeth and neonatal teeth are usually part of the normal complement of deciduous teeth; they are not supernumerary teeth and should therefore be retained if possible.

Premature eruption of permanent teeth is usually a consequence of premature loss of the preceding deciduous teeth. This becomes readily apparent when a single deciduous tooth has been prematurely lost. In the event that the entire permanent dentition is obviously erupting prematurely, the possibility of an endocrine dysfunction such as hyperthyroidism should be considered.

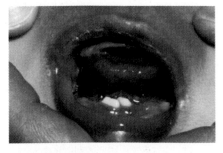

FIGURE 1-6
Natal teeth. Two normally sized mandibular incisors that were present at birth. (Courtesy Dr. Heddie O. Sedano.)

Delayed Eruption

Delayed eruption usually refers to the first appearance of deciduous teeth relative to the normal age range. This occurrence is relatively uncommon and is usually idiopathic or associated with certain systemic conditions such as rickets, cleidocranial dysplasia, or cretinism. Local factors such as gingival fibromatosis, in which dense fibrous connective tissue impedes tooth eruption, can result in delayed eruption of the deciduous dentition. Treatment of the systemic condition or the causative local factors may alleviate the eruption problem. In conditions such as cleidocranial dysplasia, the pathophysiologic basis for noneruption is unclear and there is no known treatment. Delayed eruption of permanent teeth may result from the same local and systemic conditions that give rise to the delayed eruption of deciduous teeth.

Impacted Teeth

> ■ IMPACTED TEETH: teeth that continue to form within bone but fail to erupt.

Teeth that fail to erupt because of crowding of the dental arch, a location that does not present a path of eruption, or are obstructed by some physical barrier are termed *impacted teeth*. Examples of physical barriers that impair tooth eruption and result in impaction include supernumerary teeth, odontogenic cysts (particularly odontogenic keratocysts), and odontogenic tumors (particularly odontomas). Although virtually any tooth can be impacted, the most common impacted teeth are the mandibular and maxillary third molars and maxillary cuspids, followed by the mandibular second premolars and supernumerary teeth. Impacted third molars have been classified according to their orientation within the dental arch, hence the terms *mesioangular, distoangular, horizontal,* and *vertical impactions.* Mesioangular impactions are the most common type. An impacted tooth that is totally surrounded by bone is considered to be **completely impacted** (Figure 1-7, *A*), whereas one that is partly in bone and partly in soft tissue is considered to be **partially impacted** (Figure 1-7, *B*). Partially impacted teeth, particularly mandibular third molars, may communicate with the oral cavity via an inconspicuous periodontal pocket on the distal aspect of the adjacent second molar, thus predisposing the impacted tooth to pericoronal infection and dental caries. A tooth that is completely impacted does not communicate with the oral cavity and is therefore not vulnerable to infection or dental caries. Individual teeth that fail to erupt for no apparent reason have sometimes been termed **embedded teeth;** however, this term is rarely used. Instead, all examples of delayed eruption are collectively referred to as impacted teeth.

The common complications of impacted teeth are root resorption of adjacent normal teeth, infection and associated pain, a predispositon to dentigerous cyst formation, and external resorption of the impacted tooth. External resorption in an impacted tooth usually begins in the occlusal area of the crown and radiographically resembles dental caries. The treatment of impacted teeth will vary with the involved tooth and the individual circumstances. Most impacted molars are surgically removed. Since the maxillary cuspids are important cornerstones in the maxillary dentition, special efforts are usually made to retain these teeth. To accomplish this, the crown of the impacted maxillary cuspid is first surgically uncovered; then, with the aid of an orthodontic appliance, the tooth is slowly guided into its proper position in the dental arch. If tooth impaction is caused by a physical barrier such as a cyst, tumor, or supernumerary tooth, the treatment must include the removal of the causative barrier. Whether the impacted tooth is also removed at the same time will depend on individual circumstances.

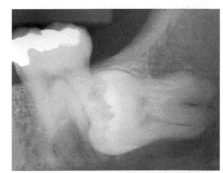

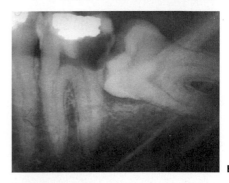

FIGURE 1-7

Impacted teeth. Completely **(A)** and partially impacted **(B)** mandibular third molars. A large area of caries is present on the distum of the adjacent molar of the partially impacted tooth.

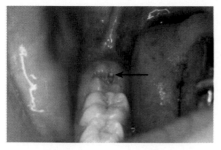

FIGURE 1-8

Eruption sequestrum. A small spicule of bone is present on the occlusal surface of the third molar (*arrow*).

Eruption Sequestrum

■ ERUPTION SEQUESTRUM: a small spicule of calcified tissue that is extruded through the alveolar mucosa that overlies an erupting molar.

An *eruption sequestrum* may arise from the small area of slightly thickened cortical bone that occupies the area of the central occlusal fossa of molars or may represent a miniature complex odontoma present in the follicular soft tissue overlying the tooth. As a molar erupts through bone into the alveolar soft tissue, bone resorption over the cusps is completed slightly ahead of the resorption over the central depression of the crown, termed the *occlusal fossa*; the net result is a small island of nonvital bone or odontoma that is pushed out ahead of the erupting molar (Figure 1-8). Although most eruption sequestra are spontaneously exfoliated and therefore require no treatment, occasionally they may remain in the alveolar mucosa for a few days and may be brought to the attention of a dentist. In this event, they can be easily removed.

DISTURBANCES IN SHAPE

Dilaceration

■ DILACERATION: a sharp bend or angulation of the root portion of a tooth.

Although occasional examples of dilaceration result from trauma during tooth development (Figure 1-9), most cases are the result of continued root formation during a curved or tortuous path of eruption. In some instances the cause of the bent or curved root is idiopathic. Dilaceration can complicate tooth extraction, underlining the importance of securing preoperative radiographs before extracting a tooth.

Taurodontism

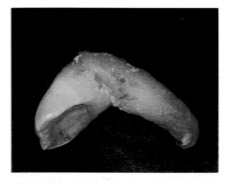
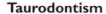

FIGURE 1-9

Dilaceration. A severely bent root of the maxillary central incisor that prevented the eruption of the tooth.

■ TAURODONTISM: a molar with an elongated crown and apically placed furcation of the roots, resulting in an enlarged rectangular coronal pulpal chamber.

Taurodontism, meaning "bull-like" teeth, is a developmental disturbance that primarily affects molars, although premolars are also occasionally affected. Both the permanent and deciduous teeth may be affected, although involvement of the permanent teeth appears to be more common. The condition is readily rec-

FIGURE 1-10

Taurodontism. A, Radiograph of a molar with an enlarged coronal pulpal chamber and lowered bifuration area of roots. **B,** Similar abnormally formed tooth that has been cut in a sagittal plane to illustrate the abnormal shape of the tooth and its pulpal chamber.

B

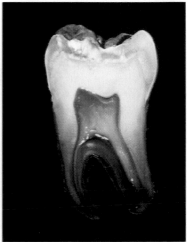

A

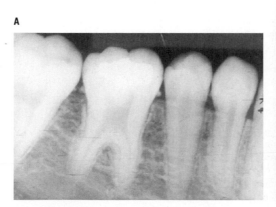

ognized radiographically and characterized by teeth that exhibit an overall rectangular shape, minimal constriction and definition of the cervical margin, and an apically displaced furcation resulting in an extremely large pulpal chamber that exhibits an exaggerated apical-occlusal height and short root pulpal canals (Figure 1-10). The unusual root shape probably results from late invagination of Hertwig's root sheath, the mechanism that determines the shape of the tooth roots. Taurodontism may also occur in patients with amelogenesis imperfecta, Klinefelter syndrome, and Down syndrome. Of anthropologic interest is the fact that taurodontism was relatively common in Neanderthal man and thus may be a form of *atavism*, the occurrence of ancestral forms. Taurodontism requires no treatment but can be a complicating factor during root canal procedures.

Dens Invaginatus

■ DENS INVAGINATUS: developmental anomaly in which a focal area of the crown of a maxillary lateral incisor is folded inward (invaginated) for various distances; when severe, this results in a conically shaped tooth with a small surface opening ("dens in dente") that quickly becomes subject to caries, pulpitis, and periapical inflammation.

Dens invaginatus, also termed **"dens in dente,"** is a developmental abnormality that primarily affects the permanent maxillary lateral incisors. A milder form of this anomaly is relatively common and is characterized by the presence of a deeply invaginated lingual pit that extends for varying distances into the substance of the tooth during development (Figure 1-11). The extent of the invagination is not always clinically visible; the external pit on the lingual surface is often inconspicuous on clinical examination but may be visible with a periapical radiograph (Figure 1-12, *A*). Dens in dente, which clinically appears as a conically shaped tooth, is an intermediate form of the anomaly. A radiograph is helpful in establishing the diagnosis (Figure 1-12, *B* and *C*). In its most extreme form

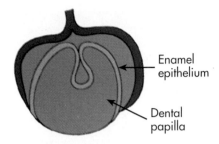

Premineralization

Enamel epithelium

Dental papilla

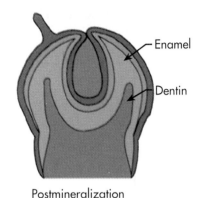

Postmineralization

Enamel

Dentin

FIGURE 1-11

Dens invaginatus. Diagram in which a focal area of the forming crown is infolded or fails to develop while the surrounding tooth continues to grow outward and over the defect.

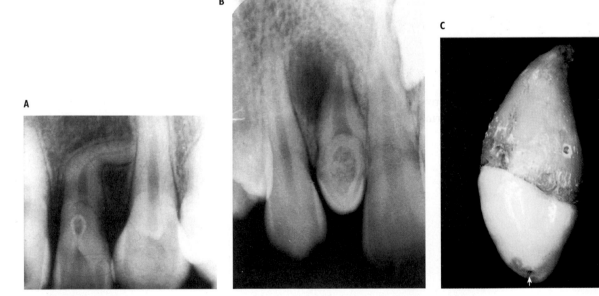

FIGURE 1-12

Dens invaginatus. Radiograph of lateral incisors exhibiting a mild form of the defect in a tooth with a dilaceration of the root **(A)** and a moderate form in which the tooth is conically shaped and exhibits the characteristic appearance of a tooth within a tooth ("dens in dente") **(B).** Both teeth have the commonly associated periapical lesions. **C,** Gross appearance of the "dens in dente" form of the anomaly with the small orifice visible at the tip of the crown *(arrow).*

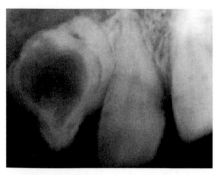

FIGURE 1-13

Dens invaginatus. Radiograph of the most severe form of this anomaly in which there is a large bulbous expansion of the root portion and a central radiolucency. This form is sometimes referred to as "dilated odontoma."

the deep invagination results in a bulbous expansion of the affected root, and it has been erroneously termed a **"dilated odontoma"** (Figure 1-13). The base of the pit or deep invagination is composed of a thin, often defective layer of enamel and dentin (Figure 1-14) that is extremely vulnerable to carious destruction soon after the tooth erupts into the oral cavity. Nearly all teeth with deep invaginations quickly undergo pulpitis, pulpal necrosis, and inflammatory periapical disease in what clinically appears to be an intact tooth. Because of their altered structure, these teeth are seldom candidates for endodontic treatment. For the deep lingual pits in otherwise normally shaped teeth, early radiologic diagnosis and restorative treatment of the abnormality are essential if pulpal and periapical disease are to be prevented. Treatment of the more severe forms of the invagination (dens in dente) is usually extraction.

Supernumerary Cusps

Occasionally, teeth exhibit extra or *supernumerary cusps*. The most common example of this phenomenon is the Carabelli cusp, which typically develops on the mesiolingual surface of permanent maxillary first molars. This particular supernumerary cusp usually presents no clinical problems and is therefore considered to simply represent a normal variation. Occasionally, however, certain teeth develop supernumerary cusps that result in clinical problems and may require treatment. Examples of such supernumerary cusps are **dens evaginatus** and **talon cusps.**

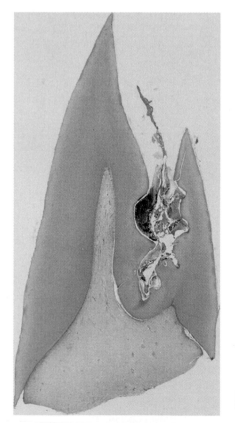

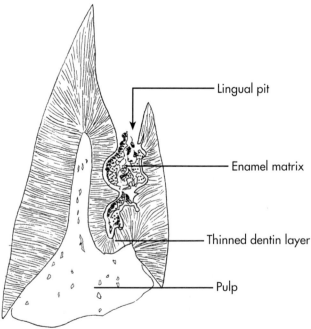

Lingual pit

Enamel matrix

Thinned dentin layer

Pulp

FIGURE 1-14

Dens invaginatus. Photomicrograph of a decalcified section of a developing tooth with a deep lingual pit. A thin layer of dentin separates the base of the invagination from the pulp.

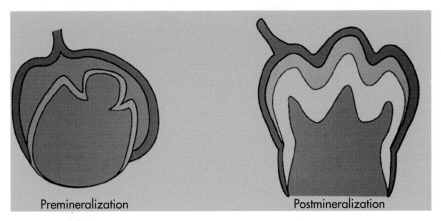

FIGURE 1-15

Dens evaginatus. Diagram of early (premineralization) and late (postmineralization) stages of tooth crown development illustrating the formation of an extra cusp or projection composed of a pulpal horn and normal layers of enamel and dentin.

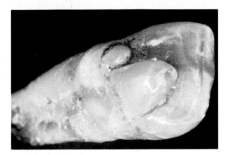

FIGURE 1-16

Dens evaginatus. Maxillary central incisor exhibiting a large and a small cuspal projection on the lingual surface.

Dens evaginatus

■ DENS EVAGINATUS: a developmental anomaly in which a focal area of the crown projects outward and produces what appears as an extra cusp or an abnormal shape to existing cuspal arrangements ("talon cusps").

Dens evaginatus is a developmental abnormality that primarily affects premolars. It is characterized by the development of an abnormal globe-shaped projection appearing as an extra cusp centrally located on the occlusal surface between the buccal and lingual cusps of premolars, although any tooth may be involved (Figures 1-15 and 1-16). It commonly occurs in Chinese, Japanese, Filipino, Northern Native, and American Indian patients, and it occasionally occurs in Caucasian patients. The clinical significance of dens evaginatus is that it can interfere with tooth eruption and result in incomplete eruption or tooth displacement. Since this extra cusp contains a pulp horn, attrition or fracture can result in pulp exposure leading to pulpal inflammation and its sequelae. As with any type of supernumerary cusp, the dentist should be aware that it contains a pulp horn that can be readily exposed if reduction or removal of the cusp is attempted.

Talon cusp

An uncommon but clinically significant form of supernumerary cusp, typically seen on the lingual aspect of maxillary central incisors, is called a *talon cusp* since its unusual shape resembles an eagle's talon. This abnormal cusp arises from the cingulum portion of the tooth and usually extends to the incisal edge as a prominent projection of enamel that imparts a T shape (Figure 1-17). Occasionally, lingual pits develop on either side of the talon cusp, where it joins the lingual surface of the tooth. If lingual pits are present, these should be restored to prevent dental caries. If the cusp interferes with normal occlusion, preventive care that includes endodontic and restorative treatment of the affected tooth may be required to achieve normal tooth form. Simple reduction of the cusp should not be attempted because the cusp contains a prominent pulp horn; therefore pulp exposure is almost certain to occur. Although this abnormality is uncommon in the general population, it has been reported to be more prevalent in patients with Rubinstein-Taybi syndrome.

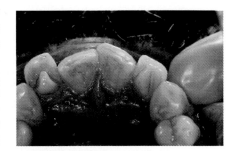

FIGURE 1-17

Talon cusp. In this specific form of dens evaginatus, cuspal projections are present bilaterally and arise from the cingulum of the lateral incisors, resembling eagle's talons.

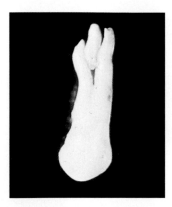

FIGURE 1-18

Supernumerary roots. Maxillary premolar with three roots rather than the usual two.

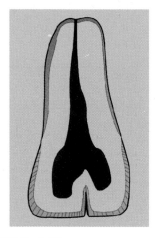

FIGURE 1-19

Gemination/fusion. Diagram of section through a tooth showing both gemination and fusion. Both may have the same microscopic appearance of a widened crown with common dentin, root, and pulpal chambers. Although both may have the same result, gemination occurs due to the partial splitting of a single tooth bud, whereas fusion results from the mingling of two adjacent tooth buds.

Supernumerary Roots

Additional roots (more than the expected number) are termed *supernumerary roots*. This is a common developmental phenomenon that is most often seen in mandibular premolars (Figure 1-18), cuspids, and maxillary and mandibular third molars. It is important to radiologically detect the presence of supernumerary roots before tooth extraction to allow for appropiate surgical planning, to facilitate root tip removal in the event that root fracture occurs, and to plan endodontic treatment.

Gemination

■ GEMINATION: abnormally shaped crown that is extra wide due to the development of two crowns from one tooth germ.

Gemination is a developmental anomaly that primarily affects anterior teeth and that clinically resembles another anomaly known as fusion (Figure 1-19). Althoughly they are clinically and microscopically similar, they result from two different developmental processes. Gemination is characterized by the partial division or "twinning" of a single tooth germ, resulting in a tooth that exhibits two separate or partly separated crowns and a single root and root canal (Figure 1-20, *A*). Gemination can affect the deciduous and permanent dentitions.

Fusion

■ FUSION: an abnormally shaped tooth that may appear as an extra wide crown, a normal crown with an extra root, or other combinations resulting from the union of two adjacent tooth germs by dentin during development.

Fusion is defined as the union of two normally separate tooth germs. The minimal criterion for fusion is that the teeth in question exhibit confluent dentin. This developmental condition can occur in the deciduous and permanent dentition. Some hereditary tendency has been reported. Fusion can be complete or incomplete, and its extent will vary with the stage of development that a tooth has reached at the time of fusion. If fusion begins before calcification, then the union will involve all components of the tooth, including enamel, dentin, cementum, and pulp. If the union begins at a later stage of tooth development, then the affected teeth may have separate crowns and the fusion may be limited

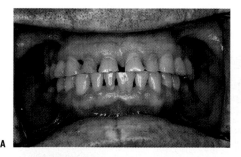
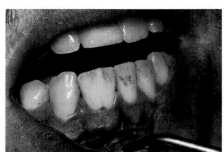

A   B

FIGURE 1-20

A, Gemination. The patient exhibits an extra wide lower central incisor that is most likely caused by gemination because there is a normal number of incisors in the arch. **B, Fusion.** Patient with an extra wide lower incisor most likely caused by fusion because the arch contains three incisors instead of four.

to the roots. The pulp canals may be either fused or separate. Fusion can be differentiated from gemination by counting the teeth in the area. In the case of fusion, there will be one less tooth present in the arch (Figure 1-20, *B*). The clinical implications of fusion include esthetic considerations, crowding when fused to a supernumerary tooth, and periodontal disease.

Concrescence

> ■ CONCRESCENCE: union of the roots of two or more normal teeth caused by confluence of their cemental surfaces.

Concrescence is a type of fusion that occurs after root formation is complete. Union of the teeth is limited to and is the result of confluent cementum (Figures 1-21 and 1-22). The condition is thought to occur as a result of traumatic injury to the area or crowding where interseptal bone is lost, allowing close proximation of the tooth roots. Concrescence can occur before or after tooth eruption and primarily involves the permanent maxillary molars. With rare exceptions, this type of union involves only two teeth. The clinical implications of concrescence relate primarily to the importance of its radiologic diagnosis before attempting tooth extraction. Failure to recognize its presence can result in the extraction of two teeth when a single extraction was intended.

Hypercementosis

Occasionally, one or more teeth exhibit excessive deposits of cementum on the tooth root. Such deposits are sometime problematic because the lower portion of the root may have a larger circumference than the upper portion, resulting in a bulbous or "pear-shaped" root (Figure 1-23). Teeth with these shapes are not easily extracted without surgically removing substantial amounts of the surrounding bone.

Hypercementosis is more common on teeth that are subject to both increased or decreased occlusal forces, on the teeth of patients with Paget's disease or hyperpituitarism, and on adjacent teeth in areas of chronic inflammation. In teeth associated with periapical inflammatory lesions, the increased cementum

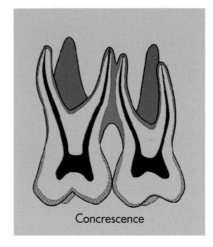

FIGURE 1-21

Concrescence. Diagram of the union of two molars due to confluence of the cementum of the roots of two adjacent teeth.

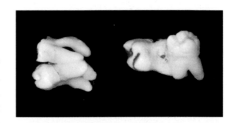

FIGURE 1-22

Concrescence. Molars adhered to each other by fusion of their cementum.

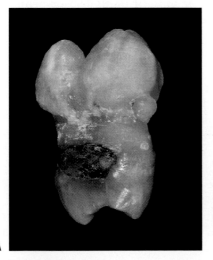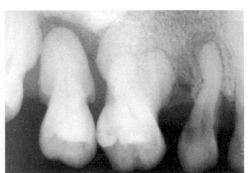

A   B

FIGURE 1-23

Hypercementosis. A, Maxillary molar exhibiting massive deposits of cementum on all roots. **B,** Radiograph of maxillary molars in an area of chronic inflammation exhibiting extensive hypercementosis.

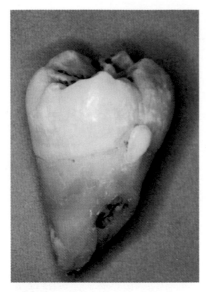

FIGURE 1-24

Ectopic enamel projections. Molar with droplet of enamel in the furcation area of the root ("enamel pearl").

commonly deposits in a band around the apical third of the root, with the tip often exhibiting some resorption. Occasionally, adjacent teeth in an area of chronic inflammation may produce excessive cementum deposits on their roots that eventually fuse at those points, resulting in a concrescence. Because these changes are clinically undetectable, radiographic evaluation is a valuable aid before tooth extraction.

Cervical Enamel Projection

Focal apical extensions of the coronal enamel beyond the normally smooth cervical margin (cementoenamel junction) and onto the root of the tooth are termed *cervical enamel projections*. These enamel projections are approximately 1 mm wide, 1 to 3 mm long, and occur primarily on maxillary and mandibular molars. Their clinical significance relates to the fact that they could contribute to periodontal pocket formation, which might progress to periodontal disease. Cervical enamel projections differ from the ectopic droplets of enamel that primarily occur in the bifurcation or trifurcation areas on the roots of molars (Figure 1-24). These are termed *enamel pearls* or *enamelomas*. These enamel pearls are relatively uncommon and can be radiographically seen as 1 to 3 mm round radiopacities. Histologically, enamel pearls may be composed largely of enamel, or they may exhibit a central core of dentin. Treatment is not recommended because it often leads to the development of root caries, external resorption, or pulpitis.

DISTURBANCES IN STRUCTURE OF ENAMEL

Acquired Disturbances

Disturbances in the structure of enamel can occur as a result of environmental or hereditary factors. Among the environmental factors are bacterial and viral infections (syphilis, scarlet fever), inflammation, nutritional deficiencies (vitamins A, C, and D and calcium), chemical injuries (fluoride), and trauma. Depending on the etiologic factor, the enamel disturbance may be localized to one or two teeth (focal), or it may affect many or all teeth (generalized). The extent of the enamel defect is generally related to the specific etiologic factor, the duration of the injury, and the stage of enamel formation at the time of the injury. Enamel defects resulting from environmental factors usually affect either the deciduous or the permanent dentition but seldom both. Unlike hereditary factors that usually affect either the enamel or the dentin, environmental factors often damage both types of hard tissues.

Focal enamel hypoplasia

Localized or *focal enamel hypoplasia* involving only one or two teeth is relatively common. Although the etiology is often unclear (idiopathic), in some cases it is readily apparent. A common form of focal enamel hypoplasia of known etiology is **"Turner tooth,"** which results from localized inflammation or trauma during tooth development. Typical examples of this phenomenon occur when a deciduous tooth develops a caries- or trauma-related abscess that damages the underlying developing permanent successor (Figure 1-25, *A*). Depending on the severity of the injury, the affected crown may have an area of enamel hypoplasia that is relatively smooth with pitted areas or is grossly deformed with a yellowish or brownish discoloration (Figure 1-25, *B*).

Generalized enamel hypoplasia

Short-term systemic environmental factors inhibit functioning ameloblasts at a specific period during tooth development and are manifested clinically as a horizontal line of small pits or grooves on the enamel surface that correspond to the

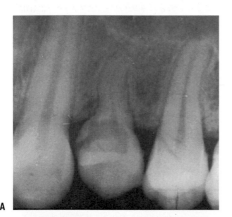

A

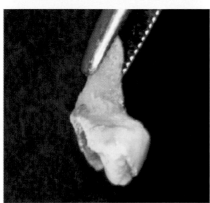

B

FIGURE 1-25

Turner tooth. A, Radiograph of first maxillary premolar exhibiting radiolucency due to hypoplasia acquired during development of the crown. **B,** Gross appearance of the tooth illustrated in **A** with a brownish-yellow, irregular shape and surface of crown.

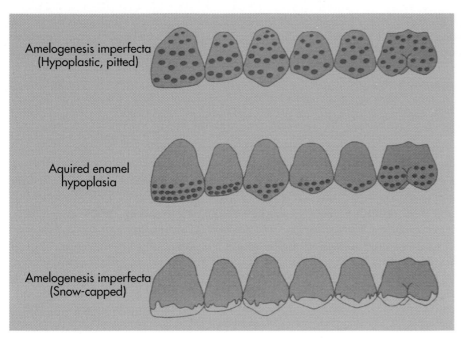

FIGURE 1-26

Acquired and hereditary enamel defects. Comparison of surface appearances of common enamel defects. The acquired type differs from the hereditary pitted hypoplastic type because the defective enamel is limited to the portions of the teeth that were forming at the time of the insult.

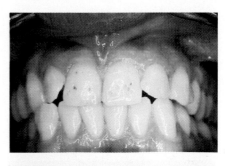
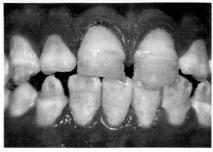

FIGURE 1-27

Acquired enamel hypoplasia. A, Maxillary central incisors with a mild form of pitted enamel. **B,** Multiple teeth with horizontal band of severe form of enamel hypoplasia.

time of development and the duration of the insult (Figure 1-26). If the duration of the environmental insult is brief, the line of hypoplasia is narrow, whereas a prolonged insult produces a wider zone of hypoplasia and may affect more teeth (Figure 1-27). A knowledge of the chronologic order of tooth development is helpful in determining the approximate time of an injurious insult. Clinical studies indicate that most cases of generalized environmental hypoplasia involve teeth that are formed in babies during the first year after birth; thus the teeth that are most often involved are the permanent incisors, cuspids, and first molars. Premolars, second molars, and third molars are seldom affected because their formation does not begin until a child is 3 years of age or older.

The enamel hypoplasia resulting from congenital syphilis affects the incisal edges of the permanent incisors (Figure 1-28) and the occlusal surfaces of the permanent first molars. The notched, "screwdriver-shaped" incisors are termed **"Hutchinson incisors,"** whereas the globular occlusal surfaces of the first molars are termed **"mulberry molars."** Not all patients with congenital syphilis exhibit the hypoplastic changes previously described. In addition, occasional patients who have no history of congenital syphilis exhibit changes that are indistinguishable from "mulberry molars" and Hutchinson incisors. A diagnosis of congenital syphilis should therefore be made only after conclusive evidence is available.

Enamel hypoplasia that results from hypocalcemia secondary to vitamin D deficiency is usually of the pitted type. It is clinically indistinguishable from enamel hypoplasia caused by exanthematous diseases such as measles, chicken pox, and scarlet fever and by vitamin A and C deficiencies.

The *neonatal line* microscopically seen in cross sections of deciduous teeth and first permanent molars can be considered a mild form of enamel hypoplasia

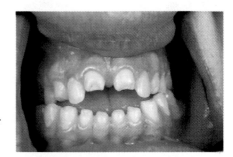

FIGURE 1-28

Acquired enamel hypoplasia. Severe generalized form of enamel hypoplasia caused by congenital syphilis. The teeth lack the formation of the central lobe of the crown, resulting in the "screwdriver" shape of the incisors.

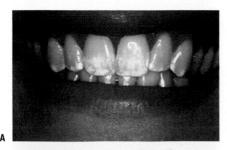

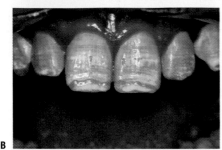

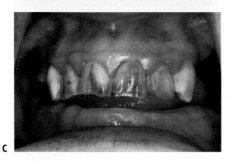

A

B

C

FIGURE 1-29

Fluorosis. A, Mild form of fluoride mottling, exhibiting white opaque flecks near the incisal edges with the surface remaining smooth and intact. **B,** Moderate form of fluoride mottling with ridges of hypoplasia and white and brownish enamel. **C,** Severe form of fluoride-induced hypoplasia and discoloration with associated cracking and chipping of the enamel.

and is indicative of the systemic insult to the teeth during birth. Clinical studies also indicate that enamel hypoplasia is more common in prematurely born children than in those born at normal term.

A well-recognized example of chemically induced generalized enamel hypoplasia results from the ingestion of fluoride. Although total fluoride intake will vary with total water consumption, fluoride-induced enamel hypoplasia **(fluoride mottling)** is usually inconspicuous at levels below 1.0 ppm in the drinking water. With increased amounts of fluoride in the drinking water, the resultant enamel hypoplasia becomes progressively evident. Increased fluoride levels interfere with ameloblastic function, which adversely affects both enamel matrix formation and enamel matrix calcification. Clinically, minimal fluoride mottling exhibits a smooth enamel surface with occasional subtle whitish flecking; mild mottling exhibits a smooth enamel surface with opaque white areas (Figure 1-29, *A*); moderate to severe mottling exhibits varying degrees of obvious pitting and brownish discoloration of the enamel suface (Figure 1-29, *B*). In severe fluoride mottling the enamel is considerably softer and weaker than normal, resulting in excessive wear and fracturing of the incisal and occlusal surfaces (Figure 1-29, *C*); conventional restorations are therefore difficult to retain. Regardless of the degree of fluoride mottling, affected teeth are largely resistant to dental caries.

Hereditary Disturbances

Amelogenesis imperfecta

> ■ A M E L O G E N E S I S   I M P E R F E C T A : a spectrum of hereditary defects in the function of ameloblasts and the mineralization of enamel matrix that results in teeth with multiple generalized abnormalities affecting the enamel layer only.

Amelogenesis imperfecta is a heterogeneous group of hereditary disorders of enamel formation affecting both the primary and permanent dentitions. These disorders are confined to the enamel; the other components of the teeth are normal. Normal enamel formation progresses through three stages: (1) enamel matrix formation (functioning ameloblasts), (2) mineralization of the enamel matrix (primary mineralization), and (3) enamel maturation (secondary mineralization). Three basic types of amelogenesis imperfecta correlate with defects in these stages: (1) the **hypoplastic** type (focal or generalized), which exhibits decreased enamel matrix formation caused by interference in the functioning of the ameloblasts; (2) the **hypocalcified** type, which exhibits a severely defective form

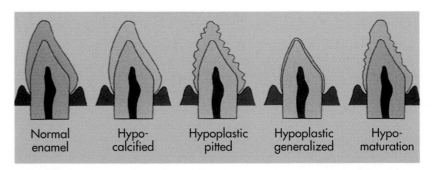

Normal enamel   Hypo-calcified   Hypoplastic pitted   Hypoplastic generalized   Hypo-maturation

FIGURE 1-30

Amelogenesis imperfecta. Diagram of enamel defects of basic types. Hypocalcified—normal thickness, smooth surface, less hardness. Hypoplastic, pitted—normal thickness, pitted surface, normal hardness. Hypoplastic, generalized—reduced thickness, smooth surface, normal hardness. Hypomaturation—normal thickness, chipped surface, less hardness, opaque white coloration.

of mineralization of the enamel matrix; and (3) the **hypomaturation** type, which exhibits less severe mineralization with focal or generalized areas of immature enamel crystallites (Figure 1-30). Utilizing this basic outline in conjunction with clinical, histologic, and genetic criteria, Witkop and Sauk classified the various types of amelogenesis imperfecta (Box 1-1).

The following are clinical features useful for differentiating the three *basic* types of amelogenesis imperfecta.

Hypoplastic type: the enamel is not of normal thickness in focal (Figure 1-31) or generalized areas (Figure 1-32); radiodensity of the enamel is greater than that of dentin.

Hypocalcified type: the enamel is of normal thickness but soft and easily removed with a blunt instrument (Figure 1-33); enamel is less radiodense than dentin.

Hypomaturation type: the enamel is of normal thickness but not of normal hardness and translucency (Figure 1-34, *A*); enamel can be pierced with the point of an explorer with firm pressure and can be chipped away from the underlying normal dentin; enamel radiodensity is about the same as dentin. The mildest form of the hypomaturation is of normal hardness and has white opaque flecks in the incisal areas of the teeth ("snow-capped" teeth) (Figure 1-34, *B*).

■ **BOX 1-1**
Witkop/Sauk Classification of Amelogenesis Imperfecta

Hypoplastic
  Pitted, autosomal dominant
  Local, autosomal dominant
  Smooth, autosomal dominant
  Rough, autosomal dominant
  Rough, autosomal recessive
  Smooth, X-linked dominant

Hypocalcified
  Autosomal dominant
  Autosomal recessive

Hypomaturation
  Hypomaturation-hypoplastic with taurodontism, autosomal dominant
  X-linked recessive
  Pigmented, autosomal recessive
  Snow-capped teeth

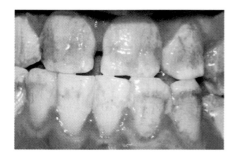

FIGURE 1-31
Focal hypoplastic amelogenesis imperfecta. The enamel is of normal thickness and hardness with diffuse pitting.

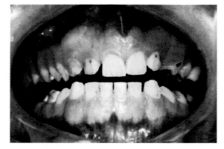

FIGURE 1-32
Generalized hypoplastic amelogenesis imperfecta. The enamel is evenly reduced in thickness but of normal hardness, resulting in spacing and alteration of the shape of teeth.

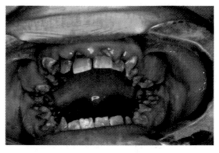

FIGURE 1-33
Hypocalcified amelogenesis imperfecta. The enamel is soft and easily chipped away, leaving exposed dentin that is easily stained, worn, and caries prone.

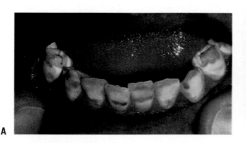

A

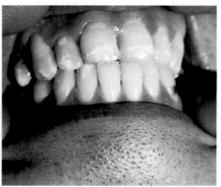

B

FIGURE 1-34
Hypomaturation amelogenesis imperfecta. A, Severe form with enamel of normal thickness but that exhibits loss of translucency and hardness, resulting in some chipping of incisal edges. **B,** In the mild form the teeth may be relatively normal but contain white flecks in the incisal third of the teeth ("snow-capped" teeth).

CLINICAL

The clinical appearance of the various types of amelogenesis imperfecta can be remarkably different. In some types, the teeth appear essentially normal, whereas in others they may be extremely unsightly and obviously abnormal. Both dentitions are commonly affected to some degree. In the X-linked subtypes the clinical appearance differs between males and females.

RADIOGRAPHIC

The radiologic appearance of amelogenesis imperfecta varies with the type. In the smooth hypoplastic type, the enamel layer is conspicuously thin and its radiodensity is greater than the adjacent dentin; in the hypocalcified type the enamel layer appears wispy or absent and is usually less radiodense than the adjacent dentin; in the hypomaturation type, the radiodensity of the enamel is almost equal to that of normal dentin.

DISTURBANCES IN THE STRUCTURE OF DENTIN

Local or systemic environmental factors that affect dentin formation also tend to affect enamel formation. Turner tooth and regional odontodysplasia are examples of disturbed dentin formation resulting from environmental factors. Generalized disturbances in dentin formation are usually hereditary and include conditions such as dentinogenesis imperfecta and dentin dysplasia. Familial hypophosphatemia (vitamin D resistant rickets) is also in this category.

Hereditary Disturbances in Dentin

There are two basic types of hereditary dentinal disturbances—dentinogenesis imperfecta and dentin dysplasia. Dentin dysplasia has a well-known subtype referred to as type II. When grossly examined in a saggital plane, the characteristic features of overall appearance and the shape of pulpal structures are useful in differentiating between the two types (Figure 1-35).

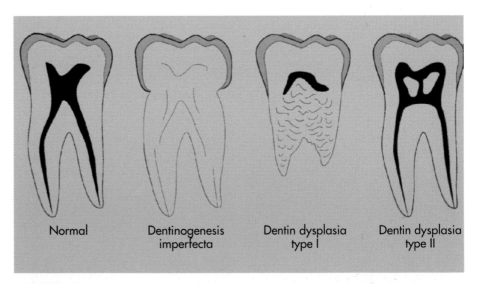

| Normal | Dentinogenesis imperfecta | Dentin dysplasia type I | Dentin dysplasia type II |

FIGURE 1-35

Hereditary disturbances of dentin. Diagram of the characteristic morphologic features of the major types of dentin disturbances. Dentinogenesis imperfecta—constricted cementoenamel junction and lack of pulpal structures. Dentin dysplasia, type I—normal crown, shortened roots, rippled dentin, chevron-shaped coronal pulp. Dentin dysplasia, type II—normal crown, normal length roots, pulpal chamber with large pulp stones.

Dentinogenesis imperfecta

> ■ DENTINOGENESIS IMPERFECTA: a hereditary defect consisting of opalescent teeth composed of irregularly formed and undermineralized dentin that obliterates the coronal and root pulpal chambers.

Dentinogenesis imperfecta (DI) is an inherited disorder of dentin formation, usually exhibiting an autosomal dominant mode of transmission. This disorder has been classified into three types:

Type I: Dentinogenesis imperfecta that occurs in patients afflicted with osteogenesis imperfecta (OI), although not all patients with OI exhibit DI. This type is usually inherited as an autosomal dominant trait. Although the teeth have the same opalescent color as type II, the patients often exhibit other features of osteogenesis imperfecta such as having a bluish tint to the sclera of the eyes (Figure 1-36).

Type II: Dentinogenesis imperfecta that is not associated with osteogenesis imperfecta. The common term for this type of DI is **hereditary opalescent dentin.** It is the most common type inherited as an autosomal dominant trait. Incidence is approximately 1:8000 persons.

Type III: Dentinogenesis imperfecta (Brandywine type) that is rare and inherited as an autosomal dominant trait that occurs in a racial isolate area in the state of Maryland. Clinically, it is the same as type I and type II except that patients exhibit multiple pulpal exposures in the deciduous dentition.

CLINICAL

In all three types, teeth of both dentitions are affected with variable clinical appearances. The teeth are opalescent with the color ranging from bluish-gray (Figure 1-37, *A*) to brown to yellowish. The dentin is abnormally soft, providing inadequate functional support to the overlying enamel. Although the enamel is normal, it fractures or chips away easily, exposing the occlusal and incisal dentin (Figure 1-37, *B*). The exposed soft dentin often undergoes rapid and severe functional attrition. Despite the exposure of dentin, teeth are not particularly prone to dental caries.

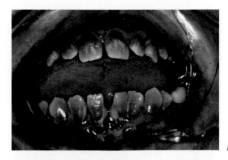

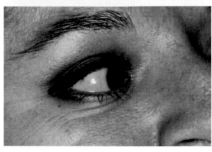

FIGURE 1-36

Dentinogenesis imperfecta associated with osteogenesis imperfecta.
A, Patient's teeth exhibit characteristic opalescent coloration. **B,** Same patient with "blue sclera" of the eye.

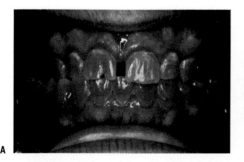

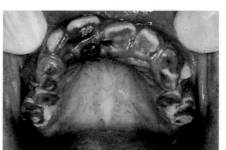

FIGURE 1-37

Dentinogenesis imperfecta (hereditary opalescent dentin). A, Patient's teeth with characteristic blue-gray (opalescent) appearance. **B,** Incisal edges reveal chipping of normal enamel, exposing soft dentin that undergoes rapid attrition.

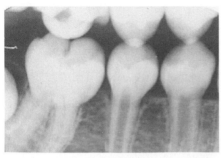

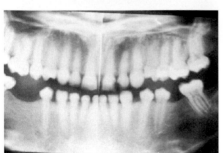

FIGURE 1-38

Dentinogenesis imperfecta. A, Radiograph of the teeth of a young patient that reveals the globe-shaped crowns caused by cervical constriction and obliteration of the coronal pulp. **B,** Panoramic radiograph indicating the coronal shape and complete obliteration of the pulpal chambers of nearly all teeth.

RADIOGRAPHIC

The teeth in types I and II are similar and exhibit bulb-shaped crowns with constricted cementoenamel junctions and thin roots (Figure 1-38, *A*). Depending on the age of the patient, the teeth will exhibit varying stages of obliteration of the coronal and root pulpal chambers (Figure 1-38, *B*). The cementum, periodontal ligament, and supporting alveolar bone appear normal. The teeth in DI (type III) may be similar to those seen in types I and II, or they may exhibit extremely large pulpal chambers surrounded by a thin shell of dentin.

HISTOPATHOLOGY

The enamel in DI is normal. The mantle dentin, a narrow zone of dentin immediately beneath the enamel, remains nearly normal, whereas the remaining dentin is severely dysplastic (Figure 1-39, *A*). Within the dysplastic dentin are focal areas of an amorphous matrix with globular and interglobular areas of mineralization. The dentinal tubules are disoriented, irregular, widely spaced, and usually larger than normal (Figure 1-39, *B*). Within the abnormal dentin, entrapped odontoblasts and degenerating cellular debris may be observed.

TREATMENT

The treatment of DI is directed toward preventing excessive loss of enamel and dentin though attrition and toward improving the teeth esthetically. This can be accomplished with appropriate restorations such as metal/porcelain crowns. Teeth do not make good abutments for partial dentures because root fractures may occur from the functional stress. In severe cases full dentures are usually inevitable.

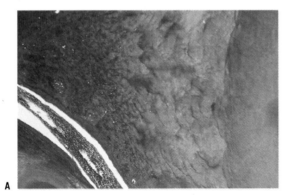

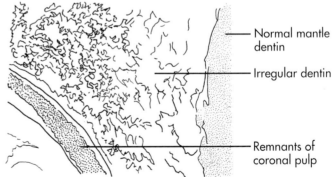

— Normal mantle dentin

— Irregular dentin

— Remnants of coronal pulp

FIGURE 1-39

Dentinogenesis imperfecta. A, Low-power photomicrograph of dentin depicting the thin zone of normal mantle dentin on the right, with dysplastic irregular dentin replacing all but a small remnant of the coronal pulp. **B,** High-power photomicrograph demonstrating the large-sized and widely spaced dentin tubules and the lack of normal density of intertubular collagen deposits.

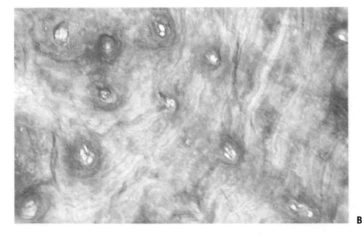

Dentin dysplasia

> ■ DENTIN DYSPLASIA: a hereditary defect in dentin formation in which the coronal dentin and tooth color is normal; the root dentin is abnormal with a gnarled pattern and associated shortened and tapered roots.

Dentin dysplasia (DD), originally termed "rootless teeth," is an autosomal dominant inherited disorder characterized by abnormal dentin formation and abnormal pulpal morphology. The disorder has been classified into type I, radicular dentin dysplasia, and type II, coronal dentin dysplasia.

Type I (radicular dentin dysplasia). Although both types of dentin dysplasia are rare, type I is far more common than type II. All teeth in both dentitions are affected. The color of the teeth is usually within the normal range (Figure 1-40). In some cases the crowns of the teeth may exhibit a slight bluish or brownish translucency in the cervical region. The teeth usually exhibit a normal eruption pattern, although occasional delayed eruption has been reported. Affected teeth often exhibit increased mobility and may exfoliate prematurely.

RADIOGRAPHIC

The roots of the teeth are usually short, blunt, bulged, conical, or absent. The mandibular molars commonly have characteristic W-shaped roots. In the deciduous dentition, teeth often exhibit total obliteration of the pulpal chambers and canals. The permanent teeth may also exhibit pulpal obliteration; however, thin crescent-shaped or chevron-shaped remnants of the pulpal chambers are often present. Periapical radiolucencies representing abscesses, granulomas, or cysts may be present in the absence of dental caries (Figure 1-41).

HISTOPATHOLOGY

The enamel and the mantle layer of dentin are normal. The remaining coronal and root dentin consist of a series of fused nodular masses composed of tubular dentin and osteodentin that present a histologic appearance, which has been described as resembling "lava flowing around boulders," "gnarled burlwood," or "a series of sand dunes" (Figure 1-42, *A*). Occasionally, slitlike remnants of pulpal

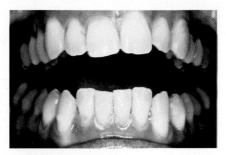

FIGURE 1-40

Dentin dysplasia, type I. Patient exhibits normally shaped and colored teeth.

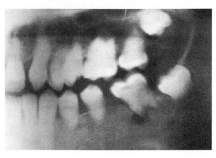

FIGURE 1-41

Dentin dysplasia, type I. Panoramic radiograph depicting the obliteration of the pulp except for the occasional "chevron" radiolucency, shortened and W-shaped roots, and periapical radiolucency.

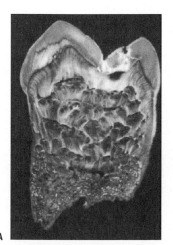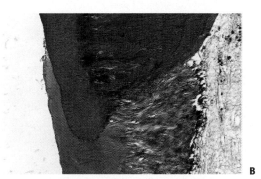

A B

FIGURE 1-42

Dentin dysplasia, type I. A, Sectioned tooth revealing the gnarled and rippling formation of dysplastic dentin occupying the root portion of the tooth. **B,** Low-power photomicrograph of the junction of normal and dysplastic dentin revealing the abrupt transition and dysplastic nature of the root dentin.

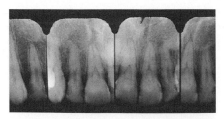

FIGURE 1-43
Dentin dysplasia, type II. Periapical radiographs indicating teeth with relatively normal roots and pulpal chambers that contain large pulp stones.

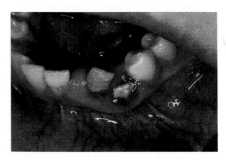

FIGURE 1-44
Regional odontodysplasia. Patient exhibiting a localized area of the mandible in which two abnormal teeth are present surrounded by an increase in the soft tissue.

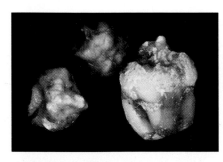

FIGURE 1-45
Regional odontodysplasia. Removed teeth reveal shortened roots and abnormally shaped crowns with a brown leathery coloration and texture.

tissue may be seen between the normal and the abnormal nodular dentin masses. The junction between normal and abnormal dentin may be abrupt. The abnormal dentin is less dense and lacks regular distribution and orientation of tubular dentin (Figure 1-42, *B*).

Type II (coronal dentin dysplasia). Both the primary and permanent dentitions are affected in this type of dentin dysplasia; however, the clinical appearance of the deciduous teeth differs from that of the succeeding permanent teeth. Clinically, the deciduous teeth exhibit a bluish-gray, brownish, or yellowish color and have the same translucent/opalescent appearance that is seen in dentinogenesis imperfecta. In contrast, the permanent teeth have a normal clinical appearance.

RADIOGRAPHIC
The deciduous teeth of DD type II exhibit obliterated pulpal chambers and canals that are similar to those seen in type I and in dentinogenesis imperfecta. The pulpal obliteration occurs after tooth eruption. The roots of the deciduous and permanent dentitions are of normal shape and length. The pulpal chambers in the permanent teeth are abnormally large, rather than obliterated, and exhibit a radicular extension that imparts a thistle or flame shape to the root portion of the pulp. *Pulpal calcifications* ("pulp stones") are visible in most of the pulpal chambers. The pulpal canals are narrow (Figure 1-43).

HISTOPATHOLOGY
The deciduous teeth exhibit a normal zone of mantle dentin that changes abruptly into a dense amorphous mass of dentin exhibiting only occasional haphazardly arranged tubules. The permanent teeth exhibit a relatively normal coronal dentin except for the pulpal third, which exhibits areas of globular and interglobular dentin. The root dentin is amorphous and largely atubular. The pulpal chamber exhibits numerous pulp stones; the pulpal canals are narrow but otherwise normal. The prognosis for teeth in DD type I varies with the severity of the disorder. If the roots of the teeth are extremely short, early tooth loss is almost inevitable and appropriate prosthetic replacements will be required. If the roots are relatively normal, tooth loss may not be a major problem. The prognosis for the permanent teeth in DD type II is essentially the same as it is for normal teeth.

REGIONAL ODONTODYSPLASIA

> ■ REGIONAL ODONTODYSPLASIA: a developmental disturbance of several adjacent teeth in which the enamel and dentin are thin and irregular and fail to adequately mineralize; surrounding soft tissue is hyperplastic and contains focal accumulations of spherical calcifications and odontogenic rests.

Regional odontodysplasia (ROD) or "ghost teeth" is a sporadically occurring nonhereditary disturbance of tooth development characterized by the defective formation of enamel and dentin in addition to abnormal pulp and follicle calcifications. Although its etiology is not fully understood, experimental evidence points to a local ischemic cause.

CLINICAL
The disturbance more commonly appears in the maxilla than the mandible; it is "regional" in that it usually affects several contiguous teeth in a single quadrant (Figure 1-44). Involvement of two quadrants of the same arch has been reported. The condition is most commonly seen in the permanent dentition. The affected

teeth exhibit a delay or a total failure to erupt. The teeth are considerably deformed with a soft "leathery" surface and are yellowish-brown (Figure 1-45).

RADIOGRAPHIC

The teeth have been described as "ghost-teeth" because of the marked decrease in radiodensity. The enamel and dentin are very thin and indistinct; the pulpal chambers are extremely large (Figure 1-46). Pulp stones may occasionally be visible.

HISTOPATHOLOGY

The dentin is dysplastic and characterized by irregular tubules, large areas of globular and interglobular dentin, and a wide predentin layer. The large pulpal chambers (Figure 1-47, *A*) exhibit numerous pulpal calcifications (pulp stones). The dental follicles are occasionally hyperplastic and exhibit significant numbers of epithelial odontogenic rests, numerous clusters of tiny droplet calcifications, and larger lamellar calcifications (Figure 1-47, *B*). Extraction of the affected teeth and replacement with a suitable prosthesis are usually required.

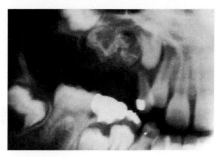

FIGURE 1-46

Regional odontodysplasia. Panoramic radiograph revealing several faint outlines of teeth in the posterior maxilla with large pulpal chambers and lacking root formation.

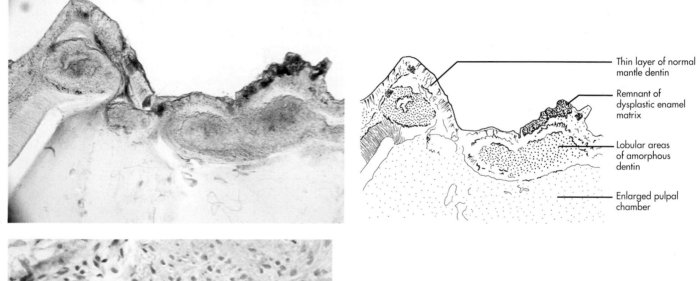

Thin layer of normal mantle dentin

Remnant of dysplastic enamel matrix

Lobular areas of amorphous dentin

Enlarged pulpal chamber

A

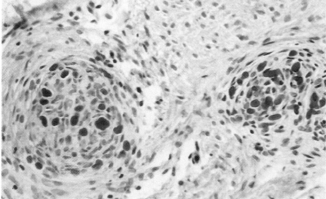

B

FIGURE 1-47

Regional odontodysplasia. A, Low-power photomicrograph through the crown of a decalcified tooth depicting a remnant of the defective enamel matrix; thin normal mantle dentin overlying severely dysplastic dentin with lobular areas of amorphous dentin and a greatly enlarged coronal pulpal chamber. **B,** Surrounding soft tissue contains nodular arrangements of connective tissue cells containing accumulations of spherical calcifications.

SOFT TISSUE

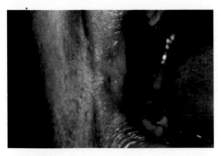

FIGURE 1-48

Congenital lip pit. An orifice of a lip pit is present in the angle (commissure) of the lips.

CONGENITAL LIP PITS

Congenital lip pits are developmental defects that may involve the paramedial portion of the vermilion of the lower and upper lip (paramedial lip pit) or the labial commissure area (commissural lip pit) (Figure 1-48). Both types of lip pits appear to be inherited as an autosomal dominant trait. The paramedial lip pit may occur as an isolated finding or may be associated with cleft lip or cleft palate (Van der Woude syndrome). The paramedial lip pit may be unilateral or bilateral and most commonly occurs on the lower lip. Lip pits are congenital invaginations that can represent blind tracts (Figure 1-49) or dilated ectopic salivary ducts. Mucus secretion is visible at the opening of those pits that communicate with salivary gland tissue. The surface opening (pore) of the paramedial lip pit usually measures 1 to 3 mm in diameter; the depth will range from 5 to 15 mm. The commissural lip pit exhibits an opening of 1 to 2 mm and a depth of 2 to 4 mm. Although lip pits usually present no clinical problems, the paramedial lip pits are occasionally excised for cosmetic reasons; commissural lip pits require no treatment.

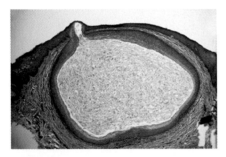

FIGURE 1-49

Congenital lip pit. Photomicrograph of removed lip pit that had become "cystic." The blind pouch is lined by a thin epithelium and contains densely packed desquamated epithelium.

DOUBLE LIP

A double lip is an anomaly characterized by a horizontal fold of redundant mucosal tissue that is usually located on the inner aspect of the upper lip, although the lower lip can also be occasionally involved. This redundant tissue can be congenital or acquired. The double lip is usually visible when the lip is tense but not when the lip is at rest. Occasionally, the double lip will be seen in association with a fold of drooping skin above the upper eyelid (blepharochalasis) and with nontoxic thyroid enlargement (Ascher syndrome). Although this redundant fold of tissue is occasionally excised for cosmetic reasons, double lip usually requires no treatment.

FRENAL TAG

The frenal tag is a redundant piece of mucosal tissue that projects from the maxillary labial frenum. Its shape and size varies from patient to patient. Although this tag of tissue has no known function, it is familial and appears to be inherited as an autosomal dominant trait. The frenal tag is often mistaken for an acquired fibrous hyperplasia caused by local injury or irritation and is therefore occasionally excised and submitted for pathologic examination. Histologically, the frenal tag consists of normal oral mucosa.

ANKYLOGLOSSIA

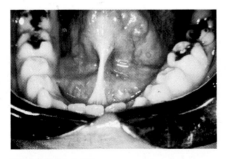

FIGURE 1-50

Ankyloglossia. The tongue of the patient has reduced mobility caused by the large band of fibrous tissue extending from the ventral tongue to the lingual gingiva of the anterior mandible.

> ■ ANKYLOGLOSSIA: lack of normal tongue mobility caused by the presence of an abnormal fibrous tissue attachment between its ventral surface and the floor of the mouth.

Ankyloglossia or "tongue-tie" is a developmental anomaly characterized by an abnormally short and anteriorly positioned lingual frenum that results in severely restricted tongue movements and impaired speech. Occasionally, the abnormal lingual frenum connects the tip of the tongue to the anterior lingual gingiva (Figure 1-50), resulting in tension of the gingival tissue that progresses to local gingival and periodontal disease in the region of the frenal attachment. Ankyloglossia is best treated by surgically repositioning the lingual frenum.

MACROGLOSSIA

Macroglossia or "large tongue" is a condition that may be congenital or secondary. Congenital macroglossia is seen in Down syndrome, Beckwith-Wiedemann syndrome, and occasionally in multiple endocrine neoplasia syndrome (type III). Secondary macroglossia can result from diffuse involvement of the tongue by tumors such as lymphangioma (Figure 1-51), hemangioma, or neurofibroma and from diffuse infiltration of the tongue by amyloid deposits in amyloidosis. Systemic conditions such as acromegaly (adult hyperpituitarism) and cretinism (congenital hypothyroidism) can also result in macroglossia.

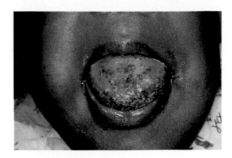

FIGURE 1-51

Macroglossia. The tongue of the young patient is excessively large due to the presence of a lymphangioma.

FORDYCE GRANULES

Collections of sebaceous glands that occur in various locations within the oral cavity are termed *Fordyce granules*. Although they are most commonly seen bilaterally on the buccal mucosa and on the vermilion of the upper lip, they occur in various other intraoral sites, including the gingiva. Fordyce granules appear as multiple small, milia-like yellowish maculopapular structures that measure 1 to 2 mm in diameter (Figure 1-52, *A*). Since it is estimated that at least 80% of adults exhibit Fordyce granules to some extent, the presence of sebaceous glands in this area must be considered normal.

HISTOPATHOLOGY

Fordyce granules of the oral mucosa are identical to the normal sebaceous glands found in skin, except they are not associated with hair. The glands are usually superficial, composed of 1 to 5 lobules, and empty into a duct that opens on the mucosal surface (Figure 1-52, *B*). No treatment is required for this condition other than informing the patient of the nature of the entity.

Rarely, a solitary sebaceous gland will undergo adenomatous hyperplasia and clinically present as a discrete, slightly elevated yellowish lesion measuring 5 to 10 mm in diameter. Histologically, these lesions are indistinguishable from Fordyce granules, except that they are larger, being composed of 15 or more sebaceous lobules (Figure 1-52, *C*). Most of these lesions appear to represent a localized focus of sebaceous hyperplasia rather than a sebaceous adenoma.

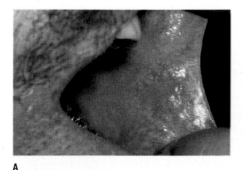
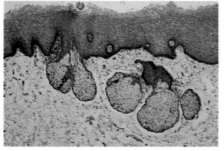
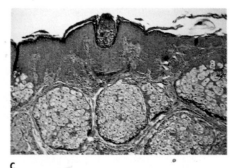

A   B   C

FIGURE 1-52

Fordyce granules. A, The buccal mucosa contains numerous yellowish small macular and papular structures that are symptomless. **B,** Photomicrograph illustrates the lobules of sebaceous glands that empty into ductal structures that communicate with the surface of the mucosa. **C,** Photomicrograph of excessive accumulations of larger lobules of sebaceous glands that often produce a noticeable submucosal swelling.

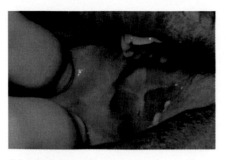

FIGURE 1-53

Leukoedema. Buccal mucosa of the patient exhibits an asymptomatic white-gray superficial layer that does not rub off.

LEUKOEDEMA

■ LEUKOEDEMA: accumulation of fluid within the epithelial cells of the buccal mucosa.

Leukoedema is an alteration of oral epithelium characterized by the intracellular accumulation of fluid (edema) within the spinous cell layer. The etiology of this condition is presently unknown. It is so common in some racial groups that it is not considered to be a disease but a variation of normal.

CLINICAL
Typically, leukoedema involves the buccal mucosa bilaterally, although the lateral borders of the tongue can also be affected. It is found in 85% to 95% of African Americans but only in 40% to 45% of Caucasians. The affected mucosa exhibits an asymptomatic, diffuse, translucent, grayish-white, filmy appearance (Figure 1-53). In extreme cases the mucosa may be wrinkled or corrugated. When stretched, the appearance is greatly decreased. Mild degrees of leukoedema are common and often overlooked.

HISTOPATHOLOGY
Leukoedema is characterized by a mild degree of parakeratosis and acanthosis and a remarkable accumulation of intracytoplasmic fluid and glycogen, which results in enlarged spinous cells with clear cytoplasm and small shrunken (pyknotic) nuclei. The associated underlying connective tissue is normal.

TREATMENT
Leukoedema is often included in the differential diagnosis of leukoplakias. Because of its bilateral locations, frequency of occurrence, and alteration in appearance when stretched, it is usually clinically recognized and does not require biopsy. No treatment is necessary.

WHITE SPONGE NEVUS

■ WHITE SPONGE NEVUS: an autosomal dominant hereditary condition in which the oral mucosa is white, thickened, and folded.

White sponge nevus, also termed "white-folded gingivostomatitis" and "oral epithelial nevus," is a relatively uncommon, autosomal dominant hereditary disorder that manifests as a white lesion of the oral mucosa. The condition exhibits a variable penetrance; some patients exhibit lesions at birth, whereas in others, lesions may not appear until early childhood or even adolescence.

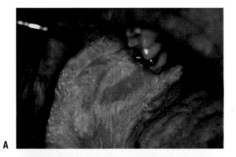

A

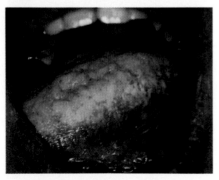

B

FIGURE 1-54

White sponge nevus. Patient with asymptomatic white folded superficial layer of the buccal mucosa **(A)** and tongue **(B)** that has been present for most of the patient's life.

CLINICAL
Lesions are asymptomatic, whitish, and often folded (corrugated). They may exhibit a translucent opalescence similar to that seen in leukoedema. Lesions may be widespread and involve various sites including the buccal mucosa, tongue (Figure 1-54), gingiva, palate, and floor of the mouth. In some patients lesions may be present on other surfaces such as the mucosa of the anus and the nares.

HISTOPATHOLOGY
White sponge nevus is characterized by a mild to moderate hyperparakeratosis, acanthosis, and intracellular edema of the spinous layer. The nuclei of the spinous cells are shrunken (pyknotic). The associated connective tissue is usually free of inflammation. The diagnosis is generally reached by combining its histopathologic features, clinical appearance, and the patient's family history.

TREATMENT

The condition requires no treatment since it is entirely benign. The patient often benefits from an explanation of the nature of the condition and its hereditary pattern so that future clinicians who observe the condition during routine examinations do not advise additional diagnostic procedures.

LINGUAL THYROID NODULE

> ■ LINGUAL THYROID NODULE: accessory accumulation of thyroid tissue that is usually functional within the body of the posterior tongue.

A lingual thyroid nodule is a rare anomaly characterized by the development of a mass of thyroid tissue on the midposterior dorsum of the tongue. Embryologically, the thyroid gland anlage arises at the site of the foramen caecum and migrates inferiorly along the thyroglossal tract to its ultimate destination in the anterior neck. If all or part of the thyroid anlage fails to migrate, remnants of thyroid tissue can develop along its path of migration; a lingual thyroid nodule represents a thyroid remnant in the region of the thyroid gland's origin. Microscopic examination of human tongues removed at autopsy reveals that despite the absence of a clinically apparent thyroid nodule, as many as 10% exhibit remnants of thyroid tissue within the tongue.

CLINICAL

A lingual thyroid nodule is far more common in females and most commonly becomes clinically apparent during puberty and adolescence. It presents as a 2 to 3 cm smooth sessile mass located on the midposterior dorsum of the tongue, in the region of the foreman caecum. The chief symptoms are dysphagia, dysphonia, dyspnea, and a feeling of tightness in the area.

HISTOPATHOLOGY

Most cases are composed of normal mature thyroid tissue, although embryonic or fetal thyroid tissue may also be seen.

TREATMENT

Before excision of a lingual thyroid nodule is planned, it should be determined if the patient possesses a functioning thyroid gland in the anterior neck with sufficient secretion to support the daily requirement when the supplementary source in the tongue is removed. If a normal thyroid gland is present, then the lingual nodules can be excised. If a subnormal thyroid gland has developed in the anterior neck as a result of the ancillary source, then thyroid replacement therapy is needed.

ORAL TONSIL

Tonsillar lymphoid tissue is primarily distributed in a circular arrangement (Waldeyer ring) in the posterior region of the mouth. It consists of three main masses of lymphoid tissue, namely the paired palatine (faucial) tonsils, the pharyngeal tonsils (adenoids), and the lingual tonsil located at the base of the tongue. The lingual tonsil often extends anteriorly along the posterolateral borders of the tongue and includes the region of the foliate papillae. Reactive lymphoid hyperplasia of the lingual tonsil in this location is sometimes termed *foliate papillitis*. In children and adolescents tonsillar tissue may also be visible as discrete, slightly elevated reddish plaques in the floor of the mouth on either side of the lingual frenum. These islands of extrapharyngeal tonsillar tissue are termed *"oral tonsils."* Oral tonsils consist of lymphoid aggregates that exhibit germinal centers surfaced by nonkeratinized squamous epithelium, with or without occasional crypts.

RETROCUSPID PAPILLA

The *retrocuspid papilla* is a 2 to 4 mm slightly raised area of mandibular alveolar mucosa located lingual to the cuspids, between the marginal gingiva and the mucogingival junction. It is commonly bilateral but can also be unilateral, and it is more prominent in children. Since retrocuspid papilla is commonly bilateral and has a very specific location, it is logical to assume that it represents a normal anatomic structure. Histologically, a retrocuspid papilla exhibits a striking resemblance to an incisive papilla; it is often composed of highly vascular fibrous connective tissue surfaced by orthokeratinized or parakeratinized squamous epithelium. Gross anatomic examination of human mandibles suggests that the retrocuspid papilla is analagous to an incisive papilla, representing a focus of fibrovascular tissue covering the osseous foramen of a nutrient blood vessel.

BONE

HEMIFACIAL HYPERTROPHY

Although most humans exhibit some degree of facial asymmetry, only individuals who exhibit significant unilateral enlargement of the face are considered to exhibit *hemifacial hypertrophy*. Although a number of factors have been proposed to explain this condition, the most plausible appears to be an increased neurovascular supply to the affected side of the face. Either side of the face can be affected, and there is a slight female predilection. Unilateral enlargement of the facial soft tissue, bones, and teeth is usually present. Specifically, the asymmetry usually involves the frontal bone, maxilla, palate, mandible, alveolar process, condyles, and associated soft tissue (Figure 1-55, *A*). On the affected side, the skin is thick and coarse, the hair is thick and abundant (hypertrichosis), and the sebaceous and sweat gland secretions are excessive. The ear and eye on the affected side may also be enlarged. Unilateral enlargement of the cerebral hemispheres may be responsible for the mental retardation seen in 15% to 20% of these patients and for the occurrence of seizures. Intraorally, a unilateral macroglossia (Figure 1-55, *B*) with an increase in the size of the fungiform papillae is often present. The roots and crowns of the teeth, particularly the permanent teeth, are often enlarged and may prematurely erupt. Because of the osseous and dental asymmetries, malocclusion is common (Figure 1-55, *C*). Patients with hemifacial hypertrophy may exhibit an increased incidence of certain visceral tumors, particularly Wilms tumor of the kidney. On rare occasions, the hypertrophy may extend beyond the face and include the entire side of the body.

The differential diagnosis of hemifacial hypertrophy should include neurofibromatosis, fibrous dysplasia, and arteriovenous malformation of the jaws. There is no specific treatment for hemifacial hypertrophy, although selective surgical treatment to improve functional and cosmetic abnormalities may be required in some cases.

HEMIFACIAL ATROPHY

Hemifacial atrophy is a rare condition characterized by a progressive decrease in the size of one side of the face. Occasionally, other parts of the body may also be affected. Although the cause of the condition is presently unknown, peripheral

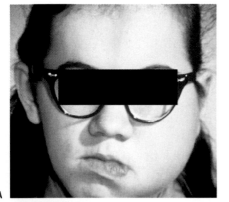
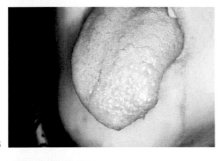
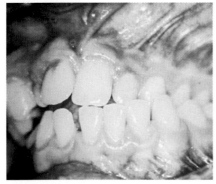

FIGURE 1-55

Hemifacial hypertrophy. The patient exhibits extensive disproportionate growth of the whole left side of the cranium, midface, and mandible **(A)**; the left side of the tongue **(B)**; and a severe malocclusion **(C)**.

nerve dysfunction, trauma, infection, heredity, and a regional unilateral progressive systemic sclerosis have been proposed as possible causes.

Clinically, the condition usually begins in the first or second decade of the patient's life. The tissues of the face, including the skin, subcutaneous tissue, muscle, and bone, are affected to varying degrees. The affected side of the face may become hyperpigmented, and a slightly depressed vertical furrow may become apparent at the midline of the forehead and brow. As the condition progresses, a hollowing of the cheek and the orbit may appear on the affected side. The left side of the face is more commonly affected than the right side. Other features that may accompany hemifacial atrophy include trigeminal neuralgia, ocular changes, facial hair loss, and contralateral jacksonian epilepsy. Intraorally, a unilateral atrophy of the lips and tongue are often present. The jaw bones and the roots of teeth on the affected side may exhibit delayed development, and tooth eruption may be retarded. There is no known treatment for hemifacial atrophy; however, progression of the condition usually ceases after a few years and remains static for the remainder of the patient's life.

CLEFT LIP AND CLEFT PALATE

■ CLEFT LIP: a developmental defect usually of the upper lip characterized by a wedge-shaped defect resulting from the failure of two parts of the lip to fuse into a single structure.

■ CLEFT PALATE: a developmental defect of the palate characterized by a lack of complete fusion of the two lateral portions of the palate, resulting in a communication with the nasal cavity.

Since cleft lip and cleft palate are developmentally related and often occur together, they will be discussed together. The etiology of cleft lip and cleft palate appears to involve both hereditary and environmental factors. Research indicates that approximately 40% of cleft lip cases, with or without cleft palate, appear to be hereditary, whereas less than 20% of isolated cleft palate cases appear to be hereditary. This type of genetic data suggests that cleft lip, with or without cleft palate, is distinct from isolated cleft palate.

A number of different studies have shown that most cleft cases are polygenic (influenced by several different genes acting together). In this context it is presumed that every individual carries some genetic liability for clefting, and only if the combined liabilities of the parents exceeds a minimum threshold does clefting occur in their offspring. Clefting occurs in numerous syndromes, which collectively represent approximately 5% of all cleft cases. In these syndromes, however, the clefting appears to be monogenic (influenced by a single gene) rather than polygenic. Although it is generally agreed that heredity is probably the most important single factor in cleft lip and cleft palate, a number of environmental factors have also been investigated.

Environmental factors that have been postulated to play an accessory role in the development of cleft lip and cleft palate include (1) nutritional factors such as deficiency of or excess of vitamin A and riboflavin deficiency; (2) physiologic, emotional, or traumatic stress; (3) relative ischemia to the area; (4) mechanical obstruction by an enlarged tongue; (5) substances such as alcohol, drugs, or toxins; and (6) infections. Experimental animal studies utilizing vitamin A deficiency, vitamin A excess, riboflavin deficiency in pregnant rats, and cortisone administration in pregnant rabbits have resulted in an increased incidence of cleft

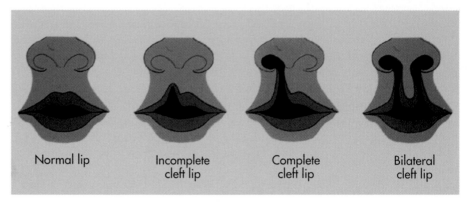

FIGURE 1-56

Cleft lip. Diagram of the common presentations of congenital defects in lip formation.

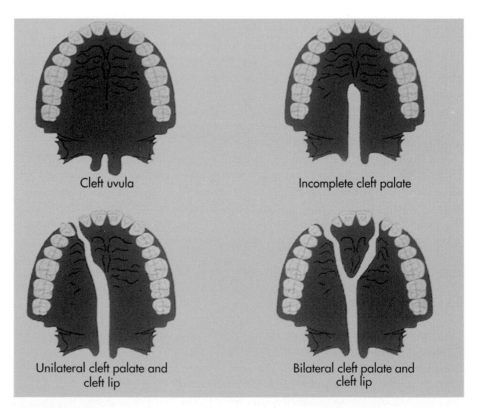

FIGURE 1-57

Cleft palate. Diagram of the common presentations of congenital defects in palate formation.

palate; no similar effects have been proven to occur in humans. Stress-induced hydrocortisone secretion in humans, analogous to cortisone administration in rabbits, has been postulated, but not conclusively proven, to result in cleft palate formation.

CLINICAL

Clefts of the lip and palate can be classified into four major categories: (1) cleft lip, (2) cleft palate, (3) unilateral cleft lip and palate, and (4) bilateral clefts of the lip and palate. Clefts of the upper lip can be classified as follows: (1) unilateral incomplete, (2) unilateral complete, (3) bilateral incomplete, and (4) bilateral complete (Figure 1-56).

Cleft deformities of the oral regions are extremely variable in complexity. They range from a minimal deformity such as a bifid uvula or a mild notch of the upper lip to severe bilateral clefts that involve the lip, alveolus, and the entire hard and soft palate (Figure 1-57). Cleft palate usually results in a direct communication between the oral and nasal cavities, resulting in significant functional impairment. Approximately 50% of isolated cleft palates are associated with other developmental abnormalities such as congenital heart disease, polydactyly and syndactyly, hydrocephalus, microcephalus, clubfoot, supernumerary ear, hypospadias, spina bifida, hypertelorism, and mental deficiency.

The incidence of the different types of clefts varies significantly. For example, clefts of the upper lip are relatively common, whereas clefts of the lower lip are extremely rare. Unilateral cleft upper lip accounts for approximately 80% of all cleft lips. The combined cleft lip and cleft palate is the most common type of cleft deformity, accounting for approximately 50% of all cleft cases. Cleft lip and cleft palate are somewhat more common in males than in females, whereas isolated cleft palate is more common in females. The incidence of cleft lip and cleft palate ranges between 1:700 and 1:1000 births. Isolated cleft lip and cleft palate each account for approximately 25% of the cases. The incidence of isolated cleft palate ranges between 1:1500 to 1:3000 births.

The **median maxillary anterior alveolar cleft** that occurs in approximately 1% of the population is unrelated to the cleft lip or cleft palate. In this particular type of cleft, the defect is limited to bone and there is no breach in the continuity of the soft tissue. The cleft can be visualized radiographically as an incomplete closure of the median fissure of the anterior maxilla. Clinically, a wide diastema is often present between the maxillary central incisors.

TREATMENT

Cleft lip is usually treated surgically during the first month of a patient's life. In most cases surgical repair achieves excellent cosmetic and functional results. Before treatment, cleft palate usually causes significant eating and drinking problems for the patient, with regurgitation of food and drink through the nose being particularly problematic. Surgical treatment of cleft palate is usually delayed until the patient is approximately 18 months of age. By this time significant growth has occurred, but speech habits have not yet been established. Surgical closure of cleft palate can be achieved in most cases; however, varying amounts of speech training may be required to overcome any functional deficiency. Therapeutic support may be needed to overcome any psychologic trauma that the patient may have experienced before treatment.

OSTEOPOROTIC BONE MARROW DEFECT

The osteoporotic bone marrow defect is an ill-defined radiolucency found in an edentulous area of the mandible that was previously occupied by a tooth. The most commonly proposed theory of pathogenesis is that following an extraction,

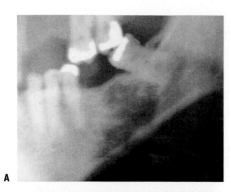

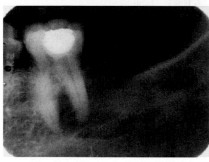

FIGURE 1-58

Osteoporotic bone marrow defect. Radiographs of edentulous areas of the posterior mandible containing an asymptomatic irregularly shaped mixed radiolucent/radiopacity **(A)** and a unilocular, mostly radiolucent area with faint wisps of bone **(B).**

the defect is replaced with hematopoietic marrow rather than the trabecular bone normal for the area.

The defect is symptomless, and no cortical expansion is found during a routine radiographic survey. It is found predominantly in middle-age females and in the mandibular molar area. The radiographic appearance is variable, ranging from a rounded, barely noticeable mixed radiolucent-radiopaque lesion to a diffuse irregularly shaped radiolucent area with faint wisps of a trabecular pattern (Figure 1-58). The microscopic appearance consists of normal hematopoietic elements with the usual spectrum of blast and mature cells in the erythrocytic, myelocytic, lymphocytic, and megakaryocytic series. This is in contrast to the adipose marrow commonly found in this location.

Since the radiographic appearance is nearly indistinguishable from more serious conditions such as Langerhans cell histiocytosis, metastatic carcinoma, and multiple myeloma, incisional biopsy is usually necessary. Once the diagnosis is confirmed, no further treatment is necessary.

CLEIDOCRANIAL DYSPLASIA

Cleidocranial dysplasia is a syndrome in which there is abnormal growth of the bones of the face, skull, and clavicles, with a concomitant tendency for failure of tooth eruption. The syndrome may be hereditary with an autosomal dominant pattern or appear as a spontaneous mutation. The degree of involvement varies widely.

The striking features in the appearance of the patients with high expressivity are the disproportionate growth of the facial and skull bones that produces the characteristic facial appearance and their ability to appose the shoulders to near the midline of the chest. The frontal and occipital skull plates are enlarged (bossing), whereas the other bones may remain relatively normal, producing an enlarged and abnormally shaped head (Figure 1-59). Radiographs of these bones

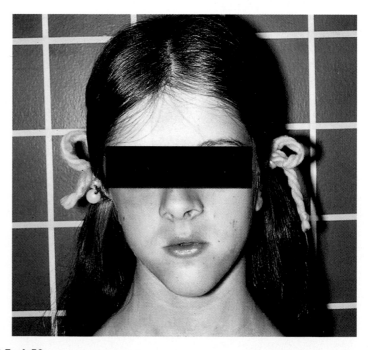

FIGURE 1-59

Cleidocranial dysplasia. Typical facies of patient exhibiting bossing of frontal bones, depressed midface, and prominent chin.   (Courtesy Dr. Richard K. Wesley.)

usually reveal tortuous suture lines ("wormian bones") and some areas in which the sutures are greatly widened caused by the lack of sufficient bone growth within the plates (Figure 1-60). This is in contrast to an underdeveloped midface and a maxilla that appears depressed, particularly in relation to the enlarged forehead. The nose is commonly flat, wide, and lacks a bridge. Although the mandible may be of normal size, it appears enlarged because of the hypoplastic maxilla. The clavicles may be bilaterally absent or may have various sizes of partial structures (Figure 1-61).

Intraorally, patients may retain the primary dentition into adulthood; radiographs reveal numerous fully formed teeth embedded within the mandible and maxilla, many of which are supernumerary (Figure 1-62). The palate is usually highly vaulted and narrow.

There is no known treatment for patients with cleidocranial dysplasia, except counseling regarding its hereditary tendency. Extraction of primary teeth does not necessarily result in eruption of the secondary dentition, although exposure combined with orthodontic procedures may be helpful in some cases.

LINGUAL MANDIBULAR SALIVARY GLAND DEPRESSION

■ LINGUAL MANDIBULAR SALIVARY GLAND DEPRESSION: a developmental concavity of the lingual cortex of the mandible, usually in the third molar area, that forms around an accessory lateral lobe of the submandibular gland and has the radiographic appearance of a well-circumscribed cystic lesion within the bone, usually below the inferior alveolar canal.

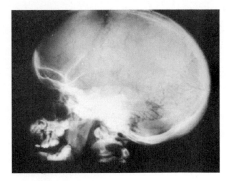

FIGURE 1-60

Cleidocranial dysplasia. Same patient as in Figure 1-59. Lateral cranial radiograph depicting the disproportionately large frontal and occipital bones, tortuous suture lines ("wormian bones"), and depressed midfacial bones.   (Courtesy Dr. Richard K. Wesley.)

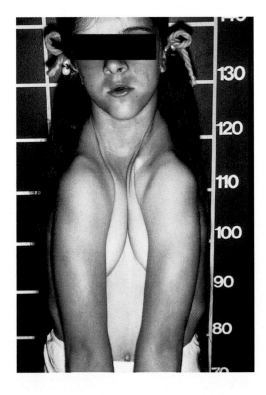

FIGURE 1-61

Cleidocranial dysplasia. Same patient as in Figure 1-59. The patient is able to proximate the shoulders as a result of aplasia or extensive hypoplasia of the clavicle bones.   (Courtesy Dr. Richard K. Wesley.)

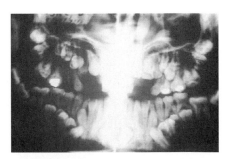

FIGURE 1-62

Cleidocranial dysplasia. Panoramic radiograph of dentition demonstrating the presence of a permanent dentition with associated supernumerary teeth embedded within the mandible and maxilla and deciduous dentition that has failed to exfoliate.

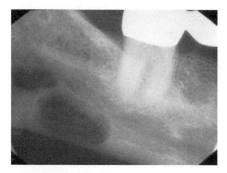

FIGURE 1-63

Lingual mandibular salivary gland depression. Radiograph of molar area of mandible revealing the presence of an oval-shaped, circumscribed radiolucency beneath the inferior alveolar canal that is not in continuity with the apices of the overlying molar. (Courtesy Dr. Heddie O. Sedano.)

The lingual mandibular salivary gland depression is also referred to by several other names such as Stafne cyst, static bone cyst, and latent bone cyst. It is a relatively uncommon entity that presents as a distinct, localized, deep concavity (depression) located on the lingual aspect of the mandible, between the mandibular canal and the inferior border of the mandible (Figure 1-63). Although most commonly seen in the molar region, this entity can occasionally involve the lingual aspect of the anterior mandible. Most reported cases of this entity have been in males. Sialography has shown that the concavities in the molar region are usually occupied by an accessory lateral lobe of the submandibular salivary gland. Surgical exploration and biopsy of the contents of these concavities generally reveals normal submandibular salivary gland tissue. Although the radiologic appearance and the anatomic location of this entity are considered to be characteristic, sialography or magnetic resonance imaging (MRI) can be utilized to confirm the salivary gland nature of this entity. No treatment is required.

ADDITIONAL READING

GENERAL

Aldred M, Crawford P. Register of developmental dental anomalies. *Br Dent J.* 1989; 167:370.

Jones ML, Mourino AP, Bowden TA. Evaluation of occlusion, trauma, and dental anomalies in African-American children of metropolitan Headstart programs. *J Clin Pediatr Dent.* 1993; 18:51-4.

MacDonald-Jankowski DS. Multiple dental developmental anomalies. *Dentomaxillofac Radiol.* 1991; 20:166-8.

Trope M, Rabie G, Tronstad L. Pulp capping of immature teeth with anatomic anomalies. *Endod Dent Traumatol.* 1991; 7:139-43.

Witkop CJ. Clinical aspects of dental anomalies. *Int Dent J.* 1976; 26:378-90.

MICRODONTIA AND MACRODONTIA

Atasu M, Atalay T, Eryilmaz A. Macrodontia: a clinical, genetic and dermatoglyphic study of a case and his family members. *J Clin Pediatr Dent.* 1994; 18:223-6.

Bazopoulou-Kyrkanidou E, Dacou-Voutetakis C, Nassi H, Tosios K and others. Microdontia, hypodontia, short bulbous roots and root canals with strabismus, short stature, and borderline mentality. *Oral Surg Oral Med Oral Pathol.* 1992; 74:93-5.

Gazit E, Lieberman MA. Macrodontia of maxillary central incisors: case reports. *Quintessence Int.* 1991; 22:883-7.

Patel JR. Transposition and microdontia. *Oral Surg Oral Med Oral Pathol.* 1993; 76:129.

Thorburn DN, Ferguson MM. Familial ogee roots, tooth mobility, oligodontia, and microdontia: Christchurch Hospital, New Zealand. *Oral Surg Oral Med Oral Pathol.* 1992; 74:576-81.

CONGENITALLY ABSENT AND SUPERNUMERARY TEETH

Clarke A, Burn J. Sweat testing to identify female carriers of X linked hypohidrotic ectodermal dysplasia. *J Med Genet.* 1991; 28:330-3.

Russell BG, Kjaer I. Tooth agenesis in Down syndrome. *Am J Med Genet.* 1995; 13;55:466-71.

Stermer Beyer-Olsen EM. Premaxillary hyperdontia in medieval Norwegians: a radiographic study. *Dentomaxillofac Radiol.* 1989; 18:177-9.

Vierucci S, Baccetti T, Tollaro I. Dental and craniofacial findings in hypohidrotic ectodermal dysplasia during the primary dentition phase. *J Clin Pediatr Dent.* 1994; 18:291-7.

TOOTH ERUPTION

Carl W, Sullivan MA. Dental abnormalities and bone lesions associated with familial adenomatous polyposis: report of cases. *J Am Dent Assoc.* 1989; 119:137-9.

Priddy RW, Price C. The so-called eruption sequestrum. *Oral Surg Oral Med Oral Pathol.* 1984; 58:321-6.

Watkins JJ. An unusual eruption sequestrum: a case report. *Br Dent J.* 1975; 138:395-6.

TAURODONTISM

Alvesalo L, Varrela J. Taurodontism and the presence of an extra Y chromosome: study of 47 XYY males and analytical review. *Hum Biol.* 1991; 63:31-8.

Houlston RS, Winter GB, Speight PM, Fairhurst J and others. Taurodontism and disproportionate short stature. *Clin Dysmorphol.* 1994; 3:251-4.

Jaspers MT. Taurodontism in the Down syndrome. *Oral Surg Oral Med Oral Pathol.* 1981; 51:632-6.

Li Y, Navia JM, MacDonald-Jankowski DS, Li TT. Taurodontism in a young adult: Chinese population. *Dentomaxillofac Radiol.* 1993; 22:140-4.

Seow WK. Taurodontism of the mandibular first permanent molar distinguishes between the tricho-dento-osseous (TDO) syndrome and amelogenesis imperfecta. *Clin Genet.* 1993; 43:240-6.

Sood PB, Sood M. Taurodontism and pyramidal molars. *J Indian Soc Pedod Prev Dent.* 1992; 10:25-7.

Varrela J, Alvesalo L. Taurodontism in females with extra X chromosomes. *J Craniofac Genet Dev Biol.* 1989; 9:129-33.

DENS INVAGINATUS (DENS IN DENTE)

Kulild JC, Weller RN. Treatment considerations in dens invaginatus. *J Endod.* 1989; 15:381-4.

Vajrabhaya L. Nonsurgical endodontic treatment of a tooth with double dens in dente. *J Endod.* 1989; 15:323-5.

DENS EVAGINATUS AND SUPERNUMERARY CUSPS

Reddy VV, Mehta DS. Talon cusp in primary lateral incisor: report of a case. *J Indian Soc Pedod Prev Dent.* 1989; 7:20-2.

Rusmah M. Talon cusp in Malaysia. *Aust Dent J.* 1991; 36:11-4.

Wong MT, Augsburger RA. Management of dens evaginatus. *Gen Dent.* 1992; 40:300-3.

Yip, WK. The prevalence of dens evaginatus. *Oral Surg.* 1974; 38:80-87.

SUPERNUMERARY ROOTS

Ferraz JA, Pecora JD. Three-rooted mandibular molars in patients of Mongolian, Caucasian and Negro origin. *Braz Dent J.* 1993; 3:113-7.

Sabala CL, Benenati FW, Neas BR. Bilateral root or root canal aberrations in a dental school patient population. *J Endod.* 1994; 20:38-42.

CERVICAL ENAMEL PROJECTION AND ENAMELOMA

Askenas BG, Fry HR, Davis JW. Cervical enamel projection with gingival fenestration in a maxillary central incisor: report of a case. *Quintessence Int.* 1992; 23:103-7.

Gaspersic D. Histogenetic aspects of the composition and structure of human ectopic enamel studied by scanning electron microscopy. *Arch Oral Biol.* 1992; 37:603-11.

ENAMEL HYPOPLASIA

Bian JY. Prevalence and distribution of developmental enamel defects in primary dentition of Chinese children 3-5 years old. *Community Dent Oral Epidemiol.* 1995; 23:72-9.

Burkes EJ, Lyles KW, Dolan EA, Giammara B and others. Dental lesions in tumoral calcinosis. *J Oral Pathol Med.* 1991; 20:222-7.

Clarkson J. Review of terminology, classifications, and indices of developmental defects of enamel. *Adv Dent Res.* 1989; 3:104-9.

Commission on Oral Health, Research and Epidemiology. A review of the developmental defects of enamel index (DDE index): report of an FDI working group. *Int Dent J.* 1992; 42:411-26.

Hargreaves JA, Cleaton-Jones PE, Roberts GJ, Williams SD. Hypocalcification and hypoplasia in primary teeth of preschool children from different ethnic groups in South Africa. *Adv Dent Res.* 1989; 3:110-3.

Horowitz HS. Fluoride and enamel defects. *Adv Dent Res.* 1989; 3:143-6.

Nunn JH, Rugg-Gunn AJ, Ekanayake L, Saparamadu KD. Prevalence of developmental defects of enamel in areas with differing water fluoride levels and socio-economic groups in Sri Lanka and England. *Int Dent J.* 1994; 44:165-73.

Suckling GW. Developmental defects of enamel: historical and present-day perspectives of their pathogenesis. *Adv Dent Res.* 1989; 3:87-94.

Woltgens JH, Etty EJ, Nieuwland WM, Lyaruu DM. Use of fluoride by young children and prevalence of mottled enamel. *Adv Dent Res.* 1989; 3:177-82.

HEREDITARY AND ENDOCRINE-RELATED TOOTH ANOMALIES

Brown MD, Aaron G. Pseudohypoparathyroidism: case report. *Pediatr Dent.* 1991; 13:106-9.

Iorio RJ, Bell WA, Meyer MH, Meyer RA. Histologic evidence of calcification abnormalities in teeth and alveolar bone of mice with X-linked dominant hypophosphatemia (VDRR). *Ann Dent.* 1979; 38:38-44.

Jensen SB, Illum F, Dupont E. Nature and frequency of dental changes in idiopathic hypoparathyroidism and pseudohypoparathyroidism. *Scand J Dent Res.* 1981; 89:26-37.

Macfarlane JD, Swart JG. Dental aspects of hypophosphatasia: a case report, family study, and literature review. *Oral Surg Oral Med Oral Pathol.* 1989; 67:521-6.

Mayhall JT, Alvesalo L. Dental morphology of 45 XO human females: molar cusp area, volume, shape and linear measurements. *Arch Oral Biol.* 1992; 37:1039-43.

Midtbo M, Halse A. Tooth crown size and morphology in Turner syndrome. *Acta Odontol Scand.* 1994; 52:7-19.

Seow WK. X-linked hypophosphataemic vitamin D-resistant rickets. *Aust Dent J.* 1984; 29:371-7.

Shaw L, Foster TD. Size and development of the dentition in endocrine deficiency. *J Pedod.* 1989; 13:155-60.

Shebib SM, Reed MH, Shuckett EP, Cross HG and others. Newly recognized syndrome of cerebral, ocular, dental, auricular, skeletal anomalies: CODAS syndrome—a case report. *Am J Med Genet.* 1991; 40:88-93.

Wright JT, Roberts MW, Wilson AR, Kudhail R. Tricho-dento-osseous syndrome: features of the hair and teeth. *Oral Surg Oral Med Oral Pathol.* 1994; 77:487-93.

AMELOGENESIS IMPERFECTA

Everett MM, Miller WA. Enamel matrix proteins in normal and abnormal amelogenesis. *J Dent Res.* 1979; 58(Spec Issue B):995-6.

Sundell S, Koch G. Hereditary amelogenesis imperfecta. *Swed Dent J.* 1983; 9:157-169.

Sundell S, Valentin J. Hereditary aspects and classification of hereditary amelogenesis imperfecta. *Community Dent Oral Epidemiol.* 1986; 14:211-216.

Winter GB, Brook AH. Enamel hypoplasia and anomalies of the enamel. *Dent Clin North Am.* 1975; 19:3-24.

Witkop CJ, Sauk JJ. Heritable defects of enamel. In: Stewart RE, Prescott GH eds, *Oral Facial Genetics.* St. Louis: Mosby; 1976:151-226.

DENTINOGENESIS IMPERFECTA

Levin LS and others. Dentinogenesis imperfecta in the Brandywine isolate (DI type III): clinical, radiologic and scanning electron microscopic studies of the dentition. *Oral Surg Oral Med Oral Pathol.* 1983; 56:267.

Shields ED, Bixler D, El-Kafrawy AM. A proposed classification of heritable human dentine defects with a description of a new entity. *Arch Oral Biol.* 1973; 18:543.

Witkop CJ. Hereditary defects of dentin. *Dent Clin North Am.* 1975; 9:25-45.

DENTIN DYSPLASIA

Steidler NE, Radden BG, Reade PC. Dentin dysplasia: a clinicopathological study of eight cases and review of the literature. *Br J Oral Maxillofac Surg.* 1984; 22:274.

Wesley RK, Wysocki GP, Mintz SM, Jackson J. Dentin dysplasia type I. *Oral Surg.* 1976; 41:516.

REGIONAL ODONTODYSPLASIA

Gardner DG. The dentinal changes in regional odontodysplasia. *Oral Surg.* 1974; 38:887-897.

Gardner DG, Sapp JP. Regional odontodysplasia. *Oral Surg.* 1973; 35:351-365.

Gardner DG, Sapp JP. Ultrastructural, electron probe and microhardness studies of the controversial amorphous areas in the dentin of regional odontodysplasia. *Oral Surg.* 1977; 44:754-766.

Neupert EA, Wright JM. Regional odontodysplasia presenting as a soft tissue swelling. *Oral Surg Oral Med Oral Pathol.* 1989; 67:193.

Reever JS, King WC. Unilateral maxillary odontodysplasia. *ASDC J Dent Child.* 1971; 38:23-8.

Sapp JP, Gardner DG. Regional odontodysplasia: an ultrastructural and histochemical study of the soft tissue calcifications. *Oral Surg.* 1973; 36:383-392.

Walton JL, Witkop CJ, Walker PO. Odontodysplasia: report of three cases with vascular nevi overlying the adjacent skin of the face. *Oral Surg Oral Med Oral Pathol.* 1978; 46:676.

LIP PITS

Baker WR. Pits of the lip commissure in caucasoid males. *Oral Surg Oral Med Oral Pathol.* 1966; 21:56.

Christian J, Gorlin RJ, Anderson VE. The syndrome of pits of the lower lip and/or palate: genetic considerations. *Clin Genet.* 1971; 2:95-103.

Ord RA, Sowray JH. Congenital lip pits and facial clefts. *Br J Oral Maxillofac Surg.* 1985; 23:391.

DOUBLE LIP

Barnett ML, Bosshardt LL, Morgan AF. Double lip and double lip with blepharochalasis (Ascher's syndrome). *Oral Surg Oral Med Oral Pathol.* 1972; 34:727.

Papanayotou PH, Hatziotis JC. Ascher's syndrome: report of a case. *Oral Surg Oral Med Oral Pathol.* 1973; 35:467.

ANKYLOGLOSSIA

Berg KL. Tongue-tie (ankyloglossia) and breastfeeding: a review. *J Hum Lact.* 1990; 6:109-12.

Chidzonga MM, Shija JK. Congenital median cleft of the lower lip, bifid tongue with ankyloglossia, cleft palate, and submental epidermoid cyst: report of a case. *J Oral Maxillofac Surg.* 1988; 46:809-12.

Fleiss PM, Burger M, Ramkumar H, Carrington P. Ankyloglossia: a cause of breastfeeding problems? *J Hum Lact.* 1990; 6:128-9.

Gorski SM, Adams KJ, Birch PH, Chodirker BN and others. Linkage analysis of X-linked cleft palate and ankyloglossia in Manitoba, Mennonite and British Columbia Native kindreds. *Hum Genet.* 1994; 94:141-8.

Lekkas C, Bruaset I. Ankyloglossia superior. *Oral Surg Oral Med Oral Pathol.* 1983; 55:556-7.

Minami K, Sugahara T, Mori Y, Mishima K. Ankyloglossia superior: report of a case. *J Oral Maxillofac Surg.* 1995; 53:588-9.

Mukai S, Mukai C, Asaoka K. Congenital ankyloglossia with deviation of the epiglottis and larynx: symptoms and respiratory function in adults. *Ann Otol Rhinol Laryngol.* 1993; 102(8 pt 1):620-4.

Notestine GE. The importance of the identification of ankyloglossia (short lingual frenulum) as a cause of breastfeeding problems. *J Hum Lact.* 1990; 6:113-5.

Patterson GT, Ramasastry SS, Davis JU. Macroglossia and ankyloglossia in Beckwith-Wiedemann syndrome. *Oral Surg Oral Med Oral Pathol.* 1988; 65:29-31.

Stanier P, Forbes SA, Arnason A, Bjornsson A and others. The localization of a gene causing X-linked cleft palate and ankyloglossia (CPX) in an Icelandic kindred is between DXS326 and DXYS1X. *Genomics.* 1993; 17:549-55.

Warden PJ. Ankyloglossia: a review of the literature. *Gen Dent.* 1991; 39:252-3.

MACROGLOSSIA

Dinerman WS, Myers EN. Lymphangiomatous macroglossia. *Laryngoscope.* 1976; 86:291-6.

Dolan EA, Riski JE, Mason RM. Macroglossia: clinical considerations. *Int J Orofacial Myology.* 1989; 15:4-7.

Gaikwad S, Varthakavi P, Chandalia M, Nihalani KD. Macroglossia: the presenting feature of primary amyloidosis. *J Assoc Physicians India*. 1993; 41:386-8.

Harada K, Enomoto S. A new method of tongue reduction for macroglossia. *J Oral Maxillofac Surg*. 1995; 53:91-2.

Katou F, Shirai N, Motegi K, Satoh R and others. Symmetrical lipomatosis of the tongue presenting as macroglossia: report of two cases. *J Craniomaxillofac Surg*. 1993; 21:298-301.

Martinez Y, Martinez R, Reynoso MC, Hernandez A and others. Autosomal dominant macroglossia: an addendum to the etiological classification. *Ear Nose Throat J*. 1995; 74:108-9.

Meares N, Braude S, Burgess K. Massive macroglossia as a presenting feature of hypothyroid-associated pericardial effusion. *Chest*. 1993; 104:1632-3.

Mixter RC, Ewanowski SJ, Carson LV. Central tongue reduction for macroglossia. *Plast Reconstr Surg*. 1993; 91:1159-62.

Myer CM, Hotaling AJ, Reilly JS. The diagnosis and treatment of macroglossia in children. *Ear Nose Throat J*. 1986; 65:444-8.

Oliver AJ. Multiple myeloma presenting with amyloid purpura and macroglossia: a case report and literature review. *Compendium*. 1994; 15:712, 714-6.

Padgham ND, Bingham BJ, Purdue BN. Episodic macroglossia in Down's syndrome. *J Laryngol Otol*. 1990; 104:494-6.

Patterson GT, Ramasastry SS, Davis JU. Macroglossia and ankyloglossia in Beckwith-Wiedemann syndrome. *Oral Surg Oral Med Oral Pathol*. 1988; 65:29-31.

Reynoso MC, Hernandez A, Lizcano-Gil LA, Sarralde A and others. Autosomal dominant congenital macroglossia: further delineation of the syndrome. *Genet Couns*. 1994; 5:151-4.

Saah D, Braverman I, Elidan J, Nageris B. Traumatic macroglossia. *Ann Otol Rhinol Laryngol*. 1993; 102:729-30.

Theetranont C, Tantachamrun T, Rangsiyanond P, Phatharakulwanich S. The exomphalos, macroglossia, gigantism (EMG) syndrome. *J Med Assoc Thai*. 1978; 61:285-93.

Vogel JE, Mulliken JB, Kaban LB. Macroglossia: a review of the condition and a new classification. *Plast Reconstr Surg*. 1986; 78:715-23.

Weiss LS, White JA. Macroglossia: a review. *J La State Med Soc*. 1990; 142:13-6.

Wittmann AL. Macroglossia in acromegaly and hypothyroidism. *Virchows Arch A Pathol Pathol Anat*. 1977; 373:353-60.

Wu NF, Kushnick T. The Beckwith-Wiedemann syndrome: the exomphalos-macroglossia-gigantism syndrome. *Clin Pediatr (Phila)*. 1974; 13:452-7.

FORDYCE GRANULES

Cashion PD, Skobe Z, Nalbandian J. Ultrastructural observations on sebaceous glands of the human oral mucosa (Fordyce's disease). *J Invest Dermatol*. 1969; 53:208-16.

Gorsky M, Buchner A, Fundoianu-Dayan D, Cohen C. Fordyce's granules in the oral mucosa of adult Israeli Jews. *Community Dent Oral Epidemiol*. 1986; 14:231-2.

Rhodus NL. An actively secreting Fordyce granule: a case report. *Clin Prev Dent*. 1986; 8:24-6.

LINGUAL THYROID NODULE

Diaz-Arias AA, Bickel JT, Loy TS, Croll GH and others. Follicular carcinoma with clear cell change arising in lingual thyroid. *Oral Surg Oral Med Oral Pathol*. 1992; 74:206-11.

Douglas PS, Baker AW. Lingual thyroid. *Br J Oral Maxillofac Surg*. 1994; 32:123-4.

Jones JA. Lingual thyroid. *Br J Oral Maxillofac Surg*. 1986; 24:58-62.

Latimer J, Lindsay KA. Case report: lingual thyroid in association with a lateral ectopic thyroid mass. *Clin Radiol*. 1995; 50:501-2.

LiVolsi VA, Perzin KH, Savetsky L. Carcinoma arising in median ectopic thyroid (including thyroglossal duct tissue). *Cancer*. 1974; 34:1303.

Potdar GG, Desai PB. Carcinoma of the lingual thyroid. *Laryngoscope*. 1971; 81:427-9.

Singh HB, Joshi HC, Chakravarty M. Carcinoma of the lingual thyroid: review and case report. *J Laryngol Otol*. 1979; 93:839-44.

Vairaktaris E, Semergidis T, Christopoulou P, Papadogeorgakis N and others. Lingual thyroid: a new surgical approach—a case report. *J Craniomaxillofac Surg*. 1994; 22:307-10.

Van der Wal N, Wiener JD, Van der Waal I. Lingual thyroid: a clinical and postmortem study. *Int J Oral Maxillofac Surg*. 1986; 15:431-6.

LEUKOEDEMA

Axell T, Henricsson V. Leukoedema: an epidemiologic study with special reference to the influence of tobacco habits. *Community Dent Oral Epidemiol*. 1981; 9:142-6.

Borghelli RF, Stirparo M, Andrade J, Barros R and others. Leukoedema in addicts to coca leaves in Humahuaca, Argentina. *Community Dent Oral Epidemiol*. 1975; 3:40-3.

Frithiof L, Banoczy J. White sponge nevus (leukoedema exfoliativum mucosae oris): ultrastructural observations. *Oral Surg Oral Med Oral Pathol*. 1976; 41:607-22.

Kaugars GE. Common white lesions of the oral cavity. *New Dent*. 1981; 11:25-8, 35.

Martin JL. Leukoedema: a review of the literature. *J Natl Med Assoc*. 1992; 84:938-40.

van Wyk CW. An investigation into the association between leukoedema and smoking. *J Oral Pathol*. 1985; 14:491-9.

van Wyk CW, Ambrosio SC. Leukoedema: ultrastructural and histochemical observations. *J Oral Pathol*. 1983; 12:319-29.

Van Wyk CW, Ambrosio SC, van der Vyver PC. Abnormal keratohyalin-like forms in leukoedema. *J Oral Pathol*. 1984; 13:271-81.

Waitzer S, Fisher BK. Oral leukoedema. *Arch Dermatol*. 1984; 120:264-6.

WHITE SPONGE NEVUS

Cox MF, Eveson J, Porter SR, Maitland N and others. Human papillomavirus type 16 DNA in oral white sponge nevus. *Oral Surg Oral Med Oral Pathol.* 1992; 73:476-8.

Duncan SC, Su WP. Leukoedema of the oral mucosa: possibly an acquired white sponge nevus. *Arch Dermatol.* 1980; 116:906-8.

Frithiof L, Banoczy J. White sponge nevus (leukoedema exfoliativum mucosae oris): ultrastructural observations. *Oral Surg Oral Med Oral Pathol.* 1976; 41:607-22.

Jorgenson RJ, Levin S. White sponge nevus. *Arch Dermatol.* 1981; 117:73-6.

McGininis JP, Turner JE. Ultrastructure of the white sponge nevus. *Oral Surg Oral Med Oral Pathol.* 1975; 40:644-51.

Morris R, Gansler TS, Rudisill MT, Neville B. White sponge nevus: diagnosis by light microscopic and ultrastructural cytology. *Acta Cytol.* 1988; 32:357-61.

Su L, Morgan PR, Thomas JA, Lane EB. Expression of keratin 14 and 19 mRNA and protein in normal oral epithelia, hairy leukoplakia, tongue biting and white sponge nevus. *J Oral Pathol Med.* 1993; 22:183-9.

RETROCUSPID PAPILLA

Buchner A, Merrel PW, Hansen LS, Leider AS. The retrocuspid papilla of the mandibular lingual gingiva. *J Periodontol.* 1990; 61:586-590.

HEMIFACIAL HYPERTROPHY AND HEMIFACIAL ATROPHY

Czarnecki ES, Carrel R. Hemifacial hypertrophy. *J Pedod.* 1982; 6:270-80.

Hume WJ. Hemifacial hypertrophy associated with endocrine disharmony. *Br Dent J.* 1975; 139:16-20.

Khanna JN, Andrade NN. Hemifacial hypertrophy: report of two cases. *Int J Oral Maxillofac Surg.* 1989; 18:294-7.

Kogon SL, Jarvis AM, Daley TD, Kane MF. Hemifacial hypertrophy affecting the maxillary dentition. *Oral Surg Oral Med Oral Pathol.* 1984; 58:549-53.

Lawoyin JO, Daramola JO, Lawoyin DO. Congenital hemifacial hypertrophy: report of two cases. *Oral Surg Oral Med Oral Pathol.* 1989; 68:27-30.

Loh HS. Congenital hemifacial hypertrophy. *Br Dent J.* 1982; 153:111-2.

Viteporn S. Surgical-orthodontic treatment in hemifacial hypertrophy: a case report. *Int J Adult Orthodon Orthognath Surg.* 1993; 8:55-62.

Whyman RA, Doyle TC, Harding WJ, Ferguson MM. An unusual case of hemifacial atrophy. *Oral Surg Oral Med Oral Pathol.* 1992; 73:564-9.

CLEFT LIP AND CLEFT PALATE

Amaratunga NA. A comparative clinical study of Pierre Robin syndrome and isolated cleft palate. *Br J Oral Maxillofac Surg.* 1989; 27:451-8.

Bhatia SN. Genetics of cleft lip and palate. *Br Dent J.* 1972; 132:95.

Brattstrom V. Craniofacial development in cleft lip and palate children related to different treatment regimes. *Scand J Plast Reconstr Surg Hand Surg Suppl.* 1991; 25:1-31.

Fraser FC. Research revisited: the genetics of cleft lip and cleft palate. *Cleft Palate J.* 1989; 26:255-7.

Gorlin RJ, Cohen MM, Levin SL. *Syndromes of the Head and Neck.* 3rd ed. New York: Oxford University Press; 1990.

Hochman N, Yaffe A, Brin I, Zilberman Y and others. Functional and esthetic rehabilitation of an adolescent cleft lip and palate patient. *Quintessence Int.* 1991; 22:401-4.

Jiroutova O, Mullerova Z. The occurrence of hypodontia in patients with cleft lip and/or palate. *Acta Chir Plast.* 1994; 36:53-6.

Lal N, Utreja A, Tewari A, Chari PS. Transverse and vertical asymmetry of bilateral craniofacial structures in repaired unilateral and bilateral complete cleft lip and palate cases. *J Indian Soc Pedod Prev Dent.* 1991; 9:41-6.

McCance A, Roberts-Harry D, Sherriff M, Mars M and others. Sri Lankan cleft lip and palate study model analysis: clefts of the secondary palate. *Cleft Palate Craniofac J.* 1993; 30:227-30.

Ranta R. Forward traction of the maxilla with cleft lip and palate in mixed and permanent dentitions. *J Craniomaxillofac Surg.* 1989; 17(suppl 1):20-2.

Ranta R. Orthodontic treatment in adults with cleft lip and palate. *J Craniomaxillofac Surg.* 1989; 17(suppl 1):42-4.

Roberts CT, Semb G, Shaw WC. Strategies for the advancement of surgical methods in cleft lip and palate. *Cleft Palate Craniofac J.* 1991; 28:141-9.

Sandham A. Classification of clefting deformity. *Early Hum Dev.* 1985; 12:81-85.

Smahel Z, Mullerova Z. Craniofacial growth and development in unilateral cleft lip and palate: clinical implications (a review). *Acta Chir Plast.* 1995; 37:29-32.

Smahel Z, Mullerova Z. Facial growth and development in unilateral cleft lip and palate from the time of palatoplasty to the onset of puberty: a longitudinal study. *J Craniofac Genet Dev Biol.* 1995; 15:72-80.

Thomson HG, Reinders FX. A long-term appraisal of the unilateral complete cleft lip repair: one surgeon's experience. *Plast Reconstr Surg.* 1995; 96:549-61.

OSTEOPOROTIC BONE MARROW DEFECT

Gordy FM, Crews KM, O Carroll MK. Focal osteoporotic bone marrow defect in the anterior maxilla. *Oral Surg Oral Med Oral Pathol.* 1993; 76:537-42.

Sa'do B, Ozeki S, Higuchi Y, Nakayama E. Osteoporotic bone marrow defect of the mandible: report of a case diagnosed by computed tomography scanning. *J Oral Maxillofac Surg.* 1992; 50:80-2.

Schneider LC, Mesa ML, Fraenkel D. Osteoporotic bone marrow defect: radiographic features and pathogenic factors. *Oral Surg Oral Med Oral Pathol.* 1988; 65:127-9.

Wilson DF, D'Rozario R, Bosanquet A. Focal osteoporotic bone marrow defect. *Aust Dent J.* 1985; 30:77-80.

CLEIDOCRANIAL DYSPLASIA

Dard M. Histology of alveolar bone and primary tooth roots in a case of cleidocranial dysplasia. *Bull Group Int Rech Sci Stomatol Odontol.* 1993; 36:101-7.

Feldman GJ, Robin NH, Brueton LA, Robertson E and others. A gene for cleidocranial dysplasia maps to the short arm of chromosome 6. *Am J Hum Genet.* 1995; 56:938-43.

Frame K, Evans RI. Progressive development of supernumerary teeth in cleidocranial dysplasia. *Br J Orthod.* 1989; 16:103-6.

Jensen BL, Kreiborg S. Dental treatment strategies in cleidocranial dysplasia. *Br Dent J.* 1992; 172:243-7.

Jensen BL, Kreiborg S. Craniofacial abnormalities in 52 school-age and adult patients with cleidocranial dysplasia. *J Craniofac Genet Dev Biol.* 1993; 13:98-108.

Jensen BL, Kreiborg S. Craniofacial growth in cleidocranial dysplasia: a roentgencephalometric study. *J Craniofac Genet Dev Biol.* 1995; 15:35-43.

Mundlos S, Mulliken JB, Abramson DL, Warman ML and others. Genetic mapping of cleidocranial dysplasia and evidence of a microdeletion in one family. *Hum Mol Genet.* 1995; 4:71-5.

Quinn PD, Lewis J, Levin LM. Surgical management of a patient with cleidocranial dysplasia: a case report. *Spec Care Dentist.* 1992; 12:131-3.

Richardson A, Deussen FF. Facial and dental anomalies in cleidocranial dysplasia: a study of 17 cases. *Int J Pediatr Dent.* 1994; 4:225-31.

Seow WK, Hertzberg J. Dental development and molar root length in children with cleidocranial dysplasia. *Pediatr Dent.* 1995; 17:101-5.

Sillence DO, Ritchie HE, Selby PB. Animal model: skeletal anomalies in mice with cleidocranial dysplasia. *Am J Med Genet.* 1987; 27:75-85.

DEVELOPMENTAL LINGUAL SALIVARY GLAND DEPRESSION

Adra NA, Barakat N, Melhem RE. Salivary gland inclusions in the mandible: Stafne's idiopathic bone cavity. *AJR Am J Roentgenol.* 1980; 134:1082-3.

Ariji E, Fujiwara N, Tabata O, Nakayama E and others. Stafne's bone cavity: classification based on outline and content determined by computed tomography. *Oral Surg Oral Med Oral Pathol.* 1993; 76:375-80.

Barker GR. A radiolucency of the ascending ramus of the mandible associated with invested parotid salivary gland material and analogous with a Stafne bone cavity. *Br J Oral Maxillofac Surg.* 1988; 26:81-4.

Barker GR. Xeroradiography in relation to a Stafne bone cavity. *Br J Oral Maxillofac Surg.* 1988; 26:32-5.

Cataldo E, Kabani S. A clinico-pathological presentation: lingual mandibular salivary gland depression. *J Mass Dent Soc.* 1985; 34:8.

Salman L, Chaudhry AP. Malposed sublingual gland in the anterior mandible: a variant of Stafne's idiopathic bone cavity. *Compendium.* 1991; 12:40, 42-3.

Sawyer DR, Nwoku AL, Elzay RP, Allison MJ and others. Two probable cases of a depression in the mandible caused by the submandibular salivary gland in Pre-Columbian Peruvians. *J Maxillofac Surg.* 1981; 9:194-6.

Smith NJ, Looh FC, Todd JM, Whaites EJ. Stafne's bone cavity: a review of the literature and report of two cases. *Clin Radiol.* 1985; 36:297-9.

Tominaga K, Kuga Y, Kubota K, Ohba T. Stafne's bone cavity in the anterior mandible: report of a case. *Dentomaxillofac Radiol.* 1990; 19:28-30.

Wolf J, Mattila K, Ankkuriniemi O. Development of a Stafne mandibular bone cavity: report of a case. *Oral Surg Oral Med Oral Pathol.* 1986; 61:519-21.

CYSTS OF THE ORAL REGIONS

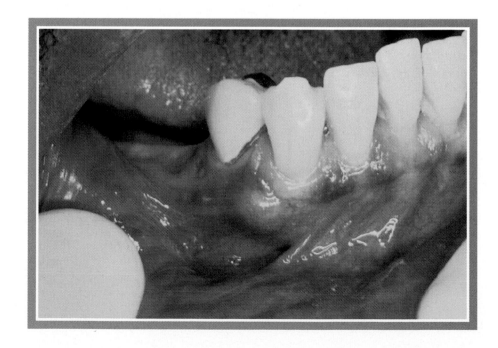

■ CYST: an abnormal cavity, lined by epithelium, containing fluid or semisolid material.

A cyst is composed of three basic structures: a central cavity (lumen), an epithelial lining, and an outer wall (capsule) (Figure 2-1). The cystic cavity usually contains fluid or semisolid material such as cellular debris, keratin, or mucus. The epithelial lining differs among cyst types and may be keratinized or nonkeratinized stratified squamous, pseudostratified, columnar, or cuboidal. The cyst wall is composed of connective tissue containing fibroblasts and blood vessels. Cysts often exhibit varying degrees of inflammation that can alter their basic morphology, sometimes obscuring their identifying features. Intense inflammation can destroy some or all of the epithelial lining. In rare instances the entire lining of a cyst may be destroyed by inflammation, allowing it to resolve completely without treatment.

Cysts are common lesions and are clinically important because they are often destructive. They produce significant signs and symptoms, particularly when they become large or infected.

Most cysts of the oral region are true cysts since they possess an epithelial lining. However, a short list of additional lesions are referred to as "cysts," although they possess no epithelial lining. The "pseudocysts" are lesions such as traumatic bone cyst, aneurysmal bone cyst, and static bone cyst, which are discussed elsewhere.

The true cysts of the oral region can be divided into those of odontogenic and developmental (nonodontogenic) origin.

ODONTOGENIC CYSTS

■ ODONTOGENIC CYST: a cyst in which the lining of the lumen is derived from epithelium produced during tooth development.

To facilitate an understanding of the origin and classification of odontogenic cysts, an understanding of odontogenesis is necessary (see Chapter 5). Odontogenic cysts are derived from the following epithelial structures: (1) **rests of Malassez**—remnants of the Hertwig epithelial root sheath that persist in the periodontal ligament after root formation is complete; (2) **reduced enamel epithelium**—residual epithelium that surrounds the crown of the tooth after enamel formation is complete; and (3) **remnants of the dental lamina (rests of Serres)**—islands and strands of epithelium that originate from the oral epithelium and remain in the tissues after inducing tooth development. These three sources of odontogenic epithelium represent logical categories on which a histogenetic classification of odontogenic cysts can be based (Box 2-1).

Making an accurate diagnosis of an odontogenic cyst requires information relative to its clinical, radiographic, and histologic findings. In many instances two cysts that are classified differently may exhibit similar histologic features. In such cases clinical and radiographic findings are necessary to make a precise diagnosis (Figure 2-2).

CYSTS DERIVED FROM RESTS OF MALASSEZ

The rests of Malassez are small islands and strands of odontogenic epithelium found in the periodontal ligament. They represent remnants of Hertwig root

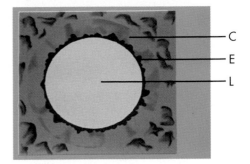

FIGURE 2-1

Diagram of a cyst consisting of an outer fibrous connective tissue capsule *(C)*, epithelial lining *(E)*, and lumen *(L)*.

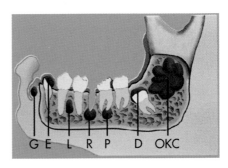

FIGURE 2-2

Diagram of odontogenic cysts based on typical clinical and radiographic features. *Left to right: G,* gingival; *E,* eruption; *L,* lateral periodontal; *R,* residual; *P,* periapical; *D,* dentigerous; *OKC,* odontogenic keratocyst.

■ **BOX 2-1**
A Histogenetic Classification of Odontogenic Cysts

Cysts Derived from Rests of Malassez
  Periapical cyst
    Residual cyst

Cysts Derived from Reduced Enamel Epithelium
  Dentigerous cyst
    Eruption cyst

Cysts Derived from Dental Lamina (Rests of Serres)
  Odontogenic keratocyst
    Multiple
  Lateral periodontal cyst
    Polycystic (botryoid)
  Gingival cyst of the adult
  Dental lamina cyst of the newborn
  Glandular odontogenic cyst

Unclassified
  Paradental cyst

sheath, an embryologic epithelial structure that surrounds a developing root. Although rests of Malassez are present along the entire length of the root, they are most plentiful at the apical region.

Periapical Cyst

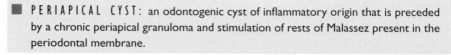

■ PERIAPICAL CYST: an odontogenic cyst of inflammatory origin that is preceded by a chronic periapical granuloma and stimulation of rests of Malassez present in the periodontal membrane.

The periapical cyst, also termed *radicular cyst* and *apical periodontal cyst*, is by far the most common type of odontogenic cyst, representing over one half of all oral cysts. It develops at the root apex of an erupted tooth whose pulp has been devitalized by dental caries or trauma (Figure 2-3). The recent decline in the incidence of dental caries has resulted in a corresponding decline in the incidence of periapical cysts. This cyst arises from the rests of Malassez, which enlarge in response to inflammation elicited by bacterial infection of the pulp or in direct response to necrotic pulpal tissue. Because epithelial cells derive their nutrients by diffusion from the adjacent connective tissues, progressive growth of an epithelial island moves the innermost cells of that island away from their nutrients. Ultimately, these innermost cells undergo ischemic liquefactive necrosis, establishing a central cavity (lumen) surrounded by viable epithelium. At this point an osmotic gradient is established across the epithelial lining (membrane) separating the connective tissue fluids from the necrotic contents of the newly formed cyst. The net effect of this osmotic gradient is a progressive increase in fluid volume within the lumen, tending to expand the cyst by the internal hydraulic pressure generated.

CLINICAL

Although most periapical cysts develop at the apex of a root, adjacent to the pulp canal opening, they can occasionally develop at the opening of large accessory pulp canals through which pulpal inflammation and products of pulpal necrosis can exit to form granulomas and stimulate the rests of Malassez located on the lateral aspect of the roots of teeth. These laterally positioned inflammatory cysts have been termed *lateral radicular (periapical) cysts*.

The size of periapical cysts is variable, but they generally measure less than 1 cm in diameter. Occasionally, however, the cyst can become much larger, especially in areas where several adjacent teeth of the anterior mandible or maxilla have been devitalized as a result of facial trauma, commonly the result of an automobile accident.

RADIOGRAPHIC

The periapical cyst appears as a rounded, well-circumscribed, often corticated radiolucency at the apex of a nonvital tooth. Cysts that develop on the lateral aspect of the root appear as semicircular radiolucencies against the root surface. Occasionally a periapical cyst that develops in the anterior maxilla in the apical region of a lateral incisor tooth will appear as a **globulomaxillary radiolucency** that may result in divergence of the roots of the lateral incisor and the adjacent cuspid. Histopathologic studies of globulomaxillary radiolucencies indicate that approximately 50% of these radiolucencies are periapical (radicular) cysts. The remaining globulomaxillary radiolucencies represent a spectrum of odontogenic and nonodontogenic lesions that include periapical granuloma, lateral periodontal cyst, odontogenic keratocyst, central giant cell granuloma, adenomatoid odontogenic tumor, calcifying odontogenic cyst, odontogenic myxoma, and ameloblastoma.

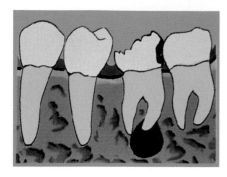

FIGURE 2-3

Periapical cyst.

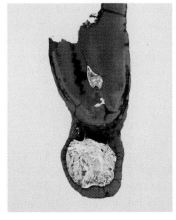
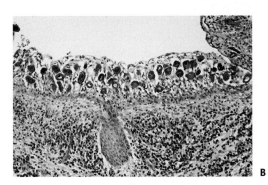

FIGURE 2-4

Periapical cyst. A, Carious root fragment with nonvital pulp and periapical cyst attached to apex. **B,** The intraepithelial reddish colored oval and crescent-shaped structures are termed Rushton bodies.

HISTOPATHOLOGY

A periapical cyst is characterized by a cavity lined with a layer of nonkeratinized squamous epithelium of variable thickness (Figure 2-4, *A*). These cysts are typically inflamed, and neutrophils are usually present within the epithelial lining. Because the inflammation is often intense, it may destroy part of the epithelial lining, leaving a zone of granulation tissue in its place. The epithelium and occasionally the connective tissues of a small percentage (5% to 10%) of odontogenic cysts exhibit collections of laminated crescent-shaped structures termed **hyaline (Rushton) bodies** (Figure 2-4, *B*). Although these curious structures appear to be unique to odontogenic cysts, they have no known biologic importance. The connective tissue wall of the periapical cyst generally exhibits a significant inflammatory infiltrate consisting of plasma cells, lymphocytes, lipid-laden histiocytes, and neutrophils. Foreign body giant cells associated with crystalline cholesterol deposits and deposits of hemosiderin are also frequently present in the cyst wall. The cystic lumen usually contains proteinaceous fluid and necrotic cellular debris.

TREATMENT

Treatment of periapical cysts depends on a number of variables. Most of these cysts are treated by enucleation after extraction or endodontic treatment of the offending tooth. Extracting the offending tooth without removing the associated cyst may result in its persistence and continued growth. A cyst that remains at the site of a previously extracted tooth is termed a **residual cyst** (Figure 2-5). Although this is the most common use of the term, it also denotes any cyst present in an edentulous area in which the origin of the epithelial lining is unknown.

CYSTS DERIVED FROM REDUCED ENAMEL EPITHELIUM

Reduced enamel epithelium refers to the layer of epithelium that remains around the tooth's crown after enamel formation is complete. This layer of epithelium is derived from the specialized epithelial components of the enamel organ (inner enamel epithelium, stratum intermedium, stellate reticulum, and outer enamel epithelium) that were active during amelogenesis (enamel formation) and collapses into a thinned dormant membrane of two or three cells in

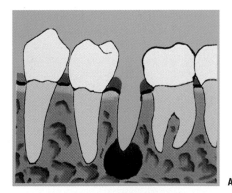
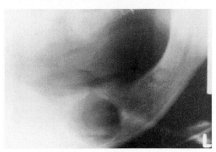

FIGURE 2-5

A, Residual cyst. **B,** Radiograph of residual cyst in an edentulous mandible.

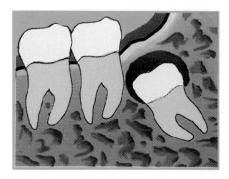

FIGURE 2-6

Dentigerous cyst.

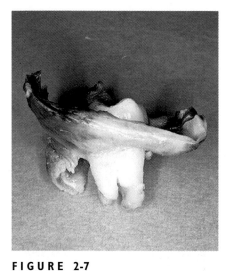

FIGURE 2-7

Dentigerous cyst. Capsule attached at cementoenamel junction exhibiting the classical appearance of the crown present within the lumen and the roots outside.

thickness. In addition, the reduced enamel epithelium may include a small population of cells derived from the dental lamina that was connected to the enamel organ during its formation. The reduced enamel epithelium therefore is a complex collection of postsecretory cells whose ratios may differ between teeth and between individuals. Whether the cellular composition of the reduced enamel epithelium affects the growth potential of individual dentigerous cysts is presently unknown.

Dentigerous Cyst

■ DENTIGEROUS CYST: an odontogenic cyst that surrounds the crown of an impacted tooth; caused by fluid accumulation between the reduced enamel epithelium and the enamel surface, resulting in a cyst in which the crown is located within the lumen and root(s) outside.

The dentigerous cyst is derived from reduced enamel epithelium that surrounds the crown of an unerupted tooth. Little is known about the stimulus that separates the reduced enamel epithelium from the enamel surface, creating a space for fluid accumulation around the crown of the tooth. These cysts are commonly associated with unerupted mandibular (Figure 2-6) or maxillary third molars or maxillary cuspids. Regardless of its size, the cyst remains attached to the cervical margin of the affected tooth. The crown of the tooth is therefore located within the lumen of the cyst and the root remains outside (Figure 2-7).

CLINICAL

A dentigerous cyst usually remains asymptomatic but may produce some swelling or pain, particularly if it is large or inflamed. Because a dentigerous cyst forms around the crown of an impacted or embedded tooth, the arch will clinically appear to be missing at least one tooth.

RADIOGRAPHIC

Dentigerous cysts are most commonly diagnosed by their radiographic appearance. They present as well-circumscribed radiolucencies surrounding the crown of a tooth (Figure 2-8). The interface with the surrounding bone is corticated, indicative of its slow and uniform growth. In the mandible this cyst may displace the associated tooth inferiorly or superiorly into the ascending ramus. In the maxilla it usually displaces the associated tooth superiorly and posteriorly.

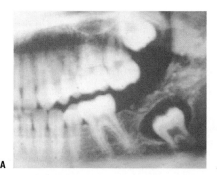

A

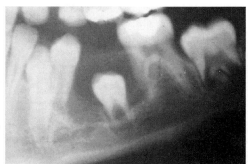

B

FIGURE 2-8

Dentigerous cyst. A, Radiograph exhibiting an unerupted molar of the left mandible with a circumscribed radiolucency around the crown. **B,** Radiograph of premolar with dentigerous cyst producing displacement of some of the adjacent teeth.

HISTOPATHOLOGY

The cystic cavity of a dentigerous cyst is lined by a relatively uniform layer of nonkeratinized, stratified, squamous epithelium measuring two to ten cells in thickness (Figure 2-9). Inflammation usually alters the epithelial lining. Depending on the type of inflammation (acute or chronic) and its severity (mild or severe), the epithelial lining may become hyperplastic, atrophic, or ulcerated. In most cases the inflammation is usually a mixture of chronic and acute inflammatory cells. Some of the incidental microscopic features seen in periapical cysts, including crystalline cholesterol deposits, hemosiderin deposits, hyaline (Rushton) bodies, and lipid-laden macrophages are also seen in dentigerous cysts. In addition, variable numbers of mucus cells are occasionally seen in the epithelial lining of this cyst. This finding has been described as either *mucus cell metaplasia* or *mucus cell prosoplasia*. Long-standing dentigerous cysts will occasionally exhibit areas of keratinization or premalignant (dysplastic) changes of their epithelial lining.

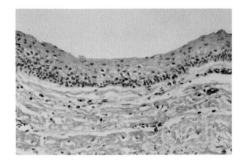

FIGURE 2-9

Dentigerous cyst. Lining exhibiting a thin stratified squamous epithelium without rete peg formation and a capsule of dense fibrous connective tissue.

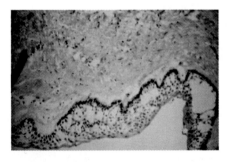

FIGURE 2-10

Ameloblastomatous change of lining epithelium of an odontogenic cystic lesion. Such changes are identical to those commonly observed in unicystic ameloblastoma.

TREATMENT

Most dentigerous cysts are treated by surgical enucleation. In the case of molar teeth the associated tooth is often extracted at the time that the cyst is enucleated. In the case of maxillary cuspid teeth the cyst may be excised or marsupialized and the tooth brought into proper alignment in the arch with the aid of an orthodontic appliance. Postsurgical recurrence of dentigerous cysts is uncommon. Although it occurs infrequently, several different epithelial neoplasms including ameloblastoma (Figure 2-10), mucoepidermoid carcinoma, and squamous cell carcinoma (Figure 2-11) can arise in dentigerous cysts. Under such circumstances the cyst and its associated neoplasm would usually require more aggressive treatment to eradicate the neoplasm.

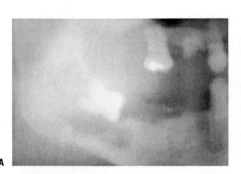

A

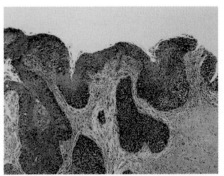

B

FIGURE 2-11

Squamous cell carcinoma arising in the wall of a dentigerous cyst. Radiographic **(A)** and microscopic features **(B).**   (From Johnson LM, Sapp JP, McIntire DN. Squamous cell carcinoma arising in a dentigerous cyst. *J Oral Maxillofac Surg.* 1994; 52:987-990.)

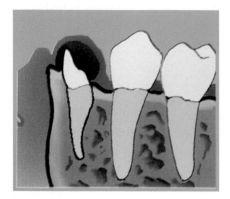

FIGURE 2-12

Eruption cyst.

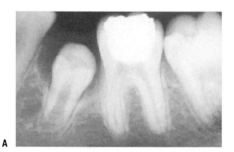

A

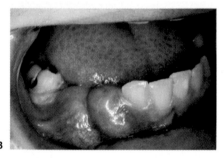

B

FIGURE 2-13

Eruption cyst. A, Radiograph of a partially erupted premolar. **B,** Clinical appearance of fluctuant soft tissue masses of lesions overlying two erupted premolars.

Eruption Cyst

■ ERUPTION CYST: an odontogenic cyst with the histologic features of a dentigerous cyst that surrounds a tooth's crown that has erupted through bone but not soft tissue and is clinically visible as a soft fluctuant mass on the alveolar ridges.

The eruption cyst is a variant of the dentigerous cyst that develops in the alveolar soft tissue around the crown of an erupting tooth (Figures 2-12 and 2-13, *A*). Because this cyst is largely confined to soft tissues, it is clinically evident as a fluctuant swelling of the alveolar ridge (Figure 2-13, *B*) rather than as an intrabony radiolucency. Mastication will occasionally induce hemorrhage in an eruption cyst, giving rise to the term "eruption hematoma" for this cyst. The cyst is derived from the reduced enamel epithelium, and its histologic features are essentially the same as those of a dentigerous cyst. Variable numbers of ghosted epithelial cells, derived from exfoliated lining cells, are often seen within the organizing hemorrhage that may be present in the lumen of these cysts. Most of these cysts require no treatment because they spontaneously rupture and become exteriorized as a result of normal mastication. For those eruption cysts that do not resolve spontaneously, the crown of the involved tooth can be surgically exposed, simultaneously treating the cyst and allowing the involved tooth to erupt.

CYSTS DERIVED FROM DENTAL LAMINA (RESTS OF SERRES)

The **dental lamina** is an embryologic strand of epithelium that carries the dental organ to its destination within the developing fetal jaws. During its functional period, the dental lamina connects the developing enamel organ to the alveolar mucosa. In its postfunctional period, the dental lamina becomes disrupted into a series of small islands and strands of epithelium that are termed **rests of dental lamina** (Figure 2-14, *A*). These rests persist into adulthood and can be found in the gingival connective tissue and within the underlying alveolar bone. These rests generally exhibit the features of squamous cells, but some accumulate significant amounts of glycogen that impart a clear or transparent appearance to their cytoplasm. The "clear" cell rests of dental lamina are termed **rests of Serres**. Although the two forms of the rests of the dental lamina are technically different, both names are commonly used interchangeably (Figure 2-14, *B*).

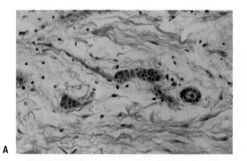

A

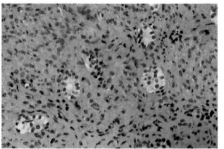

B

FIGURE 2-14

Rests of the dental lamina. A, Common form; **B,** less common clear cell variant (rests of Serres).

Odontogenic Keratocyst

■ ODONTOGENIC KERATOCYST: a cyst derived from the remnants (rests) of the dental lamina, with a biologic behavior similar to a benign neoplasm, with a distinctive lining of six to ten cells in thickness, and that exhibits a basal cell layer of palisaded cells and a surface of corrugated parakeratin.

The **odontogenic keratocyst (OKC)** is derived from remnants of the dental lamina. On occasion it also seems to arise from the lining of a dentigerous cyst. In this latter instance some believe that rather than the lining undergoing a transitional change, fusion with a nearby independent keratocyst occurs. OKC can develop at virtually any site in the jaws, with approximately two thirds of the cases occurring in the mandible, primarily in the posterior body and ramus areas (Figure 2-15). Although OKC is usually present as a single lesion, it can occasionally occur as multiple cysts that sometimes occupy all four quadrants of the jaws. OKC possesses a remarkable growth potential, greater than the other odontogenic cysts, and can attain a large size resulting in massive bone destruction (Figure 2-16, *A*). Lesions of the maxilla occur primarily in the posterior segment or in the cuspid-lateral incisor area (Figure 2-16, *B*). OKC exhibits a recurrence rate of 25% to 60%, similar to that of a neoplasm. In this respect OKC differs significantly from the other odontogenic cysts.

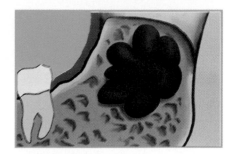

FIGURE 2-15
Odontogenic keratocyst.

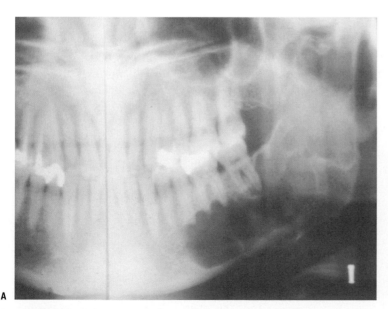

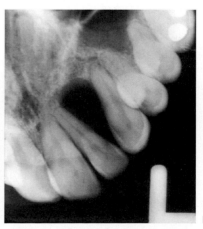

A   B

FIGURE 2-16
Odontogenic keratocyst. A, Large multilocular lesion of left mandible extending into the coronoid and condylar neck of the ascending ramus. **B,** Unilocular lesion of anterior maxilla in cuspid-lateral (globulomaxillary) area.

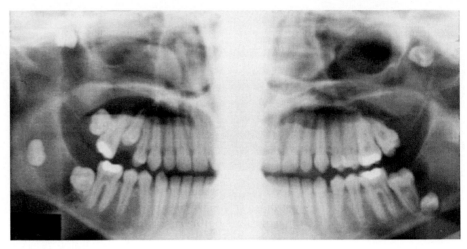

FIGURE 2-17

Nevoid basal cell carcinoma syndrome. Reveals multiple odontogenic keratocysts. Lesions are present in the posterior of all four quadrants with displaced unerupted molars.

CLINICAL

Odontogenic keratocysts occur in patients over a wide age range, from the first to the eighth decades of life; the peak incidence occurs in patients who are in the second and third decades. Multiple odontogenic keratocysts in the same patient are one of the consistent features of the **nevoid basal cell carcinoma syndrome** (Gorlin-Goltz syndrome) (Figure 2-17). Patients who exhibit multiple odontogenic keratocysts should therefore be appropriately examined to rule out this autosomal dominant syndrome. Predominant features of this syndrome, in addition to multiple OKC, bifid ribs, and basal cell carcinoma are calcification of the falx cerebri (Figure 2-18, *A*), multiple small epidermoid cysts (milia) (Figure 2-18, *B*), frontal bossing, shortened metacarpals (Figure 2-18, *C*), and medulloblastoma (Box 2-2).

RADIOGRAPHIC

The odontogenic keratocyst will appear as a well-defined, solitary lesion or as a multilocular/polycystic radiolucency exhibiting a thin corticated margin. The corticated appearance of this cyst will usually be obscured if the cyst is inflamed or has perforated the cortex of the involved bone.

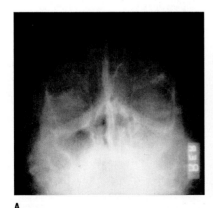

A

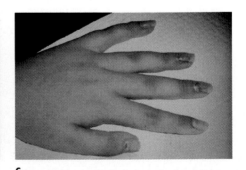

B   **C**

FIGURE 2-18

Nevoid basal cell carcinoma syndrome. Features include calcification of the falx cerebri **(A)**, forehead exhibiting frontal bossing with skin "milia" **(B)**, and shortened metacarpals **(C)**.

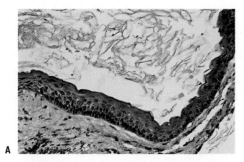
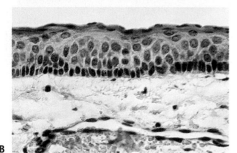
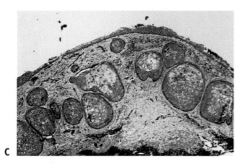
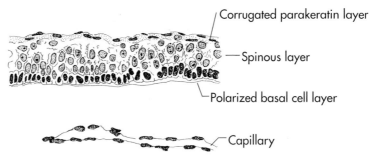

A
B
C

FIGURE 2-19

Odontogenic keratocyst. Low **(A)** and high **(B)** magnification of thin epithelial lining (six to ten cells) exhibiting the keratin-filled lumen, corrugated parakeratinizing surface, and palisaded basal cell layer that lacks rete peg formation and displays a delicate, loose connective tissue capsule. **C,** Capsule wall containing satellite (daughter) cysts.

Corrugated parakeratin layer

Spinous layer

Polarized basal cell layer

Capillary

HISTOPATHOLOGY

The microscopic appearance of odontogenic keratocysts is distinctive, characterized by (1) a thin, uniform lining of parakeratinized squamous epithelium, usually 6 to 10 cells in thickness; (2) a palisaded layer of columnar or cuboidal basal cells; (3) a corrugated (rippled) layer of parakeratin on its luminal surface; and (4) a lack of rete pegs. Commonly, there is focal separation of the epithelial lining from the adjacent connective tissue, which is often loose and fibrillar and usually free of inflammation. The cystic lumen contains variable amounts of desquamated parakeratin. Additional features that are occasionally seen include remnants of dental lamina, microcyst formation, satellite (daughter) cysts, epithelial budding from basal cell area, and a lining composed of orthokeratinized rather than parakeratinized epithelium (Figure 2-19). A summary of these features is outlined in Box 2-3.

TREATMENT

The treatment of the odontogenic keratocyst is surgical enucleation. In cases where extensive perforation of the mandible has occurred, surgical resection has occasionally been used. Marsupialization has been largely ineffective in reducing the size of keratocysts. Despite the skill of the surgeon, recurrences of this cyst can be expected, and the patient should be advised that more than one procedure may be required to eradicate the cyst. Although most recurrences will become apparent within the first 5 years following surgical removal, they may occasionally recur as long as 10 years later. Close clinical follow-up of the surgical site is therefore advisable. A notable exception to the relatively high recurrence rate of

---

■ BOX 2-3
Histologic Features of Odontogenic Keratocysts

Thin uniform lining of parakeratinized squamous epithelium of 6 to 10 cells

Corrugated parakeratin on the luminal surface

Lack of rete peg formation

Focal separation of epithelial lining from the connective tissue

Lumen containing variable amounts of desquamated parakeratin

Dental lamina rests and microcysts occasionally present in capsule wall

Generally lacks inflammatory response in capsule

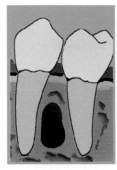

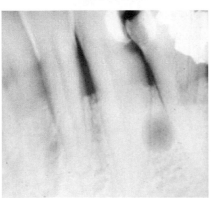

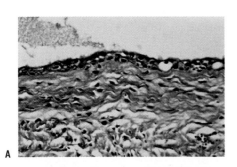

FIGURE 2-20

A, Lateral periodontal cyst. **B,** Radiograph of small lesion in premolar-cuspid area.

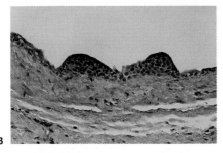

FIGURE 2-21

Lateral periodontal cyst. A, Epithelial lining consisting of cuboidal cells with occasional clear cells. **B,** Lining containing focal thickenings (plaques).

odontogenic keratocysts is the uncommon orthokeratinized variant of this cyst, which has a low recurrence rate (less than 5%).

Lateral Periodontal Cyst

> ■ LATERAL PERIODONTAL CYST: a slow-growing, nonexpansile developmental odontogenic cyst derived from one or more rests of the dental lamina, containing an embryonic lining of one to three cuboidal cells and distinctive focal thickenings (plaques).

CLINICAL

The lateral periodontal cyst is a relatively uncommon odontogenic cyst that shares a striking number of clinical and morphologic similarities with the gingival cyst of the adult. These similarities have led to the conclusion that the lateral periodontal cyst and the gingival cyst of the adult represent intraosseous and extraosseous manifestations of the same lesion, both being derived from rests of dental lamina (rests of Serres).

RADIOGRAPHIC

The lateral periodontal cyst is commonly seen as a small, well-defined, delicately corticated, solitary radiolucency located between the roots of vital teeth (Figure 2-20, *A*). The lesion is usually less than 1 cm in diameter and is most commonly found in the mandibular premolar region (Figure 2-20, *B*) and in the maxilla between the cuspid and lateral incisor. However, it occasionally occurs between any of the anterior teeth of the mandible or maxilla. The mean age of occurrence of this cyst is in patients who are approximately 50 years old.

HISTOPATHOLOGY

The typical histologic features include a thin lining of nonkeratinized epithelium measuring one to three cells in thickness, with variable numbers of glycogen-rich clear cells (Figure 2-21, *A*). Some of these cysts exhibit focal epithelial thickenings (plaques) (Figure 2-21, *B*) that exhibit cellular features seen in rests of Serres. In addition, rests of Serres in various stages of cyst formation can occasionally be seen in the wall of this cyst. This cyst is derived from dental lamina rests.

Although most lateral periodontal cysts are unicystic, they can occasionally be polycystic (Figure 2-22). This polycystic variant was originally described as the **"botryoid odontogenic cyst."** Its development seems to represent simultaneous cyst change in multiple adjacent rests of dental lamina.

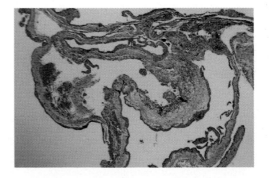

FIGURE 2-22

Lateral periodontal cyst. Polycystic variant or "botryoid odontogenic cyst."

Treatment

The treatment for this cyst is surgical enucleation. Recurrence is uncommon.

Gingival Cyst of the Adult

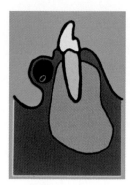

> ■ GINGIVAL CYST OF THE ADULT: a small developmental odontogenic cyst of the gingival soft tissue derived from the rests of the dental lamina, containing a lining of embryonic epithelium of cuboidal cells and distinctive focal thickenings similar to the lateral periodontal cyst.

FIGURE 2-23

Gingival cyst of the adult.

The gingival cyst of the adult is located in the gingival soft tissues outside of bone (Figure 2-23) and is derived from the rests of the dental lamina (rests of Serres), the same rests that give rise to the lateral peridontal cyst.

CLINICAL

The gingival cyst of the adult occurs as a firm but compressible, fluid-filled swelling on the mandibular or maxillary facial gingiva in the premolar/cuspid/incisor region (Figure 2-24). The clinical distribution, clinical size, age of occurrence, and histologic features of the gingival cyst of the adult are strikingly similar to those of the lateral periodontal cyst. For these reasons it has been concluded that these two cysts represent the extraosseous and intraosseous manifestations of the same entity.

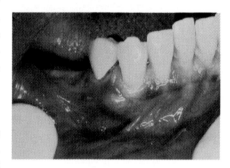

FIGURE 2-24

Gingival cyst of the adult. Lesion of the gingiva in the premolar-cuspid area.

RADIOGRAPHIC

Most gingival cysts of the adult are confined to the gingival soft tissues and are therefore not apparent on radiographs. Occasionally, however, they will cause a pressure-induced depression (saucerization) in the underlying alveolar bone that is sometimes apparent on radiologic examination.

HISTOPATHOLOGY

Lesions are often small, with the epithelial lining closely resembling the lining of the lateral periodontal cyst (Figure 2-25, *A*). It is thin, usually two to five cells in thickness, and often contains mural thickenings (plaques) (Figure 2-25, *B*). As in the lateral periodontal cyst, clear cells may be present.

TREATMENT

This cyst is easily treated with conservative surgical enucleation and has no tendency to recur.

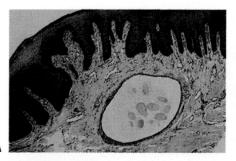 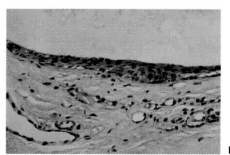

A   B

FIGURE 2-25

Gingival cyst of the adult. Small lesion of gingiva (**A**) with lining containing focal thickening (plaque) similar to lateral periodontal cyst (**B**).

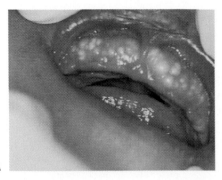

A

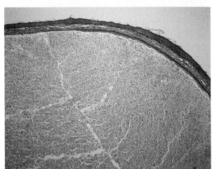

B

FIGURE 2-26

Dental lamina cysts of the newborn. A, Multiple whitish lesions of maxillary alveolar ridge of infant. **B,** Microscopic appearance consists of a large lumen filled with desquamated keratin and lined by a thinned stratified squamous epithelium.

Dental Lamina Cyst of the Newborn

> ■ DENTAL LAMINA CYST OF THE NEWBORN: uncommon superfical raised nodules on edentulous alveolar ridges of infants that resolve without treatment; derived from rests of the dental lamina and consisting of a keratin-producing epithelial lining.

The dental lamina cyst of the newborn, as the name indicates, is derived from the remnants (rests) of the dental lamina that remain in the soft tissues of the jaws. The cysts are generally seen on the alveolar ridges of newborn infants as small, often multiple swellings (Figure 2-26, *A*). The microscopic appearance consists of a superficially located thin-walled cystic lesion lined by a thin, stratified, squamous epithelium, and containing compacted desquamated keratin (Figure 2-26, *B*). Because these cysts usually resolve spontaneously in response to normal function, they require no treatment. It is of interest to note the remarkable difference in the age occurrence between the dental lamina cyst of the newborn and the gingival cyst of the adult, both of which are generally agreed to arise from dental lamina. The disparity in age of occurrence between these two cysts is probably best explained by the likelihood that the two cysts arise from different dental lamina, respectively, the "primary dental lamina," which is more superficial, and the "permanent dental lamina."

Glandular Odontogenic Cyst (Sialo-Odontogenic Cyst)

> ■ GLANDULAR ODONTOGENIC CYST: an unusually large solitary or multilocular odontogenic cyst probably derived from the rests of dental lamina, consisting of a stratified squamous epithelium containing numerous mucus-secreting cells.

The glandular odontogenic cyst was first described in 1987. It has also been referred to as *sialo-odontogenic cyst.* Because the histologic features in some examples of this cyst closely resemble those seen in the polycystic variant of lateral periodontal cyst (botryoid odontogenic cyst), both are considered to arise from dental lamina. Although the glandular odontogenic cyst shares some features with the lateral periodontal cyst, it exhibits some distinctive features. It exhibits a much greater growth potential than the lateral periodontal cyst and has a propensity to recur, thus justifying its classification as a separate entity.

RADIOGRAPHIC
The glandular odontogenic cyst occurs primarily in the mandible. The radiographic appearance is not specific, with lesions commonly being large. Cysts may appear as well-defined, unilocular, or multilocular radiolucencies.

HISTOPATHOLOGY
The histologic features that typify this unusual cyst include (1) a thin squamous epithelial lining that may be relatively uniform in thickness or may exhibit focal epithelial thickenings (plaques or eddies); (2) variable numbers of small glandular structures or microcysts within the lining epithelium; and (3) a single layer of columnar or cuboidal cells lining the glandular structures, replacing the surface layer of the stratified squamous epithelium of the cyst lining. The glandular spaces contain variable amounts of PAS-positive and mucicarmine-positive secretory product. Occasionally, mucus cells resembling goblet cells of the intestinal mucosa also are present (Figure 2-27).

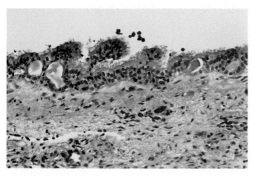

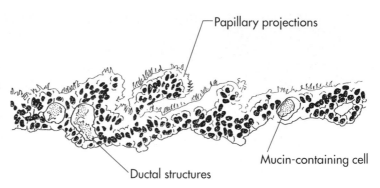

FIGURE 2-27

Glandular odontogenic cyst. Thin lining exhibiting cuboidal and columnar cells with intraepithelial microcysts containing mucoid secretion.

TREATMENT

Cases have been treated by surgical enucleation and curettage. Some of these lesions have been large and polycystic, and recurrences have been reported.

UNCLASSIFIED ODONTOGENIC CYSTS

Paradental Cyst

> ■ PARADENTAL CYST: a cyst of uncertain origin found primarily on the distal or facial aspect of a vital mandibular third molar, consisting of intensely inflamed connective tissue and epithelial lining.

The existence of the paradental cyst as a distinct entity is still controversial, and its histogenesis unresolved. Although this cyst might be derived from rests of Malassez or from reduced enamel epithelium, the possibility that it could arise from remnants of the dental lamina cannot be excluded. Additional research will be required to resolve this question. Because this cyst is virtually always intensely inflamed, inflammation is considered to play a key role in its development.

RADIOGRAPHIC

When a paradental cyst occurs on the distal aspect of a mandibular third molar, it presents as a well-circumscribed radiolucency. A paradental cyst that occurs on the facial (buccal) aspect of a mandibular molar may not be evident on routine radiographs because its image is superimposed on the associated tooth.

HISTOPATHOLOGY

The paradental cyst exhibits a striking resemblance to the periapical cyst. The lumen is lined by a hyperplastic layer of nonkeratinized squamous epithelium, and the connective tissue capsule exhibits significant inflammation.

TREATMENT

This cyst is treated by surgical enucleation; the associated molar is often extracted as part of the surgical procedure.

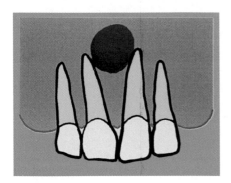

FIGURE 2-28

Nasopalatine duct cyst.

DEVELOPMENTAL CYSTS OF THE ORAL REGIONS

The term "fissural cyst" is still often used for cysts derived from epithelium present during embryonic development, but it is now considered a misnomer. Until recently it was thought that some cysts of the jaws developed from epithelium that became entrapped along embryologic lines of closure (fissures). Current thought is that epithelial entrapment does not occur in these sites during embryogenesis. As a result some of the previously held concepts of cyst formation have been modified, and terms such as "globulomaxillary cyst" and "median mandibular cyst" have been largely abandoned. The two developmental cysts that remain in this category are not of fissural derivation. They are the nasopalatine duct cyst (incisive canal cyst) and the nasolabial cyst (Klestadt cyst).

CYSTS OF VESTIGIAL DUCTS

Nasopalatine Duct Cyst

> ■ NASOPALATINE DUCT CYST: an intraosseous developmental cyst of the midline of the anterior palate, derived from the islands of epithelium remaining after closure of the embryonic nasopalatine duct.

The nasopalatine duct cyst, also termed "incisive canal cyst," arises from embryologic remnants of the nasopalatine duct. Most of these cysts develop in the midline of the anterior maxilla near the incisive foramen (Figure 2-28). Although most are intraosseous lesions, a small percentage develop at the lower end of the incisive canal entirely within the soft tissue of the anterior palate and are termed **"cyst of the incisive papilla."** On rare occasion, the nasopalatine duct remains patent and persists into adult life as small unilateral or bilateral openings on the palatal mucosa adjacent to the incisive papilla.

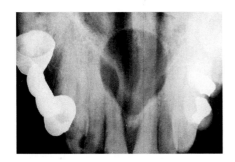

FIGURE 2-29

Nasopalatine duct cyst. Occlusal radiograph of anterior maxilla with a well-demarcated oval-shaped radiolucency of the midline extending between the roots of the central incisors.

RADIOGRAPHIC

The nasopalatine duct cyst presents as a well-circumscribed oval or heart-shaped radiolucency located in the midline of the anterior maxilla between the roots of the central incisors (Figure 2-29). In the edentulous maxilla the radiologic diagnosis may not be as obvious as in the dentate patient. Although some of these cysts are asymptomatic and discovered during routine radiologic dental examination, many are inflamed and cause pain, pressure, and swelling. Cysts of the incisive papilla are entirely within the palatal soft tissues and are not evident radiologically.

HISTOPATHOLOGY

These cysts are lined by a layer of ciliated columnar (respiratory), cuboidal (ductal), or stratified squamous epithelium or by a mixture of these epithelial types (Figure 2-30). If inflammation is present, it usually consists of an infiltrate of plasma cells and lymphocytes. The cyst capsule typically exhibits the prominent component of blood vessels and peripheral nerves that comprise normal incisive canal contents. The presence of these neurovascular elements can be helpful in reaching a histopathologic diagnosis. In addition, occasional small lobules of salivary type mucus glands may be seen in the cyst wall. Premalignant or malignant transformation of the epithelial lining in this cyst has not been reported. The histologic features of the cyst of the incisive papilla closely resemble those of the nasopalatine duct cyst.

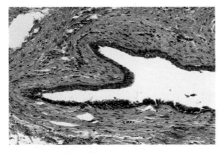

FIGURE 2-30

Nasopalatine duct cyst. Microscopic appearance of dense fibrous connective tissue capsule, surrounding a lumen lined by both stratified squamous and ciliated pseudostratified columnar epithelium.

TREATMENT

Treatment of the nasopalatine cyst is by surgical enucleation, employing a palatal approach. Recurrence of this cyst is rare.

Nasolabial Cyst

> ■ **NASOLABIAL CYST:** a developmental cyst of the soft tissue of the anterior muco-buccal fold beneath the ala of the nose, most likely derived from remnants of the inferior portion of the nasolacrimal duct.

Also known as the "nasoalveolar cyst," and eponymically as "Klestadt cyst," this rare condition occurs entirely in the soft tissues of the anterior maxillary vestibule, below the ala of the nose and deep in the nasolabial crease (Figure 2-31). Although other theories for the development of this rare cyst have been previously proposed, the most plausible and currently accepted thought points to its derivation from remnants of the inferior and anterior portions of the naso-lacrimal duct.

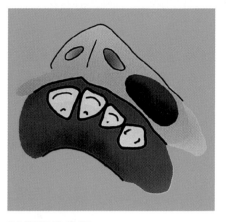

FIGURE 2-31

Nasolabial cyst.

CLINICAL

This cyst is a unilateral or occasionally bilateral painless soft tissue swelling that results in a flattening of the nasolabial crease on the skin below the ala of the nose. If the upper lip is appropriately retracted, this cyst also can be seen intra-orally as a swelling located at the depth of the maxillary vestibule. Most of these cysts occur in the fourth and fifth decades of life and have a female predilection of approximately 3 to 1. Because this cyst is located entirely within soft tissue, it is not readily apparent radiologically unless contrast medium is injected into the cystic lumen to facilitate visualization. Focal pressure-induced bone resorption (saucerization) of the anterior maxilla can occasionally be demonstrated radio-logically and is most readily seen in the edentulous patient.

HISTOPATHOLOGY

The cyst is lined by a layer of pseudostratified columnar epithelium exhibiting variable numbers of mucus (goblet) cells, or by a ductal type cuboidal epithelium (Figure 2-32). A lining of stratified squamous epithelium can be seen in some lesions. Some degree of infolding of the cyst lining and of the associated connective tissue is often seen. A narrow zone of dense, homogeneous, fibrous tissue is usually seen adjacent to the epithelial lining. Inflammation is generally absent.

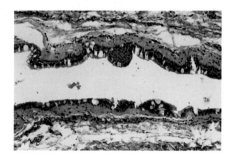

FIGURE 2-32

Nasolabial cyst. Microscopic features exhibiting loose connective tissue surrounding a lumen lined with ciliated pseudostratified columnar epithelium containing mucus (goblet) cells.

TREATMENT

A nasolabial cyst is treated by surgical enucleation with particular care being exercised to prevent the lesion's perforation and collapse. Recurrence is rare.

LYMPHOEPITHELIAL CYST

> ■ **LYMPHOEPITHELIAL CYST:** a cyst with a lumen lined by a keratinizing stratified squamous epithelium and a capsule containing multiple normal lymphoid follicles and a dense accumulation of normal lymphocytes.

Lymphoepithelial cysts are relatively uncommon lesions that occur in several areas of the head and neck, most commonly in the floor of the mouth and on the lateral aspect of the neck. Those occurring intraorally are termed **"oral lymphoepithelial cysts,"** and those occurring on the lateral aspect of the neck are termed **"cervical lymphoepithelial cysts."** Although cysts in the oral cavity are considerably smaller than those on the lateral aspect of the neck, their histopathologic features are essentially the same.

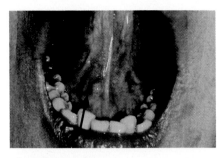

FIGURE 2-33

Oral lymphoepithelial cyst. Lesion of floor of mouth *(arrow)*.

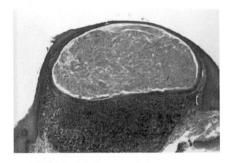

FIGURE 2-34

Oral lymphoepithelial cyst. Microscopic features exhibit cystic lumen containing desquamated keratin and lymphoid tissue with germinal centers.

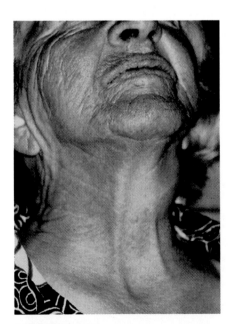

FIGURE 2-35

Cervical lymphoepithelial cyst. Lesion on left lateral neck.

Oral Lymphoepithelial Cyst

■ **ORAL LYMPHOEPITHELIAL CYST:** a lymphoepithelial cyst commonly located intraorally on the posterior lateral tongue and the anterior floor of the mouth.

The oral lymphoepithelial cyst (also termed *benign lymphoepithelial cyst*) most commonly develops where extratonsillar lymphoid tissue (oral tonsil) is found. The most common sites are the anterior floor of mouth and the posterior lateral border of the tongue. It appears to develop from epithelial invaginations (crypts) that become detached from the surface mucosa and entrapped within the lymphoid tissue; cyst formation ensues. An alternate theory suggests that the epithelium in these cysts could be derived from minor salivary ducts that traverse oral lymphoid tissue.

CLINICAL

The oral lymphoepithelial cyst is most commonly found on the anterior floor of the mouth (Figure 2-33) and on the posterior lateral borders of the tongue. However, it can occur on the ventral surface of the tongue, soft palate, tonsillar pillars, and oropharynx. It is an asymptomatic, yellowish or tan, superficial submucosal mass that usually measures less than 1 cm in diameter. Careful clinical examination of the oral mucosa overlying these cysts or gross examination of the excised lesional tissue will occasionally reveal a small pore or crypt that communicates with the cyst's lumen.

HISTOPATHOLOGY

The cyst is lined by a relatively thin layer of parakeratinized squamous epithelium surrounded by a well-defined mass of normal lymphoid tissue exhibiting variable numbers of germinal centers (Figure 2-34). The cystic lumen is usually filled with desquamated parakeratin. Occasionally, the pore or crypt that communicates between the surface mucosa and the cystic lumen can be seen microscopically. The presence of bacteria within the cystic lumen in some of these cysts is also evidence that communication with the oral cavity is present.

TREATMENT

Treatment of these cysts is by conservative surgical excision. The lesion seldom recurs.

Cervical Lymphoepithelial Cyst

■ **CERVICAL LYMPHOEPITHELIAL CYST:** an unusually large lymphoepithelial cyst located on the lateral aspect of the neck.

The cervical lymphoepithelial cyst, also commonly termed *branchial cleft cyst* or *benign cystic lymph node*, occurs on the lateral aspect of the neck, usually anterior to the sternocleidomastoid muscle. It is thought to be derived from epithelium entrapped within lymphoid tissues of the neck during embryologic development of the cervical sinuses or the second branchial clefts or pouches. An alternate theory suggests that the epithelium in this cyst might be derived from salivary duct epithelium trapped within cervical lymph nodes during embryogenesis.

CLINICAL

The cyst becomes apparent in late childhood or early adulthood as a painless swelling on the lateral aspect of the neck anterior to the sternomastoid muscle (Figure 2-35). A draining fistula that communicates between the cyst and the overlying skin surface occasionally develops.

HISTOPATHOLOGY

The cyst lumen is usually lined with a thinned, stratified squamous epithelium and contains desquamated orthokeratin. The capsule wall is thickened, consisting of a fibrous connective tissue containing large numbers of well-formed lymphoid follicles (Figure 2-36).

TREATMENT

As with its intraoral counterpart, the cervical lymphoepithelial cyst is treated by conservative surgical excision; recurrence is rare.

CYSTS OF VESTIGIAL TRACT

Thyroglossal Tract Cyst

> ■ THYROGLOSSAL TRACT CYST: a cyst located above the thyroid gland and beneath the base of the tongue, with a lumen lined by a mixture of epithelial cell types derived from remnants of the embryonic thyroglossal tract, and often containing thyroid tissue in the capsule.

The thyroglossal tract cyst is a relatively uncommon lesion derived from embryologic remnants of the thyroglossal tract. This tract extends from the foramen caecum on the middorsum of the tongue to the thyroid gland. Although these cysts can develop anywhere along the length of this tract, most (70% to 80%) occur below the hyoid bone, where the tract makes two distinct turns on its descent to the thyroid gland.

CLINICAL

This cyst occurs primarily in children and young adults and presents as an asymptomatic, slowly enlarging, mobile swelling involving the midline of the anterior neck above the thyroid gland (Figure 2-37). A small percentage of these cysts occurs within the tongue, where they can induce dysphagia. If infected or inflamed, a draining fistula that communicates between the cyst and the overlying skin surface will occasionally develop.

HISTOPATHOLOGY

This cyst is lined by stratified squamous epithelium, ciliated columnar epithelium, transitional epithelium, or a mixture of epithelial types. The cyst capsule can exhibit a number of additional findings including lymphoid aggregates, thyroid tissue (Figure 2-38), mucus glands, and sebaceous glands. Carcinoma can occasionally develop from the lining of thyroglossal tract cysts and from remnants of the thyroglossal tract.

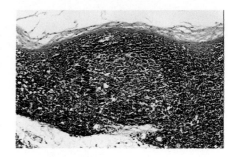

FIGURE 2-36

Cervical lymphoepithelial cyst. Cyst wall lined by keratinizing squamous cell epithelium and containing lymphoid tissue.

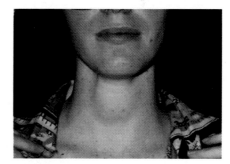

FIGURE 2-37

Thyroglossal tract cyst. Lesion located on midline of anterior neck.

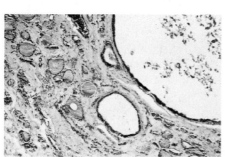

FIGURE 2-38

Thyroglossal tract cyst. Microscopic features reveal thyroid tissue in cyst wall.

TREATMENT

The treatment of the thyroglossal tract cyst requires complete surgical excision because recurrence is a distinct possibility. In an effort to minimize recurrence of cysts involving the hyoid area, it is recommended that the central portion of the hyoid bone and its associated remnants of thyroglossal tract be removed.

CYSTS OF EMBRYONIC SKIN

Dermoid Cyst

> ■ DERMOID CYST: a cyst of the midline of the upper neck or the anterior floor of the mouth of young patients, derived from remnants of embryonic skin, consisting of a lumen lined by a keratinizing stratified squamous epithelium and containing one or more skin appendages such as hair, sweat, or sebaceous glands.

The dermoid cyst represents a simple form of cystic teratoma derived from germinal epithelium entrapped during embryonic development. Most of these cysts occur in the head and neck region, primarily in the skin around the eyes and the anterior upper neck, extending superiorly into the floor of the mouth.

CLINICAL

The dermoid cyst is a lesion of young adults (teenagers). No gender predilection is seen. Cysts of the anterior upper neck or floor of the mouth present as painless swellings exhibiting a doughy consistency on palpation. Cysts that develop above the mylohyoid muscle present as a midline swelling in the sublingual/floor of the mouth area. In this location the cyst results in elevation of the tongue and can interfere with eating and speaking. Cysts that develop below the mylohyoid muscle appear as a midline swelling in the submandibular and submental region. The size of these cysts is variable, but most are 2 cm or less in diameter.

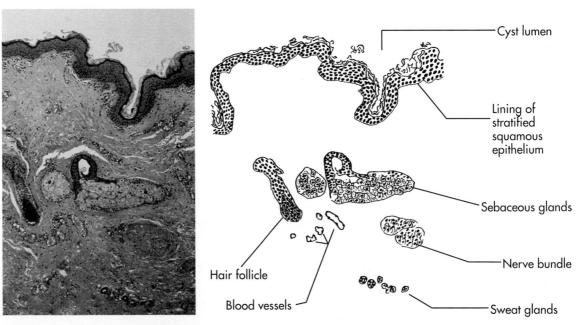

FIGURE 2-39

Dermoid cyst. Cyst lumen is lined by an orthokeratinizing stratified squamous epithelium with hair follicle, sebaceous glands, and sweat glands in the capsule.

HISTOPATHOLOGY

The cyst is lined by a layer of orthokeratinized squamous epithelium exhibiting variable numbers of dermal appendages including hair follicles, sebaceous glands, and associated erector pili muscles. The cystic lumen is generally filled with a mixture of desquamated keratin, sebum, and hair shafts. The cyst capsule is composed of a narrow zone of compressed connective tissue that is generally free of inflammation (Figure 2-39).

TREATMENT

This cyst is best treated by surgical enucleation or excision. Recurrence is uncommon.

Epidermoid Cyst

■ EPIDERMOID CYST: a cyst of skin with a lumen lined by keratinizing stratified squamous epithelium, usually filled with keratin and without skin appendages in the capsule wall.

The epidermoid cyst occurs primarily on skin. However, occasional cysts of the oral cavity exhibit the histopathologic characteristics of epidermoid cysts. The epidermoid cyst closely resembles a dermoid cyst except that the former exhibits no dermal appendages. They are lined by orthokeratinized squamous epithelium and exhibit a lumen that is generally filled with desquamated keratin (Figure 2-40). The cyst wall consists of a narrow zone of compressed fibrous connective tissue that is generally free of inflammation. This cyst is treated by surgical enucleation or excision. Recurrence is uncommon.

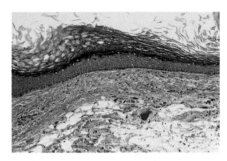

FIGURE 2-40

Epidermoid cyst. Microscopic appearance of cyst wall reveals a lumen lined by stratified squamous epithelium with a thickened layer of orthokeratin and a connective tissue capsule devoid of skin appendages.

CYSTS OF MUCOSAL EPITHELIUM

Surgical Ciliated Cyst of Maxilla

■ SURGICAL CILIATED CYST OF MAXILLA: an intrabony cyst located near the floor of the maxillary sinus lined by pseudostratified ciliated columnar epithelium, caused by implantation of normal mucus-secreting sinus epithelium during previous surgery.

The surgical ciliated cyst of the maxilla is an iatrogenic cyst that develops as a result of surgery involving the maxillary sinus, usually a Caldwell-Luc operation. The cyst develops from maxillary sinus lining that becomes implanted in the maxillary bone at the site of surgical entry into the sinus. Although this cyst is rarely seen in the United States and Europe, it is not uncommon in Japan, where its occurrence has been attributed to the management of a higher incidence of maxillary sinusitis in that country.

CLINICAL

This cyst occurs in middle-age or older adults and is discovered during radiologic investigation of pain or tenderness in the maxilla. The patient's history usually discloses a previous surgery at the site of the cyst.

RADIOGRAPHIC

The lesion presents as a well-circumscribed radiolucency in close proximity to, but separate from, the maxillary sinus.

HISTOPATHOLOGY

The cyst is lined by pseudostratified ciliated columnar epithelium exhibiting the features of maxillary sinus lining. The surrounding connective tissue may be normal or may exhibit some degree of chronic inflammation.

TREATMENT

This cyst is treated by conservative surgical enucleation and has no tendency to recur.

Heterotopic Oral Gastrointestinal Cyst

The heterotopic oral gastrointestinal cyst is a rare and unusual developmental entity that is most commonly found in the tongue or the floor of the mouth of infants or young children. Several theories have been proposed to explain the presence of gastrointestinal tract epithelium in the oral cavity. The theory of undifferentiated endodermal entrapment during the fourth or fifth week of embryonic development, followed by gastrointestinal differentiation, is a plausible explanation for the development of this cyst. This cyst is treated by surgical excision; recurrence is uncommon.

ADDITIONAL READING

ODONTOGENIC CYST

Browne RM. *Investigative Pathology of the Odontogenic Cysts.* Boca Raton, Florida: CRC Press; 1991.

Killey HC, Kay LW, Seward GR. *Benign Cystic Lesions of the Jaws: Their Diagnosis and Treatment.* 3rd ed. Churchill Livingstone; 1977.

Shear M. *Cysts of the Oral Region.* 2nd ed. Bristol: Wright PGS; 1983.

PERIAPICAL CYST

Antoh M, Hasegawa H, Kawakami T, Kage T. Hyperkeratosis and atypical proliferation appearing in the lining epithelium of a radicular cyst. *J Craniomaxillofac Surg.* 1993; 21:210-3.

Oehlers FAC. Periapical lesions and residual dental cysts. *Br J Oral Surg.* 1970; 8:103.

DENTIGEROUS CYST

Gardner DG. Plexiform unicystic ameloblastoma: a diagnostic problem in dentigerous cysts. *Cancer.* 1981; 47:1358.

Johnson L, Sapp JP, McIntire DN. Squamous cell carcinoma arising in a dentigerous cyst. *J Oral Maxillofac Surg.* 1994; 52:987-990.

Maxymiw WG, Wood RE. Carcinoma arising in a dentigerous cyst: a case report and review of the literature. *J Oral Maxillofac Surg.* 1991; 49:639-43.

ERUPTION CYST

Seward MH. Eruption cyst: an analysis of its clinical features. *J Oral Surg.* 1973; 31:31.

ODONTOGENIC KERATOCYST

Brannon RB. The odontogenic keratocyst: a clinicopathologic study of 312 cases. *Oral Surg Oral Med Oral Pathol.* 1976; 42:54.

Buch B, Dresner J, Peters E. Conservative management of an odontogenic keratocyst: a four and a half year evaluation. *J Dent Assoc S Afr.* 1988; 43:37-9.

Donatsky O, Hjorting-Hansen E. Recurrence of the odontogenic keratocyst in 13 patients with the nevoid basal cell carcinoma syndrome: a 6-year follow-up. *Int J Oral Surg.* 1980; 9:173-9.

Foley WL, Terry BC, Jacoway JR. Malignant transformation of an odontogenic keratocyst: report of a case. *J Oral Maxillofac Surg.* 1991; 49:768-71.

Gorlin RJ. Nevoid basal cell carcinoma syndrome. *Medicine.* 1987; 66:98.

Meiselman F. Surgical management of the odontogenic keratocyst: conservative approach. *J Oral Maxillofac Surg.* 1994; 52:960-3.

Shear M. The odontogenic keratocyst: recent advances. *Dtsch Zahnarztl Z.* 1985; 40:510-3.

Williams TP, Connor FA. Surgical management of the odontogenic keratocyst: aggressive approach. *J Oral Maxillofac Surg.* 1994; 52:964-6.

Woolgar JA, Rippin JW, Browne RM. The odontogenic keratocyst and its occurrence in the nevoid basal cell carcinoma syndrome. *Oral Surg Oral Med Oral Pathol.* 1987; 64:727.

Wright JM. The odontogenic keratocyst: orthokeratinized variant. *Oral Surg Oral Med Oral Pathol.* 1981; 51:609-18.

LATERAL PERIODONTAL CYST

Angelopoulou E, Angelopoulos AP. Lateral periodontal cyst: review of the literature and report of a case. *J Periodontol.* 1990; 61:126-31.

Takeda Y. Glandular odontogenic cyst mimicking a lateral periodontal cyst: a case report. *Int J Oral Maxillofac Surg.* 1994; 23:96-7.

Wysocki GP, Brannon RB, Gardner DG, Sapp P. Histogenesis of the lateral periodontal cyst and the gingival cyst of the adult. *Oral Surg Oral Med Oral Pathol.* 1980; 50:327-34.

GINGIVAL CYST OF THE ADULT

Buchner A, Hansen LS. The histomorphologic spectrum of the gingival cyst in the adult. *Oral Surg Oral Med Oral Pathol.* 1979; 48:532.

Moskow BS, Bloom A. Embryogenesis of the gingival cyst. *J Clin Periodontol.* 1983; 10:119-30.

Nxumalo TN, Shear M. Gingival cyst in adults. *J Oral Pathol Med.* 1992; 21:309-13.

Shade NL, Carpenter WM, Delzer DD. Gingival cyst of the adult: case report of a bilateral presentation. *J Periodontol.* 1987; 58:796-9.

GLANDULAR ODONTOGENIC CYST

Gardner DG, Kessler HP, Morency R, Schaffner DL. The glandular odontogenic cyst: an apparent entity. *J Oral Pathol.* 1988; 17:359.

Padayachee A, Van Wyk CW. Two cystic lesions with features of both the botryoid odontogenic cyst and central mucoepidermoid tumor: sialo-odontogenic cyst? *J Oral Pathol.* 1987; 16:499.

DENTAL LAMINA CYST OF THE NEWBORN

Cataldo E, Berkman MD. Cyst of the oral mucosa in newborns. *Am J Dis Child.* 1968; 116:44.

PARADENTAL CYST

Ackerman G, Cohen MA, Altini M. The paradental cyst: a clinicopathologic study of 50 cases. *Oral Surg Oral Med Oral Pathol.* 1987; 64:308.

Craig GT. The paradental cyst: a specific inflammatory odontogenic cyst. *Br Dent J.* 1976; 141:9.

Fowler CB, Brannon RB. The paradental cyst: a clinicopathologic study of six new cases and review of the literature. *J Oral Maxillofac Surg.* 1989; 47:243.

Vedtofte P, Praetorius F. The inflammatory paradental cyst. *Oral Surg Oral Med Oral Pathol.* 1989; 68:182-8.

Wolf J, Hietanen J. The mandibular infected buccal cyst (paradental cyst): a radiographic and histological study. *Br J Oral Maxillofac Surg.* 1990; 28:322-5.

CARCINOMA ARISING IN ODONTOGENIC CYSTS

Eversole LR, Sabes WR, Rovin S. Aggressive growth and neoplastic potential of odontogenic cysts. *Cancer.* 1975; 35:270.

Van der Waal I, Rauhamaa R, Van der Kwast WAM, Snow GB. Squamous cell carcinoma arising in the lining of odontogenic cysts: report of 5 cases. *Int J Oral Surg.* 1985; 23:450.

NASOPALATINE DUCT CYST

Abrams AM, Howell FV, Bullock WK. Nasopalatine duct cysts. *Oral Surg Oral Med Oral Pathol.* 1963; 16:306-32.

Allard RH, van der Kwast WA, van der Waal I. Nasopalatine duct cyst: review of the literature and report of 22 cases. *Int J Oral Surg.* 1981; 10:447-61.

Allard RHB, de Vries K, van der Kwast WAM. Persisting bilateral nasopalatine ducts: a developmental anomaly. *Oral Surg Oral Med Oral Pathol.* 1982; 53:24-26.

Anneroth G, Hall G, Stuge U. Nasopalatine duct cyst. *Int J Oral Maxillofac Surg.* 1986; 15:572-80.

Nortje CJ, Wood RE. The radiologic features of the nasopalatine duct cyst: an analysis of 46 cases. *Dentomaxillofac Radiol.* 1988; 17:129-32.

Swanson KS, Kaugars GE, Gunsolley JC. Nasopalatine duct cyst: an analysis of 334 cases. *J Oral Maxillofac Surg.* 1991; 49:268-71.

NASOLABIAL CYST

Adams A, Lovelock DJ. Nasolabial cyst. *Oral Surg Oral Med Oral Pathol.* 1985; 60:118-9.

Brandao GS, Ebling H, Faria e Souza I. Bilateral nasolabial cyst. *Oral Surg Oral Med Oral Pathol.* 1974; 37:480-4.

Campbell RL, Burkes EJ. Nasolabial cyst: report of case. *J Am Dent Assoc.* 1975; 91:1210-3.

Cohen MA, Hertzanu Y. Huge growth potential of the nasolabial cyst. *Oral Surg Oral Med Oral Pathol.* 1985; 59:441-5.

David VC, O'Connell JE. Nasolabial cyst. *Clin Otolaryngol.* 1986; 11:5-8.

Precious DS. Chronic nasolabial cyst. *J Can Dent Assoc.* 1987; 53:307-8.

Roed-Peterson B. Nasolabial cyst: a presentation of five patients with a review of the literature. *Br J Oral Surg.* 1970; 7:85.

Wesley RK, Scannell T, Nathan LE. Nasolabial cyst: presentation of a case with a review of the literature. *J Oral Maxillofac Surg.* 1984; 42:188-92.

LYMPHOEPITHELIAL CYST

Buchner A, Hansen LS. Lymphoepithelial cysts of the oral mucosa. *Oral Surg Oral Med Oral Pathol.* 1980; 50:441.

Chaudhry AP. A clinicopathologic study of intraoral lymphoepithelial cysts. *J Oral Med.* 1984; 39:79.

Gnepp DR, Sporck FT. Benign lymphoepithelial parotid cyst with sebaceous differentiation—cystic sebaceous lymphadenoma. *Am J Clin Pathol.* 1980; 74:683-7.

Skouteris CA, Patterson GT, Sotereanos GC. Benign cervical lymphoepithelial cyst: report of cases. *J Oral Maxillofac Surg.* 1989; 47:1106-12.

Smith FB. Benign lymphoepithelial lesion and lymphoepithelial cyst of the parotid gland in HIV infection. *Prog AIDS Pathol.* 1990; 2:61-72.

Stewart S, Levy R, Karpel J, Stoopack J. Lymphoepithelial (branchial) cyst of the parotid gland. *J Oral Surg.* 1974; 32:100-6.

Weitzner S. Lymphoepithelial (branchial) cyst of parotid gland. *Oral Surg Oral Med Oral Pathol.* 1973; 35:85-8.

Yoshimura Y, Oka M, Sugihara T, Mishima K. Lymphoepithelial (branchial) cyst and amylase. *Int J Oral Maxillofac Surg.* 1986; 15:196-200.

THYROGLOSSAL TRACT CYST

Brereton RJ, Symonds E. Thyroglossal cysts in children. *Br J Surg.* 1978; 65:507.

Castillo-Taucher S, Castillo P. Autosomal dominant inheritance of thyroglossal duct cyst. *Clin Genet.* 1994; 45:111-2.

Grabowska H. Papillary carcinoma arising from ectopic thyroid gland in the wall of a thyroglossal duct cyst. *Pathol Res Pract.* 1993; 189:1228-9.

Klin B, Serour F, Fried K, Efrati Y, Vinograd I. Familial thyroglossal duct cyst. *Clin Genet.* 1993; 43:101-3.

LiVolsi VA, Perzin KH, Savetsky L. Carcinoma arising in median ectopic thyroid (including thyroglossal duct tissue). *Cancer.* 1974; 34:1303.

McHenry CR, Danish R, Murphy T, Marty JJ. Atypical thyroglossal duct cyst: a rare cause for a solitary cold thyroid nodule in childhood. *Am Surg.* 1993; 59:223-8.

Vincent SD, Synhorst JB. Adenocarcinoma arising in a thyroglossal duct cyst: report of a case and literature review. *J Oral Maxillofac Surg.* 1989; 47:633-5.

Wampler HW, Krolls SO, Johnson RP. Thyroglossal tract cyst. *Oral Surg Oral Med Oral Pathol.* 1978; 45:32.

Yanagisawa K, Eisen RN, Sasaki CT. Squamous cell carcinoma arising in a thyroglossal duct cyst. *Arch Otolaryngol Head Neck Surg.* 1992; 118:538-41.

DERMOID CYST

Flom GS, Donovan TJ, Landgraf JR. Congenital dermoid cyst of the anterior tongue. *Otolaryngol Head Neck Surg.* 1989; 101:388-91.

Howell CJT. The sublingual dermoid. *Oral Surg Oral Med Oral Pathol.* 1985; 59:578.

Ruggieri M, Tine A, Rizzo R, Micali G and others. Lateral dermoid cyst of the tongue: case report. *Int J Pediatr Otorhinolaryngol.* 1994; 30:79-84.

EPIDERMOID CYST

Cortezzi W, De Albuquerque EB. Secondarily infected epidermoid cyst in the floor of the mouth causing a life-threatening situation: report of a case. *J Oral Maxillofac Surg* 1994; 52:762-4.

Elston DM, Parker LU, Tuthill RJ. Epidermoid cyst of the scalp containing human papillomavirus. *J Cutan Pathol.* 1993; 20:184-6.

Mehregan DA, al-Sabah HY, Mehregan AH. Basal cell epithelioma arising from epidermoid cyst. *J Dermatol Surg Oncol.* 1994; 20:405-6.

Rahbari H. Epidermoid cysts with seborrheic verruca-like cyst walls. *Arch Dermatol.* 1982; 118:326-8.

Rios-Buceta LM, Fraga-Fernandez J, Fernandez-Herrera J. Human papillomavirus in an epidermoid cyst of the sole in a non-Japanese patient. *J Am Acad Dermatol.* 1992; 27:364-6.

SURGICAL CILIATED CYST OF MAXILLA

Gregory GT, Shafer WG. Surgical ciliated cysts of the maxilla: report of cases. *J Oral Surg.* 1958; 16:251.

Hayhurst DL, Moenning JE, Summerlin DJ, Bussard DA. Surgical ciliated cyst: a delayed complication in a case of maxillary orthognathic surgery. *J Oral Maxillofac Surg.* 1993; 51:705-8.

Miller R, Longo J, Houston G. Surgical ciliated cyst of the maxilla. *J Oral Maxillofac Surg.* 1988; 46:310-2.

Smith G, Smith AJ, Basu MK, Rippin JW. The analysis of fluid aspirate glycosaminoglycans in diagnosis of the postoperative maxillary cyst (surgical ciliated cyst). *Oral Surg Oral Med Oral Pathol.* 1988; 65:222-4.

HETEROTOPIC ORAL GASTROINTESTINAL CYST

Daley TD, Wysocki GP, Lovas GL, Smout MS. Heterotopic gastric cyst of the oral cavity. *Head Neck Surg.* 1984; 7:168-171.

INFECTIONS OF TEETH AND BONE

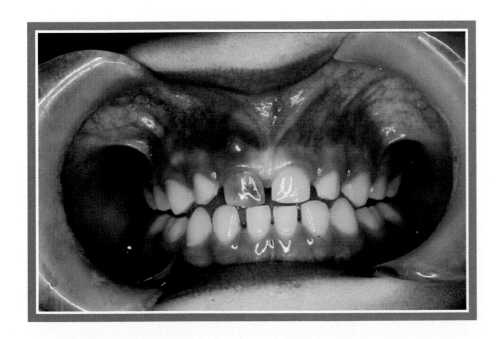

DENTAL CARIES

Dental caries is a multifaceted disease involving an interplay among the teeth, the oral host factors of saliva and microflora, and the external factor of diet. The disease is a unique form of infection in which specific strains of bacteria accumulate on the enamel surface; where they elaborate acidic and proteolytic products that demineralize the surface and digest its organic matrix. Once penetration of the enamel has occurred, the disease process progresses through the dentin to the pulp. If the process is not stopped, the tooth becomes completely destroyed. The process within the tooth can be intercepted by mechanically removing the infected tooth tissue and replacing it with an appropriate synthetic material that restores the tooth to normal form and function. Although dental caries is restricted to the hard tissue of the enamel, dentin, and cementum, if left untreated, the process will ultimately penetrate through the pulpal canal beyond the tooth into the adjacent soft tissue where it will initiate a painful and destructive inflammatory reaction. In this location it may spread into the marrow spaces of the bone and possibly the soft tissues and muscles of the face and neck.

EPIDEMIOLOGY

Although dental caries is ubiquitous, its prevalence and severity differ among the various cultures and countries throughout the world. The caries activity in a particular society or geographic area is closely correlated with the amount of sugar consumed per capita. In the more industrialized countries where diets have traditionally had a high content of refined carbohydrates, the caries rate has been considerably higher than in the less-developed countries. In recent years with the trend toward preventive measures such as fluoridated water, greater access to dental care and better oral hygiene in the industrialized countries, and the concurrent rapid increase in caries activity in the less-developed societies, the large difference in caries rates has decreased. This latter phenomenon in the less-developed countries is due to the recent increase in the consumption of sugar as a cheap source of body energy, the introduction of Western diets containing refined foods, the inability to maintain the necessary level of oral hygiene, and the unavailability of professional dental care.

In the Western world the susceptibility to dental caries differs significantly among age groups, individual teeth, and tooth surfaces. In the very young, when diets are high in sucrose and adequate prevention is not practiced, the pits and fissures of the first molars commonly become involved with caries within the first 3 years after they erupt. The second molars have the next highest susceptibility, followed by the second premolars. If the oral environmental factors are extremely cariogenic, the smooth surfaces of the molars and premolars will be affected; first the interproximal surfaces become involved, followed by the buccal and lingual surfaces. Under extraordinary circumstances the smooth surfaces of the anterior teeth also develop lesions. These surfaces are the most resistant because they are relatively self-cleansing.

CLINICAL TYPES

Clinically, dental caries is classified as *pit and fissure, smooth surface, cemental,* and *recurrent* (Box 3-1). In addition, caries may be further classified as *acute* (rampant) or *chronic.*

Pit and fissure caries is the most common type and appear at an early age on the occlusal and buccal surfaces of the molars of the primary and secondary dentition (Figure 3-1). The occlusal surfaces of the premolars and the lingual surfaces of the maxillary incisors will also become less frequently involved. This form of caries is the most destructive because it quickly goes deeply into the

■ BOX 3-1
Clinical Classification of Dental Caries

Pit and fissure
Smooth surface
Cemental
Recurrent

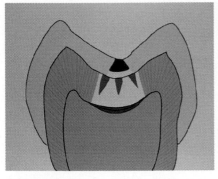
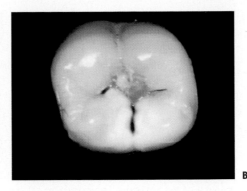

A

B

FIGURE 3-1

Pit and fissure caries. A, Diagram of the characteristic shape of lesions demonstrating a small triangle-shaped lesion in the fissure of the occlusal enamel *(brown)* that is narrow at the surface, widening at the dentoenamel junction to provide an even greater involvement of dentin *(white)*. The pulp of the tooth reacts with the deposition of reparative dentin *(blue)*. **B,** Clinical appearance of molar with fissure caries exhibiting the black areas of disintegration at the base of the fissure and the demineralized and undermined white opaque areas surrounding the enamel.

dentin, remains hidden as it undermines the enamel, and becomes clinically evident as pain due to pulpal involvement or as a large cavity when a substantial portion of the tooth crumbles.

Smooth surface caries is less common and essentially occurs on the interproximal (contact) areas of the teeth that are not self-cleansing (Figure 3-2). On occasion, the cervical regions of the buccal (Figure 3-3) and lingual surfaces of the teeth will become involved. Such occurrences are usually related to unusual circumstances.

When caries is present on the labial surfaces of the primary teeth of infants, it is nearly always caused by a habit of leaving the feeding bottle containing milk or juice in the infant's mouth when sleeping (Figure 3-4). In adults, smooth surface cervical caries is usually the result of a major alteration in the quantity or quality of the saliva. Patients who have had radiation therapy for head and neck malignancies will sustain substantial irreversible damage to the major salivary glands, which results in severely altered saliva. Patients who develop autoimmune diseases that involve the major salivary glands and patients on medications that reduce saliva production as a side effect will be similarly affected.

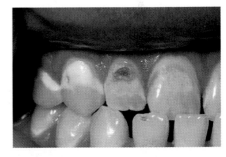

FIGURE 3-3

Smooth surface caries. Clinical appearance of white "chalky" lesions of enamel demineralization (maxillary premolar and cuspid) and cavitation (lateral incisor) in a patient with rampant caries.

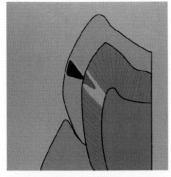
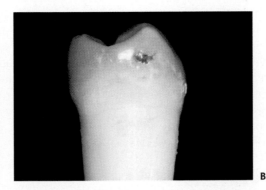

A

B

FIGURE 3-2

Smooth surface caries. A, Diagram of the characteristic triangular shape of these lesions that corresponds to the orientation of the enamel rods and the dentinal tubules. **B,** Clinical appearance of early enamel caries on the smooth interproximal surface exhibiting the central brown zone of disintegration.

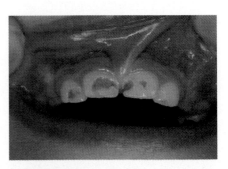

FIGURE 3-4

"Baby-bottle caries" on labial surfaces of the anterior primary teeth in a young patient.

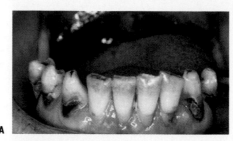
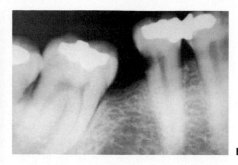

FIGURE 3-5

Cemental (root) caries. A, Multiple carious lesions on the root surfaces of mandibular teeth in a patient with extensive gingival recession. **B,** Radiograph of a mandibular premolar with deep caries on the distal root surface in close proximity to the pulpal canal.

Cemental (root) caries is nearly always exclusively found in the older population, particularly in those who have experienced substantial gingival recession. This form of caries is initiated and progresses differently than enamel and dentin caries because root surfaces are soft, thin, and subject to chemical erosion and the abrasive action incurred during toothbrushing. The combination of both acid and enzyme producing bacteria and the thin layer of dentin results in rapid progression of lesions into the pulp. This type of carious lesion presents considerable difficulties to the clinician because it is located in the soft surrounding cemental tissue in a region of the tooth where there is little tooth structure overlying the pulp (Figure 3-5).

Recurrent caries is the term applied to caries that arises around an existing restoration. Lesions usually arise as a result of an alteration in the integrity of a restoration that results in marginal "ditching" or leakage. These situations predispose the tooth to the accumulation of bacteria and food in an environment protected from the usual hygiene procedures. These carious lesions progress at variable rates depending on the extent of sclerosis of the adjacent dentin and the patient's diet and oral hygiene habits.

Acute (rampant) caries and chronic caries are infrequently used terms to denote the rate that dental caries progresses in patients. Young patients are most susceptible to *acute* or *rampant caries* because they have teeth with large pulpal chambers and wide and short dentinal tubules containing little or no sclerosis. In these patients this is often combined with a diet high in refined carbohydrates and less than adequate oral hygiene. They are capable of simultaneously developing multiple rapidly advancing carious lesions that quickly destroy tooth structure, penetrate into the pulp, and elicit severe pain. *Chronic caries* is most common in older patients whose teeth have smaller pulpal chambers, usually with additional deposits of a denser and less tubular dentin on the pulpal walls, referred to as *tertiary* or *secondary dentin*. Additionally, they have dentinal tubules that have undergone significant degrees of sclerosis, which offers some degree of resistance to the progression of the carious process. These patients may experience pain, but it is seldom of the degree that younger patients with the acute form of caries experience.

ENAMEL CARIES

Smooth surface enamel caries is most commonly located on the mesial and distal surfaces at the point of contact with the adjacent tooth ("interproximal caries"). The less common lesions on the buccal and lingual surfaces have a similar microscopic appearance. Since the enamel is composed primarily of inorganic salts, the process results in the production of a cavity due to demineralization. To achieve this end there is a prior stage of alteration in the loss and redeposition of mineralizing salts due to fluctuations in the pH in that particular location. In some situations if the pH can be stabilized in its normal range, the whole process may stop or even reverse, which is referred to as *arrested caries*. Arrested caries may also occur when an adjacent tooth is extracted (Figure 3-6) or when an undermined cusp fractures off, making the carious area self-cleansing. In some patients, a sudden and persistent improvement in oral hygiene habits can halt progression of early enamel lesions.

HISTOPATHOLOGY

Smooth surface caries progress in a cone-shaped manner, being wider at the outer surface than at the deeper advancing margin. When a thin ground section of an early lesion (before cavitation) is viewed with light microscopy, four zones can be identified (Figure 3-7): (1) *translucent zone*, the advancing front of initial demineralization; (2) *dark zone*, where the previously liberated salts are redeposited; (3) *body of lesion*, containing the region of maximal demineralization; and (4) *surface zone*, remaining relatively unaffected until it is sufficiently undermined to collapse, resulting in cavitation (Figure 3-8).

In their early stages, **pit and fissure enamel caries** have histologic zones similar to smooth surface carious lesions. The shape of the lesion differs because of the different angulations of the enamel rods. These lesions will be wider in the deeper portion and will have a wider area of involvement of the dentinal tubules at the dentinoenamel junction than at the surface. This, and the fact that the enamel is much thinner at the base of the pit or fissure, results in the lesions progressing at a much faster rate than the smooth-surface type.

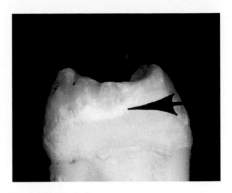

FIGURE 3-6

Smooth surface enamel caries. Example of a superficial lesion (*arrow*) capable of being arrested from further progression with the improvement of oral hygiene.

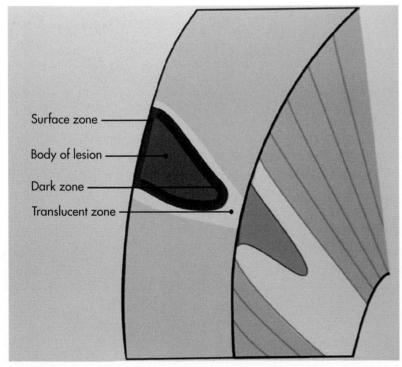

FIGURE 3-7

Enamel caries. Diagram of microscopic zones of enamel caries.

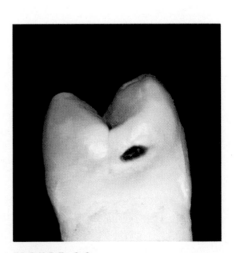

FIGURE 3-8

Enamel caries. Advanced interproximal smooth surface lesion with cavitation.

DENTIN CARIES

In general, dentin caries progresses at a much faster rate than enamel caries. It is more porous because it contains dentinal tubules and is less densely mineralized. This stage of caries progression requires a different mixture of bacterial colonies than is necessary for enamel caries. For caries to progress in dentin, bacterial strains capable of producing large amounts of proteolytic and hydrolytic enzymes are needed, rather than the acid-producing types of enamel caries. In the teeth of younger patients the dentinal tubules are less densely mineralized, shorter in length, and wider in diameter, allowing for ease of penetration and progression of the invading microorganisms. In older patients the dentinal tubules are usually narrowed by deposits of calcifying salts, making the teeth less porous. In addition, the dentin will be thicker due to the production of additional normal and abnormal secondary dentin on the pulpal walls. Because of these differences, dentinal caries in younger patients often quickly involves the pulpal tissue, which produces an acute inflammatory reaction and intense pain, whereas in older patients it has a slower course with intermittent mild pain.

HISTOPATHOLOGY

A nondecalcified cross section of a tooth with an advanced carious lesion of the dentin that has not reached the pulp will show five microscopic zones that reveal the stages of dentinal caries that eventuates in a cavity (Figures 3-9, 3-10, and 3-11).

The deepest zone, **Zone 1,** *fatty degeneration*, reflects the earliest changes of caries infection where bacterial enzymes have advanced ahead of the bacteria in the dentinal tubules, causing a breakdown of the cell membranes of the organic

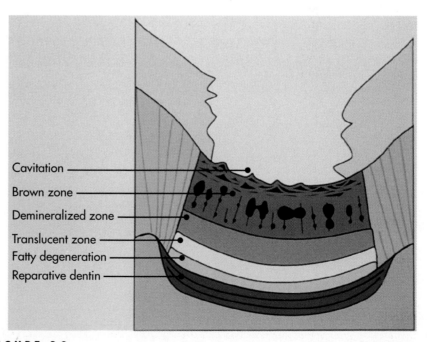

FIGURE 3-9

Dentin caries. Diagram of microscopic zones of an advanced carious lesion in dentin.

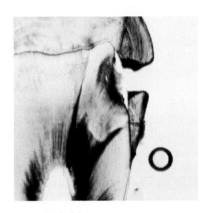

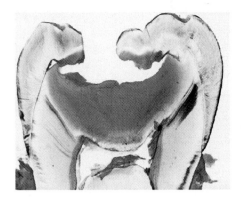

FIGURE 3-10

Dentin caries. Ground section of an advanced carious lesion of interproximal smooth surface origin.

FIGURE 3-11

Dentin caries. Ground section of an advanced carious lesion of fissure origin.

component of the dentin liberating lipid. **Zone 2,** *translucent zone,* is a band of hypermineralized dentin in which the dentinal tubules are sclerotic due to the redeposition of calcifying salts released from the demineralized zone. **Zone 3,** *demineralization,* is composed of dentin that is softer than normal due to the initial action of the bacterial enzymes. **Zone 4,** *brown discoloration,* is due to a reduction in the mineral content and the presence of distended dentinal tubules packed with bacteria. This zone is usually soft enough to be removed with a hand instrument. **Zone 5,** *cavitation,* results because no mineralization remains and the organic component is partially dissolved by the bacteria. This is the clinical base of the cavity that easily peels away in layers along the incremental lines of growth. In this zone the tubules will contain focal, dense accumulations of bacteria that form liquefaction foci, referred to as *"beading"* (Figure 3-12, *A*). These foci fuse horizontally, producing *"transverse clefts"* (Figure 3-12, *B*). These microscopic features are apparent to the clinician because of the ease with which the layers of dark brown, soft dentin present at the base of the cavity can be peeled away with a spoon excavator.

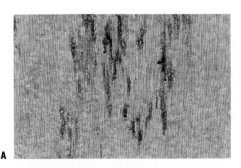

A

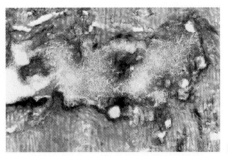

B

FIGURE 3-12

Dentin caries. Microscopic appearance of dentin exhibiting bacteria in the dentin tubules **(A)** and a large area of liquefaction of dentin caused by the horizontal fusion of the focal accumulations of bacteria within individual tubules ("transverse clefts") **(B).**

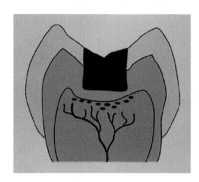

FIGURE 3-13

Reversible pulpitis. Diagram of mild transient pulpal inflammation that occurs immediately after the placement of a deep restoration.

■ **BOX 3-2**
Causes of Pupitis

Bacteria
   Caries
   Cracks in crown
   Periodontal pockets
   Malformed teeth

Trauma
   Crown fractures
   Root fractures
   Partial avulsion
   Bruxism
   Abrasion

Iatrogenesis
   Heat generation
   Depth of preparation
   Dehydration of tubules
   Pulp exposure
   Volatile/toxic disinfectants
   Filling materials

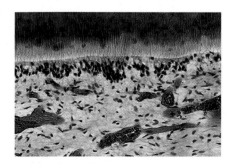

FIGURE 3-14

Reversible pulpitis. Microscopic features of dilated blood vessels and the slight disruption of the odontoblastic layer.

PULPITIS

■ PULPITIS: an inflammation of the pulpal tissue that may be acute or chronic, with or without symptoms, and reversible or irreversible.

The single most frequent diagnostic problem that clinicians confront in their daily practice is to determine the extent of the pulpal disease that has taken place within a symptomatic tooth. To make this decision, it is necessary for the clinician to be able to make an evaluation of the damage to the pulpal tissue that can be neither seen nor touched. An indirect assessment is required based on a combination of clinical tests and a knowledge of the biologic and pathologic processes that occur within pulp tissue.

The decision to be made is one of the following: (1) to conservatively restore the defective tooth structure, (2) to remove the diseased pulpal tissue, or (3) to remove the entire tooth. In making the decision the clinician is really deciding whether the disease process taking place within the pulp is a **reversible** (Figure 3-13) or an **irreversible pulpitis.**

Although there is a large number of possible causes of pulpitis (Box 3-2), the primary one is dental caries. Since dental caries destroys tooth structure, the extent to which the tooth is able to be restored plays a large part in the decision whether to treat the pulpitis without removing the pulpal tissue, to remove the diseased pulp and restore the tooth, or to remove the tooth.

Pulpitis is the name given to any inflammation of the pulp regardless of the presence of an infectious agent. Since the pulp is contained within a solid unyielding chamber with a limited blood supply through the apical foramen and no collateral support, the inflammatory process that is so beneficial in the healing process in other parts of the body often becomes a mechanism of destruction in this confined location. Inflammation is by nature an expansile process consisting of dilation of blood vessels, leakage of fluids from blood vessels into the surrounding connective tissue, and migration of cells into the immediate area. In the pulpal chamber if the inflammatory process continues for an extended period or is particularly intense, it can produce sharp and prolonged pain due to the internal pressure and strangulation of the blood supply. Without intervention, an acute form of pulpitis rapidly progresses to pulpal necrosis.

REVERSIBLE PULPITIS

The diagnosis of reversible pulpitis implies that the pulp is capable of a full recovery if the irritating factors subside or are removed. The symptoms reflect an irritated pulp tissue that reacts with the mildest and earliest forms of the inflammatory response consisting of vasodilation, some transudation, a slight infiltrate of lymphocytes, and disruption of the odontoblastic layer (Figure 3-14). The diagnosis is based on the ability of the clinician to properly assess the patient's history and clinical signs and symptoms. To differentiate between reversible and irreversible pulpitis, the following must be assessed:

1. Whether the pain is spontaneous or brought on by thermal changes
2. The duration of each episode of pain
3. The nature of the pain as described by the patient

The pain of reversible pulpitis is sharp and intense and responds to a sudden change in temperature. The pain generally remains for 5 to 10 minutes and seldom lasts longer than 20 minutes. The tooth remains without symptoms until it is stimulated again. Changes in the position of the body, such as lying down, do not generally affect the nature or the duration of the pain. The treatment of reversible pulpitis consists of protecting the pulp from further thermal stimulation and placing sedative dressings in the base of the carious defect for several weeks.

IRREVERSIBLE PULPITIS

The diagnosis of irreversible pulpitis is made when it is determined that the pulp will most likely not recover, regardless of the attempts to treat it. The pulpal tissue will exhibit a wide spectrum of acute and chronic inflammatory changes (Figure 3-15). For the patient to obtain permanent relief at this stage, the remaining pulp must be removed or the tooth must be extracted. The diagnosis is made based on the same type of clinical information used to diagnose reversible pulpitis.

The pain of an irreversible pulpitis can be of variable intensity, but it is usually less intense than that of reversible pulpitis. The main feature of irreversible pulpitis is that pain is spontaneously initiated, not the result of a sudden temperature change, and lasts for a prolonged period, usually longer than 20 minutes. The pain may be initiated or accentuated when the patient reclines. Whereas the pain from reversible pulpitis is easily localized to a particular tooth, the pain from an irreversible pulpitis may be referred to another nearby location such as the lateral aspect of the face or to other teeth in the arch (Box 3-3).

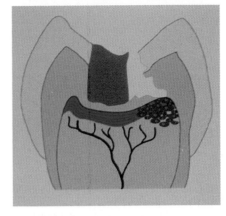

FIGURE 3-15

Irreversible pulpitis. Diagram of a focal area of acute inflammation (pulpal abscess) in a tooth with advanced recurrent caries.

■ BOX 3-3
Comparison of Pain Symptoms in Reversible and Irreversible Pulpitis

Reversible	*Irreversible*
Elicited	Spontaneous
Sharp	Dull
<20 minutes' duration	>20 minutes' duration
Unaffected by body position	Affected by body position
Easily localized	Often difficult to localize

PULPAL NECROSIS

Pulpal necrosis is the term applied to pulp tissue that is no longer living. If this is the result of a sudden traumatic event, such as a blow to the tooth in which the blood supply has been severed, the patient will often have no symptoms for a time. In other cases pulpal necrosis occurs slowly over time, as occurs during the course of an untreated irreversible pulpitis. In this latter case the patient may gradually lose the acute and chronic symptoms because the nerve fibers in the pulp degenerate from the overwhelming inflammation. In either situation the asymptomatic state is usually temporary because the pulpal tissue soon undergoes autolysis, becoming a source of irritation to the periodontal membrane tissue adjacent to the apical foramen.

In pulpal necrosis the pulpal tissue may be infected with bacteria. Infected pulpal necrosis is usually the result of dental decay, in which case the infection can quickly extend into the apical areas of the tooth and the surrounding bone. These occurrences produce a great deal of pain and other systemic reactions. Noninfected (aseptic) pulpal necrosis usually occurs after a traumatic incident and may not produce symptoms for many months. The first sign of noninfected pulpal necrosis may be a change in the coloration of the tooth (Figure 3-16).

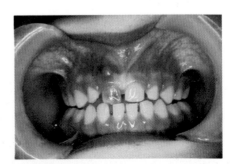

FIGURE 3-16

Pulpal necrosis. Darkened central incisor caused by penetration of the tissue remnants of nonvital pulp into the dentin tubules. The small nodule on the gingiva above the tooth (parulis) is the surface opening of a drainage tract from a periapical abscess.

This is the result of the decomposing tissue debris and break-down products of the red blood cells entering the open ends of the empty dentinal tubules and becoming distributed throughout the dentin. This process alters the translucency of the tooth. After the tooth has become nonvital, it loses its ability to rehydrate the dentin, making it more brittle and subject to cracks and fractures.

The presence of the inflammatory response in the apical periodontal membrane can produce extensive pain because of its location in a confined area between the alveolar bone and root surface. Until the surrounding bone undergoes resorption, allowing the accumulated edema and exudate to escape into the marrow spaces, the pressure from the exudate may force the tooth to extrude from the socket causing premature contact with opposing teeth. This tooth will be sensitive to even the smallest amount of pressure, including contact when chewing food.

A diagnostic tool used to determine if a tooth has undergone pulpal necrosis consists of gently tapping on several teeth in the area with a blunt instrument. A tooth that has undergone pulpal necrosis will be identified because the pressure from the tapping will produce intense pain. This is referred to as the *percussion test*.

COMMON DIAGNOSTIC TECHNIQUES

The diagnostic procedures that are commonly used to assess the status of a symptomatic tooth and pulp are as follows:

1. History and nature of the pain
2. Reaction to thermal changes
3. Reaction to mild electric stimulation
4. Reaction to percussion of the tooth
5. Radiographic examination
6. Visual clinical examination
7. Palpation of surrounding tissue

History and Nature of Pain

The history and nature of the pain relate to the circumstances of its occurrences, such as duration and the type of sensation experienced by the patient. The pain of reversible pulpitis is sharp and intense, whereas the pain of irreversible pulpitis is often described as dull, nagging, and frequently vague in its location.

Reaction to Thermal Changes

The test for a reaction to thermal changes is conducted in the dental office by placing a cold or very warm object on the tooth. In the case of a reversible pulpitis, there will be an immediate, sharp pain that will last for up to 20 minutes. If it is an irreversible pulpitis, the pain may be less sharp but may last for a much longer time.

Reaction to Electric Stimulation

The test for reaction to mild electric stimulation is conducted with a low-voltage direct current. It evaluates the degree of excitability of the nerves in the inflamed pulp. In reversible pulpitis the nerves will be easily excited and will thus respond at a lower than normal voltage level. In irreversible pulpitis the nerve tissue within the pulp is more severely damaged, and a higher level of voltage is required before the patient responds. This diagnostic test is often variable. It is particularly useful when there is no reaction at even the highest voltage level because this suggests that there is probably no live pulpal tissue.

Reaction to Percussion of Tooth

A positive reaction to percussion indicates that there is inflammation in the apical periodontal tissue of a particular tooth. This is particularly useful when the pain is vague and the offending tooth is not immediately apparent, as occurs with long-standing irreversible pulpitis.

Radiographic Examination

A radiograph is of little use in evaluating the extent of changes *within* the pulpal chambers but can be useful in determining if the inflammatory response has reached the periapical tissue. Radiographic involvement of this tissue is usually an indication that irreversible changes have taken place within the pulp. The presence of a radiolucency at the apex of a tooth is of great help in determining the cause of vague pain in a quadrant of the mandible or maxilla.

Visual Examination

A visual clinical examination may reveal an expansion of the cortical plates of the alveolar bones. This is helpful if the periapical inflammation has penetrated into the surrounding bone and is attempting to drain to the surface. Sometimes a small, raised, reddish papule or nodule (parulis) occurs over the apex of the tooth that represents the stoma (opening) of a draining sinus tract of a periapical abscess.

Palpation of Surrounding Area

Palpation of the periapical area resulting in pain to the patient signifies that the inflammation has reached the tissue surrounding the apex of the tooth. This is an indication that the pulp is necrotic and the pulpal chambers need to be filled to prevent further spreading of the inflammation to the surrounding bone.

HISTOPATHOLOGY OF PULPAL DISEASE

Correlation of the patient's clinical signs and symptoms with the degree of pulpal histopathologic changes has been difficult and inaccurate. Thus attempts to assess whether a specific instance of irreversible pulpitis is actually an acute partial pulpitis, acute total pulpitis, chronic partial pulpitis, chronic total pulpitis, fibrotic pulp, or any other severe inflammatory change should not be undertaken if the evaluation is based only on an analysis of the clinical signs and symptoms. A true evaluation of the actual degree of inflammatory pulpal changes can only be made if the tissue is actually removed and microscopically examined. Since actually sampling the pulpal tissue quickly leads to its demise, this is not possible. The major decision whether to remove the entire pulpal tissue must be based on the clinical information available. Extirpation of the pulp for examination (as a means of relieving pain or for other reasons) results in a devitalized tooth that requires the empty chamber to be filled with a synthetic material to prevent it from becoming a source of inflammation and infection to the adjacent periapical area.

Although there is not a direct correlation between the clinical and histologic disease states of the pulp, there is still a spectrum of histologic changes that takes place between a normal and a necrotic pulp. Some of the histopathologic stages fluctuate for a time (for example, acute-chronic-acute), whereas others are part of a one-way chronic progressive course that ends in fibrosis with focal or diffuse calcification or in pulpal necrosis.

Acute Pulpitis

The histopathologic features of an acute pulpitis are similar to those of an abscess in other parts of the body. Acute pulpitis may be confined to one horn of

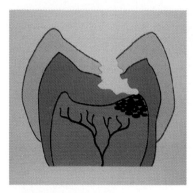

F I G U R E 3-17

Acute pulpitis. Diagram of an abscess of the pulpal horn common in teeth of young patients.

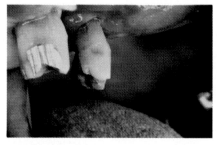

F I G U R E 3-18

Acute pulpitis. Tooth exhibiting a focal area of intrapulpal hemorrhage and acute pulpitis resulting from overheating during crown preparation.

the coronal pulp **(focal acute pulpitis)** (Figure 3-17) or involve the whole pulp **(total acute pulpitis).** The condition is usually the result of rapid bacterial invasion of large diameter (nonsclerosed) dentinal tubules and is most commonly found in the teeth of children and adolescents. For a pulpitis to remain acute, there must be no possibility of drainage of the exudate. Instead, the exudate remains within the enclosed chamber, builds pressure, and quickly extends to all parts of the healthy pulp.

An acute pulpitis can arise when the pulp becomes suddenly overheated to the extent that the blood vessels rupture, causing focal areas of hemorrhage. This may occur during crown preparation when inadequate cooling does not accompany the high-speed removal of the tooth structure (Figure 3-18).

A **pulpal abscess** is similar but not identical to an abscess in any other part of the body. The core is composed of a purulent exudate consisting of polymorphonuclear leukocytes against a background of fibrin, necrotic tissue debris, and extravasated red blood cells. This core is surrounded by a zone of granulation tissue consisting of newly forming capillary blood vessels, plump fibroblasts, plasma cells, and lymphocytes. Because the pulpal tissue is small and the process in this location is usually rapid, there is not an outer surrounding fibrous connective capsule, as occurs in other body locations. The liberated autolytic enzymes that result from tissue destruction and the exotoxins of the invading bacteria quickly spread to all parts of the remaining healthy pulp and eventually through the apical foramen into the adjacent periodontal membrane. Because of the intenseness of the irritant in the form of virulent bacteria and the lack of drainage, purulent exudate penetrates the cortical bone surrounding the apical periodontal membrane and invades the marrow spaces of the medullary bone. At this point the condition represents a form of focal acute suppurative osteomyelitis. If drainage occurs at or before this stage, the histopathologic features would quickly revert to those of the chronic form of pulpitis.

Chronic Pulpitis

The histologic features of a **chronic pulpitis** are similar to those of a chronic focal fibrosis in other parts of the body that is caused by a low-grade irritant (Figure 3-19). For chronic pulpitis to occur, there is little or no penetration by large numbers of the virulent types of bacteria. This is often the situation in older teeth because most of these teeth have had previous restorations or a slowly progressive form of caries. This form of caries allows the dentinal tubules to narrow (sclerosis) and the pulpal dentin to deposit tertiary (reparative) dentin at its interface with the pulpal soft tissue. This relatively nontubular form of dentin or

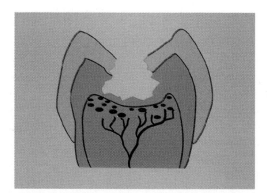

F I G U R E 3-19

Chronic pulpitis. Diagram of a large carious lesion in an older tooth in which the pulpal tissue contains a diffuse infiltrate of inflammatory cells.

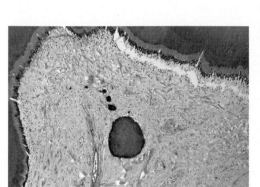
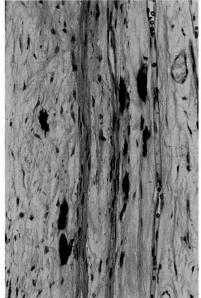

A   B

FIGURE 3-20

Chronic pulpitis. Microscopic appearance of pulp with spherical calcifications (pulp stones) **(A)** and linear (dystrophic) calcifications **(B).**

bone along with the sclerosed dentinal tubules acts as a barrier to slow the progression of bacteria and their exotoxins, allowing the pulp to develop its own immune response.

When viewed microscopically, chronic pulpitis reveals the presence of loose, delicate connective tissue with bundles of dense collagen and a severe reduction in both the size and number of the vascular structures and peripheral nerves. Throughout the pulp there is a diffuse infiltrate of lymphocytes and plasma cells. This stage of pulpal disease is referred to as **pulpal fibrosis.** If this stage persists for a time, **focal** and **diffuse calcifications** often occur. The calcifications may be in the form of **pulp stones** (spherical calcifications) (Figure 3-20, *A*) or **dystrophic calcifications** (linear calcifications) (Figure 3-20, *B*) and may be present in both the coronal and root pulpal tissues.

Eventually, prolonged chronic pulpitis leads to pulpal necrosis. The periapical lesion associated with chronic pulpitis is indolent and asymptomatic and is composed of a circumscribed nodule of fibrous tissue with a mild infiltrate of lymphocytes and plasma cells. This lesion is referred to as a *periapical granuloma*.

Chronic Hyperplastic Pulpitis

Chronic hyperplastic pulpitis is a rare condition that is primarily confined to the molars of children. It is the result of rampant acute caries in young teeth that quickly reaches the pulp before it becomes completely necrotic. In this rapid form of caries, the crown will sometimes disintegrate before the young, well-nourished pulp succumbs to infection, resulting in an open pulpitis. In patients of this young age the apical foramen is often still widely open, allowing for an ample blood supply that is able to sustain the injured pulp. The combination of an open chronic pulpitis, an ample blood supply, and the increased regenerative capacity of young pulpal tissue appears, in some instances, to stimulate the pulpal tissue to proliferate or to produce granulation tissue (Figure 3-21). Often, this hyperplastic nodule will have a surface layer of stratified squamous epithelium. In this unusual series of events the pulpal tissue may undergo excessive

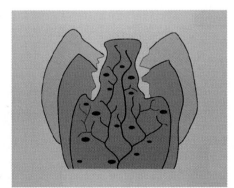

FIGURE 3-21

Hyperplastic pulpitis. Diagram of a molar in a young patient with a chronically inflamed pulp that has proliferated through the open carious defect projecting into the oral cavity.

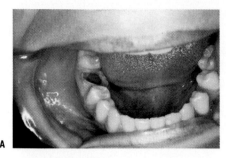

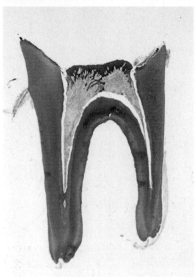

FIGURE 3-22

Hyperplastic pulpitis. A, Clinical appearance of "pulp polyp" in a grossly carious right mandibular first molar. **B,** Microscopic appearance of grossly carious tooth and fibrotic "pulp polyp" with a stratified squamous epithelium on the surface.

overgrowth (hyperplasia) and project out of the crown of the tooth (Figure 3-22). The exposed tissue and the pulp remaining within the tooth eventually become fibrotic and produce a firm nodule. Because this lesion clinically projects from the pulpal chamber, it is commonly referred to as a **pulp polyp.**

Clinically, if a pulp polyp is not covered with epithelium or becomes ulcerated, it will appear reddish. Otherwise, it has the same color as the rest of the oral tissue. Under normal circumstances these lesions produce no symptoms because they are said to be deficient in nerve fibers. If one of these polyps is found to be symptomatic, it is most likely not of pulpal origin but is instead an extension of the adjacent gingiva that is overlaying the disintegrated tooth crown.

The usual treatment of a tooth with a pulp polyp is extraction. If the molar is in the deciduous dentition, sometimes it is not extracted to maintain arch space. It should be remembered that the polyp cannot be effectively cleaned and that the remaining tooth structure will continue to decay, producing a chronic septic condition that can pose a health risk to the patient.

PERIAPICAL LESIONS

The nature and behavior of lesions that form at the apex of the tooth are a reflection of the conditions that lead to the destruction of the pulp of the associated tooth. The major factors follow.

1. Presence of an open or closed pulpitis
2. Virulence of the involved microorganisms
3. Extent of sclerosis of the dentinal tubules
4. Competency of the host immune response

When the factors are optimal (such as the presence of an open chronic pulpitis, bacteria of low virulence, an older tooth with sclerotic dentinal tubules, and a healthy patient) the changes at the apex of the tooth are mild and chronic. Multiple optimal factors are sometimes associated with little or no activation of the inflammatory response but rather act as stimulants to the fibroblastic and osteoblastic cells and scar tissue and dense bone produced in the area. When conditions are mostly adverse (such as the presence of a closed acute pulpitis, large numbers of highly virulent bacteria, and open dentinal tubules of young teeth), the inflammation at the apex of the tooth will rapidly intensify and large amounts of bacterial toxins and autolytic enzymes will be produced and disseminated. Under these circumstances there is rapid destruction of the periapical tissue and surrounding bone and the process quickly extends into the adjacent marrow spaces (Figure 3-23).

CHRONIC APICAL PERIODONTITIS

The term *chronic apical periodontitis* is used to denote the earliest radiographic evidence of extension of the inflammatory process from the pulpal chamber into the adjacent periodontal membrane around the apical foramen. Although the outline of the apical alveolar bone is still visible on a radiograph, the periodontal membrane in this region will appear to be widened. Clinically, the tooth may still exhibit some faint evidence of vitality when it is electrically stimulated, and it will usually have a positive reaction to a percussion test. The histopathologic findings are variable and will reflect the type of inflammation that existed in the pulp. This condition is merely a transitory phase between pulpitis and the more distinct forms of periapical lesions.

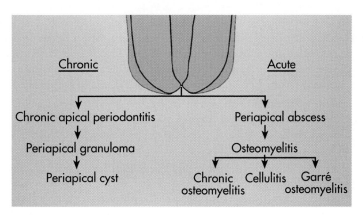

FIGURE 3-23

Periapical infections. Chronic and acute pathways that untreated infections and their accompanying clinical lesions may take depending on the type of the preceding pulpitis, virulence of the bacteria, and the presence or absence of drainage.

PERIAPICAL GRANULOMA

A periapical granuloma occurs when the contributing factors are optimal, such as when a pulpitis progresses into a periapical lesion. This is by far the most common lesion that occurs after pulpal necrosis. It is usually painless, progresses slowly, and seldom becomes very large. While a periapical granuloma is present, conditions can suddenly change. An open pulpal chamber may become blocked with food or a wooden toothpick, inhibiting drainage. When drainage of the exudate is inhibited, a periapical granuloma can be transformed into an acute periapical abscess. The most common change that occurs in a long-standing periapical granuloma is its gradual transformation into a periapical cyst. If the pulpal canal containing the necrotic tissue is not treated, a periapical cyst will gradually occur over the next several months to years.

RADIOGRAPHIC

The radiographic appearance of periapical granuloma occurs as an oval or rounded radiolucency with a well-demarcated outline located at the apex of the tooth (Figure 3-24). Rarely, the radiolucency will be located away from the apex and centered around the opening of a lateral canal. A periapical granuloma that periodically undergoes acute exacerbations will have a less distinct line of demarcation between the bone and the granulomatous tissue than a static, quiescent lesion. Frequent findings associated with a long-standing periapical granuloma are hypercementosis of the apical third of the root and resorption resulting in blunting of the root tip.

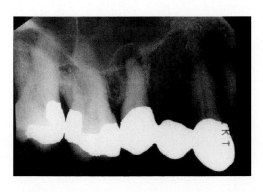

FIGURE 3-24

Periapical granuloma. Radiograph of a periapical granuloma with a prominently corticated outline of the interface with normal bone that is in continuity with the lamina dura of the associated tooth.

HISTOPATHOLOGY

A periapical granuloma is composed of an outer capsule of dense fibrous tissue and a central zone of granulation tissue (Figure 3-25). The central zone will often contain macrophages with a "foamy" cytoplasm caused by phagocytized cholesterol. Some cholesterol crystals may be present, surrounded by multinucleated giant cells. Throughout the soft tissue will be a diffuse infiltrate of lymphocytes and plasma cells. A frequent finding is the presence of irregular islands and strands of epithelium, a result of prolonged, mild stimulation of the rests of Malassez. These are the remnants of Hertwig root sheath, the epithelial membrane that outlines the shape of the roots of the teeth.

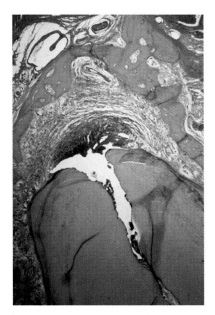
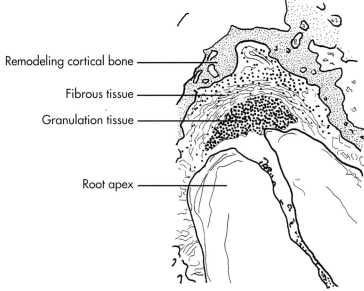

Remodeling cortical bone

Fibrous tissue

Granulation tissue

Root apex

FIGURE 3-25

Periapical granuloma. Microscopic appearance of the early stage of granuloma development exhibiting granulation tissue at the apical foramen surrounded by fibrous tissue and an outer zone of cortical bone.

The treatment of a periapical granuloma depends on the condition of the tooth as a whole. If the tooth is restorable, the root canal can be filled. If the root canal cannot be filled and the apical area is in a location accessible for surgery, an apicoectomy may be performed to remove the granuloma. Otherwise, the tooth is extracted and the periapical granuloma is curetted through the tooth socket. Failure to resolve or remove a periapical granuloma commonly results in the development of a periapical cyst.

PERIAPICAL CYST

A periapical cyst is a common development of long-standing, untreated periapical granuloma. The epithelial lining is derived from the rests of Malassez, the epithelial islands left over after root formation during odontogenesis and normally present in the apical periodontal membrane. The rests are stimulated to proliferate by the low-grade inflammation of the preceding periapical granuloma (Figure 3-26). The periapical cyst is by far the most common of the cysts of

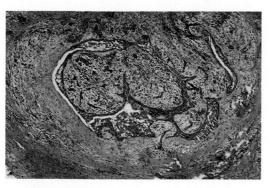
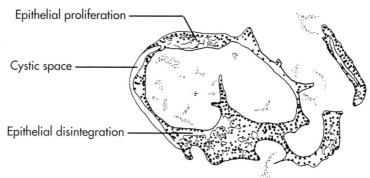

FIGURE 3-26

Periapical cyst. Microscopic appearance of developing cystic lining from proliferating rests of Malassez stimulated by the chronic inflammation of the preceding periapical granuloma.

the jaws. Since its development is the result of sequential inflammation of the tooth pulp and the adjacent surrounding apical tissue, the cyst may become inflamed and symptomatic, sometimes exhibiting acute exacerbations. Once the cyst has formed, it usually follows a slow but continuous course that can result in the destruction of a large portion of the maxilla or mandible.

RADIOGRAPHIC

The periapical cyst is well circumscribed, often with a distinct thin line of cortication separating it from the surrounding bone (Figure 3-27, *A*). It may be associated with resorption of the apices of the teeth and/or displacement of the roots. It is distinctly rounded and unilocular and may become very large, resulting in erosion of the inferior border (Figure 3-27, *B*) and bulging of the buccal and lingual cortical plates.

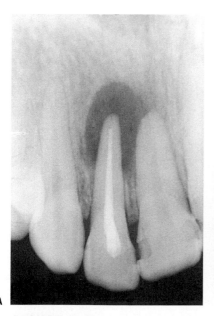
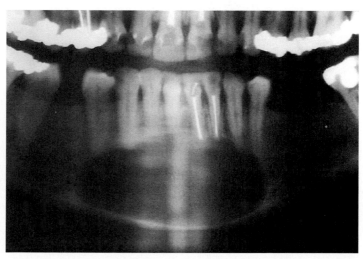

A   B

FIGURE 3-27

Periapical cyst. A, Radiograph of a small lesion surrounding the apex of a lateral incisor with the distinct line of demarcation separating the lesion from the surrounding bone. **B,** Panoramic radiograph of the anterior mandible containing a large unilocular corticated lesion involving the inferior border.

HISTOPATHOLOGY

The tissue consists of an outer dense fibrous connective tissue capsule that surrounds a central lumen containing a thick proteinaceous fluid and cellular debris. The lumen is lined by a nonkeratinized stratified squamous epithelium containing rete pegs that are generally elongated and branched. Collections of cholesterol-laden macrophages are commonly present, particularly in the early stages of cyst development (Figure 3-28, *A*). The capsule and the epithelial lining contain a diffuse infiltration of plasma cells and lymphocytes (Figure 3-28, *B*). Cholesterol crystals surrounded by foreign body giant cells are a common finding. The presence of eosinophilic refractile hyaline bodies, referred to as *Rushton bodies*, are sometimes found in the intermediate cell layer of the epithelium.

A periapical cyst that remains or forms after the offending tooth has been extracted is referred to as a **residual cyst.** It will have the same radiographic, clinical, and histopathologic features as the periapical cyst.

Periapical cysts are treated conservatively by enucleation. Recurrence is seldom a problem if the capsule is completely removed. The tissue should be microscopically examined to ensure that it is not one of the other more aggressive odontogenic cysts or a neoplastic lesion. On rare occasions, dysplastic changes and even squamous cell carcinoma have been found in the walls of long-standing cysts.

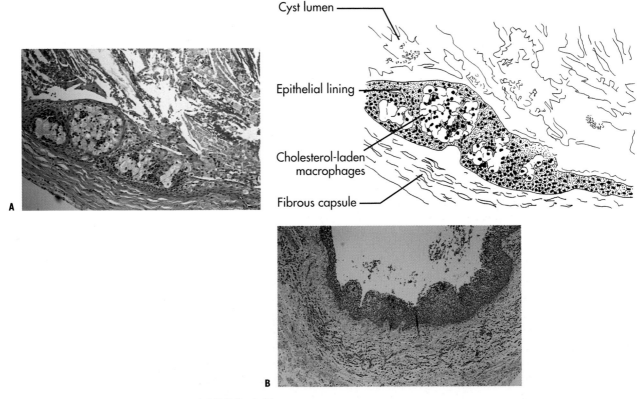

FIGURE 3-28

Periapical cyst. A, Microscopic appearance of developing cyst lining with associated cholesterol-laden macrophages within the connective tissue and the lumen. **B,** Matured stratified squamous epithelial lining and fibrous connective tissue capsule with a diffuse infiltrate of lymphocytes and plasma cells surrounding the central lumen.

ACUTE PERIAPICAL CONDITIONS

The factors leading to the development of acute lesions at the apex of a tooth are usually one or more of the following:

1. Young tooth with *open* tubules
2. *Rampant* caries
3. *Closed* acute pulpitis
4. Presence of highly *virulent* microorganisms
5. *Weakened* host defense system

Under most or all of these circumstances the ensuing inflammatory events happen quickly and cause a great deal of pain. If unchecked, infection and purulent exudate rapidly spread throughout the affected jaw into the adjacent structures and the systemic circulation where emboli of the infection could lodge in the small capillaries of a number of distant organs or anatomic locations.

PERIAPICAL ABSCESS

The periapical abscess is the initial lesion that develops when the circumstances are adverse. It is probably the most painful patient condition that confronts clinicians and is potentially one of the most dangerous. It is often a progression of an acute pulpitis that has exudate extending into the adjacent soft and hard tissues. Because it often contains one or more strains of virulent bacterial organisms, the exudate usually contains potent exotoxins and lytic enzymes capable of breaking down the tissue barriers. Additionally, an opening to allow drainage from the pulp through the crown to the oral cavity is often absent, resulting in an internal pressure within the periodontal membrane that causes extrusion of the tooth from the socket and rapid extension of the exudate throughout the underlying medullary bone.

CLINICAL

Patients with a periapical abscess are in a great deal of pain. Temperature elevation and malaise are common. In most patients the tooth associated with the abscess will extrude from the socket sufficiently to cause occlusal interference and greatly increased pain when it comes in contact with other teeth. In locations where the root apex is in close proximity to the cortex of the overlying alveolar bone, swelling and redness of the area will be present. The test that is most useful in the diagnosis of an acute periapical abscess is an intense sensitivity to percussion while the tooth is relatively insensitive or unresponsive to hot, cold, and electrical stimulation.

RADIOGRAPHIC

The area around the apex of the tooth initially exhibits a slight widening of the apical periodontal space with a gradual loss of the distinctness of the adjacent alveolar bone (lamina dura). As the exudate extends into the surrounding medullary bone, the radiographic appearance will reflect the bone loss by exhibiting a faintness of the trabecular pattern and an increased radiolucency. Because a periapical abscess is a rapid lytic process, the radiographic appearance will not exhibit a distinct line of demarcation between the inflammatory process and the normal bone.

HISTOPATHOLOGY

The microscopic features of a periapical abscess are similar to those of an abscess in other parts of the body. An outer thin capsule of fibrous tissue is infiltrated

FIGURE 3-29

Periapical abscess. Microscopic appearance of an abscess consisting of an outer fibrous wall *(bottom);* an overlying zone of granulation tissue *(center);* and a central core of purulent exudate composed of neutrophils, macrophages, fibrin, and tissue debris *(top).*

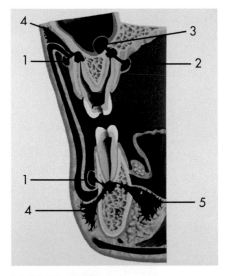

FIGURE 3-30

Diagram of the common drainage pathways of acute periapical infections. The location of the various points of drainage is determined by the anatomic location of the root apex. Common locations are: *1,* surface of gingiva (parulis); *2,* palate (palatal abscess); *3,* maxillary sinus; *4,* soft tissue spaces superior (maxilla) and inferior (mandible) to buccinator muscle (cellulitis); and *5,* floor of the mouth (Ludwig angina).

with lymphocytes and plasma cells. A wide zone of granulation tissue containing a mixture of neutrophils, lymphocytes, plasma cells, and macrophages surrounds a central core of tissue that has undergone disintegration and liquefaction and is composed of purulent exudate (Figure 3-29). In many lesions bacterial colonies are readily apparent.

OSTEOMYELITIS

■ OSTEOMYELITIS: an inflammatory process within medullary (trabecular) bone that involves the marrow spaces.

■ ACUTE OSTEOMYELITIS: a rapidly destructive inflammatory process within bone that consists of granulation tissue, purulent exudate, and islands of nonvital bone (sequestra).

ACUTE OSTEOMYELITIS

Acute osteomyelitis is a destructive lesion of the trabecular bone and bone marrow of an acute inflammatory origin and usually contains virulent strains of bacteria. It is most commonly caused by direct extension of an untreated periapical abscess. Another common cause is a minor traumatic incident involving a mandible that has had its blood supply compromised by previous high doses of radiation for the treatment of a malignancy (osteoradionecrosis). The process of acute osteomyelitis in both cases is rapid if the involved bacterial organisms are particularly virulent or the host's systemic resistance is reduced.

CLINICAL
Patients with acute osteomyelitis characteristically have intense pain and become physically ill, especially before the build up of purulent exudate has eroded through the cortical bone permitting drainage to occur. The pain will return again if the exudate continues to accumulate in the soft tissue spaces outside the bone, subsiding only when it finally erodes through the skin or mucosa. As with acute pulpitis, drainage aids resolution and results in a rapid reduction in symptoms, whereas a lack of drainage produces a rapid increase in pain with accompanying pyrexia and malaise. In the mandible the exudate with its accompanying bacterial toxins and lytic enzymes may involve the inferior alveolar canal, producing an alteration in the conductivity of the nerve (Figure 3-30). This often produces an alteration in the sensation (paresthesia) of the lower lip of the affected side. Paresthesia can cause a great deal of concern because it is also a common presenting feature when a malignant neoplasm involves the mandible.

RADIOGRAPHIC
The radiographic features of acute osteomyelitis are usually not immediately present as the exudate first progresses through the soft tissue component of the preexisting marrow spaces. It is not until the trabecular bone has undergone a significant amount of resorption that the extent of destruction will be apparent radiographically. Initially the area is faintly visible and eventually appears dif-

fusely blotchy or mottled with indistinct margins (Figure 3-31). Islands of apparently intact bone are often visible in central locations. In reality, these are fragments of dead, nonresorbed bone that are surrounded by wide zones of purulent exudate. An island of dead bone is referred to as a *sequestrum*. It is common for a sequestrum to be externalized by the body and thus appear on the mucosal surface as a loose piece of bone.

HISTOPATHOLOGY

The microscopic features of the involved bone are distinctive. They consist of granulation tissue intermixed with neutrophils, fibrin, and tissue debris surrounding spicules of bone in which the osteocytes have undergone necrosis. In the periphery near the junction with the unaffected bone, the soft tissue consists of a loose, delicate connective tissue with an infiltrate of lymphocytes and plasma cells. This latter finding is also seen in areas of affected bone that are in the early stages of transition to a chronic osteomyelitis that is in the process of resolution.

TREATMENT

The management of acute osteomyelitis is a combination of surgical intervention to establish drainage and the use of high doses of antibiotics that are targeted to the microorganisms involved, which is determined by culture and sensitivity testing.

CELLULITIS

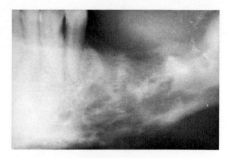

FIGURE 3-31

Acute osteomyelitis. Radiograph of posterior mandible exhibiting the mottled and blotchy pattern of radiolucent and radiopaque areas, indistinct borders, and islands of residual bone *(sequestra)*.

■ CELLULITIS: a painful swelling of the soft tissue of the mouth and face resulting from a diffuse spreading of purulent exudate along the fascial planes that separate the muscle bundles.

■ SINUS TRACT: a drainage pathway from a deep focus of acute infection through tissue and/or bone to an opening on the surface.

■ PARULIS: a sessile nodule on the gingiva at the site where a draining sinus tract reaches the surface.

■ FISTULA: a drainage pathway or abnormal communication between two epithelium-lined surfaces due to destruction of the intervening tissue.

■ LUDWIG ANGINA: cellulitis involving fascial spaces between muscles and other structures of the posterior floor of the mouth that can compromise the airway.

The term cellulitis is actually a misnomer because the process is not an inflammation of the cells but an acute condition in which purulent exudate, usually accompanied by virulent forms of bacteria, involves the fascial planes between the bundles of facial and perioral muscles. Cellulitis may occur from other causes in the head and neck area but is most commonly the result of extension of a periapical abscess into the soft tissue. This occurs when the exudate erodes through the cortical plate of the mandible or the maxilla. When the erosion pathway

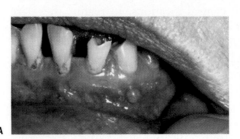
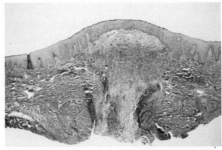

FIGURE 3-32

Parulis. A, Patient with a small nodule representing the opening of a draining sinus tract on the gingiva adjacent to a nonvital left mandibular cuspid. **B,** Microscopic appearance of a gingival nodular swelling demonstrating the central core of purulent exudate (sinus tract) exerting pressure beneath the epithelium that is near the point of rupture (Trichrome stain).

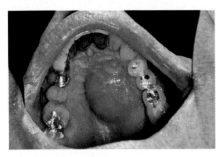

FIGURE 3-33

Palatal abscess. A large fluctuant swelling of the palate caused by the drainage of purulent exudate into the submucosal tissue from an apical area of nonvital premolars.

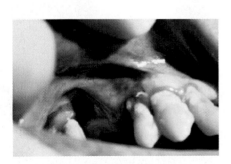

FIGURE 3-34

Oral-antral fistula. An open communication between the maxillary sinus (antrum) and the oral cavity is present on the edentulous alveolar ridge after the extraction of a molar with a long-standing periapical lesion that involved the sinus floor.

reaches the gingival surface, it results in a small nodule that enlarges until it ruptures. The site of the opening (stoma) of a sinus tract on the gingiva is commonly termed a *parulis* (Figure 3-32). Occasionally, the exudate tracks onto the palate, producing a large tumorlike mass (Figure 3-33). When a periapical abscess erodes into the maxillary sinus, destroying the intervening bone and lining, and the offending tooth is extracted, a communication between the floor of the sinus and the oral cavity may result. The tract may remain permanently patent, particularly if it becomes lined by epithelium emanating from both sinus (antrum) and oral mucosal linings. This abnormal open communication is termed an *oral-antral fistula* (Figure 3-34).

When purulent exudate emanating from a periapical abscess penetrates the alveolar bone and enters the muscle layers, the lytic enzymes from the microorganisms and the acute inflammatory process break down the fascia that normally surrounds and binds the muscle bundles. This breakdown of the fascia allows the exudate to spread throughout the immediate region, greatly increasing the magnitude of the infection. These patients exhibit extensive swelling of the affected facial region, have considerable discomfort or pain, and develop signs and symptoms of systemic involvement such as elevated temperature, malaise, lethargy, and lymphadenopathy. Involvement of the soft tissue and muscle overlying the maxilla usually results in periocular swelling and temporary loss of sight on the affected side. When the muscle layers overlying the body of the mandible are involved, patients experience a puffy, pendulous swelling on the left side of the face, closely resembling mumps. Exudate may extend lingually into the muscle spaces of the posterior floor of the mouth. Such a posterior progression can result in the swelling of the structures in and around the epiglottis. Tissue swelling in this area is life threatening because it can restrict the airway and result in suffocation if emergency measures are not undertaken immediately. The presence of cellulitis in these locations has historically been referred to as *Ludwig angina*.

Another serious complication of cellulitis is the extension of the exudate into the maxillary cavernous sinus area, resulting in thrombophlebitis. From this location fatal forms of brain abscess or acute meningitis are possible unless rapid intervention is undertaken.

CHRONIC OSTEOMYELITIS

Chronic osteomyelitis differs greatly from the acute types by inducing bone to form and become more dense. It occurs in response to a low-grade inflammatory

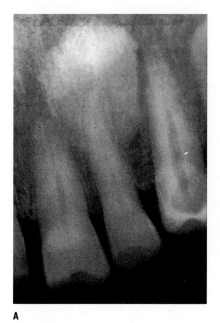
A

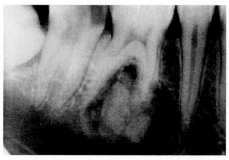
B

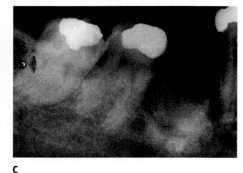
C

FIGURE 3-35

Chronic osteosclerosis. A, Radiograph of an area of uniform increase in bone density located apically to the maxillary lateral incisor. **B,** Radiograph of a localized area of radiolucency with central nodular radiopacities. **C,** Radiograph of an area of nodular radiopacities in the location of a previously existing tooth. These lesions have been also termed "focal chronic sclerosing osteomyelitis."

process rather than the intense and destructive inflammation caused by virulent bacteria. There is a great deal of variation in the chronic forms of bone inflammation. Typically there is little or no pain. In many cases the irritant may be so mild it stimulates the osteocytes inducing the trabecular bone to become more dense and even lay down additional bone, which results in a reduction of the marrow spaces. The area will radiographically appear mottled and more radiopaque than normal. This process is histologically referred to as **osteosclerosis.** It may be confined to an area around the root of a tooth (Figure 3-35, *A* and *B*) or be present where a tooth previously existed (Figure 3-35, *C*). These localized changes in the bone are referred to as **focal chronic sclerosing osteomyelitis.** In other instances the osteosclerosis may involve larger areas of bone (Figure 3-36) or edentulous areas in one or more quadrants. These conditions are referred to as **diffuse chronic sclerosing osteomyelitis.**

GARRÉ OSTEOMYELITIS

Garré osteomyelitis is an unusual hyperplastic reaction of the periosteum to a chronic osteomyelitis of the posterior mandible that is unique to young patients. The correct terminology is **chronic osteomyelitis with proliferative periostitis,** but since this descriptive term is long and cumbersome, it is seldom used clinically.

CLINICAL

In the jaws Garré osteomyelitis is most frequently associated with advanced acute caries in young patients that has progressed to pulpitis and a periapical lesion. To become a Garré osteomyelitis the inflammatory response must extend

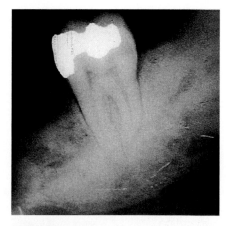

FIGURE 3-36

Diffuse chronic sclerosing osteomyelitis. A portion of a large diffuse area of radiopacity of the mandible that has indistinct boundaries indicative of increased bone density.

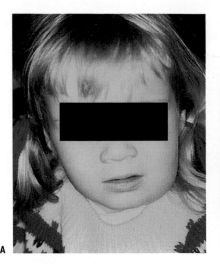

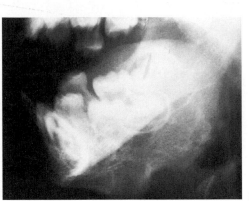

A   B

FIGURE 3-37

Garré osteomyelitis. A, Young patient with an enlargement of the left side of the face over the mandible. **B,** Lateral radiograph of the patient in *A* reveals a large mixed radiolucent/radiopaque area indicative of excess bone formation of the mandible.   (Courtesy Dr. David G. Gardner.)

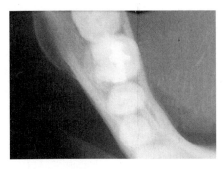

FIGURE 3-38

Garré osteomyelitis. An occlusal radiograph of excess layers of bone on the buccal plate ("onion skin") opposite partly erupted second molar.

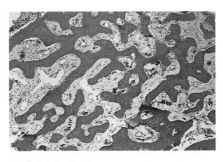

FIGURE 3-39

Garré osteomyelitis. Microscopic appearance of the periphery of excess porous bone layers with intervening cellular connective tissue and without cortex formation.

through the bone to the outer surface, stimulating the periosteum to thicken and lay down excess layers of new bone. In other situations this form of osteomyelitis occurs when the free gingival margin remains above the height of contour of the tooth, resulting in food impaction of the deepened gingival sulcus and a constant low-grade infection persists that stimulates the periosteum.

Patients who develop this form of osteomyelitis are characteristically in the age group that occurs shortly before the mixed dentition stage or immediately afterward. They slowly exhibit a diffuse or focal enlargement of an area of the mandible, usually posteriorly (Figure 3-37). The other common cause of this unique process is a molar that is unable to fully erupt (Figure 3-38). Upon palpation the area will be as hard as the normal surrounding bone and the patient will not exhibit pain when the area is slightly palpated. The area is usually asymptomatic.

RADIOGRAPHIC

A radiograph taken using an occlusal projection will demonstrate the characteristic multiple thin layers of new bone, referred to as an "onion skin" appearance. The trabecular bone will also exhibit the characteristic diffuse mottling of a chronic osteomyelitis.

HISTOPATHOLOGY

The microscopic features of the reactive bone that forms in response to the stimulated periosteum is less dense than normal cortical bone and deposited in a layered pattern. The trabecular spaces are wide and occupied with a cellular connective tissue (Figure 3-39).

TREATMENT

The condition slowly reverts back to normal after the source of infection is identified and resolved. Sometimes extraction of the offending tooth or surgical recontouring of the tissue in the molar area is necessary.

ADDITIONAL READING

DENTAL CARIES

Adriaens PA, Claeys GW, De Boever JA. Scanning electron microscopy of dentin caries: experimental in vitro studies with *Streptococcus mutans*. *Scanning Microsc*. 1987; 1:671-80.

Bjorndal L, Thylstrup A. A structural analysis of approximal enamel caries lesions and subjacent dentin reactions. *Eur J Oral Sci*. 1995; 103:25-31.

Carlsson P, Angmar-Mansson B, Redmo-Emanuelsson IM, Anderssen K. Effects on demineralization of enamel by fluoridated sucrose: a pilot study in an in situ caries model. *Adv Dent Res*. 1995; 9:9-13.

Daculsi G, LeGeros RZ, Jean A, Kerebel B. Possible physicochemical processes in human dentin caries. *J Dent Res*. 1987; 66:1356-9.

Donly K, Gomez C. In vitro demineralization-remineralization of enamel caries at restoration margins utilizing fluoride-releasing composite resin. *Quintessence Int*. 1994; 25:355-8.

Flaitz CM, Hicks MJ, Westerman GH, Berg JH and others. Argon laser irradiation and acidulated phosphate fluoride treatment in caries-like lesion formation in enamel: an in vitro study. *Pediatr Dent*. 1995; 17:31-5.

Frank RM. Structural events in the caries process in enamel, cementum, and dentin. *J Dent Res*. 1990; 69:559-66.

Garcia-Godoy F, Hicks MJ, Flaitz CM, Berg JH. Acidulated phosphate fluoride treatment and formation of caries-like lesions in enamel: effect of application time. *J Clin Pediatr Dent*. 1995; 19:105-10.

Grogono AL, Mayo JA. Prevention of root caries with dentin adhesives. *Am J Dent*. 1994; 7:89-90.

Hietala EL, Tjaderhane L, Larmas M. Dentin caries recording with Schiff's reagent, fluorescence, and back-scattered electron image. *J Dent Res*. 1993; 72:1588-92.

Ie YL, Verdonschot EH, Schaeken MJ, van't Hof MA. Electrical conductance of fissure enamel in recently erupted molar teeth as related to caries status. *Caries Res*. 1995; 29:94-9.

Kortelainen S, Larmas M. Effect of fluoride on caries progression and dentin apposition in rats fed on a cariogenic or noncariogenic diet. *Scand J Dent Res*. 1993; 101:16-20.

Nytun RB, Raadal M, Espelid I. Diagnosis of dentin involvement in occlusal caries based on visual and radiographic examination of the teeth. *Scand J Dent Res*. 1992; 100:144-8.

Schupbach P, Guggenheim B, Lutz F. Human root caries: histopathology of initial lesions in cementum and dentin. *J Oral Pathol Med*. 1989; 18:146-56.

Tagami J, Hosoda H, Burrow MF, Nakajima M. Effect of aging and caries on dentin permeability. *Proc Finn Dent Soc*. 1992; 88(suppl 1):149-54.

Takuma S, Tohda H, Watanabe K, Yama S. Size increase of dentin crystals in the intertubular matrix due to caries. *J Electron Microsc (Tokyo)*. 1986; 35:60-5.

Tveit AB, Espelid I, Fjelltveit A. Clinical diagnosis of occlusal dentin caries. *Caries Res*. 1994; 28:368-72.

Zacharia MA, Munshi AK. Microbiological assessment of dentin stained with a caries detector dye. *J Clin Pediatr Dent*. 1995; 19:111-5.

PULPITIS

Caliskan MK. Success of pulpotomy in the management of hyperplastic pulpitis. *Int Endod J*. 1993; 26:142-8.

Caliskan MK, Sepetcioglu F. Partial pulpotomy in crown-fractured permanent incisor with hyperplastic pulpitis: a case report. *Endod Dent Traumatol*. 1993; 9:71-3.

Gangarosa LP, Ciarlone AE, Neaverth EJ, Johnston CA and others. Use of verbal descriptors, thermal scores and electrical pulp testing as predictors of tooth pain before and after application of benzocaine gels into cavities of teeth with pulpitis. *Anesth Prog*. 1989; 36:272-5.

Gangarosa LP, McRae K. Fluoride iontophoresis as an aid in the diagnosis and treatment of reversible pulpitis: a case study. *Compend Contin Educ Dent*. 1985; 6:696, 698, 700-2.

Hahn CL, Falkler WA, Minah GE. Microbiological studies of carious dentine from human teeth with irreversible pulpitis. *Arch Oral Biol*. 1991; 36:47-53.

Massey WL, Romberg DM, Hunter N, Hume WR. The association of carious dentin microflora with tissue changes in human pulpitis. *Oral Microbiol Immunol*. 1993; 8:30-5.

Mendoza MM, Reader A, Meyers WJ, Foreman DW. An ultrastructural investigation of the human apical pulp in irreversible pulpitis: I: nerves. *J Endod*. 1987; 13:267-76.

Mendoza MM, Reader A, Meyers WJ, Marquard JV. An ultrastructural investigation of the human apical pulp in irreversible pulpitis: II: vasculature and connective tissue. *J Endod*. 1987; 13:318-27.

Oguntebi BR, DeSchepper EJ, Taylor TS, White CL and others. Postoperative pain incidence related to the type of emergency treatment of symptomatic pulpitis. *Oral Surg Oral Med Oral Pathol*. 1992; 73:479-83.

Piskin B, Aktener BO, Karakisi H. Neural changes in ulcerative and hyperplastic pulpitis: a transmission electron microscopic study. *Int Endod J*. 1993; 26:234-40.

Sigurdsson A, Jacoway JR. Herpes zoster infection presenting as an acute pulpitis. *Oral Surg Oral Med Oral Pathol Oral Radiol Endod*. 1995; 80:92-5.

Tzukert A. Pulpitis and root canal therapy: is a diagnostic radiograph of value? *Oral Surg Oral Med Oral Pathol*. 1986; 61:284-8.

PERIAPICAL LESIONS

PERIAPICAL GRANULOMA

Babal P, Soler P, Brozman M, Jakubovsky J and others. In situ characterization of cells in periapical granuloma by monoclonal antibodies. *Oral Surg Oral Med Oral Pathol*. 1987; 64:348-52.

Gerner NW, Hurlen B, Dobloug J, Brandtzaeg P. Endodontic treatment and immunopathology of periapical granuloma in an AIDS patient. *Endod Dent Traumatol.* 1988; 4:127-31.

Gilbert BO, Dickerson AW. Paresthesia of the mental nerve after an acute exacerbation of chronic apical periodontitis. *J Am Dent Assoc.* 1981; 103:588-90.

Lukic A, Arsenijevic N, Vujanic G, Ramic Z. Quantitative analysis of the immunocompetent cells in periapical granuloma: correlation with the histological characteristics of the lesions. *J Endod.* 1990; 16:119-22.

Marton I, Kiss C, Balla G, Szabo T and others. Acute phase proteins in patients with chronic periapical granuloma before and after surgical treatment. *Oral Microbiol Immunol.* 1988; 3:95-6.

Piattelli A, Artese L, Rosini S, Quaranta M and others. Immune cells in periapical granuloma: morphological and immuno-histochemical characterization. *J Endod.* 1991; 17:26-9.

PERIAPICAL CYST

Cassella EA, Pickett AB, Chamberlin JH. Unusual management problems in the treatment of a long-standing destructive periapical cyst: report of a case. *Oral Surg Oral Med Oral Pathol.* 1981; 51:93-8.

Fergus HS, Savord EG. Actinomycosis involving a periapical cyst in the anterior maxilla: report of a case. *Oral Surg Oral Med Oral Pathol.* 1980; 49:390-3.

George DI, Gould AR, Behr MM. Intraneural epithelial islands associated with a periapical cyst. *Oral Surg Oral Med Oral Pathol.* 1984; 57:58-62.

ACUTE PERIAPICAL CONDITIONS

PERIAPICAL ABSCESS

Brook I, Friedman EM. Intracranial complications of sinusitis in children: a sequela of periapical abscess. *Ann Otol Rhinol Laryngol.* 1982; 91:41-3.

Brook I, Grimm S, Kielich RB. Bacteriology of acute periapical abscess in children. *J Endod.* 1981; 7:378-80.

Dickens CW. Metronidazole in the treatment of chronic periapical abscess. *N Z Dent J.* 1981; 77:26.

Southard DW, Rooney TP. Effective one-visit therapy for the acute periapical abscess. *J Endod.* 1984; 10:580-3.

OSTEOMYELITIS

Adekeye EO, Cornah J. Osteomyelitis of the jaws: a review of 141 cases. *Br J Oral Maxillofac Surg.* 1985; 23:24-35.

Barak S, Rosenblum I, Czerniak P, Arieli J. Treatment of osteo-radionecrosis combined with pathologic fracture and osteomyelitis of the mandible with electromagnetic stimulation. *Int J Oral Maxillofac Surg.* 1988; 17:253-6.

Bartowski SB, Heczko PB, Lisiewicz J, Dorozynski J and others. Combined treatment with antibiotic, heparin and streptokinase—a new approach to the therapy of bacterial osteomyelitis. *J Craniomaxillofac Surg.* 1994; 22:167-76.

Bernier S, Clermont S, Maranda G, Turcotte JY. Osteomyelitis of the jaws. *J Can Dent Assoc.* 1995; 61:441-2, 445-8.

Bouquot JE, Roberts AM, Person P, Christian J. Neuralgia-inducing cavitational osteonecrosis (NICO): osteomyelitis in 224 jawbone samples from patients with facial neuralgia. *Oral Surg Oral Med Oral Pathol.* 1992; 73:307-19.

Chuong R, Piper MA, Boland TJ. Osteonecrosis of the mandibular condyle: pathophysiology and core decompression. *Oral Surg Oral Med Oral Pathol Oral Radiol Endod.* 1995; 79:539-45.

Davies HT, Carr RJ. Osteomyelitis of the mandible: a complication of routine dental extractions in alcoholics. *Br J Oral Maxillofac Surg.* 1990; 28:185-8.

Elbagoury EF, Fayed NA, Abd el Lattif ZA. Diffuse scherosing osteomyelitis of maxilla and mandible: review of the literature and case report. *Egypt Dent J.* 1988; 34:297-308.

Eversole LR, Stone CE, Strub D. Focal sclerosing osteomyelitis/focal periapical osteopetrosis: radiographic patterns. *Oral Surg Oral Med Oral Pathol.* 1984; 58:456-60.

Felsberg GJ, Gore RL, Schweitzer ME, Jui V. Sclerosing osteomyelitis of Garré (periostitis ossificans). *Oral Surg Oral Med Oral Pathol.* 1990; 70:117-20.

Groot RH, van Merkesteyn JP, van Soest JJ, Bras J. Diffuse sclerosing osteomyelitis (chronic tendoperiostitis) of the mandible: an 11-year follow-up report. *Oral Surg Oral Med Oral Pathol.* 1992; 74:557-60.

Hudson JW. Osteomyelitis of the jaws: a 50-year perspective. *J Oral Maxillofac Surg.* 1993; 51:1294-301.

Jacobsson S. Diffuse sclerosing osteomyelitis of the mandible. *Int J Oral Surg.* 1984; 13:363-85.

Kaneda T, Minami M, Ozawa K, Akimoto Y and others. Magnetic resonance imaging of osteomyelitis in the mandible: comparative study with other radiologic modalities. *Oral Surg Oral Med Oral Pathol Oral Radiol Endod.* 1995; 79:634-40.

Koorbusch GF, Fotos P, Goll KT. Retrospective assessment of osteomyelitis: etiology, demographics, risk factors, and management in 35 cases. *Oral Surg Oral Med Oral Pathol.* 1992; 74:149-54.

Krutchkoff DJ, Runstad L. Unusually aggressive osteomyelitis of the jaws: a report of two cases. *Oral Surg Oral Med Oral Pathol.* 1989; 67:499-507.

Loh FC, Yeo JF. Florid osseous dysplasia in Orientals. *Oral Surg Oral Med Oral Pathol.* 1989; 68:748-53.

Ludlow JB, Brooks SL. Idiopathic focal sclerosing osteomyelitis mimicking retained root tip. *Oral Surg Oral Med Oral Pathol.* 1990; 70:241-2.

Nortje CJ, Wood RE, Grotepass F. Periostitis ossificans versus Garré's osteomyelitis: part II: radiologic analysis of 93 cases in the jaws. *Oral Surg Oral Med Oral Pathol.* 1988; 66:249-60.

Osaki T, Nomura Y, Hirota J, Yoneda K. Infections in elderly patients associated with impacted third molars. *Oral Surg Oral Med Oral Pathol Oral Radiol Endod.* 1995; 79:137-41.

Parrish LC, Kretzschmar DP, Swan RH. Osteomyelitis associated with chronic periodontitis: a report of three cases. *J Periodontol.* 1989; 60:716-22.

Reck SF, Fielding AF, Hess DS. Osteomyelitis of the coronoid process secondary to chronic mandibular third molar pericoronitis. *J Oral Maxillofac Surg.* 1991; 49:89-90.

Rohlin M. Diagnostic vlaue of bone scintigraphy in osteomyelitis of the mandible. *Oral Surg Oral Med Oral Pathol.* 1993; 75:650-7.

Saini T. Multiple sclerotic masses of jaws. *Odontostomatol Trop.* 1991; 14:29-32.

Schneider LC, Mesa ML. Differences between florid osseous dysplasia and chronic diffuse sclerosing osteomyelitis. *Oral Surg Oral Med Oral Pathol.* 1990; 70:308-12.

Shakenovsky BN, Ripamonti U, Lownie JF. Chronic osteomyelitis of the jaws. *Int J Oral Maxillofac Surg.* 1986; 15:352-6.

Shroyer JV, Lew D, Abreo F, Unhold GP. Osteomyelitis of the mandible as a result of sickle cell disease: report and literature review. *Oral Surg Oral Med Oral Pathol.* 1991; 72:25-8.

Suei Y, Tanimoto K, Taguchi A, Wada T and others. Chronic recurrent multifocal osteomyelitis involving the mandible. *Oral Surg Oral Med Oral Pathol.* 1994; 78:156-62.

Tomaselli DL, Feldman RS, Krochtengel AL, Fernandez P. Osteomyelitis associated with chronic periodontitis in a patient with end-stage renal disease: a case report. *Periodontal Clin Investig.* 1993; 15:8-12.

van Merkesteyn JP, Bakker DJ, Van der Waal I, Kusen GJ and others. Hyperbaric oxygen treatment of chronic osteomyelitis of the jaws. *Int J Oral Surg.* 1984; 13:386-95.

van Merkesteyn JP, Groot RH, Bras J, Bakker DJ. Diffuse sclerosing osteomyelitis of the mandible: clinical radiographic and histologic findings in twenty-seven patients. *J Oral Maxillofac Surg.* 1988; 46:825-9.

van Merkesteyn JP, Groot RH, Bras J, McCarroll RS and others. Diffuse sclerosing osteomyelitis of the mandible: a new concept of its etiology. *Oral Surg Oral Med Oral Pathol.* 1990; 70:414-9.

Wannfors K, Hammarstrom L. Periapical lesions of mandibular bone: difficulties in early diagnostics. *Oral Surg Oral Med Oral Pathol.* 1990; 70:483-9.

Wood RE, Nortje CJ, Grotepass F, Schmidt S and others. Periostitis ossificans versus Garré's osteomyelitis: part I: what did Garré really say? *Oral Surg Oral Med Oral Pathol.* 1988; 65:773-7.

Yoshiura K, Hijiya T, Ariji E, Sa'do B and others. Radiographic patterns of osteomyelitis in the mandible: plain film/CT correlation. *Oral Surg Oral Med Oral Pathol.* 1994; 78:116-24.

CELLULITIS

Allan BP, Egbert MA, Myall RW. Orbital abscess of odontogenic origin: case report and review of the literature. *Int J Oral Maxillofac Surg.* 1991; 20:268-70.

Bullock JD, Fleischman JA. The spread of odontogenic infections to the orbit: diagnosis and management. *J Oral Maxillofac Surg.* 1985; 43:749-55.

Giunta JL. Comparison of erysipelas and odontogenic cellulitis. *J Endod.* 1987; 13:291-4.

Gonty AA, Costich ER. Severe facial and cervical infections associated with gas-producing bacteria: report of two cases. *J Oral Surg.* 1981; 39:702-7.

Hanna CB. Cefadroxil in the management of facial cellulitis of odontogenic origin. *Oral Surg Oral Med Oral Pathol.* 1991; 71:496-8.

Heilelman JF, Dirlam JH. Severe cellulitis of dental origin with gas-producing bacteria. *J Indiana Dent Assoc.* 1982; 61:11-3.

Kaban LB, McGill T. Orbital cellulitis of dental origin: differential diagnosis and the use of computed tomography as a diagnostic aid. *J Oral Surg.* 1980; 38:682-5.

Madden GJ, Smith OP. Lingual cellulitis causing upper airway obstruction. *Br J Oral Maxillofac Surg.* 1990; 28:309-10.

Matusow RJ. Acute pulpal-alveolar cellulitis syndrome: V: apical closure of immature teeth by infection control: the importance of an endodontic seal with therapeutic factors: part 2. *Oral Surg Oral Med Oral Pathol.* 1991; 72:96-100.

Matusow RJ. The acute primary endodontic cellulitis syndrome: etiologic, pathogenic, and therapeutic factors. *Compendium.* 1988; 9:682-4, 687-90.

Ochs MW, Dolwick MF. Facial erysipelas: report of a case and review of the literature. *J Oral Maxillofac Surg.* 1991; 49:1116-20.

Ogundiya DA, Keith DA, Mirowski J. Cavernous sinus thrombosis and blindness as complications of an odontogenic infection: report of a case and review of literature. *J Oral Maxillofac Surg.* 1989; 47:1317-21.

Soffin CB, Morse DR, Seltzer S, Lapayowker MS. Thermography and oral inflammatory conditions. *Oral Surg Oral Med Oral Pathol.* 1983; 56:256-62.

Strauss HR, Tilghman DM, Hankins J. Ludwig angina, empyema, pulmonary infiltration, and pericarditis secondary to extraction of a tooth. *J Oral Surg.* 1980; 38:223-9.

Travis RT, Steinle CJ. The effects of odontogenic infection on the complete blood count in children and adolescents. *Pediatr Dent.* 1984; 6:214-9.

Woods R. Diagnosis and antibiotic treatment of alveolar infections in dentistry. *Int Dent J.* 1981; 31:145-51.

CHAPTER

BONE LESIONS

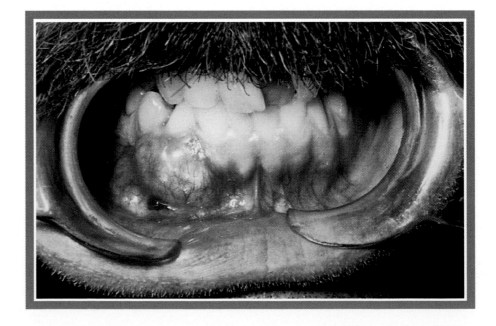

O btaining universal agreement on the classification and terminology of bone lesions of the mandible and maxilla has been difficult. For our purposes the conditions covered have been categorized under four general headings: (1) benign fibro-osseous lesions, (2) metabolic conditions, (3) benign tumors, and (4) malignant tumors. Except for the malignant tumors, this categorization may not be accurate in light of future knowledge because the nature of some of the benign fibro-osseous lesions is not yet known. Moreover, the altered biochemical pathways of many of the metabolic conditions is not completely understood, and not all the lesions designated as benign bone tumors are true neoplasms.

BENIGN FIBRO-OSSEOUS LESIONS

■ BENIGN FIBRO-OSSEOUS LESIONS: a collection of nonneoplastic intraosseous lesions that replace normal bone and consist of a cellular fibrous connective tissue within which nonfunctional osseous structures form.

Lesions that develop within the jaws by replacing normal trabecular bone and marrow with cellular fibrous tissue and randomly oriented mineralized structures have been conveniently included under the general heading of **benign fibro-osseous lesions.** Different names have been applied to the lesions in this group, attesting to the lack of knowledge of their true identity. In the mandible and maxilla, a subgroup of the most common of these lesions is collectively referred to as the **cemento-osseous dysplasias.** They are so named because they all contain a combination of spherical calcifications believed to be of cemental origin ("cementicles") and randomly oriented osseous structures resembling detached fragments of trabecular bone. The two other conditions in this category

TABLE 4-1
Comparison of Benign Fibro-Osseous Lesions of Jaws

	Clinical	Radiographic
PERIAPICAL CEMENTAL DYSPLASIA	Nonexpansile Nonsymptomatic Anterior mandible Middle-age females Vital teeth	Lucent; lucent/opaque; opaque Distinct periodontal membrane Lucent peripheral zone Periapical location only
FLORID CEMENTO-OSSEOUS DYSPLASIA	Nonexpansile Nonsymptomatic One to four jaw quadrants Middle-age African-American females	Mixed lucent/opaque lesions "Cotton ball" appearance Occupies entire jaw
FIBROUS DYSPLASIA	Expansion of cortices One or many bones Usually self-limiting Mild malocclusion	Early—lucent area Late—"ground glass" Lamina dura usually lost Movement of tooth roots
CHERUBISM	Hereditary Distinct facies Bilateral/symmetrical Childhood to late teens Self-limiting Severe malocclusion	Posterior quadrants Early—cystic lucencies Late—"ground glass" Displaced teeth and buds Expanded arches

are **fibrous dysplasia** and **cherubism.** Although the latter two conditions are far less common, they are of greater clinical significance because of their potential to acheive a large size, distort the face, and produce extensive malocclusion (Table 4-1).

CEMENTO-OSSEOUS LESIONS

> ■ CEMENTO-OSSEOUS LESIONS: benign fibro-osseous lesions of the jaws closely associated with the apices of teeth and containing amorphous spherical calcifications thought to resemble an aberrant form of cementum; lesions are usually without signs or symptoms.

Until recently, these lesions were included in the classification of odontogenic tumors of connective tissue origin. They were considered odontogenic because the spherical calcifications that are often prominent in the connective tissue were thought to be an aberrant form of cementum originating from the periodontal membrane (Figure 4-1). Although these lesions occur most commonly in the jaws, lesions with similar histologic features are found in other bones.

Periapical Cemental Dysplasia

> ■ PERIAPICAL CEMENTAL DYSPLASIA: asymptomatic diffuse periapical radiolucent and radiopaque areas, primarily of the anterior mandible, in which cemento-osseous tissue replaces the normal architecture of bone.

The term *periapical cemental dysplasia* (PCD) was first used in the 1971 World Health Organization (WHO) Classification of Odontogenic Tumors, where it was included as one of the four types of cementoma. Before that time, names such as multiple cementoma, periapical fibrous dysplasia, periapical osteofibrosis, and localized fibro-osteoma were applied to the lesion. In the 1992 WHO classification, PCD was removed from the classification of odontogenic tumors and placed among the fibro-osseous bone lesions. PCD is not a true neoplasm but a dysplastic condition in which multiple focal areas of normal bone and mar-

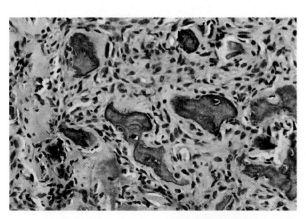
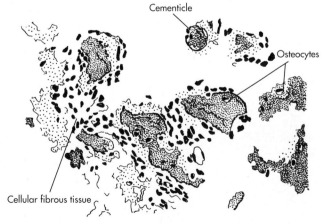

FIGURE 4-1

Cemento-osseous lesion. Microscopic features are common to all cemento-osseous lesions and demonstrate spherical ("cementicle") and irregularly shaped calcifications containing occasional osteocytes ("osseous") in a background of typical cellular loose fibrous connective tissue.

row are replaced by cellular connective tissue lesions with limited growth potential. The lesions attain a fixed size and later undergo a maturation process that culminates in the formation of multiple dense calcified (sclerotic) intraosseous nodules.

CLINICAL

PCD is usually discovered accidently during evaluation of routine radiographs or during an investigation of another problem. No symptoms or visible external alterations of the involved bone occur. Lesions are primarily found in middle-age women, with a higher incidence among African-Americans; it is rarely found in patients under 20 years of age. It is most frequently located below the apices of the mandibular incisors, but can be more widely distributed, occurring within other areas of the arch or the opposing arch. The teeth overlying the lesions remain vital. Buccal or lingual expansion of the cortices is usually absent.

RADIOGRAPHIC

Periapical cemental dysplasia has three radiographic appearances, indicating stages from early formation to maturation.

Osteolytic stage. In this early stage lesions are well-defined radiolucencies at the apex of one or more teeth. The radiolucencies surround the tip of the root and are usually indistinguishable from an inflammatory periapical lesion of pulpal origin (Figure 4-2, *A*). In most cases the teeth are free from caries or restorations but may be coincidentally involved. Thus, before endodontic treatment or extraction is performed, it is necessary to undertake pulpal evaluation of the associated teeth.

Cementoblastic stage. The cementoblastic stage displays similarly sized lesions and a demarcated border with radiolucencies containing nodular radiopaque deposits (Figure 4-2, *B*).

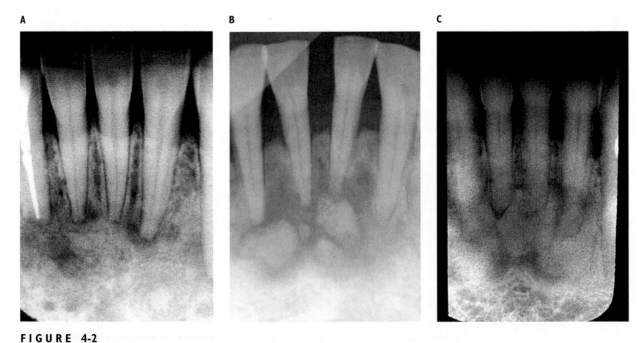

A   **B**   **C**

FIGURE 4-2

Periapical cemental dysplasia. Radiographic features of osteolytic **(A)**, cementoblastic **(B)**, and mature stages **(C)**.

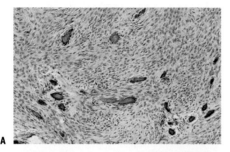

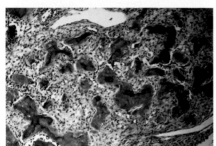

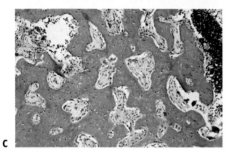

FIGURE 4-3

Periapical cemental dysplasia. Typical microscopic features correspond to the radiographic stages illustrated in Figure 4-2. **A,** Osteolytic—primarily cellular connective tissue with microscopic calcifications usually too small to be detected on radiographs. **B,** Cementoblastic—mixture of spherical and irregularly shaped calcifications large enough to be visible radiographically. **C,** Mature—primarily coalesced calcifications or dense bone with minimum connective tissue.

Mature stage. After lesions have reached this stage, they are well-defined, dense radiopacities that usually exhibit some nodularity. The periodontal membrane can be seen separating the lesion from the tooth. Each radiopaque nodule has a thin radiolucent zone around its periphery that separates it from the surrounding bone and nearby teeth (Figure 4-2, *C*).

HISTOPATHOLOGY

The histologic appearance changes with the stage of maturation. The osteolytic stage consists primarily of cellular connective tissue replacing the normal trabecular bone with calcified structures of insufficient size to be radiographically observed (Figure 4-3, *A*). The cementoblastic stage has the same connective tissue component, but displays a mixture of spherical calcifications and irregularly shaped deposits of osteoid and mineralized bone. These calcified and mineralized structures are surrounded by osteoblasts containing osteocytes (Figure 4-3, *B*). Tissue from the matured stage is composed almost entirely of coalesced spherical calcifications and sclerotic mineralized bone with little connective tissue (Figure 4-3, *C*).

TREATMENT

After a diagnosis of periapical cemental dysplasia is made, no further treatment is necessary.

Florid Cemento-Osseous Dysplasia

> ■ FLORID CEMENTO-OSSEOUS DYSPLASIA: diffuse asymptomatic radiopaque and radiolucent intraosseous areas of cemento-osseous tissue that involve one or both arches.

Florid cemento-osseous dysplasia (FCOD) is a more extensive form of PCD. It may be confined to one quadrant or involve all four quadrants. It has been added to the classification of oral disease, replacing the previous diagnosis of *diffuse sclerosing osteomyelitis* when no evidence of infection or other bone inflammation is present.

CLINICAL

Patients are most commonly middle-age African-American females, although lesions in females of other ethnic groups have occasionally been reported. It is uncommon in males. External signs or symptoms are generally absent with lesions found on routine radiographic evaluation. Patients will experience pain or discomfort if involved areas become secondarily infected as a result of periapical infection or after an extraction. The areas of dense bone have reduced vascularity and are less able to cope with the usual transient infection. On occasion, after patients become edentulous, some of the dense sclerotic bone nodules break through the surface because they do not resorb at the same rate as normally vascularized alveolar bone. These sequestra cause much discomfort and act as a portal of entry for bacteria that can cause an acute osteomyelitis.

RADIOGRAPHIC

The radiographic appearance of FCOD is dramatic, consisting of multiple radiolucent/radiopaque intraosseous lesions. The lesions are diffusely distributed and contain faint nodular radiopacities reminiscent of clouds or cotton balls. Some large, purely radiolucent areas may be interspersed among the radiopacities. Lesions occupy the complete thickness of the bone and are found from the alveolar crest to the inferior border (Figure 4-4, *A*). A solitary lesion is occasionally present, usually in a molar area. Such lesions have recently been designated as *focal cemento-osseous dysplasias* (Figure 4-4, *B*).

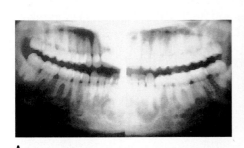
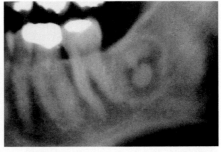

A

B

FIGURE 4-4

A, Florid cemento-osseous dysplasia. Panoramic radiograph demonstrating multiple mixed radiopaque-radiolucent intraosseous lesions throughout the mandible. **B,** Focal cemento-osseous dysplasia. Radiograph of solitary well-demarcated mixed radiopaque-radiolucent lesion in the posterior mandible.

HISTOPATHOLOGY

Tissue from the involved area is composed of cellular connective tissue containing many small and large spherical calcifications and large nodules of dense bone (Figure 4-5). A zone of connective tissue usually separates the lesions from the surrounding bone. Occasionally, areas of traumatic (hemorrhagic) bone cyst can be observed in the connective tissue of the lesions.

TREATMENT

FCOD lesions are not treated unless the dense bone nodules become secondarily infected and produce osteomyelitis in the area. Treatment of the complicating osteomyelitis consists of debridement, drainage, and antibiotics.

FIBROUS DYSPLASIA

■ FIBROUS DYSPLASIA: an asymptomatic regional alteration of bone in which the normal architecture is replaced by fibrous tissue and nonfunctional trabeculae-like osseous structures; lesions may be monostotic or polyostotic, with or without associated endocrine disturbances.

Fibrous dysplasia is a poorly understood benign fibro-osseous lesion that occurs within a single bone (monostotic) or multiple bones (polyostotic), replacing the normal internal trabecular pattern and altering its size and shape. **Fibrous dysplasia** is not a neoplasm because it is self-limiting. It begins as a fibrous replacement of the medullary bone, which in turn is gradually replaced by a metaplastic woven bone that eventually matures into dense lamellar bone. The condition is commonly found in juveniles and young adults, but an adult-onset form is occasionally encountered. **Polyostotic fibrous dysplasia** occurs as part of **McCune-Albright syndrome,** a condition that also includes skin pigmentations and endocrinopathies. When, on rare occasions, the polyostotic form occurs in the absence of endocrine disturbances, it has been termed **Jaffe syndrome** (Box 4-1).

Juvenile Fibrous Dysplasia

In the head and neck area, **monostotic juvenile fibrous dysplasia** is the most common type of regional deformity. It is a slow-growing regional distortion that enlarges proportionately with the affected bone. The regional overgrowth continues until general body growth ceases in the late teens or early twenties. An

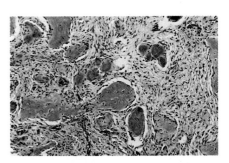

FIGURE 4-5

Florid cemento-osseous dysplasia. Microscopic features consisting of a cellular connective tissue containing spherical and irregular calcified structures similar to other cemento-osseous lesions.

■ **BOX 4-1**
Clinical Forms of Fibrous Dysplasia of Jaw

Monostotic
  Juvenile
  Juvenile, aggressive
  Adult

Polyostotic
  Craniofacial
  McCune-Albright syndrome
  Jaffe syndrome

FIGURE 4-6

Juvenile fibrous dysplasia. A, Facial asymmetry due to expansile lesion of right maxilla. **B,** Diffuse buccal and lingual expansion of right alveolar process exhibiting displacement of first premolar and retained primary molar. (Courtesy Dr. Alan M. Coote and Dr. Douglas W. Stoneman.)

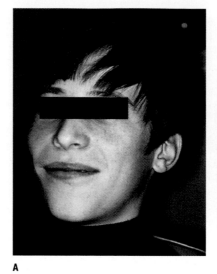
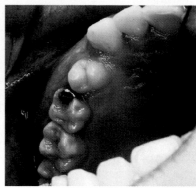

A   B

uncommon form known as *aggressive juvenile fibrous dysplasia* grows at an even faster rate producing major, often grotesque deformity that results in loss of function of the affected bone. Another uncommon form of fibrous dysplasia is *craniofacial fibrous dysplasia*, a component of polyostotic fibrous dysplasia in which lesions occur in the bones of the jaws and cranium.

CLINICAL

Juvenile fibrous dysplasia begins in early to late childhood. Initially it may go unnoticed because the asymmetry may be so mild as to be considered within normal ranges (Figure 4-6). The maxilla is affected more often than the mandible. Eventually the lesion becomes noticeable, although pain or discomfort is absent. Teeth are often displaced, rotated, or malaligned. This results in a severe malocclusion that often requires orthodontic intervention, even though treatment of the bone enlargement is unnecessary. The aggressive form of juvenile fibrous dysplasia becomes symptomatic if the lesion is traumatized and ulcerated because of impingement by the teeth during mastication. In the maxilla the aggressive form often extends to the floor of the orbit and the nasal passages, interfering with both sight and breathing. Treatment to alleviate gross distortion and to restore function is often required in these lesions.

RADIOGRAPHIC

The radiographic appearance varies with the stage of maturity of the lesion. In early lesions the area may be radiolucent, becoming more radiopaque as more bone is formed. A mature lesion retains none of the normal architecture of trabecular bone, having replaced it with abnormal bone that produces a "ground glass" or "orange peel" pattern on radiographs (Figure 4-7). There is no line of demarcation because the lesion blends with the surrounding bone. Expansion of the cortical plates and displacement of tooth roots is common. The lamina dura is usually obscured and the cortical plates thinned.

HISTOPATHOLOGY

The composition of the tissue differs throughout the various stages until maturity is reached. Initially it is composed of cellular connective tissue that has replaced the normal trabeculae and marrow. Gradually irregular islands of metaplastic bone emerge from the fibrous tissue background (Figure 4-8). The new bone has a woven pattern when viewed with polarized light. In the jaws, some

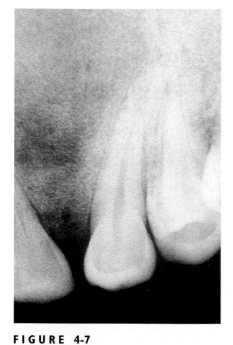

FIGURE 4-7

Juvenile fibrous dysplasia. Radiograph of maxillary alveolar process exhibiting "ground glass" or "orange peel" appearance.

spherical calcifications may be included with the abnormal bone formation. Eventually the bony component predominates the lesion with much of the bone-collagen matrix developing a lamellar pattern. By adulthood, the lesion usually matures and bone may be somewhat normal.

TREATMENT

Treatment is pursued only when lesions are cosmetically unacceptable or interfere with sight, breathing, mastication, or speech. Some clinicians believe that constant surgical osteoplasty of a lesion will accelerate it from an indolent to an aggressive course, resulting in greater distortion than might otherwise occur. It is important to biopsy lesions, because other, more serious diseases may have a similar clinical and radiographic appearance. Most lesions of the normal form of juvenile fibrous dysplasia do not require treatment until the patient has reached early adulthood. At this time the degree of cosmetic improvement that can be accomplished by surgery is assessed. Lesions should not be treated by radiotherapy in an attempt to halt growth, because the risk of a malignancy in later life is greatly enhanced.

Adult Monostotic Fibrous Dysplasia

This rare form of fibrous dysplasia occurs spontaneously in adults. It resembles an ossifying fibroma in many ways but must be separated from it because treatment is very different.

CLINICAL

Adult monostotic lesions resemble those of mature juvenile fibrous dysplasia. The affected area presents as an asymptomatic diffuse expansion of the cortices (Figure 4-9). Some movement of teeth within the area may occur.

RADIOGRAPHIC

The radiographic appearance of adult lesions is usually less homogeneous than juvenile fibrous dysplasia, exhibiting a mixed radiolucent-radiopaque "cotton ball" pattern. As with other forms of the disease, individual lesions blend with the surrounding bone. Expansion and thinning of the cortical plates is usually evident (Figure 4-10).

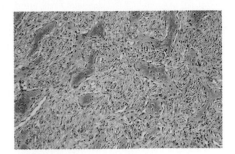

FIGURE 4-8

Juvenile fibrous dysplasia. Microscopic appearance of cellular fibrous connective tissue with irregularly shaped islands of osteoid and bone.

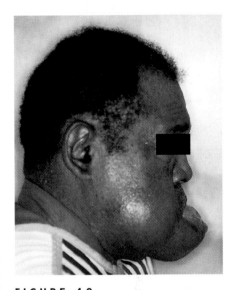

FIGURE 4-9

Adult monostotic fibrous dysplasia. Clinical appearance of an unusually large lesion of the mandible.

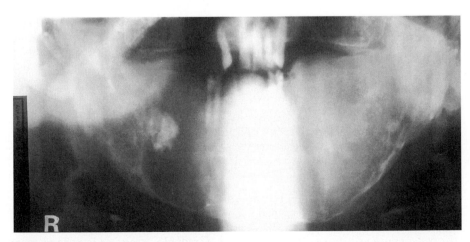

FIGURE 4-10

Adult monostotic fibrous dysplasia. Panoramic radiograph of lesion in Figure 4-9 revealing massive expansion of the mandible and the "ground glass" appearance of the involved bone.

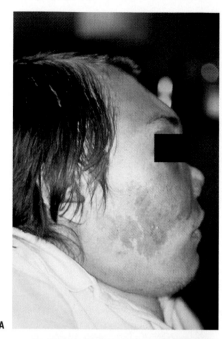

A

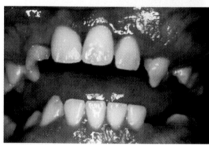

B

FIGURE 4-11

Polyostotic fibrous dysplasia. A, Clinical appearance of patient exhibiting disproportionate bone growth caused by multiple fibrous lesions of the craniofacial bones and café au lait pigmentations. **B,** Expansile lesions of the mandible and maxilla are evident in all quadrants.

HISTOPATHOLOGY

The tissue contains some areas in which cellular fibrous connective tissue predominates, and other areas dominated by immature metaplastic bone with a woven pattern. Of diagnostic importance is the blending of lesional tissue with surrounding normal bone and the cortical plates, a feature that separates it from ossifying fibroma.

TREATMENT

Treatment of adult monostotic fibrous dysplasia differs from the juvenile form because it is not self-limiting. In adults, attempts are made to completely remove smaller lesions and halt the progression of larger ones with continuous conservative treatment.

Polyostotic Fibrous Dysplasia

Polyostotic fibrous dysplasia is usually accompanied by skin pigmentation and endocrine dysfunction. Bone lesions may be confined to the craniofacial area or distributed diffusely throughout the skeleton.

CLINICAL

The presence of expansile lesions in multiple bones (particularly the craniofacial bones) gives the patient an unpleasant appearance. Many patients will also have large light-brown pigmentations termed *café au lait spots* on the torso, particularly the back, buttocks, and sacral areas. The pigmented areas have a jagged periphery, in contrast to pigmented skin areas found in multiple neurofibromatosis, where the periphery is smooth (Figure 4-11). The bones most commonly involved are the ribs, cranium, maxilla, femur, tibia, and humerus. When endocrine dysfunction is present (McCune-Albright syndrome), manifestations often begin in early childhood. The most notable and concerning is precocious sexual development in young women consisting of premature vaginal bleeding, breast development, and emergence of axillary and pubic hair. Other endocrine dysfunctions are related to the pituitary, thyroid, and parathyroid glands. Fortunately, McCune-Albright syndrome is uncommon.

HISTOPATHOLOGY

The microscopic appearance of bone lesions of polyostotic fibrous dysplasia is identical to that of monostotic disease.

TREATMENT

It is impossible to treat all lesions and remove all pigmentations. Surgical management is primarily directed toward alleviating functional disturbances. In mild afflictions cosmetic surgery to improve appearance is sometimes possible.

CHERUBISM

■ CHERUBISM: autosomal dominant fibro-osseous lesion of the jaws involving more than one quadrant that stabilizes after the growth period, usually leaving some facial deformity and malocclusion.

Cherubism is the name applied to a hereditary form of benign fibro-osseous lesions thought to be inherited as an autosomal dominant trait with a great deal of variability in its expressivity. It is found only in the jaws, where it mainly involves the mandible in a bilateral symmetrical manner. The maxilla is less commonly involved. The condition's name is derived from the clinical appearance of many of the young patients, particularly those who have involvement of all four quadrants. When expansile lesions are present in the mandible and maxilla, they give the face a "chubby" appearance and often produce some elevation of the floor of the orbits, causing the pupils to be elevated upward. This angelic appearance is reminiscent of the cherub of Romanesque art.

CLINICAL
Lesions begin in early childhood as slow-growing expansions of the posterior portions of the mandible or maxilla (Figure 4-12). Expansion is asymptomatic and not limited to the buccal and lingual cortical plates. The ramus may be expanded anteriorly and the other arches superiorly and inferiorly. In addition to obvious facial deformity, concern is directed to interference in mastication and speech development, random alignment of teeth, and resultant severe malocclusion. Lesions continue to enlarge until the patient reaches puberty, at which time the lesions stabilize. Eventually, the involved bones may undergo some reduction in size. At this time surgical recontouring can make the disfigurement less noticeable.

RADIOGRAPHIC
The radiographic appearance is striking, especially during the active growth phases. The overall appearance consists of large areas of radiolucency in the bones that exhibit massive expansion (Figure 4-13). Both erupted and unerupted teeth are randomly distributed within the enlarged arches. Faint radiopacities resembling residual or new bone are sometimes present. As the lesion matures, the radiographic appearance gradually changes with more radiopaque structures becoming evident. After stabilization, the involved areas exhibit a "ground glass" radiographic appearance similar to that found in stabilized fibrous dysplasia.

HISTOPATHOLOGY
Tissue findings vary extensively in accordance with the different stages the lesions undergo until stabilization occurs. In the early stages lesions are composed almost entirely of giant cell tissue in which numerous multinucleated giant cells are present in a background of mononuclear cells (Figure 4-14, *A*). During this stage, the tissues are identical to those of a benign giant cell tumor, a much more

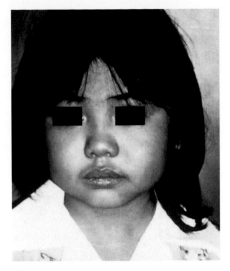

FIGURE 4-12

Cherubism. Facial features resemble a cherub due in part to symmetric bilateral enlargement of the posterior mandible.

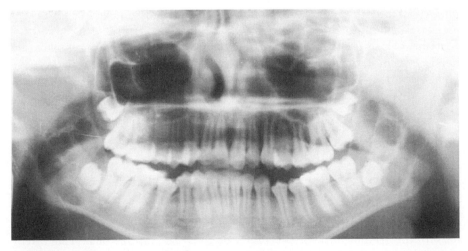

FIGURE 4-13

Cherubism. Panoramic radiograph of patient in Figure 4-12 revealing bilateral expansion of the rami and multilocular intraosseous radiolucencies.

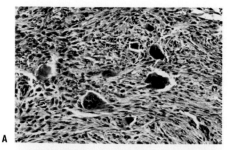

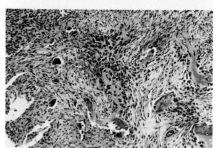

FIGURE 4-14

Cherubism. A, Microscopic appearance of an early-stage lesion containing giant cell tissue with little evidence of fibrous tissue and bone formation. **B,** Mature stage in older patient reveals a reduction in the proportion of giant cell tissue and an increase in fibrous tissue and bone formation.

serious condition that requires immediate surgical management. As individual lesions mature, the giant cell component is gradually replaced by cellular fibrous tissue in which randomly oriented spicules of metaplastic woven bone develop that resemble those found in fibrous dysplasia (Figure 4-14, *B*). After lesions become stabilized, the bone dominates the lesion, becoming lamellar and reoriented for structure and function.

TREATMENT

Treatment is directed toward maintaining speech and mastication. Because the condition is self-limiting, with regression and remodeling taking place after puberty, evaluation and cosmetic surgery are delayed until that time. Care must be exercised that the lesions are not mistaken for multiple giant cell tumors and disfiguring surgery unnecessarily performed.

METABOLIC CONDITIONS

Bones provide structure and strength to the anatomy and determine overall body size. Of equal importance are their roles as reservoirs for essential metabolic minerals and envelopes to house the necessary tissues for blood and immune cell production. To carry out these roles, bone cells and their precursors react to the influences of circulating hormones and other regulating substances. Thus the bones are particularly sensitive to physiologic and genetic derangements that can result in alterations to their structure and mineral content. Four conditions that produce changes in the jaws and other craniofacial bones will be discussed.

PAGET'S DISEASE

■ **PAGET'S DISEASE:** uncoordinated increase in the osteoclastic and osteoblastic activity of the bone cells of older adults producing larger but weaker bones, extensive pain, high levels of serum alkaline phosphatase and urinary hydroxyproline, and an increased tendency to develop malignant bone neoplasms.

Paget's disease (osteitis deformans) is a focal alteration in the histology and morphology of bone. It can be confined to one bone or be distributed in multiple regions throughout the body. It consists of a simultaneous increase in the resorption and apposition mechanisms of bone. Initially the process is dominated by bone resorption, primarily mediated by hyperactivity of osteoclasts. Excessive bone formation follows, with a net increase in volume but a decrease in strength. During a period of exacerbation, both osteoclastic resorption and osteoblastic apposition occur simultaneously on the same side of a section of bone. This uncoordinated function of osteoclastic and osteoblastic activity results in numerous tortuous "cement" or "reversal" lines that give the bone a characteristic *mosaic* pattern when viewed microscopically.

The etiology of Paget's disease is still unknown. In Sir James Paget's original description of the condition, the process was considered inflammatory and given the name *osteitis deformans*. This etiology has now been largely discounted, with a coincident drift away from the use of that name. At present, most of the prominent theories center around factors capable of altering osteoclast behavior. Changes in the osteoclast, in turn, produce secondary effects in other bone cells, their precursors, and the blood vessels. Intranuclear viral inclusion bodies have been found within some of the multiple nuclei of pagetic osteoclasts. Because the inclusion bodies are not present in all nuclei, it has been postulated that they remain in some of the cells' permanent nuclei and not in transient nuclei. The viruslike structures have antibodies against two of the paramyxoviruses—the measles and canine distemper virus—and the respiratory syncytial virus. Inclusion bodies have not been found in other bone or marrow cells. It is postulated that the regional, rather than generalized, distribution of the areas affected by Paget's disease is attributable to a requirement for concomitant local factors.

CLINICAL

Paget's disease is seldom found in patients younger than 40 years of age. Its exact incidence is difficult to assess because most cases are asymptomatic and often detected only during a postmortem examination. The prevalence varies throughout the world, being more common in the Western countries. Even within countries, great variability in regional prevalence is seen. Occasionally families are found that have a much higher incidence than normal for their region, with several members being affected simultaneously.

The disease may be confined to one bone (monostotic) or simultaneous in multiple bones (polyostotic). When multiple bones are involved, most patients develop some degree of incapacity, altered physical appearance, pain, and joint disease. Involvement of the skull is common, resulting in a net increase in head size and shape and in the thickness of the cranial bones. A frequent presenting symptom is a gradual increase in hat size caused by increased cranial circumference. Of more serious concern is the involvement of the base of the skull. In this location encroachment on the various foramina can result in compression of the spinal cord and cranial nerves and lead to paralysis and loss of hearing and sight.

In the jaws the maxilla is more commonly involved than the mandible. The arch may exhibit complete or partial involvement, giving it either a diffuse enlargement or tumorous appearance (Figure 4-15). Because symptoms are absent, the first sign of involvement may be the gradual appearance of regional or generalized spaces between the teeth. In the edentulous patient a denture may become tight and uncomfortable.

Because all elements of bone turnover are heightened in Paget's disease, many bone metabolism markers can be used to make a diagnosis and monitor the disease's progress. The most informative is the assessment of osteoblastic activity as measured by the serum level of **alkaline phosphatase.** Separation of bone-derived alkaline phosphatase from its extraskeletal counterpart is possible but not always necessary in patients with normal liver function and no other disease processes. Normal alkaline phosphatase levels are approximately 63 IU/L, but in Paget's disease they may approach 1000 to 5000 IU/L in patients with a polyostotic distribution and 200 to 500 IU/L when a monostotic lesion is present. In monitoring osteoclastic activity, elevated levels of **urinary hydroxyproline** are indicative of increased resorptive activity. The relationship between these two factors is important in the staging and monitoring of the disease. Although considerable calcium loss from bone occurs, serum calcium usually remains within normal levels.

When bones are seriously affected, they often become painful and subject to fracture. Bones that are close to the skin surface (such as the skull and tibia) will exhibit an elevated surface temperature due to the increase in bone vascularity. Increase in peripheral vascularity, particularly when the vessels are encased within bone, often gives rise to high-output heart failure, a major cause of death in these patients.

The most severe complication of Paget's disease is the increased incidence of sarcoma. Sixty percent of patients over the age of 50 with osteosarcoma have an associated polyostotic form of Paget's disease. The next most common neo-

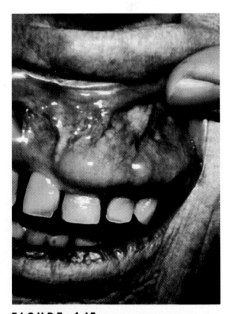

FIGURE 4-15

Paget's disease. Maxillary enlargement with associated separation of teeth. (Courtesy Dr. Gordon Rick.)

FIGURE 4-16

Paget's disease. A, Mandible, maxilla, and part of cranium exhibiting a mottled mixture of radiopaque and radiolucent bone formation ("cotton ball" appearance). **B,** Periapical radiograph of teeth exhibiting hypercementosis and loss of lamina dura.

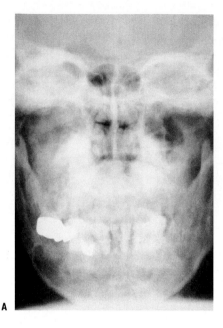

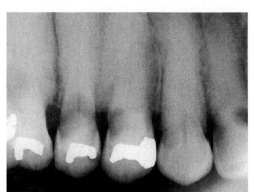

A

B

plasm is fibrosarcoma, found in 20% of cases. Benign and malignant giant cell tumors (either solitary or multiple) are also found.

RADIOGRAPHIC

Radiographic and scintigraphic findings are important in the diagnosis of Paget's disease. Radiographs provide more detailed information regarding the general architecture and extent of damage, regardless of the degree of disease activity at the time the patient was examined. The radiographic appearance of Paget's disease varies extensively. In the early osteolytic stage the bone may exhibit a diffuse radiolucency, but in some late or less active stages a diffuse area of increased bone density is present. The most common radiographic appearance is a combination of radiolucent/radiopaque lesions resembling cotton balls in a diffusely defined radiolucent area (Figure 4-16, *A*). The area is contained within a region of bone that has enlarged and displays thickened but less dense outer cortices. The skull is strikingly involved, with some patients having "cotton ball" cranial cortical plates several centimeters thick. The maxilla and mandible are often greatly enlarged and exhibit loss of the lamina dura. Often teeth in the area exhibit hypercementosis of their roots (Figure 4-16, *B*).

Scintigraphy does not replace radiographs but is useful in surveying the body for incipient lesions and evaluating the degree of cellular activity of all lesions. The scanning agents are isotopes that are taken up by cells are actively metabolizing or undergoing rapid mitotic activity. In some cases "hot spots" are found in areas that are normal on radiographs. Although these areas of increased isotope uptake may represent unrelated activities, they often indicate early lesions of Paget's disease that have not produced enough osteolysis to be radiographically apparent (Figure 4-17).

HISTOPATHOLOGY

The histopathologic features are essentially the same throughout Paget's disease, consisting of an increase in osteoclasts, osteoblasts, and blood vessels and a replacement of the normal dense lamellar bone with a less dense bone having a mosaic pattern (Figure 4-18, *A*). The phases differ only in the degree of osteoclastic bone resorption and osteoblastic apposition taking place at a given time.

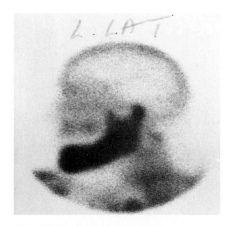

FIGURE 4-17

Paget's disease. Scintigraphy demonstrates notable increases in uptake of isotope ("hot spots") in mandible, vertebrae, and clavicle of patient with active disease.

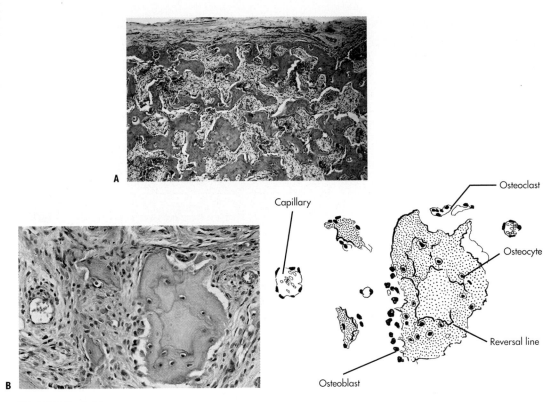

Capillary

Osteoclast

Osteocyte

Reversal line

Osteoblast

FIGURE 4-18

Paget's disease. A, Replacement of normal cortical lamellar bone by a thickened layer of irregular bone fragments surrounded by fibrous tissue with increased numbers of osteoblastic and osteoclastic cells. **B,** High-power photomicrograph of fragment of "pagetoid" bone exhibiting reversal lines caused by multiple alterations of osteoblastic and osteoclastic activity, resulting in a characteristic mosaic pattern.

During the *osteolytic* phase, osteoclasts are numerous and large, containing 50 to
100 nuclei. They are present throughout the bone in deep indentations of resorption, with relatively few osteoblasts laying down new woven bone within the
region. When the disease is in the *osteosclerotic* phase, osteoblasts predominate
and the woven bone matures to dense lamellar bone, with little resorption taking
place. The mixed phase consists of zones in which each end of the spectrum is
present simultaneously. The mosaic pattern is a prominent feature of the residual matured lamellar bone that is found in the mixed and osteosclerotic phases of
the disease, with the lines reflecting the many reversals in bone cell activity (Figure 4-18, *B*).

TREATMENT

Treatment is not routinely administered to patients with Paget's disease because
many are elderly and asymptomatic. Those who become immobilized or have
severe pain, preexisting cardiac failure, renal calculi, or severe neurologic deficits
are considered for treatment. The most effective therapeutic agents are calcitonin and diphosphonates such as disodium etidronate. These compounds inhibit bone resorption through their inhibitory effect on osteoclasts. This provides the bone-forming cells a chance to keep pace with bone resorption and
produce an environment approaching that of normal bone. Treatment does not
stop the process but does slow it considerably and produces stronger, less fragile
bone. Surgery is to be avoided as much as possible. Osteolytic bone is prone to
hemorrhage and the osteosclerotic bone prone to a difficult-to-manage os-

teomyelitis. Surgery is used only to relieve severe pain caused by pressure on nerves and the spinal cord and for open reduction procedures during fracture fixation.

HYPERPARATHYROIDISM

■ HYPERPARATHYROIDISM: loss of bone mineralization (osteoporosis) because of increased PTH secretion (primary) or increased demand for serum calcium (secondary), resulting in multiple systemic complications, loss of alveolar bone architecture, and occasionally giant cell tumor ("brown tumor").

Hyperparathyroidism may be primarily caused by excessive secretion of parathyroid hormone (PTH) or secondarily by kidney disease. In both, resultant hypercalcemia and hypophosphatemia can give rise to associated disturbances in ion metabolism, depletion of bone minerals, kidney stones, gastrointestinal disorders, and muscle weakness. The hypersecretion in **primary hyperparathyroidism** is most commonly due to the presence of one or more adenomas of the parathyroid gland. If the adenomas are discovered early and surgically removed, the patient quickly reverts to normal. However, not all excess parathormone secretion is due to adenomas. In some patients the gland may be reacting secondarily to other alterations in the body, with the increased secretion part of a compensatory mechanism. This form of the disease is termed **secondary hyperparathyroidism.** The most common alteration is renal disease in which chronic loss of circulating phosphate ion is due to damage to the kidneys' distal tubules. The depleted serum phosphate ion causes a constant demand for calcium to maintain the electrolyte balance. Increased amounts of PTH are required to liberate calcium from the bone reservoir through osteolysis. Less commonly, patients may have an idiopathic hyperplasia of all four parathyroid glands. This form of the disease is more common when the condition is familial. Regardless of the cause, the resulting manifestations of hyperparathyroidism are the same in all patients.

CLINICAL

In patients over 60 years of age, some degree of hyperparathyroidism is found in 1:500 females and 1:1000 males. Most patients are asymptomatic, and treatment is unnecessary. They are monitored for kidney stones and for the extent of their osteolysis. Hypercalcemia is the most common manifestation of hyperparathyroidism and is diagnosed when serum calcium is above the normal range of 8.6 to 10.4 mg/100 ml. A lowered serum phosphate level also is helpful in confirming the diagnosis. Levels of urinary phosphate may be elevated. In most cases, the serum alkaline phosphatase and urinary hydroxyproline are not elevated unless the condition is severe. This finding indicates rapid bone turnover with a net loss of bone structure that should be visible on radiographs. Because many causes other than excessive PTH secretion can lead to hypercalcemia, immunoassays for PTH are often performed to confirm the diagnosis.

RADIOGRAPHIC

Bone changes consist of either a subtle generalized reduced bone density (osteoporosis) or mottled areas of radiolucency with thinning of the cortical plates and the medullary bone (osteitis fibrosa cystica). In the mandible and maxilla, the normal trabecular pattern may be lost, and some lack of distinctness of the lamina dura occurs in the late stages of chronic or severe disease (Figure 4-19). Occasionally, a large destructive radiolucency may be present, indicative of a giant cell tumor of hyperthyroidism ("brown tumor"). These lesions are reversible if the condition predisposing the patient to hyperparathyroidism can be corrected.

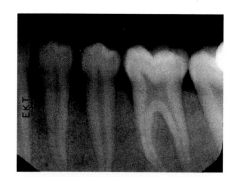

FIGURE 4-19

Hyperparathyroidism. Radiograph of mandibular alveolar process demonstrating generalized lack of bone density, indistinct trabecular pattern, and loss of distinct lamina dura surrounding tooth roots.

HISTOPATHOLOGY

Microscopic findings are generally subtle and nonspecific, consisting of increased osteoclastic activity, thinning of the trabecular bone, and wide zones of osteoid rimmed with activated osteoblasts. Some replacement of marrow with loose cellular connective tissue may occur. On rare occasions destructive lesions that are histologically identical to other forms of giant cell bone lesions may be present.

TREATMENT

The treatment of hyperparathyroidism depends on the cause. Surgery can correct excessive PTH secretions when they are due to hyperplasia or neoplasia of the parathyroid glands. Medical management is usually preferred in milder forms of the disease if the patient is over 50 years old and progressive bone loss has not occurred. Patients who are difficult to manage otherwise may benefit from dietary phosphate supplements. In others, vitamin D supplements have been beneficial. Patients who are being treated medically need to be carefully monitored because mineral and vitamin supplements may trigger other, more severe problems.

OSTEOPETROSIS

■ OSTEOPETROSIS: generalized hereditary condition consisting of excessive bone mineralization, resulting in altered stature, frequent fractures, lack of bone marrow hematopoietic function, and a tendency for severe osteomyelitis of the jaws.

Osteopetrosis is a generalized hereditary condition in which the bones become substantially denser than normal. Many hormonal, metabolic, dietary, or hereditary disorders can produce osteopetrosis. The two most common forms are hereditary, consisting of an autosomal dominant "benign" type that has few symptoms and an autosomal recessive "malignant" type that is fatal in early life. In general the mechanism involves genetic defects that lead to less effective osteoclast function and a resultant reduction in resorption and remodeling even as the osteoblasts continue to deposit more bone. The most serious features are lack of resorption of calcified cartilage during endochondral growth, reduced marrow space for red and white blood cell development, and overly deposited and mineralized bones. The defects result in patients of short stature who are highly susceptible to infection and hemorrhage and who are reluctant to participate in vigorous activities because of the high frequency of bone fracture. The exact location of the gene defect in each hereditary pattern is unknown.

CLINICAL

Patients with severe osteopetrosis have symptoms that begin in infancy with breathing and hearing difficulties due to oversized facial and mastoid bones. These are followed by functional defects in the ocular and trigeminal nerves as they become compressed by sclerosis of the foramina of the base of the skull. Eventually the patients develop an enlarged cranium with prominent frontal bossing. Delayed eruption of teeth is a common oral finding. The long bones are shortened and extremely fragile, and they exhibit replacement of marrow with dense bone. This results in depletion of platelets, leukocytes, and erythrocytes, which produces a tendency for spontaneous hematomas, multiple infections, and anemia. Patients with severe osteopetrosis usually die from complications of marrow depletion before they reach 10 years of age.

In the more benign forms, reduced stature occurs less commonly and nerve deficits are less severe. Teeth erupt but have a tendency for ankylosis. Routine extraction and periapical infection from advanced caries often result in a persis-

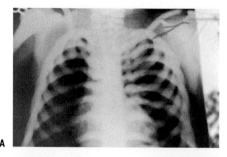

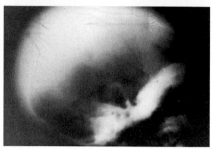

FIGURE 4-20

Osteopetrosis. A, Ribs, humerus, and clavicles exhibit increased bone density. **B,** Increase in bone density of cranial and base-of-skull bones.

tent osteomyelitis caused by dense avascular bone and limited connective tissue unable to initiate an adequate healing response.

RADIOGRAPHIC

The condition is characterized by a generalized increase in bone density with obliteration of normal internal architecture. It is particularly severe in the enchondral areas of long bone. The cartilaginous portion of the ribs also exhibits an uncharacteristic increase in opacity (Figure 4-20, *A*). The cranial plates are thickened, and the base is affected to a greater degree than the other bones (Figure 4-20, *B*). Sinus cavities are greatly reduced in size. Fracture of the long bones is common. Embedded or unerupted teeth are common in the severe forms of the disease (Figure 4-21).

HISTOPATHOLOGY

The bone is dense and sclerotic, with most of the marrow spaces replaced with bone or fibrous tissue. In some forms a normal number of osteoclasts are present but do not display a ruffled border and clear zone that are present in normal functioning cells during resorption. In other forms of the disease the number of osteoclasts is greatly reduced. The bone is somewhat avascular and in some cases islands of calcified cartilage are found that are normally resorbed during development.

TREATMENT

Treatment depends on the form of the condition. Transplantation of allogenic bone marrow has been helpful in relieving some of the hematologic and neurologic problems in some forms of the disease and has helped restore a population of competent osteoclasts. In other forms marrow transplants have been of little use. Oral calcitriol combined with a calcium-deficient diet has provided improvement. Osteomyelitis that occurs in the jaws has been successfully treated with hyperbaric oxygen.

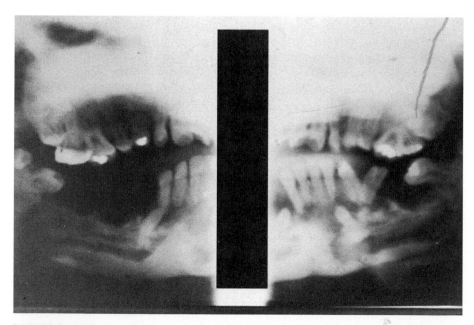

FIGURE 4-21

Osteopetrosis. Panoramic radiograph demonstrating unerupted teeth and areas of increased bone density of the mandible and maxilla.

OSTEOGENESIS IMPERFECTA

■ OSTEOGENESIS IMPERFECTA: a spectrum of diseases of bone due to a basic alteration in the formation of bone connective tissue matrix, resulting in an inability of the matrix to fully mineralize, a tendency for multiple broken bones, blue sclera of the eyes, and associated dentinogenesis imperfecta.

In contrast to osteopetrosis, osteogenesis imperfecta (OI) is a bone disease characterized by defective matrix formation and lack of mineralization. The net result is similar to osteopetrosis in that there is bone fragility, multiple fractures, and hearing defects. Of importance is the close association of OI with dentinogenesis imperfecta. The previous categorizations of OI congenita and OI tarda indicating the age when fractures begin and the disease's severity are no longer used. In 1988 a classification of OI was developed based on specific phenotypes, biochemical data, and hereditary patterns. It classifies OI into four types according to onset and lethality: (1) **neonatal lethal;** (2) **severe nonlethal;** (3) **moderate and deforming;** and (4) **mild nondeforming.** Many patients share clinical features with other hereditary connective tissue diseases such as Ehlers-Danlos syndrome and Marfan syndrome. These conditions are thought to have defective translation of the genes responsible for type I collagen.

CLINICAL
The neonatal lethal form of OI occurs in 10% of cases, with patients suffering multiple fractures during gestation and delivery. Most die within weeks if they survive birth. The severe nonlethal form occurs in 20% of patients; they also have multiple fractures at birth. There is fragility and generalized deformity of all bones, blue sclera of the eyes, and dentinogenesis imperfecta. Patients are confined to a wheelchair. Patients with the moderate and deforming type are less severely affected than the other two, but have a high incidence of blue sclera (Figure 4-22) and dentinogenesis imperfecta. The mild nondeforming type affects 60% of patients. Little evidence of the condition is present at birth, but the ease of bone fractures appears as the child begins to walk. The incidence of fractures declines at puberty. All patients have some degree of blue sclera, but only 25% will have dentinogenesis imperfecta. Some joint laxity is present, and 70% will have hearing impairment.

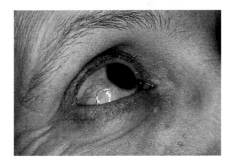

FIGURE 4-22

Osteogenesis imperfecta. Characteristic blue sclera of the moderate, deforming type of the disease.

RADIOGRAPHIC
The radiographs exhibit shortened, deformed extremities with large areas of cystlike radiolucencies. The midshaft areas are narrowed with bulbous metaphyseal-epiphyseal zones. Multiple fractures and healed fractures are apparent. Nearly all forms exhibit some spinal scoliosis. The teeth exhibit the usual changes of dentinogenesis imperfecta with bulbous crowns, obliteration of the pulpal chambers, and shortened roots. Unilocular radiolucencies that occupy both sides of the mandible have been found. They are similar surgically and microscopically to traumatic bone cysts.

HISTOPATHOLOGY
The bones of patients with severe forms of OI have markedly thinned cortices composed of immature woven bone. The trabeculae are short, thin, widely spaced, and disorganized. Bones display an increased number of osteoblasts, osteoclasts, and osteocytes, as well as decreased mineral content.

TREATMENT
At present, no therapy is capable of altering the course of the disease. Correction of deformities and the prevention of additional fractures is usually all that can be attempted.

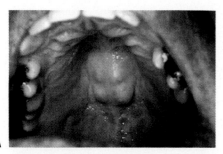

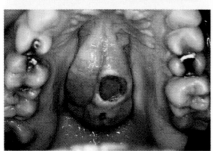

FIGURE 4-23

Torus palatinus. A, Typical presentation as four lobes of dense bone located in the midline of the hard palate. **B,** A common complication of unremoved lesions is chronic ulceration that often leads to focal osteomyelitis.

BENIGN TUMORS

Other than odontogenic tumors, the number of *true* neoplasms arising within the jaws is small. Although some are locally destructive, most of the common tumorous lesions such as tori, exostoses, and peripheral and even most central giant cell lesions are not true neoplasms. Other neoplasms occurring in and around the mandible and maxilla are derived from tissue that gives rise to blood vessels and lymphatics, nerves and lymphocytes, and myelogenous and erythrocyte series of cells and will be discussed in Chapters 9 and 12.

TORUS/EXOSTOSIS/OSTEOMA

■ TORUS: rounded, smooth-surfaced, nonneoplastic growth of nodular dense bone found in the midline of the palate and lingual surfaces of the mandible.

A torus commonly occurs in two specific intraoral locations—on the midline of the hard palate, termed **torus palatinus,** and on the lingual of the mandible in the cuspid/premolar region, termed **torus mandibularis.** Histologically identical lesions occurring on the alveolar bone of the mandible and maxilla in other regions of the gingiva are termed **exostoses.** Similar lesions arising on the periosteal surfaces, but not in the previously mentioned locations, are termed **osteomas.** Whereas tori and exostoses are thought to be reactions to bone stresses, the osteomas are considered benign neoplasms.

CLINICAL

Torus Palatinus

■ TORUS PALATINUS: an exophytic nodular growth of dense cortical bone located in the midline of the hard palate.

Torus palatinus is found on the midpalate of over 20% of adults. It is not present in young patients, developing only after puberty in susceptible individuals. Once begun, lesions usually grow slowly over the patient's entire life. Growths commonly consist of four evenly spaced lobes composed of dense bone with a thin layer of mucosa tightly stretched over the surface (Figure 4-23, *A*). Lesions can grow large, sometimes becoming pedunculated. Larger tori interfere with speech, placement of prosthetic appliances, and oral hygiene maintenance and may develop nonhealing ulcers (Figure 4-23, *B*) that progress to chronic osteomyelitis.

Torus Mandibularis

■ TORUS MANDIBULARIS: an exophytic nodular growth of dense cortical bone located in the cuspid/premolar area of the lingual mandible.

Torus mandibularis is commonly found bilaterally in the cuspid area of the lingual mandible (Figure 4-24). In some racial groups such as northern native peoples it occurs in over 30% of adults. The tori are slow-growing, usually multiple-lobed, and may become very large. Larger growths may interfere with tongue movement, oral hygiene maintenance, and the ability to wear an intraoral prosthesis. They are easily lacerated and slow to heal.

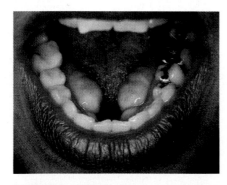

FIGURE 4-24

Torus mandibularis. Unusally large lesions located on the lingual cortical bone in the cuspid/premolar area of the mandible.

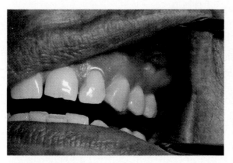

FIGURE 4-25

Exostoses. Lesions commonly occur on the buccal cortical bone in premolar and molar areas.

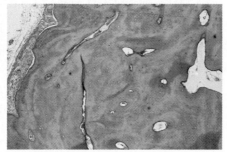

FIGURE 4-26

Exostoses. Photomicrograph of periphery of bone nodule consisting of dense cortical bone exhibiting sclerosis, loss of marrow spaces, and increased periosteal cellularity.

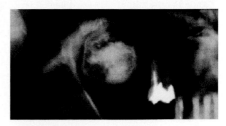

FIGURE 4-27

Osteoma. Solitary lesion of posterior maxilla.

Exostosis

■ EXOSTOSIS: an exophytic nodular growth of dense cortical bone commonly located on maxillary or mandibular buccal alveolar bone, usually in the bicuspid/molar area.

Exostoses are found randomly in adult patients, usually occurring on the attached gingiva over the apices of teeth. They most commonly appear on the buccal plate over the biscupids (Figure 4-25) as multiple rounded or oval nodules of dense bone (Figure 4-26). They are of little consequence to the patient unless they are cosmetically unacceptable or interfere with the placement of a prosthesis.

Osteoma

■ OSTEOMA: an exophytic nodular growth of dense cortical bone on or within the mandible or maxilla in locations other than those occupied by tori or exostoses.

Osteomas are found at nearly any age and may be solitary (Figure 4-27) or multiple. They may be located either superficially or intraosseously on any bone of the cranium or face or within the sinus cavities. When multiple, they are often associated with **Gardner syndrome,** a hereditary condition with an autosomal dominant pattern (Figure 4-28). The syndrome consists of multiple intestinal polyps with malignant potential, unerupted normal and supernumerary teeth, and cysts and fibromas of the skin.

HISTOPATHOLOGY

Each of the lesions is composed of dense cortical bone with a lamellar pattern. The cortical bone is sclerotic and relatively avascular. The medullary bone is denser than normal with reduced marrow spaces. The periosteal layer is often more active in osteoma than in tori or exostoses.

TREATMENT

Lesions are only treated if the patient encounters problems or a prosthetic appliance is necessary. Treatment of tori and exostoses consists of surgically reducing the lesions to the level of the surrounding bone. Surface osteomas are similarly treated but may recur. Removal of intraosseous lesions is only pursued if embedded teeth are to be removed or brought into positions to allow them to fully erupt.

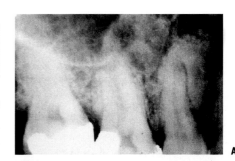

A

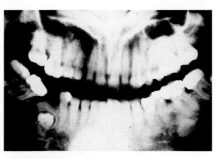

B

FIGURE 4-28

Multiple osteomas of Gardner syndrome. A, Periapical radiograph of intraosseous and superimposed extraosseous osteomas. **B,** Panoramic radiograph of mixed intraosseous and extraosseous osteomas and associated unerupted teeth.

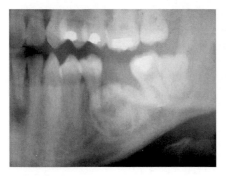

FIGURE 4-29

Osteoblastoma. Panoramic radiograph of a well-demarcated expansile lesion exhibiting faint central radiolucency.

OSTEOID OSTEOMA/OSTEOBLASTOMA

■ OSTEOID OSTEOMA/OSTEOBLASTOMA: benign intraosseous lesions with similar clinical, radiographic, and histopathologic features consisting of well-demarcated, rounded intraosseous swellings, each with an active cellular central nidus surrounded by a wide zone of osteoid, with pain upon palpation.

CLINICAL

Osteoid osteoma and osteoblastoma share many common clinical and histological features with each other and with cementoblastoma. All produce swelling and pain (particularly when pressure is applied), and all occur in young patients. A similar histologic pattern is common to all lesions, consisting of a central nidus of increased vascularity with extremely active osteoblasts and osteoclasts surrounded by cellular bone that contains a wide zone of osteoid. They differ in that osteoid osteoma is small (0.5 to 2 cm), and osteoblastomas and cementoblastomas are large (>2 cm). Cementoblastoma also differs because it surrounds and is in continuity with the root cementum of a molar. The three lesions are considered variations of the same process.

RADIOGRAPHIC

The radiographic features of osteoid osteoma and osteoblastoma are distinctive and pathognomonic. They are rounded, with a well-defined central radiolucency (nidus) surrounded by a zone of increased radiopacity (Figure 4-29).

HISTOPATHOLOGY

All lesions pass through several phases. Initially, a small focus of active osteoblasts is followed by a period in which wide zones of osteoid are deposited. In the matured stage, the osteoid becomes well calcified, creating an atypical form of bone. The center usually remains vascular with increased numbers of plump osteoblasts and large osteoclasts (Figure 4-30). The density and size of the cellular component is often of concern and can be confused as a sign of malignancy.

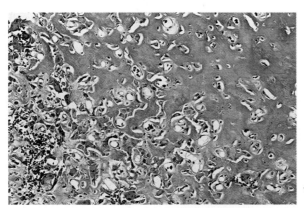
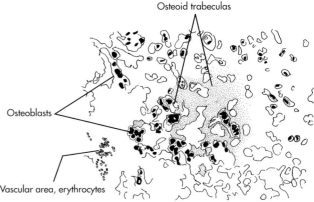

Osteoid trabeculas

Osteoblasts

Vascular area, erythrocytes

FIGURE 4-30

Osteoblastoma. Microscopic features display characteristic wide peripheral zone of cellular osteoid and bone *(right)* and central nidus of vascular connective tissue containing increased numbers of osteoblasts and osteoclasts and reduced bone formation *(left)*.

Treatment

Treatment of osteoid osteoma is directed at removal of the radiolucent nidus or active cellular area of the lesion. In some this has been successfully accomplished with curettage, but others require block resection. Osteoblastoma often requires a large surgical enblock specimen because of the size of the lesion.

CEMENTO-OSSIFYING FIBROMA

> ■ CEMENTO-OSSIFYING FIBROMA: a well-demarcated, encapsulated, expansile intraosseous lesion of the jaws composed of cellular fibrous tissue containing spherical calcifications and irregular, randomly oriented bony structures.

The cemento-ossifying fibroma (COF) is also widely known as **ossifying fibroma,** a term applied to lesions of extragnathic bones that do not contain the spherical calcification commonly found in the jaw lesions. Although jaw and nonjaw lesions may or may not contain the spherical calcifications thought by some to be an aberrant form of cementum ("cementicles"), the incidence is far higher in the mandible and maxilla. In some jaw lesions, the calcifications are exclusively "cementicles" and the lesions are termed **cementifying fibroma.** Studies have shown that the biologic behavior of all histologic variants is identical, causing expansion of the cortical plates, replacement of normal bone with neoplastic cellular fibrous tissue, and formation of spherical calcifications and irregular, randomly oriented bony structures. The histologic features of many COFs closely resemble those of fibrous dysplasia. It is separated from fibrous dysplasia primarily by its clinical and radiographic features and the finding that the neoplastic tissue does not blend with the surrounding bone but is sharply demarcated from it by a thin zone of fibrous tissue. A faster growing and more destructive variant of COF sometimes occurs in patients under age 15 and is termed **juvenile (aggressive) ossifying fibroma.**

Clinical

Cemento-ossifying fibroma is most often located in the mandible posterior to the canines and only occasionally in the maxilla and other locations. It occurs twice as often in females and primarily in the 20- to 30-year age group. The lesion is usually painless and grows slowly, exhibiting marked buccal and lingual bony expansion (Figure 4-31).

Radiographic

The radiographic appearance is of utmost importance in the diagnosis of COF because it is often needed to separate it from other fibro-osseous lesions. The lesions may be either unilocular or multilocular. In the early stages the lesions are small and usually completely radiolucent. As they enlarge, increased amounts of irregularly shaped radiopacities appear within the radiolucent area. In the later more matured stage, the radiopaque structures enlarge and coalesce, often forming a nearly radiopaque lesion with a thin rim of radiolucency separating it from the surrounding normal bone. Root resorption and displacement of teeth are frequent findings (Figure 4-32).

Histopathology

The microscopic findings mirror the radiographic findings. The more radiolucent lesions are composed of cellular fibrous connective tissue, frequently in a whorled pattern. Spherical amorphous calcifications of various sizes ("cementicles") are often present and randomly distributed (Figure 4-33, *A*). Irregularly shaped calcified structures containing osteocytes and a wide zone of osteoid and

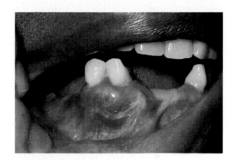

FIGURE 4-31

Cemento-ossifying fibroma. Expansile lesion of right mandible.

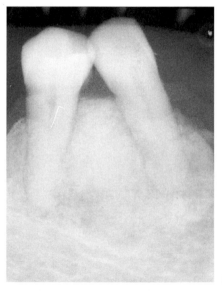

A

B

FIGURE 4-32

Cemento-ossifying fibroma. A, Periapical radiograph of patient in Figure 4-31 exhibiting a unilocular radiopaque lesion with a well-demarcated periphery and displacement of roots of involved teeth. **B,** Panoramic radiograph of large expansile radiopaque lesion of posterior mandible revealing molar impaction, root resorption, and displacement of posterior teeth.

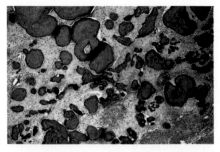

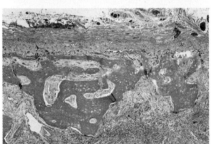

FIGURE 4-33

Cemento-ossifying fibroma. Photomicrographs of characteristic cellular fibrous connective tissue containing coalesced calcified structures **(A)** and periphery showing a well-formed fibrous capsule separating lesional tissue from the surrounding normal tissue *(top)* **(B)**.

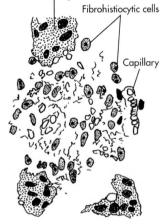

> ■ **BOX 4-2**
> **Lesions of the Jaws Containing**
> **Giant Cell Tissue**
>
> Central giant cell granuloma/tumor
> Peripheral giant cell granuloma
> Cherubism
> Aneurysmal bone cyst
> "Brown tumor" of hyperparathyroidism

osteoblasts are frequently intermingled. A thin outer zone of fibrous connective tissue is usually present, separating the fibro-osseous tissue from the surrounding normal bone (Figure 4-33, *B*).

TREATMENT

Treatment is surgical removal with the extent depending on the size and location of the individual lesion. Lesions have been successfully removed with curettage, local excision, and block resection.

GIANT CELL LESIONS

Many lesions of the mandible and maxilla contain giant cell tissue. They include peripheral giant cell granuloma, central giant cell granuloma/tumor, aneurysmal bone cyst, "brown tumor" of hyperparathyroidism, and early stage cherubism (Box 4-2). In all of these lesions the giant cell tissue has the same histopathologic composition—accumulations of multinucleated giant cells in a background of mononuclear fibrohistiocytic cells, plump fibroblasts, and extravasated red blood cells (Figure 4-34).The histologic features of each of these lesions are markedly similar, although they vary substantially in their clinical behavior. They are designated as separate entities based on a combination of their microscopic features, location, and associated clinical features.

Controversy still exists over whether the central giant cell lesion that occurs in the jaws is a true neoplasm, identical to those that occur in the long bones. Many believe that intraosseous jaw lesions are not as aggressive as their long bone counterparts and prefer the term **central giant cell granuloma.** The majority of investigators now acknowledge that although most are not aggressive, lesions do occasionally occur in the jaws that are identical to the aggressive, high-grade lesions that are sometimes found in the extremities; when this type occurs, the lesion should be referred to as **central giant cell tumor.** The occurrence of a true undisputed neoplastic giant cell lesion of the jaws has been documented in the reported case of a young patient with a malignant central giant cell lesion of the mandible who died with radiographic evidence of pulmonary metastasis.

Peripheral giant cell granuloma, central giant cell granuloma/tumor, and aneurysmal bone cyst will be discussed in this chapter; the other previously mentioned lesions are discussed elsewhere.

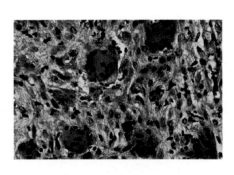

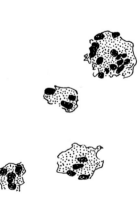

FIGURE 4-34

Giant cell tissue. Photomicrograph of basic histopathologic features of all giant cell lesions—large multinucleated cells surrounded by mononuclear fibrohistiocytic cells, matured fibroblasts, and extravasated red blood cells. Individual lesions will vary in the proportion of each of the components.

Peripheral Giant Cell Granuloma

■ PERIPHERAL GIANT CELL GRANULOMA: most common of the giant cell lesions of the jaws, arising from the periosteum or periodontal membrane as a purplish-red nodule consisting of multinucleated giant cells in a background of mononuclear cells and red blood cells.

CLINICAL

The peripheral giant cell granuloma (PGCG) is the most common giant cell lesion occurring in the jaws, arising from the connective tissue of the periosteum and periodontal membrane. It occurs throughout life, with peaks in the incidence during the mixed dentition years and the 30- to 40-year-old age group. It is more common among females. PGCG most often appears as a sessile focal purplish nodule on the gingiva. Lesions can become large, some attaining 2 cm in size. They are usually exophytic and may encompass one or more teeth (Figure 4-35), spreading through penetration of the periodontal membrane. Occasionally, lesions arise from the periosteum overlying edentulous areas.

RADIOGRAPHIC

There may be little radiographic evidence of some lesions in teeth-bearing areas because lesions may be small and primarily in the soft tissues. Larger lesions exhibit a superficial erosion of the cortical bone and may demonstrate some widening of the adjacent periodontal space. Close examination of the area may reveal small spicules of bone extending vertically into the base of the lesion (Figure 4-36, A). In edentulous areas, the cortical bone exhibits a concave area of resorption beneath the lesion, often referred to as "saucerization" (Figure 4-36, B). Radiographs are important to determine if the lesion is of gingival origin or of central origin with extension to the surface. If the lesion is of central origin, other predisposing conditions must be ruled out before a definitive diagnosis can be made.

HISTOPATHOLOGY

PGCG is composed of nodules of multinucleated giant cells in a background of mononuclear cells and extravasated red blood cells. The nodules are surrounded by bands of fibrous connective tissue stroma containing small sinusoidal spaces, especially in the periphery (Figure 4-37). Osteoid deposits or spicules of new

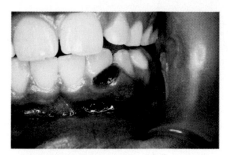

FIGURE 4-35

Peripheral giant cell granuloma. Lesion of mandibular gingiva exhibiting a focal area of ulceration on the upper surface.

A
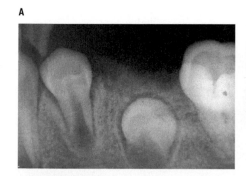
B
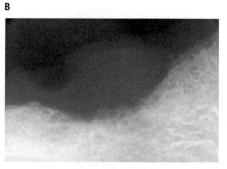

FIGURE 4-36

Peripheral giant cell granuloma. A, Periapical radiograph of mixed dentition area illustrating the lesion's extraosseous nature, lack of involvement of the underlying bone, erupting teeth, and presence of small bone spicules extending into the base of the lesion. **B,** Radiograph of bone beneath a lesion in an edentulous area of a patient who wears a denture, exhibiting the concave area of bone resorption ("saucerization").

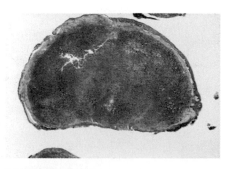

FIGURE 4-37

Peripheral giant cell granuloma. Low-power photomicrograph of trichrome-stained tissue demonstrating the lack of mature collagen *(blue-green)* and the abundance of cells *(red).*

bone are often present in the base of the lesion. Accumulations of hemosiderin are found throughout.

TREATMENT

Most lesions of PGCG respond well to thorough surgical curettage that exposes all bony walls. When the periodontal membrane is involved, the associated teeth may need to be extracted to accomplish complete removal. Occasionally, lesions may recur. This is not an indication for more radical treatment.

Central Giant Cell Lesion

> ■ CENTRAL GIANT CELL LESION: an intraosseous destructive lesion of the anterior mandible and maxilla in which larger lesions expand the cortical plates, cause movement of teeth, and produce root resorption; composed of multinucleated giant cells in a background of mononuclear fibrohistiocytic cells and red blood cells.

The giant cell lesion that occurs centrally within the mandible and maxilla is generally less aggressive and destructive compared to those occurring in the long bones and has been termed **central giant cell granuloma** (CGCG). The more aggressive lesions commonly found in the long bones are rare in the jaws. However, lesions resembling the less destructive granulomatous jaw form of the disease can occasionally be found in the other skeletal bones.

CLINICAL

Central giant cell granuloma/tumor occurs far less commonly than peripheral giant cell granuloma. The majority of lesions are found in patients in the 10- to 30-year-old age group. Lesions occur in the anterior mandible and maxilla (Figure 4-38) with nearly 75% located in the mandible and crossing the midline. Expansion of the buccal and lingual cortical plates is common. Some lesions exhibit cortical perforation and resorption of root apices. In other lesions a much less aggressive behavior is observed.

RADIOGRAPHIC

The radiographic appearance of CGCG is not specific for this condition. It consists of a radiolucency (usually relatively large) with an indistinct line of demar-

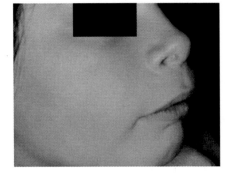

FIGURE 4-38

Central giant cell granuloma. Young patient with large lesion of anterior maxilla producing a midface deformity.

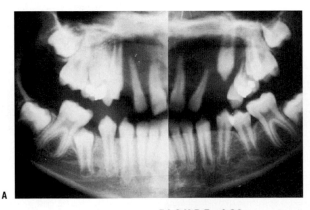
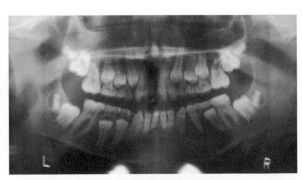

FIGURE 4-39

Central giant cell granuloma. Panoramic radiographs of patient in Figure 4-38 revealing large area of ill-defined radiolucency of anterior maxilla, displacement of teeth, and resorption of root apices **(A)** and more common location of the anterior mandible in which the patient exhibits a lesion extending from the left cupsid to the right first molar **(B)**.

cation with the adjacent normal bone. Buccal and lingual expansion is usually observed on occlusal radiographs, which often exhibit complete cortical bone loss. Movement of associated teeth and resorption of tooth roots is commonly observed (Figure 4-39).

HISTOPATHOLOGY

Tissue from the lesions is composed of giant cells, usually containing 5 to 20 nuclei, against a background of mononuclear cells and fibrous tissue (Figure 4-40). In less aggressive lesions, the giant cells are within distinct nodules separated by wide zones of cellular fibrous tissue. In the more granulomatous lesions, foci of new bone formation are evidenced by osteoid and woven bone. In the more aggressive lesions, the proportion of mononuclear cells and giant cell tissue is greatly increased, mature fibrous tissue is decreased, and foci of bone formation are lacking. Although grading the degree of aggressiveness is possible to a certain extent based on an assessment of the features of the lesion, it is difficult in most cases.

TREATMENT

Most cases of CGCG are successfully treated by curettage. Occasionally, lesions will recur and require one or more retreatments. Recent reviews of reports containing large numbers of patients indicate that the younger the patient, the greater the tendency of recurrence. Block resection is sometimes required due to the size, initial presentation, or anatomic location of the lesion. Radiotherapy is contraindicated.

Aneurysmal Bone Cyst

■ ANEURYSMAL BONE CYST: an uncommon lesion located primarily in the posterior mandible and maxilla with clinical features similar to central giant cell lesion; it contains many large blood-filled spaces separated by connective tissue septa containing giant cell tissue.

The aneurysmal bone cyst (ABC) is uncommon and is considered a variant of CGCG. It differs primarily by containing many large blood-filled spaces separated by bands of fibrous tissue containing giant cells. Blood flows through the spaces at pressure levels too low to produce the bruit sounds that can sometimes be heard in the similar-appearing intraosseous hemangioma. ABC is commonly found in association with other intraosseous lesions, giving credence to the popular hypothesis that ABC is a secondary phenomenon to other events occurring in bone. The most commonly associated conditions are benign and malignant bone tumors, fibrous dysplasia, traumatic bone cyst, and intraosseous hemangioma.

CLINICAL

In the jaws, aneurysmal bone cyst occurs in the first three decades of life, with a peak incidence in patients in the 10- to 19-year-old age group. Most lesions occur in the posterior mandible and often extend into the ramus. The occasional lesion that occurs in the maxilla is also confined to the molar area (Figure 4-41). Lesions are firm, diffuse swellings that produce facial deformity and malocclusion. ABC grows rapidly and may perforate the cortex.

RADIOGRAPHIC

The radiographic features are not distinctive, consisting of an oval or fusiform expansile radiolucency in which the cortex is thinned or eroded. Teeth are often moved and roots resorbed. Lesions are usually unilocular with some exhibiting faint trabeculation.

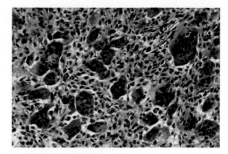

FIGURE 4-40

Central giant cell granuloma. Microscopic features include large multinucleated cells in a fibrohistiocytic background.

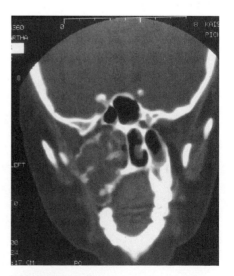

FIGURE 4-41

Aneurysmal bone cyst. Computed tomography of large lesion of posterior right maxilla exhibits extension into the sinus and right nasal passage.

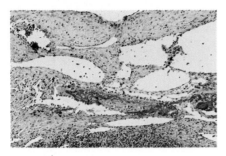

FIGURE 4-42

Aneurysmal bone cyst. Microscopic appearance reveals multiple sinusoidal spaces without an endothelial cell lining, separated by cellular fibrous septa, containing fibrohistiocytic cells and islands of bone formation. Some lesions also will contain foci of multinucleated giant cells.

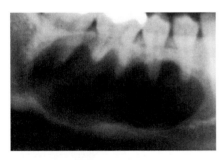

FIGURE 4-43

Traumatic bone cyst. Radiograph of mandible demonstrating a large well-circumscribed radiolucency extending superiorly between the roots of the teeth, producing a characteristic scalloped appearance.

HISTOPATHOLOGY

ABC tissue consists of large blood-filled spaces separated by fibrous septa. The septa are composed of connective tissue containing osteoid deposits, spicules of woven bone, and deposits of hemosiderin (Figure 4-42). Varying numbers of multinucleated giant cells may be observed.

TREATMENT

ABC is usually treated by curettage. Lesions recur in 20% of cases and are retreated in the same manner. Treatment is often coordinated with that of the associated lesion.

TRAUMATIC BONE CYST

■ TRAUMATIC BONE CYST: asymptomatic intraosseous empty cavity of young patients located primarily within the mandible, lined by a thin loose connective tissue membrane and is adequately treated when blood enters the space during an intraosseous biopsy.

The traumatic bone cyst, also termed "simple bone cyst," "hemorrhagic bone cyst," and "idiopathic bone cavity," is an intrabony cavity that spontaneously occurs in the mandible of young patients. Although the etiology of this lesion is unclear, it is commonly thought that it occurs after a traumatic injury in which faulty resolution or lysis of the intramedullary hemorrhage results in the formation of an empty bone cavity.

CLINICAL

The predominant site of occurrence is the molar/premolar region of the mandible. Most lesions occur in patients under 20 years of age. A slight female predilection has been reported. Lesions are asymptomatic and are generally discovered during routine radiographic examination. Surgical exploration of the lesion reveals a cavity that may be empty or contain a small amount of serous or serosanguinous fluid.

RADIOGRAPHIC

Traumatic bone cyst appears as a well-circumscribed, solitary radiolucency of variable size. Larger lesions frequently extend between the roots of the associated teeth to produce a scalloped appearance that is characteristic of this lesion (Figure 4-43). Although buccal or lingual cortical expansion of the mandible is usually absent, it has been reported in some cases.

HISTOPATHOLOGY

Tissue obtained from the wall of the lesion reveals a thin layer of loose and delicate connective tissue overlying a zone of reactive bone that exhibits remodeling. Often the soft tissue luminal surface contains a thin layer of fibrin (Figure 4-44, *A*). In areas where healing is taking place, the connective tissue will contain mineralized deposits of new bone with a distinctive lamellar pattern (Figure 4-44, *B*).

TREATMENT

Surgical hemorrhage induced during diagnostic exploration and curettage of the cavity is usually all that is required to achieve complete resolution of the lesion. Some lesions are compartmentalized by a thin membrane, requiring penetration of the individual spaces and curettage of the walls to induce hemorrhage in all cavities. Caution is required in large lesions to prevent severance of the neu-

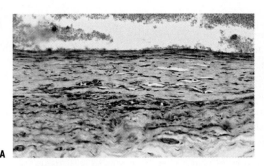
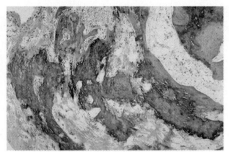

A   B

FIGURE 4-44

Traumatic bone cyst. A, Photomicrograph of active lesion reveals a thinned connective tissue lining surrounding a lumen that contains a thin layer of fibrin on the luminal surface and deposits of hemosiderin. **B,** In areas in which healing has begun, the tissues display a distinctive lamellar pattern of mineralization and new bone formation within the regenerating connective tissue.

rovascular bundles extending from the inferior alveolar nerve to the area's vital teeth. The frequency of this lesion in patients younger than 25 years and its rarity after that time suggest that most lesions resolve spontaneously because not all lesions are found and treated. Surgical exploration is still advised to rule out more serious disease and to facilitate healing.

LANGERHANS CELL HISTIOCYTOSIS

> ■ **LANGERHANS CELL HISTIOCYTOSIS:** a probable neoplastic proliferation of Langerhans type of histiocytic cells with a wide spectrum of biological behavior ranging from a single lesion of the mandible to diffusely distributed bone lesions in combination with organ and other soft tissue lesions; consists of S-100 positive histiocytes containing Birbeck granules and accumulations of eosinophils.

The principal cells of the histiocytic system are the mononuclear phagocyte, the dendritic Langerhans cell, and the lymph node follicular dendritic cell. The cell type most commonly involved in a proliferative disorder is the Langerhans cell, and the disease is designated as Langerhans cell histiocytosis (LCH). It is estimated that LCH occurs at the rate of 0.2 to 0.5 cases per 100,000 children per year. Controversy regarding the etiology and pathogenesis of LCH is reflected in the many and varied names applied to it. Lesions with the same basic histopathologic features were originally considered three separate diseases—Letterer-Siwe disease, Hand-Schüller-Christian disease, and eosinophilic granuloma. The hypothesis that all three conditions were essentially one disease process with multiple clinical manifestations led to a variety of names, the most prevalent being *histiocytosis X* because it acknowledged both the proliferation of histiocytes and the unknown etiological factor ("X"). More recently, terms such as idiopathic histiocytosis, Langerhans cell granuloma, and Langerhans cell disease have been used to indicate that the cause is unknown but the process is most likely a condition of immune cells. The term now used—Langerhans cell histiocytosis—reflects the consensus regarding the basic etiology as published in 1987 by the Histiocyte Society. The studies leading to these conclusions used DNA technology on cells from each of the clinical disease types and determined that the cells were a single clonal proliferation of the CD1a-positive Langerhans cell. The single clonality of the cell type is strong evidence that the disease process is neoplastic rather than a polyclonal immunoreactive process.

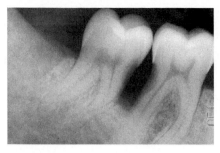

FIGURE 4-45

Langerhans cell histiocytosis. Periapical radiograph of intraosseous lesion of chronic focal form ("eosinophilic granuloma") located in crestal bone between molars.

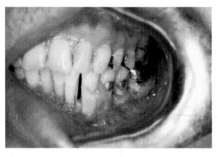

FIGURE 4-46

Langerhans cell histiocytosis. Lesion affecting the crestal bone in localized area presenting clinically as an area of advanced periodontal disease.

CLINICAL

Langerhans cell histiocytosis has a wide clinical spectrum of prognosis and severity of involvement. Depending on the patient's age of onset and distribution of the lesions, it has been clustered into three clinical syndromes, all of which may have the same histopathologic tissue findings. Assessing the degree of cellularity and atypia of the lesional tissue has not shown a reliable indication of prognosis. More accurate information is obtained by a determination of the number of affected bones and organs and other bodily dysfunctions.

Based on the clinical findings, LCH is grouped into three categories for treatment and prognostic purposes: **chronic focal**—usually a solitary lesion in one bone but occasionally in multiple bones, with no soft tissue or organ involvement (previously termed eosinophilic granuloma); **chronic disseminated**—involving multiple bones, organs, lymph nodes, and occasionally skin (previously designated as Hand-Schüller-Christian disease); and **acute disseminated**—involving most organs, lymph nodes, bone marrow, and skin of infants (previously referred to as Letterer-Siwe disease).

RADIOGRAPHIC

In the oral cavity the chronic focal form of LCH ("eosinophilic granuloma") occurs with the greatest frequency. It commonly appears in teenagers and young adults as an area of discomfort in which radiographs reveal a solitary intraosseous punch-out lesion around and beneath the teeth roots (Figure 4-45). The lesions may involve several teeth (Figure 4-46) and appear as focal areas of advanced periodontal disease in which the teeth seem to be "floating in space" because of the lack of surrounding bone (Figure 4-47). In edentulous or non–tooth-bearing areas, the lesion presents as a demarcated radiolucency (Figure 4-48). In other areas the lesion closely resembles a large periapical abscess with teeth erroneously treated endodontically. The discovery of one lesion should be followed by a survey of the rest of the jaws, skull, ribs, vertebrae, and skeletal bones to determine if multiple bones are involved. The chronic dissem-

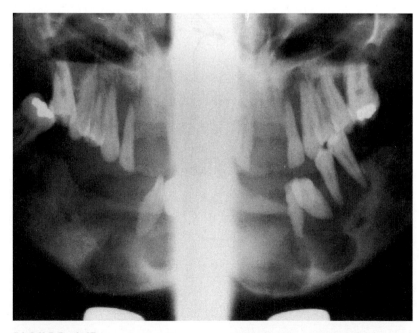

FIGURE 4-47

Langerhans cell histiocytosis. Panoramic radiograph of mandibular involvement in patient with chronic disseminated disease in which the teeth appear to be "floating in space."

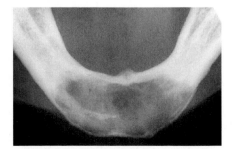

FIGURE 4-48

Langerhans cell histiocytosis. Occlusal radiograph of large lesion of focal chronic form of the disease in anterior mandible of edentulous patient.

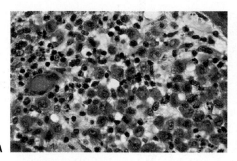
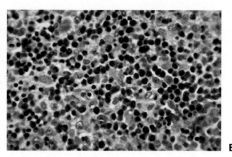

FIGURE 4-49

Langerhans cell histiocytosis. Photomicrographs of large sheets of Langerhans histiocytic cells **(A)** and histiocytic and eosinophilic cells **(B).**

inated form (Hand-Schüller-Christian disease) has bone lesions similar to the chronic focal form and also soft tissue lesions. This form tends to occur most commonly in patients under 10 years of age. The status of the acute disseminated form (Letterer-Siwe disease) is in question, because many believe that cases attributed to this form may represent other disease processes such as acute forms of lymphoma. Patients are usually infants who follow a rapidly fatal course because of extensive involvement of skin and visceral organs by anaplastic cells.

HISTOPATHOLOGY

Except for the acute disseminated form of the disease, the microscopic features of the tissue have a remarkable similarity. The tissue contains sheets of large histiocytic cells with eosinophilic cytoplasm and centrally placed nuclei with occasional multinucleated cells interspersed with other inflammatory cells (Figure 4-49, *A*). Of particular note is the presence of abundant focal concentrations of eosinophils (Figure 4-49, *B*), a histopathologic feature useful in differentiating common periapical and periodontal inflammatory lesions of the jaws from LCH.

The presence of Birbeck granules when viewed with electron microscopy confirms a diagnosis of LCH. These intracytoplasmic structures are unique in mononuclear Langerhans histiocytic cells and appear either as elongated thin rods or tennis-racket–shaped (Figure 4-50). Using immunohistochemistry, the mononuclear histiocytic cells are S-100 and CD1a-positive (Figure 4-51).

TREATMENT

For the focal chronic forms ("eosinophilic granuloma") that are easily accessible to surgical intervention, thorough curettage is the treatment of choice. For more diffusely located inaccessible lesions, chemotherapy with cytotoxic agents is commonly used. Recurrence and the development of new lesions is often problematic, requiring long-term follow-up.

MALIGNANT TUMORS

OSTEOGENIC SARCOMA

■ OSTEOGENIC SARCOMA: most common of the malignant neoplasms derived from bone cells that in the jaws exhibit radiographic widening of periodontal membrane of teeth and histologically exhibit a wide spectrum of findings, all of which contain atypical osteoblasts and abnormal bone or osteoid formation.

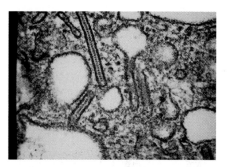

FIGURE 4-50

Langerhans cell histiocytosis. Ultrastructure of Langerhans histiocytes reveals rods and tennis-racket–shaped intracytoplasmic structures.

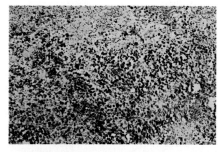

FIGURE 4-51

Langerhans cell histiocytosis. Photomicrograph of positive staining *(brown)* of histiocytes with S-100 immunostain.

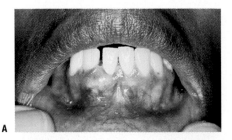

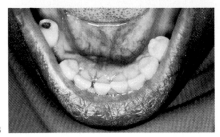

FIGURE 4-52

Osteogenic sarcoma. Lesion of anterior mandible exhibiting buccal **(A)** and lingual swelling and separation of teeth **(B).**

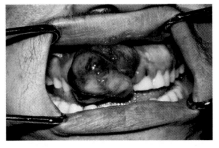

FIGURE 4-53

Juxtacortical osteogenic sarcoma. Exophytic lesion of anterior maxilla.

Osteogenic sarcoma is the most common malignant bone tumor, occurring in 1 of every 100,000 people. Of the malignancies arising in bones, it is second only to multiple myeloma. Osteogenic sarcoma most commonly occurs in the long bones and has a predilection for the distal and proximal areas of the femur, tibia, and humerus. Approximately 7% of osteogenic sarcomas occur in the head and neck area. Many conditions predispose individuals to osteogenic sarcoma. Some lesions may originate through the same gene mutation associated with retinoblastoma because a substantial increase in incidence of osteogenic sarcoma occurs in patients with this condition. Retinoblastoma is caused by gene deletion on chromosome 13 at the 13q14 location. Lesions also commonly develop in bones beneath soft tissue that has received radiation treatments. The incidence of osteogenic sarcoma is substantially increased in older patients with a history of Paget's disease of bone.

CLINICAL

The peak incidence of osteogenic sarcoma of the jaws is 10 years later than the peak in the long bones, having a mean onset age of 33 years rather than 24 years of age. Lesions of the mandible and maxilla are usually first noticed as bony-hard swellings of the buccal and lingual cortices, with or without pain and often associated with separation of teeth (Figure 4-52). In some patients lesions occur as exophytic hard nodules on the attached gingiva, appearing as soft tissue epulides (Figure 4-53). Such lesions are uncommon and have been termed **juxtacortical osteogenic sarcomas.** These lesions were previously separated into parosteal and periosteal variants. This distinction is now considered unnecessary because the lesions seem to be variations of the same entity. Both arise in tissues external to the bone (either in or near the periosteum) rather than from the usual endosteal origin.

RADIOGRAPHIC

The radiographic appearance of osteogenic sarcoma varies considerably depending on the specific histopathologic type. Some lesions, such as the telangiectatic or fibrohistiocytic types, have little bone formation and are radiolucent. Lesions of the well-differentiated osteoblastic and chondroblastic types of osteogenic sarcoma form large amounts of mineralized bonelike tissue, producing large areas of radiopacity within a diffuse nondefined radiolucent background. A characteristic finding in jaw lesions is widening of the periodontal membrane in adjacent teeth (Figure 4-54). Although this finding is not unique to osteogenic

FIGURE 4-54

Osteogenic sarcoma. Periapical radiograph of lesions in Figure 4-52 **(A)** and Figure 4-53 exhibiting mottling of alveolar bone and characteristic widening of the periodontal membrane **(B).**

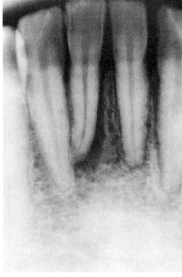

A

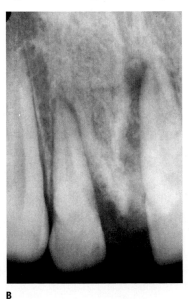

B

sarcoma, it is sufficiently consistent to be of diagnostic value. An occlusal radiograph usually reveals a sunburst pattern of radiopacity radiating from the periosteum (Figure 4-55). Although this pattern is also not exclusive to osteogenic sarcoma, it assists in the diagnosis.

HISTOPATHOLOGY

Four *intraosseous* variants and one *juxtacortical* histologic variant of osteogenic sarcoma have been described. Osteogenic sarcoma lesions must contain normal or abnormal osteoid or bone that is closely associated with the malignant connective tissue cells to distinguish them from other forms of sarcoma. (Figure 4-56).

Intraosseous variants are separated according to the variability in the sarcomatous component and the amount and nature of the hard tissue component (Box 4-3). The *osteoblastic* type is the most common (particularly in the extremities) and contains a relatively equal distribution of the pleomorphic and hyperchromatic sarcomatous cell component and the hypercellular trabecular bone. The *chondroblastic* type contains deposits of hypercellular cartilage and abnormal osteoid and bone. This variant is common in the jaws. *Fibroblastic osteogenic* sarcoma is composed of sarcomatous spindle-shaped cells with little malignant osteoid. On radiographs, these lesions may appear completely radiolucent. *Telangiectatic* lesions have a reduced hard tissue component and a greatly increased number of enlarged blood vessels and giant cells.

Juxtacortical (parosteal) lesions are located above the periosteum and are low-grade osteoblastic lesions containing large separate areas of malignant cartilage. Lesion are usually nodular and may only contact the cortical bone in focal areas.

TREATMENT

Treatment is usually a combination of surgical resection that produces a wide margin of normal bone followed by extensive chemotherapy. The prognosis seems to be better in the mandible than in the rest of the skeleton. Patients with juxtacortical osteogenic sarcoma fare much better in both skeletal and jaw locations.

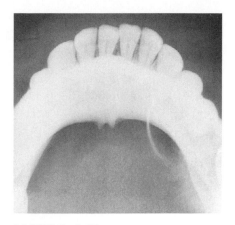

FIGURE 4-55
Osteogenic sarcoma. Occlusal radiograph of lesion in posterior right mandible with commonly observed sunburst pattern of radiopacity.

■ **BOX 4-3**
Histologic Variants of Intraosseous Osteosarcoma

Osteoblastic
Chondroblastic
Fibroblastic
Telangiectatic

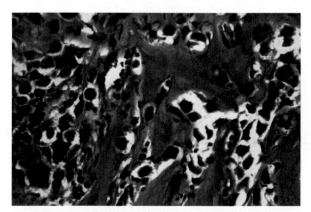

FIGURE 4-56
Osteogenic sarcoma. Photomicrograph of malignant cells surrounding and within abnormal bone.

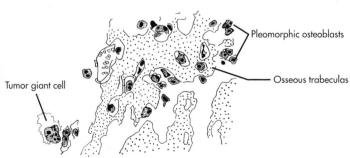

Tumor giant cell

Pleomorphic osteoblasts

Osseous trabeculas

CHONDROSARCOMA

> ■ CHONDROSARCOMA: uncommon malignant bone neoplasm in the jaws, usually of the anterior maxilla, consisting of a proliferation of plump chondroblasts or spindle-shaped mesenchymal cells and abnormal cartilage but no osteoid or bone.

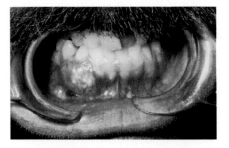

FIGURE 4-57

Chondrosarcoma. Lesion of anterior right mandible with minor movement of teeth.

Chondrosarcomas are malignant bone tumors in which the malignant cells produce abnormal cartilage exclusively, and no osteoid or bone. Lesions may be *primary chondrosarcomas* (arising directly from bone cells as malignant neoplasms) or *secondary chondrosarcomas* (arising in a preexisting benign cartilaginous lesion such as enchondroma or osteochondroma). Lesions have been associated with Paget's disease, Ollier disease (multiple enchondromatosis), and Maffucci syndrome (multiple enchondromatosis, hemangiomas, and fibromas). In the jaws nearly all chondrosarcomas arise de novo without the preexistence of benign chondromas.

CLINICAL

Chondrosarcoma of the jaws occurs at any age but has a peak incidence in patients in the 30- to 40-year-old age group. Nearly all lesions are confined to the anterior maxilla, where preexisting nasal cartilage is present, and the premolar areas of the mandible, the site of the embryonically derived Meckel cartilage.

Lesions are expansile masses that produce distortion of the areas (Figure 4-57). In the larger lesions pain and paresthesia may occur. In the anterior maxilla, nasal obstruction and breathing difficulties are often presenting signs.

RADIOGRAPHIC

The radiographic appearance can be variable depending on the extent of calcification of the cartilaginous component. Commonly, it appears as an expansile "moth-eaten" radiolucent area with indistinct boundaries containing flecks or blotchy radiopacities throughout (Figure 4-58). Widening of the periodontal membrane of associated teeth is a common finding.

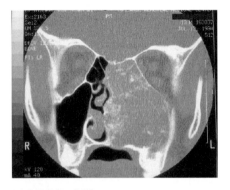

FIGURE 4-58

Chondrosarcoma. Computed tomography of large lesion of left maxilla containing flecks of radiopacities.

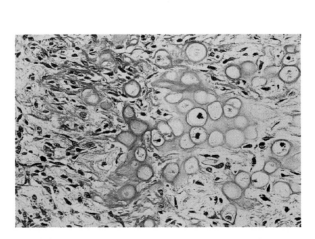

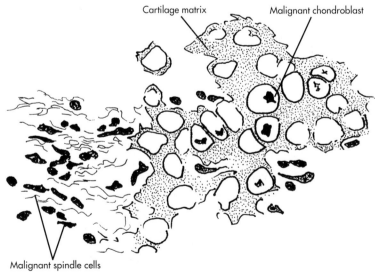

FIGURE 4-59

Chondrosarcoma. Photomicrograph exhibiting malignant cells both within and surrounding deposits of abnormal cartilage.

HISTOPATHOLOGY

A great deal of variability may occur in the histologic features of chondrosarcoma, because they may be well-differentiated and resemble a benign cartilaginous lesion or they may be anaplastic, composed of spindled cells with little evidence of cartilage formation. Most lesions exhibit a combination of abnormal cartilage surrounded by neoplastic cells (Figure 4-59). Lesions are graded I to III depending on the amount and maturity of the cartilage and the proportion and anaplasticity of the connective tissue cells. In grades II and III areas of myxoid tissue and cystic degeneration are present.

TREATMENT

Treatment consists of wide surgical excision. The extent of the surgical margin depends on the size and grade of the lesion. Metastasis is usually to the lungs and other bones. The prognosis for jaw lesions is worse than for lesions occurring in other locations.

EWING SARCOMA

> ■ EWING SARCOMA: rare malignant bone neoplasm of uncertain cell origin in young patients; the lesion is composed of anaplastic small, dark, round cells containing glycogen granules and intermediate filaments.

Ewing sarcoma is a highly malignant bone tumor thought to arise from primitive bone cells. The cell of origin and histogenesis is still unresolved. The lesions consist of densely packed, small, darkly stained round cells without prominent nucleoli or distinct cell borders. It comprises 10% of the malignant bone tumors. It is rarely seen in Chinese, African, and African-American patients. It has been found in family clusters and in patients with birth defects. Ewing sarcoma is most common in the femur and pelvic bones, with only 1% of lesions affecting the jaws. The exact incidence is difficult to determine because lesions closely resemble non–Hodgkin lymphoma and neuroblastoma.

CLINICAL

Ewing sarcoma has a predilection for younger patients, usually children and adolescents, and is rarely seen in patients more than 30 years old. Patients usually have slight to moderate fever, leukocytosis, and increased sedimentation rates. In the area of involvement pain is concurrent with rapid swelling. In the jaws there is usually loosening of teeth and in later stages, focal ulceration. It is present in the craniofacial bones in approximately 4% of cases. The mandible is affected more often than the maxilla, cranial base, and skull.

RADIOGRAPHIC

The involved bone appears "moth-eaten," simulating an osteomyelitis with indistinct margins. The periosteum often has a lamellar layering referred to as an "onion-skin" reaction.

HISTOPATHOLOGY

The histologic features are sufficiently nonspecific that routine light microscopic evaluation is insufficient for diagnosis. It usually requires additional stains, electron microscopy, or immunohistochemical markers. Individual cells may be of two types: small and round with darkly staining nuclei and a visibly delineated cytoplasm; and larger cells with a finely granular nucleus and a faint ill-defined cytoplasm. Both cell types are undifferentiated, small, dark, round cells (Figure 4-60) similar to those present in many other primary or metastatic

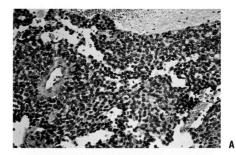

A

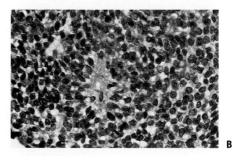

B

FIGURE 4-60

Ewing sarcoma. A, Low-power photomicrograph reveals sheets of small, dark, rounded cells with scant amounts of stromal tissue. **B,** High-power photomicrograph displays malignant cells with rounded nuclei and ill-defined cytoplasm in characteristic cluster arrangement around vascular structure.

undifferentiated neoplasms that occur in bone. Silver nitrate staining reveals septa surrounding lobules of cells. Both PAS stains and ultrastructural studies demonstrate characteristic glycogen granules in neoplastic cells. Immunomarkers are used to rule out other tissues of origin and establish the presence of vimentin-positive intermediate filaments.

TREATMENT
The anaplastic nature of the neoplastic cells makes it sensitive to both chemotherapy and radiotherapy. Surgery is sometimes employed for small lesions in conjunction with the other modalities. Lesions metastasize early to lungs and other bones. Prognosis depends on the extent of metastasis and the effectiveness of chemotherapy. In general, there is a 30% local recurrence rate within 5 years. Lesions of the mandible have the most favorable survival rate of any site in the body.

ADDITIONAL READING

PERIAPICAL CEMENTAL DYSPLASIA

Sedano HO, Kuba R, Gorlin RJ. Autosomal dominant cemental dysplasia. *Oral Surg Oral Med Oral Pathol.* 1982; 54:642-6.

Summerlin DJ, Tomich CE. Focal cemento-osseous dysplasia: a clinicopathologic study of 221 cases. *Oral Surg Oral Med Oral Pathol.* 1994; 78:611-20.

Tanaka H, Yoshimoto A, Toyama Y, Iwase T and others. Periapical cemental dysplasia with multiple lesions. *Int J Oral Maxillofac Surg.* 1987; 16:757-63.

Thakkar NS, Horner K, Sloan P. Familial occurrence of periapical cemental dysplasia. *Virchows Arch A Pathol Anat Histopathol.* 1993; 423:233-6.

Waldron CA. Fibro-osseous lesions of the jaws. *J Oral Maxillofac Surg.* 1993; 51:828-35.

FLORID CEMENTO-OSSEOUS DYSPLASIA

Ariji Y, Ariji E, Higuchi Y, Kubo S and others. Florid cemento-osseous dysplasia: radiographic study with special emphasis on computed tomography. *Oral Surg Oral Med Oral Pathol.* 1994; 78:391-6.

Gingrass DJ, Sadeghi EM, Eslami A. Florid osseous dysplasia: clinical, histopathologic, and therapeutic considerations. *Compendium.* 1986; 71:731-6.

Loh FC, Yeo JF. Florid osseous dysplasia in Orientals. *Oral Surg Oral Med Oral Pathol.* 1989; 68:748-53.

Musella AE, Slater LJ. Familial florid osseous dysplasia: a case report. *J Oral Maxillofac Surg.* 1989; 47:636-40.

Rhodus NL, Kuba R. Hereditary hemorrhagic telangiectasia with florid osseous dysplasia: report of a case with differential diagnostic considerations. *Oral Surg Oral Med Oral Pathol.* 1993; 75:48-53.

Schneider LC, Mesa ML. Differences between florid osseous dysplasia and chronic diffuse sclerosing osteomyelitis. *Oral Surg Oral Med Oral Pathol.* 1990; 70:308-12.

Wolf J, Hietanen J, Sane J. Florid cemento-osseous dysplasia (gigantiform cementoma) in a Caucasian woman. *Br J Oral Maxillofac Surg.* 1989; 27:46-52.

FIBROUS DYSPLASIA

Bohay RN, Daley T. Osteosarcoma and fibrous dysplasia: radiographic features in the differential diagnosis: a case report. *J Can Dent Assoc.* 1993; 59:931-4.

Casselman JW, De Jonge I, Neyt L, De Clercq C, D'Hont G. MRI in craniofacial fibrous dysplasia. *Neuroradiology.* 1993; 35:234-7.

Dal Cin P, Sciot R, Speleman F, Samson I and others. Chromosome aberrations in fibrous dysplasia. *Cancer Genet Cytogenet.* 1994; 77:114-7.

Daly BD, Chow CC, Cockram CS. Unusual manifestations of craniofacial fibrous dysplasia: clinical, endocrinological and computed tomographic features. *Postgrad Med J.* 1994; 70:10-6.

Ferguson BJ. Fibrous dysplasia of the paranasal sinuses. *Am J Otolaryngol.* 1994; 15:227-30.

Greene GS. Polyostotic fibrous dysplasia. *Clin Nucl Med.* 1984; 9:600-2.

Liens D, Delmas PD, Meunier PJ. Long-term effects of intravenous pamidronate in fibrous dysplasia of bone. *Lancet.* 1994; 343:953-4.

Pensler JM, Langman CB. Metabolic changes in osteoclasts isolated from children with fibrous dysplasia. *Cell Biol Int.* 1993; 12:411-4.

Ruggieri P, Sim FH, Bond JR, Unni KK. Malignancies in fibrous dysplasia. *Cancer.* 1994; 73:1411-24.

Shenker A, Weinstein LS, Sweet DE, Spiegel AM. An activating Gs alpha mutation is present in fibrous dysplasia of bone in the McCune-Albright syndrome. *J Clin Endocrinol Metab.* 1994; 79:750-5.

Tanaka Y, Tajima S, Maejima S, Umebayashi M. Craniofacial fibrous dysplasia showing marked involution postoperatively. *Ann Plast Surg.* 1993; 3071-6.

Yano M, Tajima S, Tanaka Y, Imai K and others. Magnetic resonance imaging findings of craniofacial fibrous dysplasia. *Ann Plast Surg.* 1993; 30:371-4.

CHERUBISM

Chomette G, Auriol M, Guilbert F, Vaillant JM. Cherubism: histo-enzymological and ultrastructural study. *Int J Oral Maxillofac Surg.* 1988; 17:219-23.

Dunlap C, Neville B, Vickers RA, O'Neil D and others. The Noonan syndrome/cherubism association. *Oral Surg Oral Med Oral Pathol.* 1989; 67:698-705.

Faircloth WJ, Edwards RC, Farhood VW. Cherubism involving a mother and daughter: case reports and review of the literature. *J Oral Maxillofac Surg.* 1991; 49:535-42.

Friedman E, Eisenbud L. Surgical and pathological considerations in cherubism. *Int J Oral Surg.* 1981; 10:52-7.

Katz JO, Dunlap CL, Ennis RL. Cherubism: report of a case showing regression without treatment. *J Oral Maxillofac Surg.* 1992; 50:301-3.

Kaugars GE, Niamtu J, Svirsky JA. Cherubism: diagnosis, treatment, and comparison with central giant cell granulomas and giant cell tumors. *Oral Surg Oral Med Oral Pathol.* 1992; 73:369-74.

Levine B, Skope L, Parker R. Cherubism in a patient with Noonan syndrome: report of a case. *J Oral Maxillofac Surg.* 1991; 49:1014-8.

Pina-Neto JM, Moreno AF, Silva LR, Velludo MA and others. Cherubism, gingival fibromatosis, epilepsy, and mental deficiency (Ramon syndrome) with juvenile rheumatoid arthritis. *Am J Med Genet.* 1986; 25:433-41.

Zohar Y, Grausbord R, Shabtai F, Talmi Y. Fibrous dysplasia and cherubism as an hereditary familial disease: follow-up of four generations. *J Craniomaxillofac Surg.* 1989; 17:340-344.

PAGET'S DISEASE

Carrillo R, Morales A, Rodriguez-Peralto JL, Lizama J and others. Benign fibro-osseous lesions in Paget's disease of the jaws. *Oral Surg Oral Med Oral Pathol.* 1991; 71:588-92.

Carter LC. Paget's disease: important features for the general practitioner. *Compendium.* 1990; 11:662, 664, 668-9.

Kaplan FS, Horowitz SM, Quinn PD. Dental complications of Paget's disease: the need for hard facts about hard tissues. *Calcif Tissue Int.* 1993; 53:223-4.

Marks JM, Dunkelberger FB. Paget's disease. *J Am Dent Assoc.* 1980; 101:49-52.

Otis LL, Terezhalmy GT, Glass BJ. Paget's disease of bone: etiological theories and report of a case. *J Oral Med.* 1986; 41:214-9, 273.

Penfold CN, Evans BT. Giant cell lesions complicating Paget's disease of bone and their response to calcitonin therapy. *Br J Oral Maxillofac Surg.* 1993; 31:267.

Smith BJ, Eveson JW. Paget's disease of bone with particular reference to dentistry. *J Oral Pathol.* 1981; 10:233-47.

HYPERPARATHYROIDISM

Phelps KR, Bansal M, Twersky J. Jaw enlargement complicating secondary hyperparathyroidism in three hemodialysis patients. *Clin Nephrol.* 1994; 41:173-9.

van Damme PA, Mooren RE. Differentiation of multiple giant cell lesions, Noonan-like syndrome, and (occult) hyperparathyroidism: case report and review of the literature. *Int J Oral Maxillofac Surg.* 1994; 23:32-6.

OSTEOPETROSIS

Ruprecht A, Wagner H, Engel H. Osteopetrosis: report of a case and discussion of the differential diagnosis. *Oral Surg Oral Med Oral Pathol.* 1988; 66:674-9.

Shaff MI, Mathis JM. Osteomyelitis of the mandible: an initial feature in late-onset osteopetrosis. *Arch Otolaryngol.* 1982; 108:120-1.

OSTEOGENESIS IMPERFECTA

Jones AC, Baughman RA. Multiple idiopathic mandibular bone cysts in a patient with osteogenesis imperfecta. *Oral Surg Oral Med Oral Pathol.* 1993; 75:333-7

Lukinmaa PL, Ranta H, Ranta K, Kaitila I and others. Dental findings in osteogenesis imperfecta: II: dysplastic and other developmental defects. *J Craniofac Genet Dev Biol.* 1987; 7:127-35.

TORI/EXOSTOSES/OSTEOMA

Cutilli BJ, Quinn PD. Traumatically induced peripheral osteoma: report of a case. *Oral Surg Oral Med Oral Pathol.* 1992; 73:667-9.

Kaplan I, Calderon S, Buchner A. Peripheral osteoma of the mandible: a study of 10 new cases and analysis of the literature. *J Oral Maxillofac Surg.* 1994; 52:467-70.

Rezai RF, Jackson JT, Salamat K. Torus palatinus, an exostosis of unknown etiology: review of the literature. *Compend Contin Educ Dent.* 1985; 6:149-52, 147.

Richards HE, Strider JW, Short SG, Theisen FC and others. Large peripheral osteoma arising from the genial tubercle area. *Oral Surg Oral Med Oral Pathol.* 1986; 61:268-71.

Schneider LC, Dolinsky HB, Grodjesk JE. Solitary peripheral osteoma of the jaws: report of case and review of literature. *J Oral Surg.* 1980; 38:452-5.

OSTEOID OSTEOMA/OSTEOBLASTOMA

Miller AS, Rambo HM, Bowser MW, Gross M. Benign osteoblastoma of the jaws: report of three cases. *J Oral Surg.* 1980; 38:694-7.

Slootweg PJ. Cementoblastoma and osteoblastoma: a comparison of histologic features. *J Oral Pathol Med.* 1992; 21:385-9.

Smith RA, Hansen LS, Resnick D, Chan W. Comparison of the osteoblastoma in gnathic and extragnathic sites. *Oral Surg Oral Med Oral Pathol.* 1982; 54:285-98.

Storkel S, Wagner W, Makek MS. Psammous desmo-osteoblastoma: ultrastructural and immunohistochemical evidence for an osteogenic histogenesis. *Virchows Arch A Pathol Anat Histopathol.* 1987; 411:561-8.

van der Waal I, Greebe RB, Elias EA. Benign osteoblastoma or osteoid osteoma of the maxilla: report of a case. *Int J Oral Surg.* 1983; 12:355-8.

CEMENTO-OSSIFYING FIBROMA

Kenney JN, Kaugars GE, Abbey LM. Comparison between the peripheral ossifying fibroma and peripheral odontogenic fibroma. *J Oral Maxillofac Surg.* 1989; 47:378-82.

Langdon JD, Rapidis AD, Patel MF. Ossifying fibroma—one disease or six: an analysis of 39 fibro-osseous lesions of the jaws. *Br J Oral Surg.* 1976; 14:1-11.

Slootweg PJ, Panders AK, Koopmans R, Nikkels PG. Juvenile ossifying fibroma: an analysis of 33 cases with emphasis on histopathological aspects. *J Oral Pathol Med.* 1994; 23:385-8.

PERIPHERAL/CENTRAL GIANT CELL GRANULOMA

Auclair PL, Cuenin P, Kratochvil FJ, Slater LJ and others. A clinical and histomorphologic comparison of the central giant cell granuloma and the giant cell tumor. *Oral Surg Oral Med Oral Pathol.* 1988; 66:197-208.

Bonetti F, Pelosi G, Martignoni G, Mombello A and others. Peripheral giant cell granuloma: evidence for osteoclastic differentiation. *Oral Surg Oral Med Oral Pathol.* 1990; 70:471-5.

Burkes EJ, White RP. A peripheral giant-cell granuloma manifestation of primary hyperparathyroidism: report of case. *J Am Dent Assoc.* 1989; 118:62-4.

Cohen MA, Hertzanu Y. Radiologic features, including those seen with computed tomography, of central giant cell granuloma of the jaws. *Oral Surg Oral Med Oral Pathol.* 1988; 65:255-6.1

Dayan D, Buchner A, David R. Myofibroblasts in peripheral giant cell granuloma: light and electron microscopic study. *Int J Oral Maxillofac Surg.* 1989; 18:258-61.

Eisenbud L, Stern M, Rothberg M, Sachs SA. Central giant cell granuloma of the jaws: experiences in the management of thirty-seven cases. *J Oral Maxillofac Surg.* 1988; 46:376-84.

Ficarra G, Sapp JP, Eversole LR. Multiple peripheral odontogenic fibromas, World Health Organization type, and central giant cell granuloma: a case report of an unusual association. *J Oral Maxillofac Surg.* 1993; 51:325-8.

Horner K. Central giant cell granuloma of the jaws: a clinico-radiological study. *Clin Radiol.* 1989; 40:622-6.

Katsikeris N, Kakarantza-Angelopoulou E, Angelopoulos AP. Peripheral giant cell granuloma: clinicopathologic study of 224 new cases and review of 956 reported cases. *Int J Oral Maxillofac Surg.* 1988; 17:94-9.

Kaw YT. Fine needle aspiration cytology of central giant cell granuloma of the jaw. *Acta Cytol.* 1994; 38:475-8.

Lovely FW, Blankstein KC, Lovely GF. Definitive treatment of recurring reparative central giant cell granuloma: a 10-year follow-up. *J Can Dent Assoc.* 1986; 52:323-4.

Slootweg PJ. Comparison of giant cell granuloma of the jaw and non-ossifying fibroma. *J Oral Pathol Med.* 1989; 18:128-32.

Stimson PG, McDaniel RK. Traumatic bone cyst, aneurysmal bone cyst, and central giant cell granuloma—pathogenetically related lesions? *J Endod.* 1989; 15:164-7.

Swanson AE. Conservative treatment of central giant cell granuloma of the mandible: report of a case with a 10-year follow-up. *J Can Dent Assoc.* 1988; 54:523-5.

Tallan EM, Olsen KD, McCaffrey TV, Unni KK and others. Advanced giant cell granuloma: a twenty-year study. *Otolaryngol Head Neck Surg.* 1994; 110:413-8.

Wolfson L, Tal H, Covo S. Peripheral giant cell granuloma during orthodontic treatment. *Am J Orthod Dentofacial Orthop.* 1989; 96:519-23.

ANEURYSMAL BONE CYST

Dahlin DC, McLeod RA. Aneurysmal bone cyst and other non-neoplastic conditions. *Skeletal Radiol.* 1982; 8:243-50.

Eveson JW, Moos KF, MacDonald DG. Aneurysmal bone cyst of the zygomatic arch. *Br J Oral Surg.* 1978; 15:259-64.

Medeiros PJ, Sampaio R, Almeida F, Andrade M. Aneurysmal bone cyst of the maxilla: report of a case. *J Oral Maxillofac Surg.* 1993; 51:184-8.

Motamedi MH, Yazdi E. Aneurysmal bone cyst of the jaws: analysis of 11 cases. *J Oral Maxillofac Surg.* 1994; 52:471-5.

Struthers PJ, Shear M. Aneurysmal bone cyst of the jaws: I: clinicopathological features. *Int J Oral Surg.* 1984; 13:85-91.

Struthers PJ, Shear M. Aneurysmal bone cyst of the jaws: II: Pathogenesis. *Int J Oral Surg.* 1984; 13:92-100.

TRAUMATIC BONE CYST

Chapman PJ, Romaniuk K. Traumatic bone cyst of the mandible: regression follo ing aspiration. *Int J Oral Surg.* 1985; 14:290-4.

Freedman GL, Beigleman MB. The traumatic bone cyst: a new dimension. *Oral Surg Oral Med Oral Pathol.* 1985; 59:616-8.

Kaffe I, Littner MM, Begleiter A, Mintz S and others. Traumatic bone cyst of the maxilla—a rarity? *Clin Prev Dent.* 1983; 5:11-2.

Kaugars GE, Cale AE. Traumatic bone cyst. *Oral Surg Oral Med Oral Pathol.* 1987; 63:318-24.

Precious DS, McFadden LR. Treatment of traumatic bone cyst of mandible by injection of autogeneic blood. *Oral Surg Oral Med Oral Pathol.* 1984; 58:137-40.

Sapp JP, Stark ML. Self-healing traumatic bone cysts. *Oral Surg Oral Med Oral Pathol.* 1990; 69:597-602.

Stimson PG, McDaniel RK. Traumatic bone cyst, aneurysmal bone cyst, and central giant cell granuloma—pathogenetically related lesions? *J Endod.* 1989; 15:164-7.

LANGERHANS CELL HISTIOCYTOSIS

Favara BE. Histiocytosis syndromes: classification, diagnostic features and current concepts. *Leuk Lymphoma.* 1990; 2:141-50.

Favara BE. Langerhans' cell histiocytosis: pathobiology and pathogenesis. *Semin Oncol.* 1991; 18:3-7.

Grois N, Barkovich AJ, Rosenau W, Ablin AR. Central nervous system disease associated with Langerhans' cell histiocytosis. *Am J Pediatr Hematol Oncol.* 1993; 15:245-54.

Hage C, William CL, Favara BE, Isaacson PG. Langerhans' cell histiocytosis (histiocytosis X): immunophenotype and growth fraction. *Hum Pathol.* 1993; 24:840-5.

MacMillan AR, Oliver AJ, Radden BG, Lacy MF. Langerhans cell disease associated with pathological fracture of the mandible. *Aust Dent J.* 1991; 36:451-5.

Schaumburg-Lever G, Rechowicz E, Fehrenbacher B, Moller H and others. Congenital self-healing reticulohistiocytosis—a benign Langerhans cell disease. *J Cutan Pathol.* 1994; 21:59-66.

Thorbecke GJ, Belsito DV, Bienenstock AN, Possick LE and others. The Langerhans cell, as a representative of the accessory cell system, in health and disease. *Immunobiology.* 1984; 168:313-24.

Willman CL, Busque L, Griffith BB, Favara BE and others. Langerhans'-cell histiocytosis (histiocytosis X): a clonal proliferative disease. *N Engl J Med.* 1994; 331:154-60.

OSTEOGENIC SARCOMA

Ajagbe HA, Junaid TA, Daramola JO. Osteogenic sarcoma of the jaw in an African community: report of twenty-one cases. *J Oral Maxillofac Surg.* 1986; 44:104-6.

Bertoni F, Dallera P, Bacchini P, Marchetti C and others. The Istituto Rizzoli-Beretta experience with osteosarcoma of the jaw. *Cancer.* 1991; 68:1555-63.

Bras JM, Donner R, van der Kwast WA, Snow GB and others. Juxtacortical osteogenic sarcoma of the jaws: review of the literature and report of a case. *Oral Surg Oral Med Oral Pathol.* 1980; 50:535-44.

Chan CW, Kung TM, Ma L. Telangiectatic osteosarcoma of the mandible. *Cancer.* 1986; 58:2110-5.

Clark JL, Unni KK, Dahlin DC, Devine KD. Osteosarcoma of the jaw. *Cancer.* 1983; 51:2311-6.

Dahlin DC. Osteosarcoma of bone and a consideration of prognostic variables. *Cancer Treat Res.* 1978; 62:189-92.

Dahlin DC. Pathology of osteosarcoma. *Clin Orthop.* 1975; 111:23-32.

Dahlin DC. The problems in assessment of new treatment regimens of osteosarcoma. *Clin Orthop.* 1980; 81:5.

deFries HO, Kornblut AD. Malignant disease of the osseous adnexae: osteogenic sarcoma of the jaws. *Otolaryngol Clin North Am.* 1979; 12:129-34.

Delgado R, Maafs E, Alfeiran A, Mohar A and others. Osteosarcoma of the jaw. *Head Neck,* 1994; 16:246-52.

Grodjesk JE, Dolinsky HB, Schneider LC, Doyle JL. Osteosarcoma of the jaw: report of a case. *J NJ Dent Assoc.* 1979; 50:41-2.

Ivins JC, Ritts RE, Pritchard DJ, Gilchrist GS and others. Transfer factor versus combination chemotherapy: a preliminary report of a randomized postsurgical adjuvant treatment study in osteogenic sarcoma. *Ann N Y Acad Sci.* 1976; 277:558-74.

Maldonado AR, Spratt JS. Osteogenic sarcoma of the mandible and maxilla. *South Med J.* 1986; 79:1453-5.

Millar BG, Browne RM, Flood TR. Juxtacortical osteosarcoma of the jaws. *Br J Oral Maxillofac Surg.* 1990; 28:73-9.

Schulz A, Baerker R, Delling G. Ultrastructural study of tumor cell differentiation in osteosarcoma of jaw bones. *J Oral Pathol.* 1978; 7:69-84.

Slootweg PJ, Muller H. Osteosarcoma of the jaw bones: analysis of 18 cases. *J Maxillofac Surg.* 1985; 13:158-66.

Tanzawa H, Uchiyama S, Sato K. Statistical observation of osteosarcoma of the maxillofacial region in Japan: analysis of 114 Japanese cases reported between 1930 and 1989. *Oral Surg Oral Med Oral Pathol.* 1991; 72:444-8.

Vener J, Rice DH, Newman AN. Osteosarcoma and chondrosarcoma of the head and neck. *Laryngoscope.* 1984; 94:240-2.

CHONDROSARCOMA

Ajagbe HA, Daramola JO, Junaid TA. Chondrosarcoma of the jaw: review of fourteen cases. *J Oral Maxillofac Surg.* 1985; 43:763-6.

Anwar R, Ruddy J, Ghosh S, Lavery KM and others. Chondrosarcoma of the maxilla. *J Laryngol Otol.* 1992; 106:53-5.

Christensen RE. Mesenchymal chondrosarcoma of the jaws. *Oral Surg Oral Med Oral Pathol.* 1982; 54:197-206.

Garrington GE, Collett WK. Chondrosarcoma: II: chondrosarcoma of the jaws: analysis of 37 cases. *J Oral Pathol.* 1988; 17:12-20.

Hackney FL, Aragon SB, Aufdemorte TB, Holt GR and others. Chondrosarcoma of the jaws: clinical findings, histopathology, and treatment. *Oral Surg Oral Med Oral Pathol.* 1991; 71:139-43.

Sato K, Nukaga H, Horikoshi T. Chondrosarcoma of the jaws and facial skeleton: a review of the Japanese literature. *J Oral Surg.* 1977; 35:892-7.

Takahashi K, Sato K, Kanazawa H, Wang XL and others. Mesenchymal chondrosarcoma of the jaw: report of a case and review of 41 cases in the literature. *Head Neck.* 1993; 15:459-64.

EWING SARCOMA

Arafat A, Ellis GL, Adrian JC. Ewing's sarcoma of the jaws. *Oral Surg Oral Med Oral Pathol.* 1983; 55:589-96.

Bacchini P, Marchetti C, Mancini L, Present D and others. Ewing's sarcoma of the mandible and maxilla: a report of three cases from the Istituto Beretta. *Oral Surg Oral Med Oral Pathol.* 1986; 61:278-83.

Baker CG, Tishler JM. Malignant disease in the jaws. *J Can Assoc Radiol.* 1977; 28:129-41.

Gupta SC. Ewing's sarcoma of the upper jaw. *Ear Nose Throat J.* 1987; 66:176-7.

Khanna S, Khanna NN, Gupta OP, Tripathi FM and others. Primary tumours and tumour-like conditions of the mandible. *J Surg Oncol.* 1981; 6:365-70.

Khanna S, Khanna NN, Varanasi MS. Primary tumors of the jaws in children. *J Oral Surg.* 1979; 37:800-4.

Lam KH, Wong J, Lim ST, Ong GB. Primary sarcomas of the jaw. *Aust N Z J Surg.* 1979; 49:668-75.

Wood RE, Nortje CJ, Hesseling P, Grotepass F. Ewing's tumor of the jaw. *Oral Surg Oral Med Oral Pathol.* 1990; 69:120-7.

ODONTOGENIC TUMORS

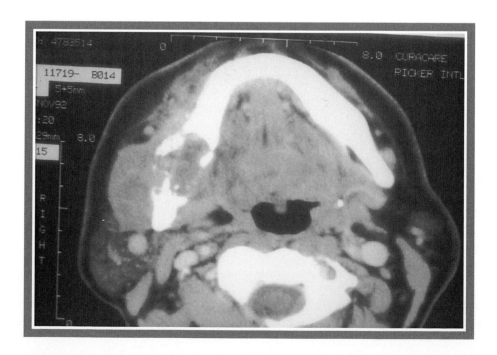

O dontogenic tumors are unique to the jaws and originate from tissue associated with tooth development. The abnormal tissue in each of these tumors can often be correlated with similar tissue in normal odontogenesis from inception to tooth eruption. The following brief review of odontogenesis will aid the understanding of these tumors.

REVIEW OF ODONTOGENESIS

Tooth formation originates during embryogenesis, arising from the oral epithelium covering the maxillary and mandibular alveolar processes. It begins as a "budding" of the basal cell layer over each specific location where teeth will occur. The epithelial bud elongates in the form of a solid tubelike structure that penetrates the connective tissue, a process known as *invagination* (Figure 5-1, *A*). The elongated epithelial structure is referred to as the *dental lamina* and is the dentition's source of all future activity and differentiation relative to development. When the appropriate depth is reached, the basal cell layer at the tip of the dental lamina thickens, forming a concavity. This structure represents the *cap stage* of tooth development (Figure 5-1, *B*). As odontogenesis proceeds, the cap-shaped structure enlarges and the bottom layer of epithelium (*inner enamel epithelium*) separates from the top layer (*outer enamel epithelium*). The intervening zone is composed of loosely arranged star-shaped epithelial cells (*stellate reticulum*). There is a concurrent elongation of the periphery of the epithelial structure, shaping the future crown of the tooth specific for that location. This stage is referred to as the *early bell stage* (Figure 5-1, *C*). This specialized epithelium induces the adjacent connective tissue to be modified into a circumscribed zone of embryonic and myxomatous connective tissue that may be further inducted to form dentin or pulp tissue. The altered connective tissue around which the future tooth root will form is termed the *dental papilla*. Induction of the connective tissue surrounding the whole embryonic tooth structure also occurs at this stage of odontogenesis. This outer zone of connective tissue that encapsulates the developing tooth bud is dense and fibrous and is referred to as the *dental follicle*. The dental follicle remains around the tooth until it erupts; the

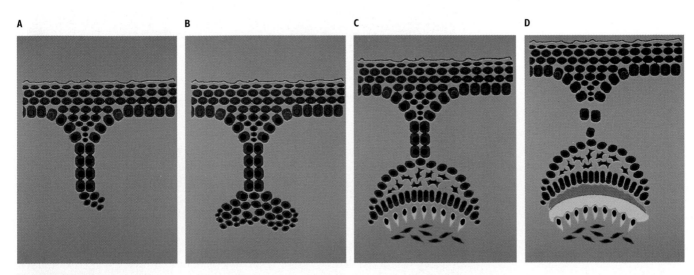

A   B   C   D

FIGURE 5-1

Diagram of early stages of odontogenesis. **A,** Invagination. **B,** Cap stage. **C,** Early bell stage. **D,** Late bell stage.

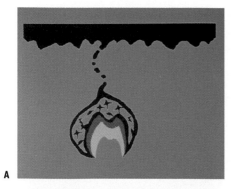

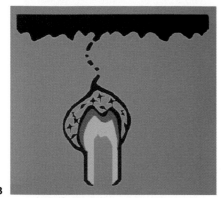

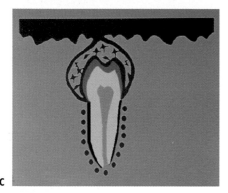

FIGURE 5-2

Diagram of later stages of odontogenesis. **A,** Crown formation and remnants of dental lamina. **B,** Root formation. **C,** Preeruption completed tooth formation and rests of Malassez *(red dots).*

crown portion of the follicle becomes part of the connective tissue of the free marginal gingiva, and the root portion becomes the periodontal ligament that separates the bone from the cememtum.

During the *late bell stage* (Figure 5-1, *D*) the cells of the inner enamel epithelium become elongated and palisaded. Concurrent migration of the nucleus away from the basement membrane occurs, a process referred to as *reverse polarization.* This event indicates the cells' change to presecretory ameloblasts. Reverse polarization induces the undifferentiated cells in the adjacent dental papilla to differentiate into presecretory odontoblasts that align in a palisaded manner against the basement membrane opposite the presecretory ameloblasts. As the ameloblasts mature, the odontoblasts are stimulated to secrete dentin matrix which in turn initiates the deposition of enamel matrix on the opposite side of the basement membrane. During this stage of odontogenesis, the dental lamina begins to break up and forms small islands in the connective tissue. These islands of residual epithelium are inactive and referred to as *rests of the dental lamina* or *rests of Serres.*

After the specific shape of a tooth crown has been completed (Figure 5-2, *A*), the epithelium that forms the outer rim of the bell-shaped enamel organ elongates, forming the shape and length of the roots (Figure 5-2, *B*). This epithelium forms a thin transient membrane referred to as *Hertwig root sheath.* In this location odontoblasts form to produce the dentin necessary to form the tooth root. When the root is nearly complete, the continuity of the epithelial root sheath begins to break down, first becoming porous and eventually becoming completely fragmented. This allows the connective tissue cells from the dental follicle adjacent to the root to come in contact with the newly formed dentin. The dentin stimulates these cells to differentiate into *cementoblasts.* Cementoblasts are responsible for generating the calcified layer over the dentin, referred to as *cementum.* Cementum serves to anchor the collagen fibers of the dental follicle and periodontal ligament to the tooth root and to seal the outer side of the dentinal tubule. The epithelial remnants of Hertwig root sheath remain in the periodontal ligament after tooth formation is complete and are referred to as *rests of Malassez* (Figure 5-2, *C*).

EPITHELIAL ODONTOGENIC TUMORS

AMELOBLASTOMA

> ■ AMELOBLASTOMA: a locally aggressive neoplasm of odontogenic epithelium that has a wide spectrum of histologic patterns resembling early odontogenesis.

Ameloblastoma is a benign neoplasm derived from residual epithelial components of tooth development. Its growth pattern recapitulates many of the embryonic structures and tissue that occur before hard tissue formation. An ameloblastoma can arise from any of the multiple sources of odontogenic epithelium that remain within the alveolar soft tissue and bone. These include (1) remnants of the dental lamina (rests of Serres), (2) reduced enamel epithelium, (3) rests of Malassez, and (4) the basal cell layer of overlying surface epithelium (Figure 5-3). For many years ameloblastoma had been regarded as a single, distinct clinical entity with a broad spectrum of histologic features. The tumor is slow growing, locally aggressive, and capable of causing large facial deformities. Ameloblastomas have a high recurrence rate if they are not widely and carefully excised. Metastasis is rare. Over the last 60 to 70 years nearly all metastases have occurred in patients who have had multiple or extensive surgical treatments of their lesions.

In recent years experience has shown that not all lesions with histologic features of ameloblastoma have the same potential for destruction, recurrence, and even metastasis. As additional information is compiled, it appears that for *management* purposes, not all ameloblastomas require the same surgical treatment, but a correlation of the clinical, radiographic, and histologic features of each individually encountered lesion is required to determine the clinical subtype. Although not all lesions fall neatly into the different clinical categories, many do; for these lesions, treatment can be modified to prevent unnecessarily extensive surgery. Three clinical subtypes of ameloblastomas are generally recognized for treatment purposes: (1) the **common (polycystic) ameloblastoma**, (2) the **unicystic ameloblastoma**, and (3) the rarely encountered **peripheral (extraosseous) ameloblastoma** (Figure 5-4).

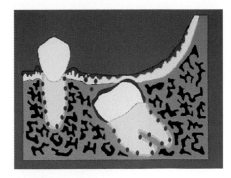

FIGURE 5-3

Diagram of possible epithelial sources of ameloblastoma *(represented by red color):* remnants of the dental lamina *(dots above crown of molar);* reduced enamel epithelium *(on surface of molar crown);* rests of Malassez *(dots in periodontal membrane);* surface epithelium.

A
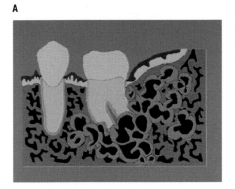

B
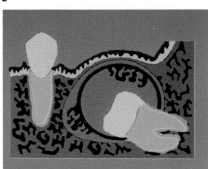

C
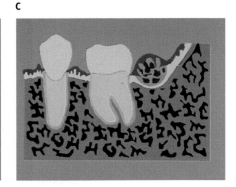

FIGURE 5-4

Ameloblastoma. Diagram of three clinical subtypes. **A,** Common (polycystic). **B,** Unicystic. **C,** Peripheral (extraosseous).

Common Ameloblastoma

The **common ameloblastoma**, sometimes referred to as *simple* or *follicular* ameloblastoma, is the most prevalent form of this lesion, and nearly all occur in patients over 25 years of age. Most common ameloblastomas originate de novo, but some may evolve from the other two clinical subtypes that have remained untreated for a prolonged period.

CLINICAL

The common form of ameloblastoma may produce extensive, even grotesque, deformities of the mandible and maxilla (Figure 5-5). It is most commonly located in the mandible, with 75% occurring in the molar and ascending ramus areas. Lesions of the maxilla are concentrated in the molar area where they often extend into the maxillary sinus and floor of the nose. The majority occur in patients between 20 to 40 years of age, although they can occur at any age. There is no significant sex or race predilection. A feature of this form of ameloblastoma is the tendency to expand the bony cortices because their slow growth allows time for the periosteum to produce a thin shell of bone ahead of the expanding lesion. This thinned outer shell of bone cracks easily when palpated—a diagnostic sign referred to as "eggshell cracking."

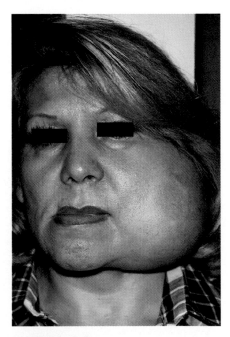

FIGURE 5-5

Ameloblastoma. Patient with large lesion of left posterior mandible.

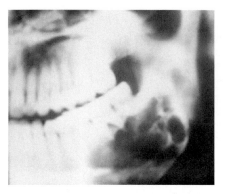

FIGURE 5-6
Ameloblastoma. Radiograph exhibiting multilocular ("soap bubble") appearance.

RADIOGRAPHIC

Multiloculation characterizes the larger lesions and gives the radiograph a "soap bubble" appearance (Figure 5-6). The actual size of the lesion is usually difficult to determine because lesions do not exhibit a distinct line of demarcation with the normal bone. Root resorption is uncommon but is occasionally observed in some rapidly growing lesions (Figure 5-7).

HISTOPATHOLOGY

The classic microscopic appearance of an ameloblastoma consists of epithelium in which the basal cell layer contains columnar or palisaded cells that have a tendency for the nucleus to move from the basement membrane to the opposing end of the cell, a process referred to as *reverse polarization* (Figure 5-8). The cytoplasm adjacent to the basement membrane assumes a clear zone that is reminiscent of the change that occurs in the cells of the inner enamel epithelium before they undergo transition to presecretory ameloblasts. This histologic feature

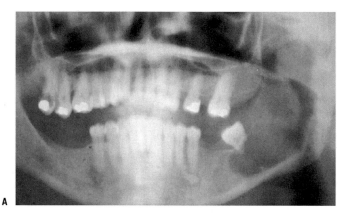
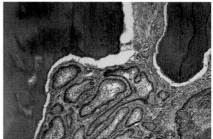

A   B

FIGURE 5-7
Ameloblastoma. A, Radiograph illustrating extensive polycystic lesion of left mandible with resorption of roots of the molar. **B,** Photomicrograph of neoplastic cells in close proximity to resorbed roots of molar tooth *(left).*

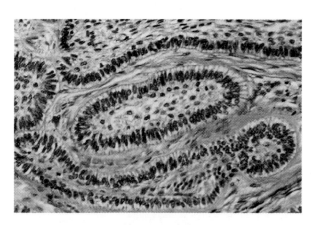
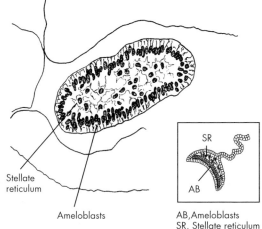

Stellate
reticulum

Ameloblasts

AB, Ameloblasts
SR, Stellate reticulum

FIGURE 5-8
Ameloblastoma. Classic microscopic features of the common follicular form of ameloblastoma that demonstrate movement of the nucleus from basement membrane pole of basal cells to opposite pole ("reverse polarization"), resulting in outer cells resembling presecretory ameloblasts. *Inset:* tumor recapitulates cap/early bell stage of odontogenesis.

is present in other odontogenic lesions, such as calcifying odontogenic cysts and odontogenic keratocysts. In ameloblastoma, the reverse polarization of the basal cell layer must be part of one of the specific architectural patterns of epithelium that is known to be associated with locally aggressive behavior. The two most common are the *follicular* and *plexiform* patterns.

The **follicular pattern** is the most prevalent, recapitulating the earlier stages of tooth development. It consists of epithelium in the form of islands, strands, and medullary arrangements against a background stroma of fibrous connective tissue. The epithelial arrangements have an outer border composed of the palisaded ameloblast-like cells in which reversed polarization has occurred; the remainder consists of loosely arranged and widely separated triangular-shaped cells that are similar to those of the stellate reticulum found in the bell stage of odontogenesis. Occasionally, there is a distinctive zone of hyalinization surrounding the epithelial islands. This zone is believed to be an inductive effect of odontogenic epithelium on the connective tissue. In some islands the stellatelike cells of the central areas degenerate, forming central microcysts (Figure 5-9, *A*). Large and small cysts within the epithelium are not considered a separate histologic variant because nearly all islands contain varying degrees of cell lysis, which is probably due to ischemic degeneration within the large islands of epithelial proliferation. In other islands the central cells are transformed to squamous cells that produce keratin within individual cells or in the form of **"keratin pearls."** When this occurs the histologic variant is referred to as the **acanthomatous pattern** (Figure 5-9, *B*). The central cells less commonly appear swollen and densely packed with eosinophilic granules that are ultrastructurally considered lysomal elements. This pattern has been termed the **granular cell variant** (Figure 5-9, *C*). Most patterns of ameloblastoma exhibit cyst formation, particularly when follicles become large.

The **plexiform pattern** differs considerably from the follicular pattern because it does not recapitulate a recognized stage of odontogenesis. It consists of epithelium that proliferates in a "fishnet" or mesh arrangement (Figure 5-9, *D*). In many areas the basal or bordering cells do not resemble ameloblasts because they lack the distinctive reversed polarization of the nucleus. The general pattern consists of thin strands of epithelium that are in continuity. Large and small cystlike areas are present that are not necessarily caused by the degeneration of the epithelium but are the result of the strangulation and degeneration of connective tissue stroma by the proliferating epithelium.

Other histologic variations of the common ameloblastoma are less frequently encountered. One type is the **basal cell variant,** in which there is only densely packed, large proliferating cuboidal-shaped basaloid cells in narrow strands without stellate reticulum or other forms of centrally located epithelial cells (Figure 5-10, *A*). Another identifiable pattern is the **desmoplastic ameloblastoma,** in which the epithelial islands and strands are small and have cuboidal and darkly stained cells. The epithelial component is widely separated by fibrous tissue that is dense and scarlike (Figure 5-10, *B*). This variant has a

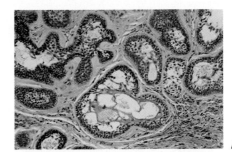
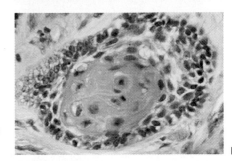
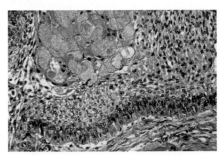
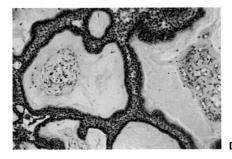

FIGURE 5-9

Ameloblastoma. Microscopic features of various histologic patterns. **A,** Follicular. **B,** Acanthomatous. **C,** Granular cell. **D,** Plexiform.

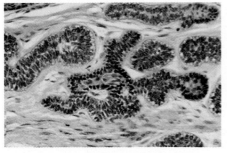
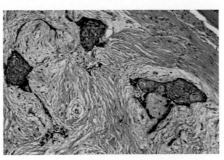

A

B

FIGURE 5-10

Ameloblastoma. Microscopic features of less common histologic patterns. **A,** Basal cell. **B,** Desmoplastic.

mixed radiolucent/opaque radiographic appearance that resembles a fibro-osseous lesion. Desmoplastic ameloblastoma is usually more difficult to treat because it appears to have a particular predilection for penetrating the surrounding trabecular bone and remaining undetected. As a result, finding the exact interface of the lesion with normal bone is especially difficult during surgical management.

TREATMENT

In general, all histologic variants of common ameloblastomas have similar biologic behavior and are not managed differently because of their microscopic features. There is a propensity to penetrate the adjacent trabecular spaces of bone without immediately causing the hard tissue to resorb; therefore radiographs and other bone imaging techniques are not always able to delineate the lesion's boundary. The best chance of completely removing the lesion is with marginal (block) resection. Since this lesion has difficulty penetrating dense cortical bone, the inferior border of the mandible can sometimes be preserved. If the inferior border is involved, segmental resection is necessary and results in the loss of bone continuity. Hemimandibulectomy or hemimaxillectomy are nearly always required in very large lesions. All lesions are treated surgically because they are relatively radioresistant.

Unicystic Ameloblastoma

The designation of **unicystic ameloblastoma** as a distinct clinical entity is a relatively new concept that has gained wide acceptance because it provides a basis for pursuing a more conservative surgical approach to treatment of a special form of ameloblastoma. Most of these lesions are found during microscopic examination of a large unilocular cyst commonly associated with the crown of an impacted tooth in a young patient (Figure 5-11). Whether the lesion represents a transformation from a normal cystic lining or arises de novo from preexisting odontogenic epithelial remnants cannot be determined. In many lesions, areas of a normal cystic lining are adjacent to the ameloblastomatous tissue; in other lesions, normal epithelial lining cannot be found.

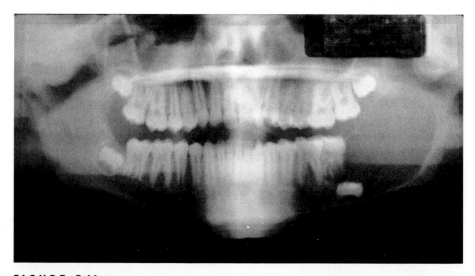

FIGURE 5-11

Unicystic ameloblastoma. Radiograph of young patient with large lesion of left mandible, exhibiting inferiorly displaced partly formed molar and expansion of ramal cortical plates.

CLINICAL

Lesions of unicystic ameloblastoma most commonly occur in patients who are 16 to 20 years of age; occasionally, lesions occur in younger patients. Rarely, lesions have been found in patients up to the age of 40. The peak occurrence of unicystic ameloblastoma appears to be 20 years earlier than for common ameloblastoma. With few exceptions, the unicystic ameloblastoma occurs in a dentigerous cyst relationship and is usually associated with a severely displaced third molar. In rare instances lesions occur in the mandibular premolar area, which is the common site of lateral periodontal cysts, and others occur in the posterior mandible beyond the tooth-bearing areas. Lesions more commonly occur in the mandible than in the maxilla.

RADIOGRAPHIC

The radiographic appearance is important in the diagnosis because it determines whether the lesion is unilocular, a necessary criterion for unicystic ameloblastoma. Lesions are usually well demarcated and may even be corticated. A tooth is often present within the radiolucency. When lesions are located in the premolar area, the roots of adjacent teeth may be displaced.

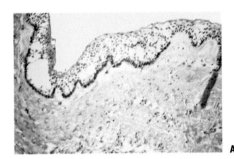

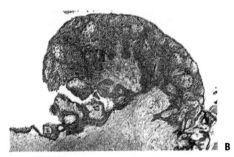

HISTOPATHOLOGY

The lesion consists of a dense uniformly thickened fibrous connective tissue capsule, surrounding a solitary large fluid-filled lumen. The epithelial lining of the lumen is uniform in thickness and has a slightly hyperchromatic layer of palisaded basal cells, most of which exhibit reversed polarization of the nucleus. The remaining layers resemble stellate reticulum (Figure 5-12, A). Some lesions will contain areas in which the epithelium is thickened with papillary projections extending into the lumen. This histologic pattern is referred to as **intraluminal unicystic ameloblastoma** (Figure 5-12, B). When the thickened lining penetrates the adjacent capsular tissue, it is termed a **mural unicystic ameloblastoma** (Figure 5-12, C). In some dentigerous cysts a slightly different histologic pattern occurs. The pattern consists of intraluminal nodular projections that contain a network or mesh pattern of epithelium without the distinctive ameloblast-like changes of the basal cell layer. This pattern is referred to as **plexiform unicystic ameloblastoma** (Figure 5-12, D).

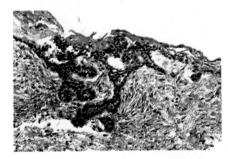

TREATMENT

The treatment of unicystic ameloblastoma depends on the histologic pattern. When the intraluminal or the plexiform pattern is present, enucleation is usually sufficient. If the lesion contains a mural component that extends into the wall to the level of interface with the bone, marginal resection is necessary to ensure adequate removal.

Peripheral Ameloblastoma

Peripheral (extraosseous) ameloblastoma is a very uncommon odontogenic tumor that histologically resembles the intraosseous common ameloblastoma but is limited to the soft tissues of the gingiva. It is believed to arise directly from the overlying epithelium or from of the remnants of the dental lamina located in the extraosseous soft tissue. Separation of this lesion from *odontogenic hamartoma* and *peripheral odontogenic fibroma* is sometimes difficult. The odontogenic hamartoma is a collection of inactive odontogenic rests, and the peripheral odontogenic fibroma is primarily a fibrous lesion containing occasional strands of odontogenic rests. Peripheral ameloblastoma is easier to diagnose when the lesion exhibits the classic histologic patterns of the intraosseous common ameloblastoma and has a history of continuous growth.

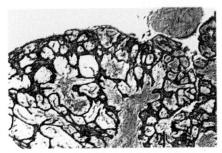

FIGURE 5-12

Unicystic ameloblastoma. Microscopic features of typical lining exhibit features of ameloblastoma **(A)**, intraluminal papillary projection **(B)**, intracapsular mural penetration **(C)**, and the plexiform pattern sometimes found **(D)**.

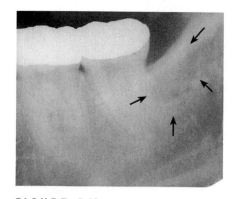

FIGURE 5-13

Peripheral ameloblastoma. Radiograph of lesion of retromolar pad exhibiting "saucerization" *(arrows)* of cortical bone.

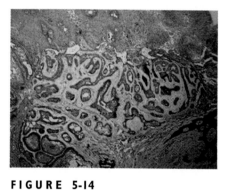

FIGURE 5-14

Peripheral ameloblastoma. Microscopic appearance exhibiting islands of follicular ameloblastoma in close proximity to surface epithelium.

CLINICAL

Lesions usually appear as firm sessile nodules of the gingiva that range in size from 0.5 to 2.0 cm, and they have a smooth surface and normal coloration. If the lesions originate from surface epithelium, they may be erythematous or ulcerated. Patients have been documented from 23 to 82 years of age, and lesions occur on the mandible twice as often as on the maxilla.

RADIOGRAPHIC

Since the lesions are primarily extraosseous, bone changes are seldom present. Occasionally, there will be a superficial saucerization of the cortical plate (Figure 5-13) that appears as a cup-shaped radiolucency beneath the elevated nodule due to the pressure the lesion exerts on the bone. If the lesion is located in the interdental papilla area, some tooth separation may occur.

HISTOPATHOLOGY

The tissue is composed of islands and strands of odontogenic epithelium, usually resembling the follicular pattern of intraosseous common ameloblastoma. The epithelial islands commonly exhibit the acanthomatous variant of this pattern with central areas of keratin formation or the cystic pattern. In some lesions the epithelial strands are in continuity with the surface epithelium and appear to arise from this source (Figure 5-14). The epithelial islands and strands are usually surrounded by fibrous tissue. Small lesions have an inferior margin that is usually above the cortical bone. Large lesions have a "pushing" margin that produces a cup-shaped resorption of the cortical plate.

TREATMENT

The recommended treatment for peripheral ameloblastoma differs from the treatment for other forms of ameloblastoma because the tumor is usually small and remains localized to the superficial soft tissue. Most lesions are successfully managed with local excision that includes a small margin of normal tissue. The inferior margin should include periosteum to ensure that bone penetration has not occurred.

CALCIFYING EPITHELIAL ODONTOGENIC TUMOR

■ CALCIFYING EPITHELIAL ODONTOGENIC TUMOR: a locally aggressive tumor consisting of strands and medullary patterns of squamous and clear cells that are often accompanied by spherical calcifications and amyloid-staining hyalin deposits.

The calcifying epithelial odontogenic tumor (CEOT) is frequently referred to by the eponym "Pindborg Tumor." It is rare, representing less than 1% of all odontogenic tumors. The lesion is locally aggressive with a biologic behavior similar to the common form of intraosseous ameloblastoma. It originates from the epithelial rests of the dental lamina and/or the reduced enamel epithelium that overlies the crowns of the teeth. The neoplastic component of CEOT is reminiscent of epithelial and calcified structures normally found around the crowns of teeth. It differs from ameloblastoma by being composed of epithelial cells that do not resemble ameloblasts and by usually containing spherical and diffuse calcifications within the epithelial islands and the connective tisssue stroma. CEOT occurs as either a **central** (intraosseous) or **peripheral** (extraosseous) lesion.

CLINICAL

Central CEOT occurs in patients between the ages of 20 and 60 years, with a mean age of 40. Two thirds of the lesions are in the mandible. In both jaws most lesions occur in the molar area followed in frequency by the premolar area. The remainder of the lesions are equally distributed throughout the rest of the jaws. The tumor presents as a slowly enlarging painless mass. Nasal airway obstruction, epistaxis, and proptosis are sometimes experienced in the maxilla.

Peripheral CEOT most commonly occurs in the anterior part of the mouth. It presents as a superficial soft tissue swelling of the gingiva in tooth-bearing and edentulous areas of the jaws.

RADIOGRAPHIC

Since calcifications are usually small, lesions tend to occur as a diffuse radiolucency with faint flecks of calcified structures (Figure 5-15, *A*). CEOT less commonly appears radiographically as a mixture of radiolucent/radiopaque areas (Figure 5-15, *B*). The radiopaque areas can be either diffuse and faint or discrete round structures. Intraosseous lesions may occur over unerupted and/or displaced teeth. Small lesions are often unilocular radiolucencies. Similar to common ameloblastoma, lesions have indistinct lines of demarcation with the surrounding bone. Since CEOT usually occurs over unerupted teeth and may be a radiolucent or mixed unilocular lesion, the radiographic differential diagnosis of CEOT includes dentigerous cyst, adenomatoid odontogenic tumor, and ameloblastic fibro-odontoma. The peripheral lesions are commonly radiolucent. Sometimes lesions exhibit superficial cortical erosion.

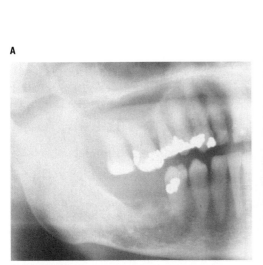

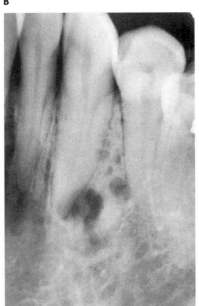

FIGURE 5-15

Calcifying epithelial odontognic tumor. A, Panoramic radiograph of lesion of right posterior mandible that occurs as a diffuse radiolucency extending to the inferior border. Faintly visible focal radiopacities are present.   (Courtesy Dr. Heddie O. Sedano.) **B,** Periapical radiograph exhibiting mixed radiolucent/opaque intraosseous lesion lacking demarcation of its boundaries.

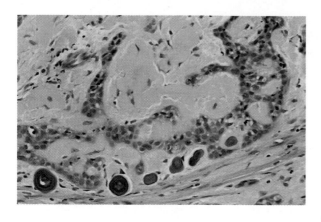
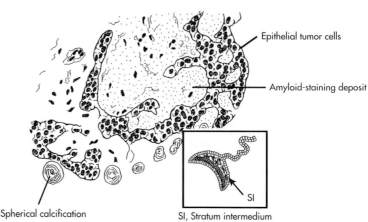

Epithelial tumor cells

Amyloid-staining deposit

SI

SI, Stratum intermedium

Spherical calcification

FIGURE 5-16

Calcifying epithelial odontogenic tumor. Characteristic microscopic features of sheets and strands of polyhedral epithelial cells, homogeneous eosinophilic deposits that stain positive for amyloid, and spherical calcifications. *Inset:* tumor cells recapitulate stratum intermedium layer of the early bell stage of odontegenesis.

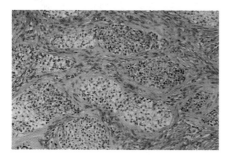

FIGURE 5-17

Calcifying epithelial odontogenic tumor. Characteristic microscopic features of the clear cell variant exhibiting lobular patterns of clear cells and eosinophilic cells. This variant has less tendency for formation of spherical calcifications and amyloid-staining hyaline deposits.

HISTOPATHOLOGY

The tumor exhibits considerable variation in its histologic appearance. The most common histologic pattern consists of sheets of polyhedral cells with prominent intercellular bridges. The cells may exhibit pleomorphism, multinucleation, prominent nucleoli, and occasionally hyperchromatism. Although these cells may have an atypical appearance, mitotic figures are rarely found. Pools of homogeneous eosinophilic material are often found within and between the epithelial sheets, along with spherical calcifications (Figure 5-16). The spherical calcifications are scattered throughout the epithelium and connective tissue; proportions vary considerably between lesions. Lesions also contain varying proportions of epithelial cells with clear cytoplasms. When clear cells dominant the epithelial component, the lesion is referred to as *clear cell variant of CEOT* (Figure 5-17). This is a particularly common histologic feature of peripheral lesions. Peripheral lesions have less tendency for calcifications. The nature of the eosinophilic deposits has been controversial. Because the substance is often positive with amyloid stains such as congo red or thioflavin T, it is believed to be a form of amyloid. Another interpretation is that the deposits are abnormal forms of tissue degeneration, enamel matrix, keratin, or basal lamina.

TREATMENT

Because of the sparsity of cases with long term follow-up, the biologic behavior of CEOT is not well understood. The lesion is locally invasive and without capsule formation. Since a few recent cases with multiple occurrences exhibited malignant features, resection that includes a margin of normal soft tissue or bone is recommended.

ADENOMATOID ODONTOGENIC TUMOR

■ ADENOMATOID ODONTOGENIC TUMOR: a well-circumscribed lesion derived from odontogenic epithelium that usually occurs around the crowns of unerupted anterior teeth of young patients and consists of epithelium in swirls and ductal patterns interspersed with spherical calcifications.

The adenomatoid odontogenic tumor (AOT) is sometimes termed *odontogenic adenomatoid tumor*. Its name reflects the characteristic histologic feature of duct-like structures interspersed throughout the epithelial component, giving the lesion a glandular or "adenomatous" appearance. Its usual clinical location around the crown of a tooth combined with the findings of ultrastructural and histochemical studies suggests that the lesion most probably originates from the reduced enamel epithelium of the postsecretory phase of enamel organ development. Because the lesion is biologically nonaggressive and requires conservative treatment, its recognition and differentiation from the other epithelial odontogenic lesions, particularly ameloblastoma, is of utmost importance.

CLINICAL
The AOT is usually associated with an impacted tooth and is often a cause of failure of the tooth to erupt. The lesion occurs during the second decade of life, commonly in patients 14 to 15 years of age; females are affected more frequently than males. It most often occurs in the anterior mouth, usually around an impacted cuspid. Occasionally, these lesions have been associated with other teeth, including molars. The common presentation is in a patient who exhibits an area of swelling over an unerupted tooth.

RADIOGRAPHIC
The radiographic appearance of AOT is usually as a unilocular lesion with well-corticated borders that contains a tooth. Most lesions are radiolucent, but some contain faint flecks of radiopacities. Lesions often surround the crown of an impacted tooth, similar to that found in a dentigerous cyst. Close examination reveals that the lesion differs from a dentigerous cyst because the radiolucency usually extends apically beyond the cementoenamel junction (Figure 5-18).

HISTOPATHOLOGY
AOT is composed of an outer capsule of fibrous connective tissue surrounding a nodular pattern of epithelial cells. The rest of the tissue may be solid or contain focal cystic areas. The nodules are composed of spindled epithelial cells that are often in a swirled pattern. Scattered throughout most lesions are ductal structures composed of a circular arrangement of columnar cells with interposed deposits of periodic acid-Schiff (PAS) positive eosinophilic material (Figure 5-19).

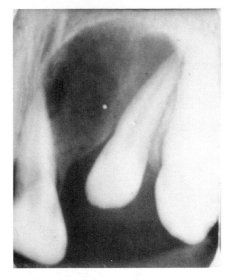

FIGURE 5-18

Adenomatoid odontogenic tumor. Radiograph demonstrating a well-demarcated mixed radiolucent/opaque lesion surrounding an impacted maxillary lateral incisor.

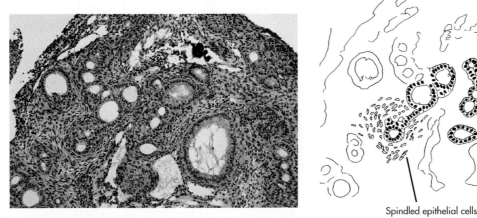
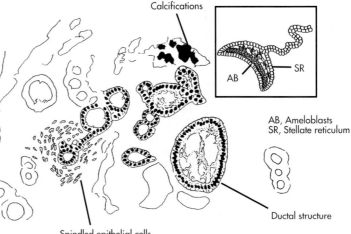

Calcifications

AB, Ameloblasts
SR, Stellate reticulum

Ductal structure

Spindled epithelial cells

FIGURE 5-19

Adenomatoid odontogenic tumor. Microscopic features reveal the nodular pattern of spindled cells, ductal structures, and a focal area of calcification *(upper center),* which is characteristic of this lesion. *Inset:* tumor cells recapitulate presecretory ameloblasts and stellate reticulum of the cap/early bell stage of odontogenesis.

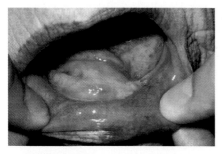

FIGURE 5-20

Calcifying odontogenic cyst. Patient exhibits extensive buccal and lingual expansion of the cortical plates of the right mandible.

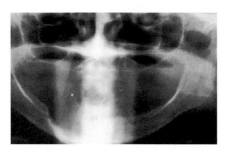

FIGURE 5-21

Calcifying odontogenic cyst. Radiograph of patient in Figure 5-20 that demonstrates a large radiolucent cup-shaped defect of the anterior right mandible with sharp line of demarcation with surrounding bone.

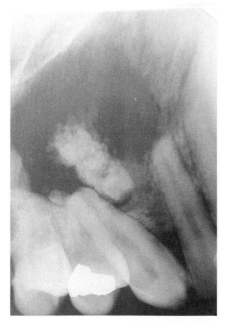

FIGURE 5-22

Calcifying odontogenic cyst. Radiograph of large lesion of maxilla with odontoma included within the lesion.

This is considered to be a form of basement membrane. Spherical calcifications are often scattered throughout the epithelium but are not a consistent finding. The stroma may occasionally contain diffuse areas of hyaline material.

TREATMENT
AOT is successfully treated with curettage and usually requires the removal of associated teeth. Recurrences are rare.

CALCIFYING ODONTOGENIC CYST

■ CALCIFYING ODONTOGENIC CYST: a rare, well-circumscribed, solid or cystic lesion derived from odontogenic epithelium that resembles follicular ameloblastoma but contains "ghost cells" and spherical calcifications.

The calcifying odontogenic cyst (COC) is an uncommon odontogenic lesion with a somewhat wide spectrum of histologic features. Because the lesion often appears as a solid noncystic lesion, it is no longer classified as an odontogenic cyst but as an odontogenic tumor. In addition to the purely cystic and solid forms, it may be associated with an odontoma.

CLINICAL
The COC can occur in any part of the tooth-bearing areas of the mouth but has a slightly increased incidence in the areas anterior to the first molar. Lesions occur at any age but have a predilection for patients in the second decade and may occur in an extraosseous or intraosseous location. Extraosseous lesions appear as focal localized swellings, whereas intraosseous lesions produce a generalized expansion of the buccal and lingual cortices (Figure 5-20). Pain is usually absent.

RADIOGRAPHIC
Lesions most commonly appear as well-circumscribed unilocular radiolucencies (Figure 5-21) containing flecks of indistinct radiopacities. In some lesions the flecks and small nodular radiopacities are confined to the periphery, with larger toothlike structures more centrally located (Figure 5-22). In younger patients lesions may closely resemble a developing odontoma or ameloblastic fibro-odontoma.

HISTOPATHOLOGY
The microscopic appearance of COC varies. Some lesions have a cystic center, and others are solid. The epithelial component resembles that found in ameloblastoma and is common to all lesions. The epithelial component consists of an outer layer of palisaded columnar basal cells and an inner layer reminiscent of stellate reticulum. Greatly enlarged eosinophilic epithelial cells without visable nuclei, referred to as **"ghost cells,"** are present within the stellate reticulum-like areas. Multiple spherical and diffuse calcifications within the epithelium and the connective tissue are also included (Figure 5-23). In some COCs, the ameloblastomatous epithelium may extend into the capsular wall. Linear deposits of hyalinized material are located within the connective tissue beneath the epithelium.

TREATMENT
Lesions of COC require conservative treatment, usually enucleation. Recurrences are uncommon.

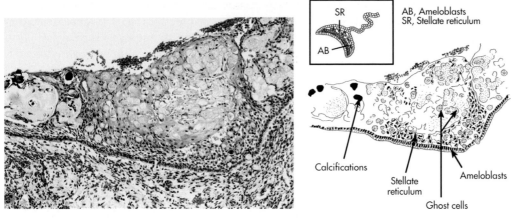

FIGURE 5-23

Calcifying odontogenic cyst. Microscopic features reveal a thick epithelial layer lining a cystic space consisting of palisaded columnar basal cells, accumulations of enlarged eosinophilic epithelial cells without nuclei ("ghost cells"), and spherical calcifications. *Inset:* tumor cells recapitulate the early bell stage of odontogenesis.

SQUAMOUS ODONTOGENIC TUMOR

> ■ SQUAMOUS ODONTOGENIC TUMOR: a rare, sometimes multifocal, potentially aggressive lesion derived from odontogenic epithelium, consisting of islands of stratified squamous epithelium that commonly contain microcysts and calcifications in a dense fibrous background.

The squamous odontogenic tumor (SOT) was first described in 1975. Its inclusion as a separate entity in a classification of odontogenic tumors is based on its characteristic histologic features and distinct biologic activity. The cases reported and the experiences of some clinicians resulted in the expansion of the original description of SOT. The available information seems to indicate that the lesion can be multifocal and have a somewhat aggressive potential if not treated in its early stages. SOT may originate from the remnants of the dental lamina, rests of Malassez, or overlying epithelium.

CLINICAL
Lesions of SOT usually occur anterior to the molars and are equally distributed between the mandible and maxilla. Lesions occur in patients at any age, with a peak incidence in the third decade. Lesions are first detected as either a painless swelling or as looseness of teeth in a region (Figure 5-24). Initially the lesions are slow growing, and patients indicate that the swelling or mild symptoms have been present for 1 or more years.

RADIOGRAPHIC
Small lesions appear as unilocular radiolucencies (Figure 5-25), whereas large ones are multilocular and have an indistinct border. Tooth separation is common with smaller lesions when they are located in the bone that is coronal to the root apices. Resorption of roots is usually absent.

HISTOPATHOLOGY
Lesions of SOT consist of rounded and elongated islands of relatively normal-appearing stratified squamous epithelium against a cellular fibrous connective

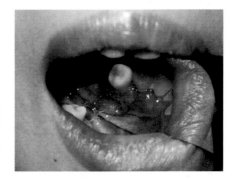

FIGURE 5-24

Squamous odontogenic tumor. Patient with multiple small nodules on lingual gingiva in mandibular premolar area.

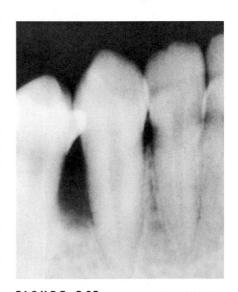

FIGURE 5-25

Squamous odontogenic tumor. Radiograph of patient in Figure 5-24 that reveals loss of interproximal alveolar bone.

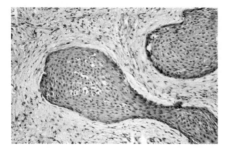

FIGURE 5-26

Squamous odontogenic tumor. Microscopic features reveal a background of cellular fibrous connective tissue containing multiple islands of inactive-appearing squamous epithelium with central areas exhibiting a tendency to become cystic.

tissue background. The epithelial islands vary in size and have a basal cell layer of inactive-appearing cuboidal cells. The remainder of the islands are composed of matured intermediate cells with prominent desmosomal bridges (Figure 5-26). Many of the epithelial islands have central areas of microcyst formation, whereas others contain spherical or irregularly shaped calcified structures. Similar calcifications can also be found in the connective tissue stroma.

TREATMENT

Most small lesions can be controlled with local curettage; large lesions require block resection.

CONNECTIVE TISSUE ODONTOGENIC TUMORS

ODONTOGENIC FIBROMA

■ ODONTOGENIC FIBROMA: a peripheral or intraosseous (central) benign neoplasm derived from connective tissue of odontogenic origin containing widely scattered islands and strands of embryonic odontogenic epithelium and calcifications.

The concept of odontogenic fibroma is presently in transition. Originally, the name was applied to any intraosseous tumor composed predominantly of fibrous connective tissue that was located within the tooth-bearing areas of the jaws. Some of these lesions were relatively acellular and were composed of dense bundles of collagen in a fascicular pattern with few spindled fibroblasts. Others were composed of a mixture of acellular connective tissue that contained islands and strands of odontogenic epithelium surrounded by zones of myxomatous tissue, hyalin deposits, and calcifications. The latter lesion (containing odontogenic epithelium) was featured in the *World Health Organization Classification of Odontogenic Tumors* as an example of a true odontogenic fibroma. The former lesion (without odontogenic epithelium) is presently considered an intraosseous form of *desmoplastic fibroma*. Both intraosseous forms of odontogenic fibroma are rare; the peripheral lesion is relatively common.

Intraosseous Desmoplastic Fibroma

The intraosseous desmoplastic fibroma is considered to be derived from the dental follicle and a more mature and fibrous form of another connective tissue lesion, the odontogenic myxoma. It is sometimes mistaken for the nonneoplastic *hyperplastic dental follicle* that commonly forms around an unerupted tooth.

CLINICAL

The intraosseous desmoplastic fibroma occurs primarily in young patients who are in the first and second decades of life. It presents as a painless swelling of the face and when examined intraorally reveals extensive cortical expansion of the buccal and lingual plates. Nearly all reported lesions have been in the mandible.

RADIOGRAPHIC

The large lesions are multilocular and may be associated with impacted or displaced teeth that appear similar to the common ameloblastoma. Resorption of the roots of the teeth is usually absent.

HISTOPATHOLOGY

The tissue is composed of a consistent homogeneous pattern of relatively acellular hyalinized connective tissue in a scarlike pattern. The fibroblasts are spindled and the collagen is in the form of interlacing fascicles. There is an absence of mitosis, epithelial islands, and calcifications.

TREATMENT

Although small lesions have been controlled by enucleation, recurrences have been reported. Large multilocular lesions appear to be best treated with block resection.

Peripheral Odontogenic Fibroma

The peripheral odontogenic fibroma is the most common form of odontogenic fibroma and appears to be derived from the overlying gingival epithelium or the rests of the dental lamina remaining in an extraosseous location. The epithelial component resembles the dental lamina formed during the early stages of odontogenesis. The lesion provides some evidence that it originates from a recapitulation of dental lamina because the epithelium is capable of producing inductive changes in the connective tissue that are similar to changes in the dental lamina during odontogenesis. Differentiation of this lesion from a gingival hamartoma or a peripheral ameloblastoma is often required and is usually done by evaluating the epithelial element.

CLINICAL

The peripheral odontogenic fibroma has a similar appearance to other focal growths of the gingiva, such as peripheral fibroma (with or without ossification). It may be of normal coloration or erythematous when ulceration occurs (Figure 5-27). Interdental lesions often cause tooth separation.

RADIOGRAPHIC

Since small lesions are located in the gingival soft tissue, radiographic alteration of the bone is not usually apparent. When lesions contain numerous calcifications within the cellular connective tissue, some small radiopaque flecks may be visible. Large lesions may reveal saucerization of the cortical bone or some widening of the cervical portion of the periodontal space.

HISTOPATHOLOGY

The lesion is composed of a mixture of somewhat dense connective tissue that separates localized zones of myxomatous or loose connective tissue. Small epithelial islands can be found near the surface adjacent to thin elongated rete pegs and in the deep areas of myxomatous change (Figure 5-28). In these areas they are located adjacent to irregularly shaped hyalinized deposits, many of which have undergone some degree of mineralization. The epithelial islands will often contain "clear cells."

TREATMENT

Although local excision is the treatment of choice, attempts to superficially remove the lesion without extending the deep margin to the underlying bone or into the periodontal ligament often results in recurrence.

Central Odontogenic Fibroma

The central odontogenic fibroma is a relatively uncommon odontogenic tumor that is described in the World Health Organization (WHO) classification of odontogenic tumors. Before that time, lesions with the specific histologic fea-

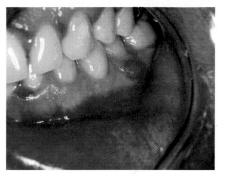

FIGURE 5-27

Peripheral odontogenic fibroma. The lesion of the mandibular buccal gingiva is raised and firm and has an erythematous surface caused by chronic irritation.

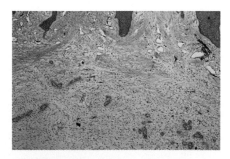

FIGURE 5-28

Peripheral odontogenic fibroma. Photomicrograph reveals a basically fibrous lesion containing multiple small islands and strands of odontogenic epithelium resembling remnants of the dental lamina. The connective tissue immediately adjacent to the epithelial islands is less dense and myxomatous.

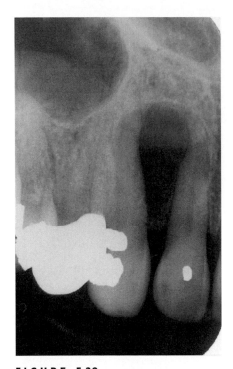

FIGURE 5-29

Central odontogenic fibroma (WHO type). Radiograph of an intraosseous lesion in the anterior maxilla exhibiting a circumscribed radiolucency.

tures ascribed to this tumor were probably diagnosed as either atypical forms of CEOT, ameloblastoma, or cementifying fibroma, depending on the amount of epithelial and calcifying elements present.

CLINICAL

Lesions are usually asymptomatic, painless swellings commonly located in the mandible.

RADIOGRAPHIC

The radiographic appearance is that of a nonspecific radiolucency, unilocular and well circumscribed in some (Figure 5-29) and multilocular in others. Some faint radiopaque flecks are sometimes observed.

HISTOPATHOLOGY

The central odontogenic fibroma differs from desmoplastic fibroma by being composed of a cellular connective tissue that contains numerous thin strands of odontogenic epithelium (Figure 5-30). The epithelial component closely resembles dental lamina and often contains cells with clear cytoplasm. Some lesions will contain varying amounts of spherical and diffuse calcifications that are usually associated with the odontogenic epithelial strands. Recently there have been several cases described in which central odontogenic fibroma contained histologic components of central giant cell lesions. The significance of this finding is not known.

TREATMENT

The number of reported cases of odontogenic fibroma described by the WHO is still small, so accurately predicting prognosis is not possible. Most cases have responded to conservative treatments such as curettage, and reports indicate that lesions separate from the surrounding bone with ease. There have been some recurrences after several years.

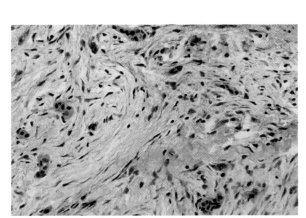

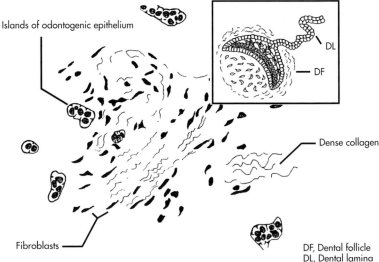

Islands of odontogenic epithelium

Dense collagen

Fibroblasts

DL

DF

DF, Dental follicle
DL, Dental lamina

FIGURE 5-30

Central odontogenic fibroma (WHO type). Microscopic features consist of a cellular fibrous connective tissue containing multiple small islands and strands of odontogenic epithelium. *Inset:* tumor recapitulates cells of dental follicle and dental lamina of the early stages of odontogenesis.

ODONTOGENIC MYXOMA

■ ODONTOGENIC MYXOMA: an aggressive intraosseous lesion derived from embryonic connective tissue associated with odontogenesis and primarily consisting of a mucoid ground substance with widely scattered undifferentiated spindled mesenchymal cells.

The odontogenic myxoma is an uncommon intraosseous lesion that has a distinct histologic appearance and a locally aggressive behavior. It has aroused considerable interest, with a few exceptions, as have nearly all lesions found in the jaws. Occasionally, lesions have been found in the ramus and other non–tooth-bearing areas of the jaws and in other facial bones. Additionally, lesions with identical histologic features are found in the soft tissues. Studies have been undertaken on the jaw lesions in an effort to prove an odontogenic origin. This effort has been somewhat unsuccessful.

CLINICAL
Lesions are nearly equally distributed between the mandible and maxilla. Maxillary lesions occur equally in all areas and frequently erode into the sinus, often crossing the midline and into the opposing sinus cavity. Mandibular lesions are most commonly found in the molar/premolar areas and often extend into the ramus.

Most lesions are painless, slowly enlarging swellings of the involved bone that sometimes displaces teeth. Patients are often aware of these lesions for several years before seeking attention.

RADIOGRAPHIC
The large lesions have a somewhat distinct radiographic appearance consisting of a multilocular radiolucency with a "soap bubble" or "honeycomb" pattern (Figure 5-31, A). In some areas coarse or angular trabeculations are noted. In general the radiographic appearance resembles that of common ameloblastoma, diffuse without a distinct demarcation with uninvolved bone. Root resorption is

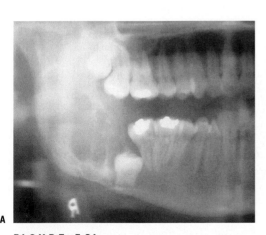
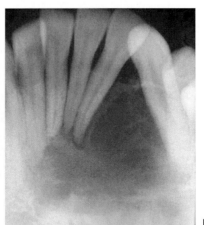

A   B

FIGURE 5-31

Odontogenic myxoma. A, Panoramic radiograph of posterior mandible and ramus exhibiting the characteristic "honeycomb" pattern, indistinct radiolucency, faint residual fragments of trabecular bone, and expansion of cortical plates. **B,** Periapical radiograph of anterior mandible revealing a mottled radiolucency with indistinct margins and containing wisps of residual bone.

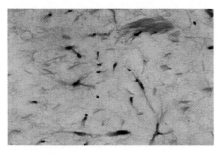

FIGURE 5-32

Odontogenic myxoma. Microscopic features reveal a background of mucoid ground substance containing widely separated spindled mesenchymal cells and occasional strands of collagen.

not a feature of myxoma, although some tooth displacement occurs (Figure 5-31, *B*). Small lesions are often unilocular and appear as nonspecific radiolucencies.

HISTOPATHOLOGY

The microscopic appearance of an odontogenic myxoma consists of widely separated spindle or angular-shaped cells against a background of a mucoid, nonfibrillar ground substance (Figure 5-32). In some odontogenic myxomas there are focal areas of fine strands of collagen, and the blood vessels will often exhibit a thin outer zone of hyalinization. In the periphery the myxomatous tissue penetrates the trabecular spaces, producing islands of residual bone. This feature accounts for the difficulty in conservatively removing the lesion. Islands of odontogenic epithelium and focal calcifications have been observed.

Occasionally, lesions have been observed containing large amounts of a mature cellular fibrous tissue. These lesions are referred to as *myxofibroma*.

TREATMENT

Some small unilocular lesions have been treated successfully with local curettage followed by chemical cautery of the bony walls, but most lesions require block resection. Because of the gelatinous nature of the lesion, it is important to remove an intact specimen to reduce the chances of recurrence.

CEMENTOBLASTOMA

■ **CEMENTOBLASTOMA:** a benign, well-circumscribed neoplasm of cementum-like tissue growing in continuity with the apical cemental layer of a molar or premolar that produces expansion of cortical plates and pain.

Some lesions, such as periapical cemental dysplasia and cementifying fibroma (formerly included under the classification of odontogenic tumors), have recently been reclassified by the WHO and are discussed in Chapter 4. Cementoblastoma still remains classified as an odontogenic tumor because it is considered to be a true benign neoplasm of cementoblasts. Although its histologic features are remarkably similar to osteoblastoma and osteoid osteoma, the fact that its growth pattern is in continuity with the cemental layer of the apical third of a tooth and that it remains separated from bone by a continuation of the periodontal membrane is considered evidence that it is of tooth tissue origin.

CLINICAL

The cementoblastoma is an uncommon lesion occurring in patients in the second and third decades, with a peak incidence in patients around the age of 19. Nearly all tumors occur in the molar/premolar area, with lesions attached to the apical third of one of the roots. The lesions grow as true neoplasms, uniformly expanding both the buccal and lingual cortical plates. The cementoblastoma is distinctive among the odontogenic tumors, because in nearly all cases patients complain of pain that becomes more intense if the area is palpated. The teeth usually remain vital.

RADIOGRAPHIC

Lesions are unilocular and well demarcated. They may be completely radiolucent, mixed radiolucent/radiopaque, or completely radiopaque. Nonradiolucent lesions exhibit a peripheral zone of radiolucency continuous with the normal periodontal ligament space of the unaffected areas of the tooth. Roots adjacent to the expanding lesion often exhibit resorption of their apical third.

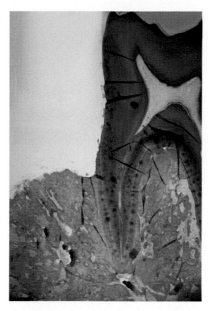

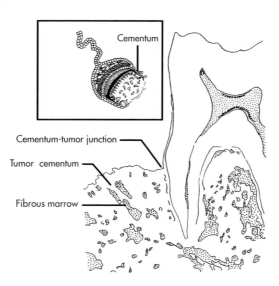

FIGURE 5-33

Cementoblastoma. Photomicrograph of a molar in which the cemental tissue of the lesion is continuous with the normal cementum of the root. *Inset:* tumor recapitulates cementum deposition during root formation in the late stage of odontogenesis.

HISTOPATHOLOGY

The lesion is characterized by a deposition of unmineralized eosinophilic matrix rimmed by plump cementoblasts that are continuous with the normal cementum layer of one of the tooth roots (Figure 5-33). The periodontal ligament that is adjacent to the normal cementum follows the bulbous periphery of the lesion, becoming integrated with the capsular fibrous tissue that separates it from the normal bone. The peripheral zone of the lesion is relatively acellular (Figure 5-34, *A*), whereas the central zone is composed of more mineralized tissue with intervening areas of soft tissue that is loose, very cellular, and exhibits an increase in vascularity. Multinucleated cells are abundant in the cellular central areas and are associated with active resorption. The mineralized tissue exhibits increased numbers of reversal lines, which is indicative of extensive remodelling during the growth of the lesion (Figure 5-34, *B*). The root of the involved normal tooth sometimes extends to the center of the lesion, and the neoplastic cemental tissue is continous with the normal cemental layer.

TREATMENT

Regardless of size, treatment of the lesion requires removal of the associated tooth. Since this lesion is well encapsulated, enucleation of the lesion from its bony crypt is usually easily accomplished. Recurrences have not been reported.

MIXED ODONTOGENIC TUMORS

Mixed odontogenic tumors contain a combination of the epithelial and connective tissue elements found in all stages of odontogenesis. In the ameloblastic fibroma, the two tissue components represent an early stage of odontogenesis, before the formation of the calcified structures of enamel and dentin. The odontoma represents the opposing end stage of odontogenesis, containing primarily

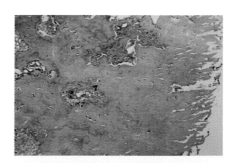

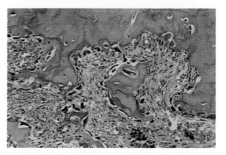

FIGURE 5-34

Cementoblastoma. Microscopic features of periphery exhibiting wide zone of hyalinized matrix ("cementoid") **(A)** and central area of increased activity of osteoblasts and osteoclasts in cellular fibrous connective tissue **(B)**.

mature enamel, dentin, and pulp. There is also an intermediate lesion, the ameloblastic fibro-odontoma, in which the tissues of all stages of odontogenesis are represented.

AMELOBLASTIC FIBROMA

■ AMELOBLASTIC FIBROMA: a circumscribed lesion predominantly located over unerupted molars in young patients; the epithelium and connective tissue recapitulate the cap and bell stages of odontogenesis.

The ameloblastic fibroma is a true histologic biphasic tumor because the epithelial and mesenchymal components are part of the neoplastic process. Questions have arisen regarding the exact nature of the tumor because some sources have suggested that it may be the most immature form of an odontoma. This suggestion has recently been largely disregarded because further studies of odontogenic lesions indicated that the age groups for the two lesions were identical, and the incidences and sex predilection of the two lesions differed, factors that should be the same if ameloblastic fibroma evolves into odontoma.

CLINICAL
The ameloblastic fibroma most commonly occurs in young patients with an average age of 14 years. It has occasionally occurred in older patients up to the age of 40. It is slow growing and commonly located in the mandibular molar area, often over an unerupted tooth. If the ameloblastic fibroma is near the surface, slight buccal and lingual cortical expansion is evident. Other symptoms are frequently missing.

RADIOGRAPHIC
Lesions are most often over an unerupted tooth. They are unilocular or multilocular radiolucencies (Figure 5-35) that are well corticated and vary considerably in size.

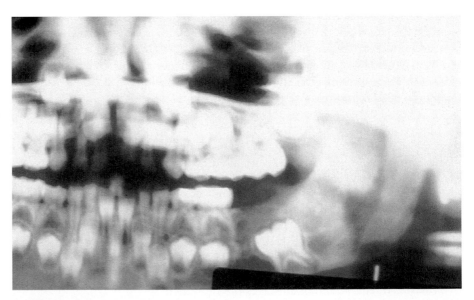

FIGURE 5-35

Ameloblastic fibroma. Panoramic radiograph of multilocular radiolucent lesion superior to the crown of an impacted mandibular first molar.

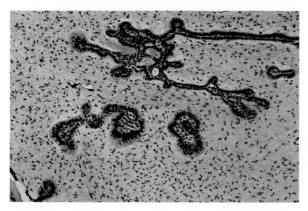

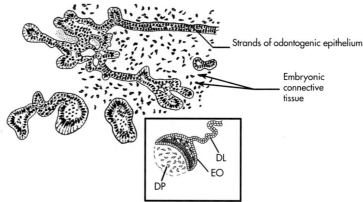

Strands of odontogenic epithelium

Embryonic connective tissue

DL, Dental lamina
EO, Enamel organ
DP, Dental papilla

FIGURE 5-36

Ameloblastic fibroma. Microscopic features consist of strands and islands of odontogenic epithelium resembling the dental lamina and cap stage of odontogenesis. *Inset:* tumor recapitulates the invagination of the dental lamina and cap stage of the earliest phases of odontogenesis.

HISTOPATHOLOGY

The microscopic appearance consists of thin strands and cords of odontogenic epithelium that resemble the dental lamina and the cap and bell stages of early odontogenesis. The background is composed of embryonic connective tissue containing randomly oriented and widely separated fibroblasts (Figure 5-36). Zones of hyalinization, sometimes with associated focal areas of calcification, are often found surrounding the epithelial component of the lesion.

TREATMENT

The lesion is well encapsulated and easily separated from the surrounding bony crypt. There have been a relatively high number of recurrences for a benign lesion. As the lesion is well circumscribed, recurrences are considered to be due to inadequate initial removal of what are frequently multiloblular lesions.

ODONTOMA

> ■ ODONTOMA: a usually hamartomatous lesion commonly found over unerupted teeth, containing enamel, dentin, pulp, and cementum in either recognizable tooth shapes (compound) or a solid gnarled mass (complex).

Odontomas are composed of mature enamel, dentin, and pulp and may be *compound* or *complex*, depending on the extent of morphodifferentiation or on their resemblance to normal teeth. Because most occur during the period of normal tooth development and often reach a fixed size, they are not considered true neoplasms, but *hamartomas*.

CLINICAL

Odontomas are by far the most common noncystic odontogenic lesions, representing nearly 70% of all odontogenic tumors. Nearly all are found in patients who are in the first and second decades. Odontomas more commonly occur in

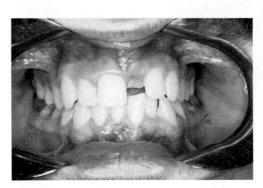

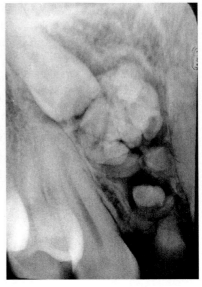

FIGURE 5-37

Odontoma. A, Common clinical finding in patients with an odontoma is the retention of a deciduous tooth and the failure of the permanent tooth to erupt. **B,** Radiograph of same patient revealing the presence of multiple individual toothlike structures in a well-demarcated bone cavity impeding the eruption of the permanent central incisor.

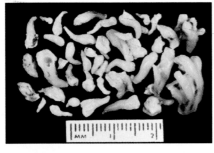

FIGURE 5-38

Compound odontoma. Multiple conical and irregularly shaped miniature teeth removed from within the capsule of a large lesion.

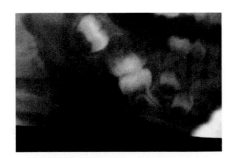

FIGURE 5-39

Complex odontoma. Radiograph of posterior mandible containing a dense structureless radiopacity preventing the eruption of an impacted molar in a young patient.

the maxilla than the mandible. Lesions are usually discovered because a tooth fails to erupt at its scheduled time (Figure 5-37, *A*). When the associated tooth is able to erupt around the odontoma, an asymptomatic swelling may be the only clinical evidence that a lesion is present.

RADIOGRAPHIC

Compound odontomas are usually located in the anterior part of the mouth, either over the crowns of unerupted teeth or between the roots of erupted ones. Lesions are usually unilocular, containing multiple radiopaque structures that resemble miniature teeth (Figure 5-37, *B*). Compound odontomas may contain as few as 2 to 3 miniature toothlike structures or as many 20 to 30 (Figure 5-38).

Complex odontomas are found in the posterior parts of the mandible over impacted teeth and can attain sizes up to several centimeters. They appear as a solid radiopaque mass exhibiting some nodularity and are surrounded by a thin radiolucent zone (Figure 5-39). The lesions are unilocilar and separated from normal bone by a distinct line of cortication. Individual toothlike structures are absent.

HISTOPATHOLOGY

The enamel, dentin, and pulpal tissue of the toothlike structures of compound odontoma are arranged in an orderly pattern. Within the surrounding capsule, each miniature conical tooth is separated by a thin band of follicular connective tissue. Complex odontoma differs by being composed of a single, gnarled, disorganized mass of enamel, dentin, and pulp with no recognizable tooth shapes (Figure 5-40). Both compound and complex forms may also contain reduced enamel epithelium, secretory ameloblasts, and functional odontoblasts. Islands of odontogenic rests and spherical calcifications are common in the surrounding connective tissue.

TREATMENT

Both forms of odontoma are well encapsulated and easily enucleated from the surrounding bone. No recurrences have been recorded.

AMELOBLASTIC FIBRO-ODONTOMA

■ **AMELOBLASTIC FIBRO-ODONTOMA:** an expansile growth in young patients that contains the soft tissue components of ameloblastic fibroma and the hard tissue components of complex odontoma.

The ameloblastic fibro-odontoma is a recently defined entity in which both ameloblastic fibroma and complex odontoma appear to be combined into one lesion. It has many clinical features in common with complex odontoma but differs significantly by having a greater potential for growth and local destruction. Care must be taken not to confuse this lesion with the *odontoameloblastoma*, an extremely rare form of ameloblastoma in which toothlike structures occur.

CLINICAL

The ameloblastic fibro-odontoma occurs in the first and second decades, the same age group as both odontoma and ameloblastic fibroma. It is primarily located in the posterior areas of the mandible but may be found in other locations. It appears as a slowly developing swelling of the affected portion of the jaw, usually in the area of an unerupted tooth. Pain is rarely associated with this lesion.

RADIOGRAPHIC

The radiograph exhibits a large, unilocular, well-circumscribed, mixed radiolucent/radiopaque lesion. The amount of soft and hard tissue components can vary extensively because both components are capable of dominating the lesion. The opacities are usually diffuse and nodular and present as a single large area or as several smaller dispersed deposits (Figure 5-41). Most lesions also contain an impacted tooth.

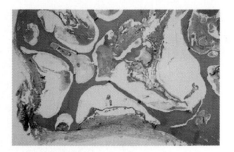

FIGURE 5-40

Complex odontoma. Microscopic appearance reveals irregular spaces containing residual elements of enamel matrix surrounded by septae of dentin interspersed with occasional areas of pulpal tissue. A fibrous connective tissue capsule is present in the periphery.

■ **BOX 5-1**
Odontogenic Tumors Predominantly Occurring in Young Patients

Odontoma
Cementoblastoma
Ameloblastic fibroma
Adenomatoid odontogenic tumor

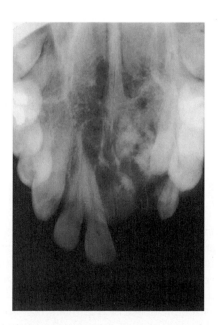

FIGURE 5-41

Ameloblastic fibro-odontoma. Radiograph of mixed radiolucent/opaque lesion of anterior maxilla preventing the eruption of the central incisor.

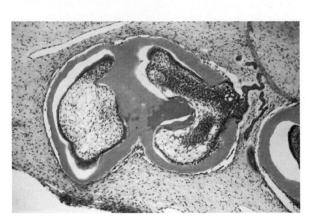

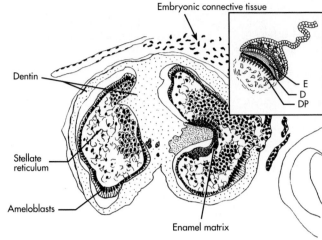

EO, Enamel organ
D, Dentin
E, Enamel
DP, Dental papilla

FIGURE 5-42

Ameloblastic fibro-odontoma. Photomicrograph of the irregularly shaped dentin deposits, enamel matrix, and odontogenic epithelium against a background of fibrillar connective tissue containing randomly oriented spindled cells. *Inset:* tumor recapitulates cells from all phases of tooth development, including enamel and dentin production as found in the late bell stage of odontogenesis.

HISTOPATHOLOGY

The radiolucent areas are composed of soft tissue that resembles ameloblastic fibroma. These areas consist of strands and cords of epithelium that resemble dental lamina against a background of embryonic connective tissue composed of randomly oriented fibroblasts. In adjacent areas, both mature and immature forms of complex odontoma can be found (Figure 5-42). The lesion may be slightly lobular but is always surrounded by a well-formed capsule.

TREATMENT

Ameloblastic fibro-odontoma is treated in the same manner as ameloblastic fibroma. Careful enucleation is required because the possibility of recurrence exists if lesional tissue remains.

■ BOX 5-2
Odontogenic Tumors Commonly Exhibiting Calcifications

Adenomatoid odontogenic tumor
Ameloblastic fibroma
Cementoblastoma
Odontoma
Calcifying odontogenic cyst
Ameloblastic fibro-odontoma
Calcifying epithelial odontogenic tumor

MALIGNANT ODONTOGENIC TUMORS

Since several of the odontogenic tumors can be locally destructive and even life threatening, particularly when located in the maxilla, the designation of malignancy is best reserved for those in which *metastasis* has occurred. It is also used to predict the anticipated future behavior of some odontogenic lesions that have cytologic features that are associated with malignancy. Even when using both of these criteria, the reported incidence of true malignant odontogenic tumors has been extremely low. The following is one classification of malignant epithelial odontogenic tumors. The lesions are in ascending order according to degree of malignancy.

MALIGNANT AMELOBLASTOMA

> ■ MALIGNANT AMELOBLASTOMA: a lesion with the histopathologic features of common ameloblastoma in which a metastasis has occurred.

A small number of ameloblastomas that appear cytologically benign have been documented in which a metastasis has occurred to regional lymph nodes or to other distant sites, the lungs being most common. In many cases these ameloblastomas recurred repeatedly, requiring multiple surgical procedures; in other cases, the metastasis occurred when the lesion was first discovered. Thus presence of a documented metastasis in an otherwise cytologically benign-appearing ameloblastoma has been termed *malignant ameloblastoma*.

AMELOBLASTIC CARCINOMA

> ■ AMELOBLASTIC CARCINOMA: an aggressive neoplasm of the mandible or maxilla in which the epithelial cells exhibit cytologic features of common ameloblastoma and malignancy.

The ameloblastic carcinoma differs from malignant ameloblastoma in that portions of its epithelial component are composed of cytologically malignant cells, yet the lesion is still readily recognizable as ameloblastoma (Figure 5-43). The histologic features portend the aggressive behavior of the lesion. If metastasis has not already occurred at the time of discovery, surgery (more aggressive than usual for ameloblastoma) is required to prevent this eventuality.

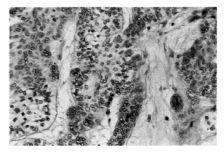

FIGURE 5-43

Ameloblastic carcinoma. Microscopic findings reveal features of ameloblastoma *(left bottom)* and cellular atypia of malignancy *(center and right).*

ODONTOGENIC CARCINOMA

> ■ ODONTOGENIC CARCINOMA: an aggressive and destructive intraosseous lesion of the mandible or maxilla that consists of poorly differented epithelial cells and clear cells in a pattern that is reminiscent of early odontogenesis.

The odontogenic carcinoma is an uncommon intraosseous epithelial malignancy that has features that are indicative of an odontogenic origin but not specific

FIGURE 5-44

Odontogenic carcinoma. A, Panoramic radiograph exhibiting a diffuse, multilocular mottled radiolucency of posterior mandible. **B,** Microscopic features consist of islands and lobular accumulations of clear and eosinophilic epithelial cells exhibiting atypia and an infiltrative pattern.

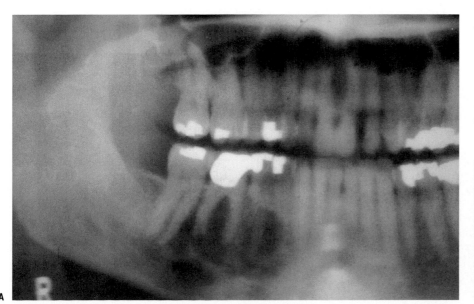

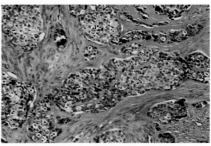

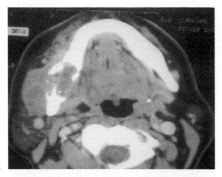

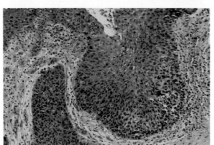

FIGURE 5-45

Primary intraosseous carcinoma. A, Computed tomograph (CT) of posterior mandible demonstrating a large area of bony destruction. **B,** Photomicrograph of squamous cell carcinoma within body of mandible with features that indicate origination from the epithelial lining of a cyst.

enough to relate it to a particular benign odontogenic tumor. The radiographic appearance exhibits a diffuse honeycomb radiolucency, features that are consistent with an aggressive destructive intraosseous lesion (Figure 5-44, *A*). Most lesions have a significant portion of their neoplastic element composed of islands and strands of "clear cells" (Figure 5-44, *B*). The nonclear cell component resembles cells of the dental lamina. The epithelial structures are usually surrounded by zones of myxomatous connective tissue that are reminiscent of the inductive activity that occurs in odontogenesis. The usual features of malignancy (such as high mitotic index, hyperchromatism, and pleomorphism) are not usually found in these lesions. Their cytologically benign appearance often masks their true identity. Odontogenic carcinoma is difficult to cure because it is very infiltrative and has a high rate of recurrence.

PRIMARY INTRAOSSEOUS CARCINOMA

■ **PRIMARY INTRAOSSEOUS CARCINOMA:** a squamous cell carcinoma within the mandible or maxilla with no indication that it originated from surface epithelium or that it metastasized from another site.

When located within the jaws, particularly when there is no breach of the overlying mucosa, the lesion is considered a malignant neoplasm of odontogenic origin because the remnants of odontogenesis are the only source of intraosseous epithelium once a metastasis from a distant site has been ruled out. In the maxilla, assuming an odontogenic origin is much more difficult because epithelium is present in the lining of the sinuses and in nasopalatine duct cysts. The primary intraosseous carcinoma behaves like any other intraosseous malignancy, destroying large areas of bone (Figure 5-45, *A*), resorbing roots of teeth, invading nerve trunks, and metastasizing regionally and to distant organs. In many intraosseous carcinomas, evidence of their origination from the lining of a preexisting odontogenic cyst, most commonly a dentigerous cyst, can be found (Figure 5-45, *B*).

Treatment is usually aggressive and often requires regional neck dissection followed by radiation and/or chemotherapy.

ADDITIONAL READING

GENERAL

Kramer IRH, Pindborg JJ, Shear M. Histologic typing of odontogenic tumours. In: *WHO International Histological Classification of Tumours.* 2nd ed. New York: Springer-Verlag; 1992.

AMELOBLASTOMA

Cowan PW. Cystic ameloblastoma. *J Ir Dent Assoc.* 1987; 33: 22-4.

Gardner DG. Radiotherapy in the treatment of ameloblastoma. *Int J Oral Maxillofac Surg.* 1988; 17:201-5.

Joseph BK, Savage NW. Maxillary ameloblastoma: case report and review of the literature. *Aust Dent J.* 1992; 37:98-102.

Kaffe I, Buchner A, Taicher S. Radiologic features of desmoplastic variant of ameloblastoma. *Oral Surg Oral Med Oral Pathol.* 1993; 76:525-9.

Nauta JM, Panders AK, Schoots CJ, Vermey A and others. Peripheral ameloblastoma: a case report and review of the literature. *Int J Oral Maxillofac Surg.* 1992; 21:40-4.

Ng KH, Siar CH. Peripheral ameloblastoma with clear cell differentiation. *Oral Surg Oral Med Oral Pathol.* 1990; 70: 210-3.

Philipsen HP, Ormiston IW, Reichart PA. The desmo- and osteoplastic ameloblastoma: histologic variant or clinicopathologic entity? *Int J Oral Maxillofac Surg.* 1992; 21:352-7.

Redman RS, Keegan BP, Spector CJ, Patterson RH. Peripheral ameloblastoma with unusual mitotic activity and conflicting evidence regarding histogenesis. *J Oral Maxillofac Surg.* 1994; 52:192-7.

Williams TP. Management of ameloblastoma: a changing perspective. *J Oral Maxillofac Surg.* 1993; 51:1064-70.

Yoshimura Y, Saito H. Desmoplastic variant of ameloblastoma: report of a case and review of the literature. *J Oral Maxillofac Surg.* 1990; 48:1231-5.

CALCIFYING EPITHELIAL ODONTOGENIC TUMOR

Chomette G, Auriol M, Guilbert F. Histoenzymological and ultrastructural study of a bifocal calcifying epithelial odontogenic tumor: characteristics of epithelial cells and histogenesis of amyloid-like material. *Virchows Arch A Pathol Anat Histopathol.* 1984; 403:67-76.

Damm DD, White DK, Drummond JF, Poindexter JB and others. Combined epithelial odontogenic tumor: adenomatoid odontogenic tumor and calcifying epithelial odontogenic tumor. *Oral Surg Oral Med Oral Pathol.* 1983; 55:487-96.

Ficarra G, Hansen LS, Stiesmeyer EH. Intramural calcifying epithelial odontogenic tumor. *Int J Oral Maxillofac Surg.* 1987; 16:217-21.

Hicks MJ, Flaitz CM, Wong ME, McDaniel RK and others. Clear cell variant of calcifying epithelial odontogenic tumor. *Head Neck.* 1994; 16:272-7.

Maranda G, Gourgi M. Calcifying epithelial odontogenic tumor (Pindborg tumor): review of the literature and case report. *J Can Dent Assoc.* 1986; 52:1009-12.

Morimoto C, Tsujimoto M, Shimaoka S, Shirasu R and others. Ultrastructural localization of alkaline phosphatase in the calcifying epithelial odontogenic tumor. *Oral Surg Oral Med Oral Pathol.* 1983; 56:409-14.

Nelson SR, Schow SR, Read LA, Svane TJ. Treatment of an extensive calcifying epithelial odontogenic tumor of the mandible. *J Oral Maxillofac Surg.* 1992; 50:1126-31.

Okada Y, Mochizuki K, Sugimura M, Noda Y and others. Odontogenic tumor with combined characteristics of adenomatoid odontogenic and calcifying epithelial odontogenic tumors. *Pathol Res Pract.* 1987; 182:647-57.

Pindborg JJ, Vedtofte P, Reibel J, Praetorius F. The calcifying epithelial odontogenic tumor. *APMIS Suppl.* 1991; 23:152-7.

Schmidt-Westhausen A, Philipsen HP, Reichart PA. Clear cell calcifying epithelial odontogenic tumor. *Int J Oral Maxillofac Surg.* 1992; 21:47-9.

Takeda Y, Suzuki A, Sekiyama S. Peripheral calcifying epithelial odontogenic tumor. *Oral Surg Oral Med Oral Pathol.* 1983; 56:71-5.

ADENOMATOID ODONTOGENIC TUMOR

Aldred MJ, Gray AR. A pigmented adenomatoid odontogenic tumor. *Oral Surg Oral Med Oral Pathol.* 1990; 70:86-9.

Philipsen HP, Reichart PA, Zhang KH, Nikai H and others. Adenomatoid odontogenic tumor: biologic profile based on 499 cases. *J Oral Pathol Med.* 1991; 20:149-58.

Philipsen HP, Samman N, Ormiston IW, Wu PC and others. Variants of the adenomatoid odontogenic tumor with a note on tumor origin. *J Oral Pathol Med.* 1992; 21:348-52.

CALCIFYING ODONTOGENIC CYST

Buchner A. The central (intraosseous) calcifying odontogenic cyst: an analysis of 215 cases. *J Oral Maxillofac Surg.* 1991; 49:330-9.

Buchner A, Merrell PW, Carpenter WM, Leider AS. Central (intraosseous) calcifying odontogenic cyst. *Int J Oral Maxillofac Surg.* 1990; 19:260-2.

Buchner A, Merrell PW, Hansen LS, Leider AS. Peripheral (extraosseous) calcifying odontogenic cyst: a review of forty-five cases. *Oral Surg Oral Med Oral Pathol.* 1991; 72:65-70.

Gunhan O, Celasun B, Can C, Finci R. The nature of ghost cells in calcifying odontogenic cyst: an immunohistochemical study. *Ann Dent.* 1993; 52:30-3.

Hong SP, Ellis GL, Hartman KS. Calcifying odontogenic cyst: a review of ninety-two cases with reevaluation of their nature as cysts or neoplasms, the nature of ghost cells, and subclassification. *Oral Surg Oral Med Oral Pathol.* 1991; 72: 56-64.

Kaugars CC, Kaugars GE, DeBiasi GF. Extraosseous calcifying odontogenic cyst: report of case and review of literature. *J Am Dent Assoc.* 1989; 119:715-8.

Shamaskin RG, Svirsky JA, Kaugars GE. Intraosseous and extraosseous calcifying odontogenic cyst (Gorlin cyst). *J Oral Maxillofac Surg.* 1989; 47:562-5.

SQUAMOUS ODONTOGENIC TUMOR

Baden E, Doyle J, Mesa M, Fabie M and others. Squamous odontogenic tumor: report of three cases including the first extraosseous case. *Oral Surg Oral Med Oral Pathol.* 1993; 75:733-8.

Batsakis JG, Cleary KR. Squamous odontogenic tumor. *Ann Otol Rhinol Laryngol.* 1993; 102:823-4.

Goldblatt LI, Brannon RB, Ellis GL. Squamous odontogenic tumor: report of five cases and review of the literature. *Oral Surg Oral Med Oral Pathol.* 1982; 54:187-96.

Hopper TL, Sadeghi EM, Pricco DF. Squamous odontogenic tumor: report of a case with multiple lesions. *Oral Surg Oral Med Oral Pathol.* 1980; 50:404-10.

Leider AS, Jonker LA, Cook HE. Multicentric familial squamous odontogenic tumor. *Oral Surg Oral Med Oral Pathol.* 1989; 68:175-81.

Leventon GS, Happonen RP, Newland JR. Squamous odontogenic tumor. *Am J Surg Pathol.* 1981; 5:671-7.

Saxby MS, Rippin JW, Sheron JE. Case report: squamous odontogenic tumor of the gingiva. *J Periodontol.* 1993; 64:1250-2.

Schwartz-Arad D, Lustmann J, Ulmansky M. Squamous odontogenic tumor: review of the literature and case report. *Int J Oral Maxillofac Surg.* 1990; 19:327-30.

Tatemoto Y, Okada Y, Mori M. Squamous odontogenic tumor: immunohistochemical identification of keratins. *Oral Surg Oral Med Oral Pathol.* 1989; 67:63-7.

ODONTOGENIC FIBROMA

Buchner A. Peripheral odontogenic fibroma: report of 5 cases. *J Craniomaxillofac Surg.* 1989; 17:134-8.

Ficarra G, Sapp JP, Eversole LR. Multiple peripheral odontogenic fibroma, WHO type, and central giant cell granuloma: a case report of an unusual association. *J Oral Maxillofac Surg.* 1993; 51: 325-28.

Gardner DG. The peripheral odontogenic fibroma: an attempt at clarification. *Oral Surg Oral Med Oral Pathol.* 1982; 54: 40-8.

Handlers JP, Abrams AM, Melrose RJ, Danforth R. Central odontogenic fibroma: clinicopathologic features of 19 cases and review of the literature. *J Oral Maxillofac Surg.* 1991; 49:46-54.

Kaffe I, Buchner A. Radiologic features of central odontogenic fibroma. *Oral Surg Oral Med Oral Pathol.* 1994; 78:811-8.

Shiro BC, Jacoway JR, Mirmiran SA, McGuirt WF and others. Central odontogenic fibroma, granular cell variant: a case report with S-100 immunohistochemistry and a review of the literature. *Oral Surg Oral Med Oral Pathol.* 1989; 67: 725-30.

ODONTOGENIC MYXOMA

Cuestas-Carnero R, Bachur RO, Gendelman H. Odontogenic myxoma: report of a case. *J Oral Maxillofac Surg.* 1988; 46:705-9.

Zachariades N, Papanicolaou S. Treatment of odontogenic myxoma: review of the literature and report of three cases. *Ann Dent.* 1987; 46:34-7, 40.

CEMENTOBLASTOMA

Cannell H. Cementoblastoma of deciduous tooth. *Oral Surg Oral Med Oral Pathol.* 1991; 71:648.

Jelic JS, Loftus MJ, Miller AS, Cleveland DB. Benign cementoblastoma: report of an unusual case and analysis of 14 additional cases. *J Oral Maxillofac Surg.* 1993; 51:1033-7.

Slootweg PJ. Cementoblastoma and osteoblastoma: a comparison of histologic features. *J Oral Pathol Med.* 1992; 21:385-9.

Ulmansky M, Hjorting-Hansen E, Praetorius F, Haque MF. Benign cementoblastoma: a review and five new cases. *Oral Surg Oral Med Oral Pathol.* 1994; 77:48-55.

AMELOBLASTIC FIBROMA

Becker J, Reichart PA, Schuppan D, Philipsen HP. Ectomesenchyme of ameloblastic fibroma reveals a characteristic distribution of extracellular matrix proteins. *J Oral Pathol Med.* 1992; 21:156-9.

ODONTOMA

Baker WR, Swift JQ. Ameloblastic fibro-odontoma of the anterior maxilla: report of a case. *Oral Surg Oral Med Oral Pathol.* 1993; 76:294-7.

Carr MM. Compound odontoma: case report and brief review. *Ont Dent.* 1990; 67:24-6.

Gallien GS, Schuman NJ, Sharp HK, McIlveen LP. Odontoma of a maxillary central incisor in a 10-year-old black male. *J Pedod.* 1986; 10:352-5.

Kaugars GE, Zussmann HW. Ameloblastic odontoma (odontoameloblastoma). *Oral Surg Oral Med Oral Pathol.* 1991; 71:371-3.

Kerebel LM, Kerebel B. Dysplastic enamel in odontoma: a light microscopic, microradiographic and SEM study. *J Oral Pathol.* 1984; 13:137-46.

Kitano M, Tsuda-Yamada S, Semba I, Mimura T and others. Pigmented ameloblastic fibro-odontoma with melanophages. *Oral Surg Oral Med Oral Pathol.* 1994; 77:271-5.

Piattelli A, Trisi P. Morphodifferentiation and histodifferentiation of the dental hard tissues in compound odontoma: a study of undemineralized material. *J Oral Pathol Med.* 1992; 21:340-2.

AMELOBLASTIC FIBRO-ODONTOMA

Baroni C, Farneti M, Stea S, Rimondini L. Ameloblastic fibroma and impacted mandibular first molar: a case report. *Oral Surg Oral Med Oral Pathol.* 1992; 73:548-9.

Blankestijn J, Panders AK, Wymenga JP. Ameloblastic fibroma of the mandible. *Br J Oral Maxillofac Surg.* 1986; 24:417-21.

Cataldo E, Giunta JL. A clinico-pathological presentation: ameloblastic fibroma. *J Mass Dent Soc.* 1984; 33:158.

Farman AG, Gould AR, Merrell E. Epithelium-connective tissue junction in follicular ameloblastoma and ameloblastic fibroma: an ultrastructural analysis. *Int J Oral Maxillofac Surg.* 1986; 15:176-86.

Slootweg PJ. An analysis of the interrelationship of the mixed odontogenic tumors: ameloblastic fibroma, ameloblastic fibro-odontoma, and the odontomas. *Oral Surg Oral Med Oral Pathol.* 1981; 51:266-76.

Takeda Y. Granular cell ameloblastic fibroma: ultrastructure and histogenesis. *Int J Oral Maxillofac Surg.* 1986; 15:190-5.

MALIGNANT AMELOBLASTOMA

Eliasson AH, Moser RJ, Tenholder MF. Diagnosis and treatment of metastatic ameloblastoma. *South Med J.* 1989; 82:1165-8.

Laughlin EH. Metastasizing ameloblastoma. *Cancer.* 1989; 64:776-80.

Matear DW, Crewe TC. Malignant ameloblastoma: a case report and review of literature outlining problems in diagnosis and treatment. *J R Nav Med Serv.* 1991; 77:5-10.

Pradhan SA, Soman CS, Patel A. Well differentiated metastasizing ameloblastoma: report of a case with review of literature. *Indian J Cancer.* 1989; 26:255-9.

Sheppard BC, Temeck BK, Taubenberger JK, Pass HI. Pulmonary metastatic disease in ameloblastoma. *Chest.* 1993; 104:1933-5.

AMELOBLASTIC CARCINOMA

Bruce RA, Jackson IT. Ameloblastic carcinoma: report of an aggressive case and review of the literature. *J Craniomaxillofac Surg.* 1991; 19:267-71.

Corio RL, Goldblatt LI, Edwards PA, Hartman KS.

Ameloblastic carcinoma: a clinicopathologic study and assessment of eight cases. *Oral Surg Oral Med Oral Pathol.* 1987; 64:570-6.

Gandy SR, Keller EE, Unni KK. Ameloblastic carcinoma: report of two cases. *J Oral Maxillofac Surg.* 1992; 50:1097-102.

Lee L, Maxymiw WG, Wood RE. Ameloblastic carcinoma of the maxilla metastatic to the mandible: case report. *J Craniomaxillofac Surg.* 1990; 18:247-50.

McClatchey KD, Sullivan MJ, Paugh DR. Peripheral ameloblastic carcinoma: a case report of a rare neoplasm. *J Otolaryngol.* 1989; 18:109-11.

Muller S, DeRose PB, Cohen C. DNA ploidy of ameloblastoma and ameloblastic carcinoma of the jaws: analysis by image and flow cytometry. *Arch Pathol Lab Med.* 1993; 117:1126-31.

Nagai N, Takeshita N, Nagatsuka H, Inoue M and others. Ameloblastic carcinoma: case report and review. *J Oral Pathol Med.* 1991; 20:460-3.

Slootweg PJ, Muller H. Malignant ameloblastoma or ameloblastic carcinoma. *Oral Surg Oral Med Oral Pathol.* 1984; 57:168-76.

ODONTOGENIC CARCINOMA

Bang G, Koppang HS, Hansen LS, Gilhuus-Moe O and others. Clear cell odontogenic carcinoma: report of three cases with pulmonary and lymph node metastases. *J Oral Pathol Med.* 1989; 18:113-8.

Fan J, Kubota E, Imamura H, Shimokama T and others. Clear cell odontogenic carcinoma: a case report with massive invasion of neighboring organs and lymph node metastasis. *Oral Surg Oral Med Oral Pathol.* 1992; 74:768-75.

Grodjesk JE, Dolinsky HB, Schneider LC, Dolinsky EH and others. Odontogenic ghost cell carcinoma. *Oral Surg Oral Med Oral Pathol.* 1987; 63:576-81.

Milles M, Doyle JL, Mesa M, Raz S. Clear cell odontogenic carcinoma with lymph node metastasis. *Oral Surg Oral Med Oral Pathol.* 1993; 76:82-9.

Waldron CA, Small IA, Silverman H. Clear cell ameloblastoma: an odontogenic carcinoma. *J Oral Maxillofac Surg.* 1985; 43:707-17.

Yoshida T, Shingaki S, Nakajima T, Suzuki M and others. Odontogenic carcinoma with sarcomatous proliferation: a case report. *J Craniomaxillofac Surg.* 1989; 17:139-42.

PRIMARY INTRAOSSEOUS CARCINOMA

Elzay RP. Primary intraosseous carcinoma of the jaws: review and update of odontogenic carcinomas. *Oral Surg Oral Med Oral Pathol.* 1982; 54:299-303.

Minic AJ. Primary intraosseous squamous cell carcinoma arising in a mandibular keratocyst. *Int J Oral Maxillofac Surg.* 1992; 21:163-5.

Muller S, Waldron CA. Primary intraosseous squamous carcinoma: report of two cases. *Int J Oral Maxillofac Surg.* 1991; 20:362-5.

Ruskin JD, Cohen DM, Davis LF. Primary intraosseous carcinoma: report of two cases. *J Oral Maxillofac Surg.* 1988; 46:425-32.

Suei Y, Tanimoto K, Taguchi A, Wada T. Primary intraosseous carcinoma: review of the literature and diagnostic criteria. *J Oral Maxillofac Surg.* 1994; 52:580-3.

To EH, Brown JS, Avery BS, Ward-Booth RP. Primary intraosseous carcinoma of the jaws: three new cases and a review of the literature. *Br J Oral Maxillofac Surg.* 1991; 29:19-25.

Waldron CA, Mustoe TA. Primary intraosseous carcinoma of the mandible with probable origin in an odontogenic cyst. *Oral Surg Oral Med Oral Pathol.* 1989; 67:716-24.

EPITHELIAL DISORDERS

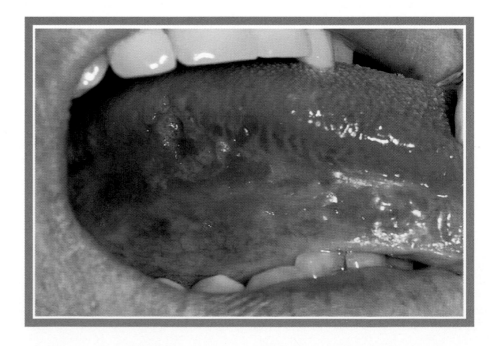

T he anatomic structures that surround the oral cavity are covered by a membrane composed of stratified squamous epithelium. The epithelium acts as both a cover for the oral soft tissue and a barrier to the passage of external pathogenic factors. The stratified squamous epithelium may have a superficial layer of orthokeratin, parakeratin, or be nonkeratinized. Depending on the specific intraoral site, the overall thickness will also vary. For example, the epithelium of the hard palate is normally thick, with the surface layer composed of orthokeratin, whereas the soft palate is thin, with the outer layer nonkeratinized. Detailed knowledge of the normal microscopic features of the epithelium in the various intraoral sites is essential when tissue is microscopically evaluated for the presence of abnormal findings.

An important component in diagnosing diseases of epithelium is an evaluation of the melanocytes. These cells are normally present in the basal cell layer where their numbers usually correspond with an individual's hereditary tendencies for skin pigmentation. Whether oral pigmentation is clinically visible depends on the amount of melanin granules elaborated by the melanocytes. In light-skinned individuals, the oral mucosa normally exhibits a uniform pink coloration. Individuals who are dark-skinned will often exhibit some pigmentation of the oral mucous membranes. Such intraoral pigmentation has been termed *physiologic* or *racial pigmentation* and may be most conspicuous on the labial gingiva but is also observed on the buccal and labial mucosa.

Multiple local and systemic factors can affect the oral epithelium and alter its normal clinical and microscopic appearances. Chronic local physical irritants such as tobacco smoke can act on the thin, normally nonkeratinized squamous epithelium to induce excessive thickening of the keratin and/or spinous cell layer. Additionally, constituents of tobacco smoke can stimulate the melanocytes to induce both local and generalized pigmentation of the oral mucosa ("smoker's melanosis").

Because numerous local and systemic factors affect the oral mucous membranes, a broad spectrum of hamartomatous, reactive, inflammatory, autoimmune, infectious, pigmented, dysplastic, and neoplastic lesions of epithelial origin are found in this anatomic location. These lesions may be local or diffuse and may appear clinically as macules, papules, papillary, white (leukoplakic), red (erythroplakic), ulcers, blue-black lesions, or as large ulcerated tumor masses. In this chapter the diseases that affect the epithelium are discussed under the general categories of benign, hyperplastic, and malignant lesions.

BENIGN EPITHELIAL LESIONS

SQUAMOUS PAPILLOMA

■ SQUAMOUS PAPILLOMA: a benign *exophytic* papillary growth of stratified squamous epithelium.

Squamous papilloma is a benign epithelial growth with etiology that has not been completely elucidated. It has been shown that in most cases benign papillary growths of the oral mucosa are caused by the human papilloma virus (HPV). Because it is not always possible to detect the virus within the epithelial cells, there is a belief that on occasion a focal papillary epithelial growth is a true benign epithelial neoplasm. A papillary lesion lacking evidence of HPV infection is referred to as squamous papilloma or *papilloma*. Some investigators contend that because these lesions also exhibit a number of the morphologic features seen in

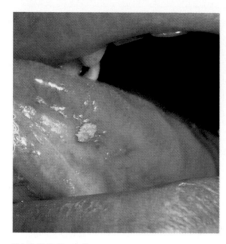

FIGURE 6-1

Papilloma of the left ventral surface of the tongue.

FIGURE 6-2

Papilloma. Low-power microscopic appearance with a diagrammatic inset illustrating the papillary projections composed of epithelium with thickened parakeratin and spinous cells layers and a central core of fibrous tissue with enlarged vascular structures.

verruca vulgaris and condyloma acuminatum, both of which are known to be caused by HPV, they still may be of viral etiology with the virus in undetectable numbers when using present research methodologies.

CLINICAL

The squamous papilloma is an exophytic papillary lesion that usually measures less than 1 cm. It may be sessile or pedunculated, white (keratinized), or pink (nonkeratinized). Most lesions are solitary and commonly occur on the soft palate, uvula, and ventral and dorsal surfaces of the tongue, gingiva, and buccal mucosa (Figure 6-1).

HISTOPATHOLOGY

The squamous papilloma is characterized by a thick papillary layer of keratinized or nonkeratinized squamous epithelium and a central core of fibrovascular connective tissue (Figure 6-2). The papillary projections may be either long and fingerlike or short, rounded, and blunt. The epithelium generally exhibits a normal maturation pattern, although a mild degree of basilar hyperplasia is sometimes seen. The histolologic variations seen in squamous papilloma may represent the normal morphologic spectrum of a single lesion, or it may be an indication that squamous papilloma is a heterogeneous group of papillary lesions with different etiologies. The latter possibility is likely since three of the lesions, once lumped within the spectrum of squamous papilloma (oral verruca vulgaris, oral condyloma acuminatum, and focal epithelial hyperplasia [Heck disease]), are now considered separate and distinct entities because they harbor subtypes of HPV (see Chapter 7).

TREATMENT

The treatment of squamous papilloma consists of surgical excision of the base of the lesion and a small area of surrounding normal tissue. Recurrence is uncommon.

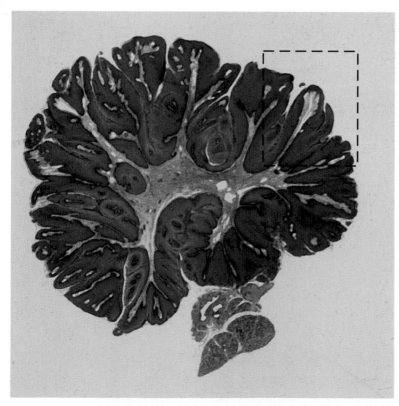

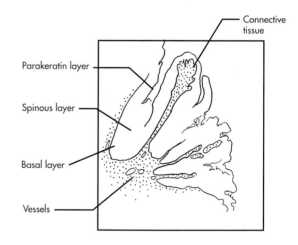

Connective tissue

Parakeratin layer

Spinous layer

Basal layer

Vessels

KERATOACANTHOMA

> ■ **KERATOACANTHOMA**: a benign *endophytic* epithelial growth appearing as a well-circumscribed keratin-filled crater on sun-exposed skin; often mistaken for squamous cell carcinoma.

The keratoacanthoma (KA) is a benign epithelial neoplasm that primarily occurs on sun-exposed skin, especially on the faces of patients 50 years of age and older. The male to female ratio for this tumor is approximately 2:1. Although most lesions occur on hair-bearing skin (cheeks, nose, eyelids, and ears), they also occur on the lower lip. It is believed that the neoplasm arises from the hair-follicle epithelium above the sebaceous glands. On the lower lip it probably arises from the superficial epithelium of sebaceous ducts or from the hair-follicle epithelium of adjacent skin.

CLINICAL
Most keratoacanthomas develop rapidly over a period of 1 to 2 months and occur as sharply circumscribed, bud-shaped nodules exhibiting a central keratin plug or keratin-filled crater (Figure 6-3). Its clinical appearance, rapid growth, and histologic appearance are all suggestive of squamous cell carcinoma. However, its frequent spontaneous regression (without treatment) suggests it is benign.

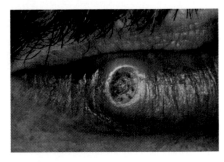

FIGURE 6-3
Keratoacanthoma of the lower lip. (Courtesy Dr. R.J. Achterberg.)

HISTOPATHOLOGY
When viewed with low power the microscopic appearance of keratoacanthoma resembles a well-differentiated squamous cell carcinoma. However, on closer observation, several important distinguishing features reveal its benign nature. These include a central plug of keratin surrounded by a sharply demarcated, cup-shaped buttress of normal epidermis (Figure 6-4); epithelium exhibiting a pseudocarcinomatous rather than a true carcinomatous growth pattern; epithelium composed of well-differentiated spinous cells with abundant cytoplasm and minimal nuclear pleomorphism, infrequent mitotic figures, and an absence of abnormal mitotic figures. The surrounding connective tissue usually exhibits a moderate to marked infiltrate of chronic inflammatory cells.

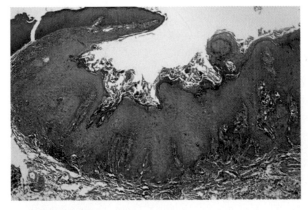

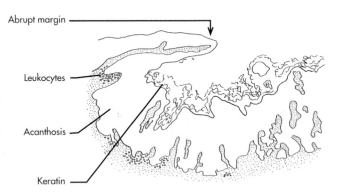

Abrupt margin

Leukocytes

Acanthosis

Keratin

FIGURE 6-4

Keratoacanthoma. Distinguishable microscopic features of one edge of the lesion demonstrating the cup-shaped appearance with a depressed center containing a keratin plug and the pseudocarcinomatous growth pattern of the basal cell layer.

TREATMENT

Although keratoacathomas regress spontaneously if left untreated, in most cases, the lesions are treated surgically before they reach their maximum size of 2.0 to 2.5 cm. Additionally, untreated lesions that regress on their own usually leave a depressed scar, which may be cosmetically unacceptable. Surgical excision of the lesion is considered the treatment of choice because this procedure is simultaneously curative, cosmetically acceptable, and provides a good tissue specimen to microscopically confirm the diagnosis.

BENIGN PIGMENTED LESIONS

A spectrum of pigmented lesions can occur within the oral cavity. The lesions described in this section are benign, and their pigmentation is largely due to the production and extracellular deposition of melanin. Melanin is produced by melanocytes, a specialized population of dendritic cells that normally populates the basal cell region of squamous epithelium in skin and mucous membranes. Increases in the number of melanocytes or amount of melanin produced by these cells usually result in increased clinically visible pigmentation. Depending on the amount and distribution of melanin present in the skin or mucosa, the color of a lesion will range between shades of brown, gray, black, and dark blue. Explanations for the differences in the coloration of pigmented lesions are (1) lesions with melanin confined to the basal cells appear brown, (2) lesions with melanin in the keratin and in the spinous cells appear black, and (3) lesions with melanin in the connective tissues appear blue.

MELANOTIC MACULES

■ MELANOTIC MACULE: physiologic or reactive small, flat, brown areas of the mucosal surfaces caused by an increase in the production of melanin granules but not in the number of melanocytes.

Small, pigmented macules occasionally occur on the lips and oral mucous membranes. The lip lesion is termed a **labial melanotic macule** and the intraoral lesion an **oral melanotic macule.** Although many melanotic macules of the mucosa represent foci of postinflammatory pigmentation, some may represent true ephelides (freckles).

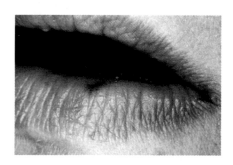

FIGURE 6-5
Labial melanotic macule of lower lip.

CLINICAL

The **labial melanotic macule** is an asymptomatic, small, flat, brown to brownish-black lesion that is primarily found on the vermilion border of the lower lip (Figure 6-5). Lesions can occur in patients at any age and are usually solitary but occasionally multiple. Most macules measure less than 5 mm in diameter and tend to occur near the midline of the lip.

An **oral melanotic macule** is the same lesion as the labial melanotic macule, except that it occurs within the confines of the oral cavity (Figure 6-6). Most oral melanotic macules are less than 1 cm in diameter and occur on the gingiva, buccal mucosa, and soft palate.

On rare occasions, solitary or multiple lesions varying in color from dark brown to black and ranging in size from 5 mm to over 2 cm in diameter have occurred on the buccal mucosa and palate of 20- to 40-year-old African-American patients. These lesions are referred to as **oral melanoacanthomas.** The lesions

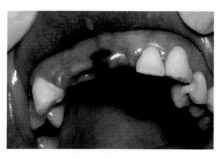

FIGURE 6-6
Oral melanotic macule. Darkly pigmented area on the anterior maxillary alveolar ridge.

are characterized by a proliferation of melanin-laden dendritic melanocytes; many present above the basal layer in an area of focally thickened epithelium. The epithelium exhibits extensive acanthosis and a mild parakeratosis. Oral melanoacanthomas can develop within a few months and occasionally resolve without treatment.

HISTOPATHOLOGY

The histologic features of the labial and oral melanotic macules are identical. They are characterized by an increase in the amount of melanin granules in the basal cell layer (Figure 6-7). The melanocytes are generally confined to the basal cell region and are usually within the normal numeric range. Occasionally, the melanocytes exhibit a conspicuous clear cytoplasm; however, nuclear atypia is absent. The basilar region of the epithelium and the superficial connective tissue often exhibit a mild infiltrate of lymphocytes and histiocytes. Small granular deposits of melanin, some within tissue histiocytes, are often visible in the superficial connective tissue. The leakage of melanin from the melanin-containing cells into the underlying connective tissue is often referred to as *melanin incontinence*.

TREATMENT

Although many melanotic macules arise slowly over time, some develop relatively quickly. Because a precise diagnosis may not be attainable through clinical examination alone, melanotic macules that arise within a short period should be excised to establish the actual diagnosis and to rule out the possibility of melanoma.

SMOKER'S MELANOSIS

> ■ SMOKER'S MELANOSIS: irregularly shaped brownish macular pigmentations of oral tissue that are associated with prolonged tobacco smoking.

Cigarette and pipe smoking commonly cause varying degrees of pigmentation of the oral mucosa. The increased pigmentation appears to be related to a constituent of tobacco smoke, which stimulates increased melanin production. A mild degree of smoker's melanosis is common in both male and female smokers and may be difficult to detect clinically, especially in individuals who exhibit significant amounts of normal physiologic pigmentation. Since some female hormones are known to amplify melanin pigmentation, a more intense mucosal pigmentation may occur in female smokers who use contraceptive pills.

CLINICAL

Smoker's melanosis is usually most conspicuous on the maxillary and mandibular anterior labial gingiva. Other intraoral sites commonly affected include the buccal mucosa, the floor of mouth, and the soft palate (Figure 6-8). It has been reported that smoker's melanosis of the soft palate should be viewed with concern because it has sometimes occurred in association with smoking-related diseases such as emphysema and bronchogenic carcinoma.

HISTOPATHOLOGY

A biopsy from an area of smoker's melanosis exhibits histologic features similar to those found in melanotic macule. There are increased melanin deposits within basal epithelial cells, and the underlying connective tissue exhibits a mild infiltrate of lymphocytes and histiocytes (Figure 6-9). The presence of melanin granules in the phagocytic cells of the superficial connective tissue is common.

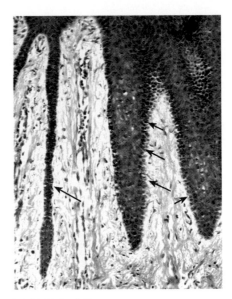

FIGURE 6-7

Melanotic macule. Microscopic features reveal an increase in the density of melanin granules in the basal cell layer *(arrows)*.

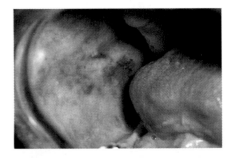

FIGURE 6-8

Smoker's melanosis of the buccal mucosa in an elderly patient who has smoked for many years.

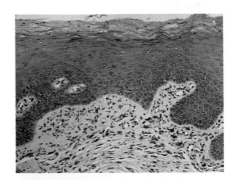

FIGURE 6-9

Smoker's melanosis. Microscopic features of melanin granules phagocytized by macrophages within the connective tissue in addition to the abundant granules present in the basal cells.

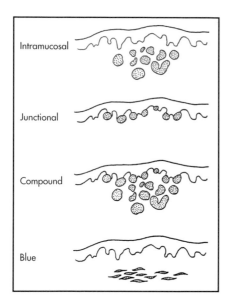

FIGURE 6-10

Diagram of the four histologic types of intra-oral nevi based on the location and shape of the nevus cells relative to the epithelium and the connective tissue.

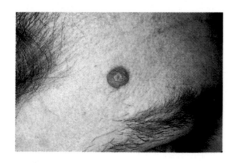

FIGURE 6-11

Intramucosal nevus presenting as a pigmented lesion of the palate.

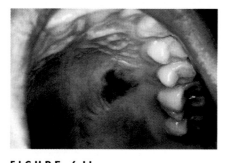

FIGURE 6-12

Lightly pigmented intradermal nevus of the skin of the forehead.

TREATMENT

The most effective treatment for smoker's melanosis is to stop smoking. This will usually result in elimination of the pigmentation within a few months. If the pigmentation persists after a period of not smoking, a biopsy to assess the lesion is advisable.

NEVI

> ■ **N E V U S :** a benign, exophytic, usually pigmented, congenital lesion of the skin or mucosa composed of focal collections (nests) of rounded melanocytes (nevus cells); depending on the location of the nevus cells, specific lesions are classified as **intradermal (mucosal), junctional,** or **compound;** a macular form, usually of the hard palate and composed of fusiform cells, is termed **blue nevus.**

The term "nevus" has several meanings. The common lay term for nevus is "mole." Most nevi occur on the skin; however, they occasionally occur on mucous membranes, including the oral cavity. Although intraoral nevi can occur in various sites, the majority are found on either the hard palate or the gingiva. Nevi are usually pigmented. Based on the distribution and morphology of nevus cells, nevi have been classified as *intramucosal (intradermal), junctional, compound,* and *blue* (Figure 6-10).

Intramucosal (Intradermal) Nevus

The terms **intramucosal nevus** and **intradermal nevus** are synonymous. The former occurs on mucosal surfaces, and the latter occurs on skin.

CLINICAL

Intradermal nevus occurs in young patients and is one of the most common lesions that occurs on the skin, where it is commonly referred to as a "mole." By comparison the intramucosal nevus in the oral cavity is a relatively uncommon occurrence. The intramucosal nevus of the oral cavity occurs as an asymptomatic, pigmented, brown to black, slightly elevated papule or flat macule on the hard palate or gingiva (Figure 6-11). The lesion grows very slowly and generally measures less than 1 cm in diameter.

On the skin the lesion can be raised or flat and tan or dark brown. It will often contain more hair than the skin in the surrounding area (Figure 6-12).

HISTOPATHOLOGY

The intramucosal nevus is characterized by nests (theques) and/or cords of nevus cells confined to the connective tissue (Figure 6-13). The morphology of the cells in the intradermal nevus is variable, and include epithelioid, lymphocyte-like, spindle, and multinucleated types. The amount and distribution of melanin is variable; some lesions have scant amounts. Mitotic figures are usually absent. A feature of the intramucosal nevus is the presence of a fibrous connective tissue zone, free of nevus cells, that separates the nevus cell theques from the overlying epithelium.

TREATMENT

As a general rule all solitary pigmented papules or nodules of the oral cavity should be excised and submitted for histopathologic evaluation. Intramucosal nevi are included in this category. Once excised, intramucosal nevi do not tend to recur.

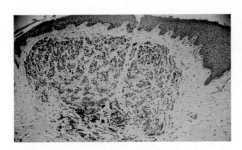
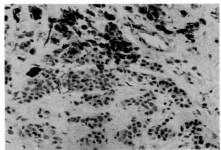

A   B

FIGURE 6-13

Intramucosal nevus. A, Low-power microscopic appearance of the nevus cells confined to a
circumscribed area and separated from the epithelium by a band of fibrous tissue. **B,** Higher magnification exhibiting the rounded or epithelioid form of the nevus cells arranged in characteristic
clusters or nests ("theques") with sporadic melanin production.

Junctional Nevus

CLINICAL

The junctional nevus is a benign, brown to black lesion that occurs primarily on
the skin and occasionally on the oral mucosa. This type of nevus is considerably
less common than the intramucosal (intradermal) nevus. Within the oral cavity
it usually appears as a pigmented macular lesion on the hard palate or gingiva.

HISTOPATHOLOGY

The junctional nevus is characterized by the presence of nevus cell nests in the
basilar region of the epithelium, primarily at the tips of the epithelial rete pegs.
There are no nevus cells in the adjacent connective tissue (Figure 6-14). Careful
examination of the individual cells is extremely important in the junctional nevus because a similar type of "junctional activity" occurs in the early phases of
melanoma—a malignant neoplasm consisting of melanocytes. It is important to
note that a junctional nevus can occasionally undergo malignant transformation
to a melanoma.

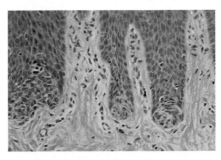

FIGURE 6-14

Junctional nevus. Microscopic appearance
demonstrating the clusters of nevus cells
confined to the basal cell layer of the epithelium.

TREATMENT

For the previously mentioned reasons, a solitary pigmented lesion of the oral
mucosa, particularly on the hard palate, should be excised and submitted for
histopathologic examination. Once excised, a junctional nevus does not tend to
recur.

Compound Nevus

The compound nevus has the combined characteristics of the intramucosal nevus and the junctional nevus, exhibiting nevus cells in the basal region of the epithelium and in the adjacent connective tissue (Figure 6-15). As is true of the
other nevi, the compound nevus is far more common on the skin than it is on the
oral mucosa. Within the oral cavity it also tends to occur as a pigmented papule
or macule on the hard palate or gingiva. As with other solitary pigmented oral
lesions the compound nevus is treated by an excisional biopsy, which simultaneously serves as a diagnostic and therapeutic procedure.

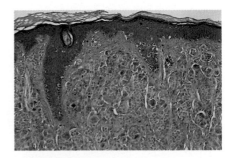

FIGURE 6-15

Compound nevus. Microscopic appearance exhibiting features of the intramucosal
and junctional nevus.

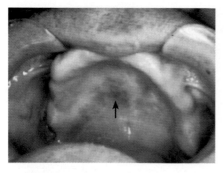

FIGURE 6-16

Blue nevus. The bluish lesion *(arrow)* is located in the middle of the hard palate, its most common intraoral location.

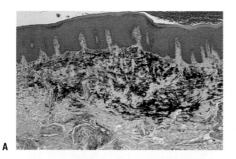

FIGURE 6-17

Blue nevus. A, Low-power microscopy illustrating the presence of melanin-laden cells confined to the connective tissue. **B,** High-power microscopy of lesion demonstrating the separated elongated spindle-shaped cells in their typical orientation parallel to the surface epithelium.

Blue Nevus

CLINICAL

The blue nevus is a benign pigmented lesion that presents as a dark blue dome-shaped papule or as a flat macule on the skin or mucosa. Within the oral cavity the blue nevus occurs most commonly on the hard palate (Figure 6-16).

HISTOPATHOLOGY

The melanin-producing cells of a blue nevus differ from those of the nevi previously discussed. In the blue nevus the pigment-producing cells are spindled and fusiform dendritic cells rather than rounded or epithelioid. The spindled dendritic nevus cells are confined to the connective tissue (Figure 6-17, *A*) . Instead of being arranged in rounded clusters (theques), they tend to be separated and parallel to the normal overlying epithelium (Figure 6-17, *B*). Variable numbers of melanin-containing macrophages (melanophages) are often present among the dendritic nevus cells. The blue nevus has no tendency to undergo malignant transformation.

TREATMENT

Because a blue nevus can clinically resemble a melanoma, a diagnostic excisional biopsy is usually performed, which also serves as the definitive treatment for this lesion.

LEUKOPLAKIA

> ■ LEUKOPLAKIA: a clinical term used to denote mucosal conditions that produce a whiter than normal coloration of the mucous membranes.

The term *leukoplakia* literally means "white patch. " It is used as a clinical term only to describe a variety of white mucosal lesions. Some diagnosticians prefer to restrict this term to those lesions that cannot be easily removed by gently rubbing the superficial mucosa, thus excluding lesions that produce a pseudomembrane (slough). In 1978 the World Health Organization (WHO) modified the concept even further by defining leukoplakia as "a white patch on the oral mucosa that can neither be scraped off *nor classified as any other diagnosable disease.*" In various parts of the world and among various diagnosticians, the term may be used slightly differently.

CLINICAL

Leukoplakic lesions have an occurrence rate of 1.5% to 12%, depending on the specific populaton studied. In general, approximately 5.4% of the lesions will eventuate in squamous cell carcinoma. If the patient is a smoker, this incidence can increase to 16%. Lesions can vary from flat, smooth, and slightly translucent macular areas to thick, firm, rough-surfaced, and fissured, raised plaques. The most common intraoral sites for leukoplakia are the buccal mucosa (Figure 6-18), the floor of the mouth, the labial commissures, the lateral borders of the tongue, and the mandibular and maxillary alveolar ridges.

Although leukoplakic lesions occasionally occur in nonsmokers, the use of smoked and smokeless tobacco is considered a strong etiologic factor in their development. Other factors that are known to play an etiologic role in some leukoplakias include premalignant changes, EBV infection in HIV-positive patients, chronic irritation caused by ill-fitting dentures, chronic infection by *Candida albicans*, chronic lichen planus, and some genetic disorders (Box 6-1).

HISTOPATHOLOGY

Because the designation "leukoplakia" does not indicate the exact nature of the tissue changes, a microscopic evaluation of the spectrum of the alterations that can be found within the mucosal epithelium must be undertaken. The epithelial alterations range from normal physiologic reactions to benign, premalignant, and malignant changes. The most common epithelial alterations are an increase in the thickness of the keratin layer (hyperorthokeratosis or hyperparakeratosis) and an increase in the thickness of the spinous layer (acanthosis). Hyperorthokeratosis is the most consistent microscopic finding in a leukoplakic lesion and occurs in many premalignant and malignant epithelial lesions.

A number of tissue alterations contribute to the white appearance of epithelium. Because stratified squamous epithelium is an avascular tissue, its constituents, keratin and spinous cells, tend to be white. The presence of a thickened layer of hyperorthokeratosis, hyperparakeratosis, or acanthosis acts as an added optical barrier that obscures the blood vessels in the underlying connective tissue. The development of a malignant proliferation of one or more of the epithelial layers also produces a similar clinical appearance. Changes in the underlying connective tissue can also impart a whitish appearance to the oral mucosa. This is usually due to a decrease in the vascularity and an increase in the collagen content of the underlying connective tissue, such as occurs in scar formation and areas of focal fibrous hyperplasia (traumatic fibroma).

DIAGNOSIS

Because clinical leukoplakic lesions can represent a diagnostic spectrum ranging from an inflamatory reaction to benign or malignant changes, determining the appropriate treatment for a particular lesion is an important clinical decision. The most effective way to make this decision is to obtain one or more biopsies of the lesion and to request a histopathologic evaluation by a qualified pathologist who has experience with lesions of this anatomic area.

■ **BIOPSY:** the removal of a sample of living tissue for laboratory examination.

A biopsy of a leukoplakic lesion is necessary to more clearly understand the nature of the disease process. This is accomplished by evaluating the histopathologic process in the tissue. If the lesion is small, the entire lesion is removed and submitted for microscopic examination, which is termed an **"excisional biopsy."** If the lesion is large, a small portion of the lesion is removed and submitted for microscopic examination, which is termed an **"incisional biopsy."** When performing an incisional biopsy of a large lesion, it is important to exercise good judgement and obtain a sample that is most likely to lead to an accurate diagnosis. If the lesion is multifocal, it is generally prudent to obtain more than one biopsy specimen for laboratory examination.

TREATMENT

The treatment of a leukoplakia is based on the exact nature of the lesion, which is determined by histopathologically evaluating the tissue. If the lesion is not premalignant or malignant, in most cases attempts are made to remove possible local factors that may be causing the hyperplasia. If the lesion exhibits moderate to severe dysplasia, steps should be taken to remove it completely.

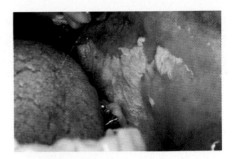

FIGURE 6-18

Leukoplakia. Clinical white patch of unknown origin on the buccal mucosa.

■ **BOX 6-1**
Common Mucosal Conditions Presenting as Leukoplakia

Reactive
  Hyperkeratosis (Ortho-, Para-)
  Acanthosis
  Actinic cheilitis
  Snuff dipper's keratosis
  Nicotine stomatitis
  Heat/chemical burns

Neoplastic
  Epithelial dysplasia
  Carcinoma in situ
  Squamous cell carcinoma
  Verrucous carcinoma

Infections
  Chronic hyperplastic candidiasis
  Hairy leukoplakia
  Syphilitic mucous patch

Immune-mediated
  Lichen planus
  Lupus erythematosus

Hereditary
  Leukoedema
  White sponge nevus

Idiopathic
  Hairy tongue
  Geographic tongue

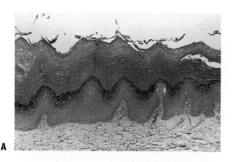

FIGURE 6-19

A, Hyperorthokeratosis. The keratin layer is without residual nuclei and is greatly thickened with an uneven surface. **B,** Hyperparakeratosis. The thickened keratin layer contains residual nuclei.

EPITHELIAL HYPERPLASIA

HYPERKERATOSIS

■ HYPERKERATOSIS: excessively thickened layer of the stratum corneum composed of orthokeratin (hyperorthokeratosis) or parakeratin (hyperparakeratosis).

Hyperkeratosis is commonly used to denote any excessive thickening of the stratum corneum. Because the superficial layer can be composed of orthokeratin or parakeratin, excessive amounts are more precisely termed **"hyperorthokeratosis"** and **"hyperparakeratosis."** On histopathologic examination the majority of leukoplakias are found to be hyperorthokeratosis (Figure 6-19, *A*) or hyperparakeratosis (Figure 6-19, *B*).

TABLE 6-1		
Characteristics of Normal Epithelium in Various Intraoral Sites		
Epithelial type	**Thickness**	**Site**
Orthokeratinized	Thick	Hard palate
		Gingiva
		Alveolar mucosa
		Dorsal tongue
Parakeratinized	Thick	Gingiva
		Alveolar mucosa
		Dorsal tongue
Nonkeratinized	Thick	Buccal mucosa
		Buccal vestibule
		Labial mucosa
		Labial vestibule
Nonkeratinized	Thin	Floor of mouth
		Ventral tongue
		Lateral tongue
		Soft palate
		Gingival sulcus

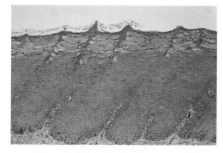

FIGURE 6-20

Smoker's keratosis. A unique tobacco-associated leukoplakia sometimes occurs on the labial mucosa, consisting of an increase in the orthokeratin or parakeratin layer and containing "chevron" or "church-spire" formations.

Depending on the specific intraoral site, normal mucosal epithelium can be either nonkeratinized, orthokeratinized, or parakeratinized (Table 6-1). **Orthokeratin** is nonnucleated keratin, whereas **parakeratin** exhibits shrunken (pyknotic) residual nuclei. Keratin functions as a protective barrier on normal skin or mucosa. Various stimuli, such as chronic frictional irritation caused by an ill-fitting denture, smoking, or the use of smokeless (chewing) tobacco, will usually induce keratinization of nonkeratinized epithelium and additional keratin formation in keratinized epithelium. The term **"smoker's keratosis"** is sometimes used to refer to a hyperkeratosis (ortho- or para-) that is induced by either cigarette, cigar, or pipe smoking. In many cases the hyperkeratosis is characterized by a uniform thickening of the keratin layer. In other cases, particularly on the labial mucosa, smoker's keratosis clinically appears as a series of slightly elevated delicate white striations. Histologic sections of the striated tissue exhibit a characteristic chevron or "church-spire" organization of the parakeratin (Figure 6-20).

ACANTHOSIS

> ■ **ACANTHOSIS**: excessive thickening of the intermediate cell layer resulting in broadening and elongation of the rete pegs.

> ■ **PSEUDOEPITHELIOMATOUS HYPERPLASIA**: excessively elongated rete pegs composed of normal keratinocytes that extend into the immediately adjacent connective tissue, giving a false impression of a squamous cell carcinoma.

Acanthosis is a benign hyperplasia of squamous epithelium characterized by an increase in the thickness of the intermediate cell layer (Figure 6-21). Acanthosis may occur alone or, more commonly, in association with hyperkeratosis. In either case the thickened squamous epithelium obscures the coloration of the underlying blood vessels and is clinically seen as an area of leukoplakia. Like hyperkeratosis, acanthosis usually develops in response to chronic irritants, such as ill-fitting dentures, smoking or chewing tobacco, and infections such as chronic candidiasis. In most cases the architectural pattern of the acanthosis conforms to that of normal epithelium. Under certain conditions, however, acanthosis can cause the rete pegs to assume an irregular and exaggerated downward growth pattern that resembles squamous cell carcinoma. This type of acanthosis is termed **"pseudoepitheliomatous hyperplasia" (PEH)** (Figure 6-22). Oral conditions in which pseudoepitheliomatous hyperplasia is commonly seen include inflammatory papillary hyperplasia (denture papillomatosis), granular cell tumor, and blastomycosis.

NICOTINE STOMATITIS

> ■ **NICOTINE STOMATITIS**: a diffuse white change of the palate and/or buccal mucosa caused by a combination of hyperkeratosis and acanthosis, frequently containing multiple small dimpled nodules; found in heavy smokers.

Nicotine stomatitis is a term used to describe a specific type of epithelial hyperplasia that primarily involves the hard palate of long-term pipe smokers. On rare occasions it is found in a cigar or cigarette smoker.

CLINICAL
The palate of patients with nicotine stomatitis is usually whiter than normal, exhibiting multiple, small circular papules with tiny umbilicated red centers on the soft palate portion (Figure 6-23). The white background may have a roughened

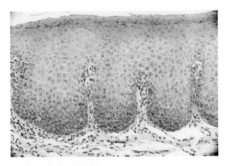

FIGURE 6-21
Acanthosis. The intermediate cell layer of stratified squamous epithelium is extensively hyperplastic, resulting in both elongated and broadened rete pegs.

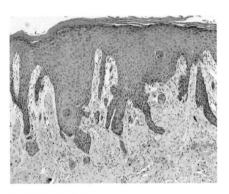

FIGURE 6-22
Pseudoepitheliomatous hyperplasia. The epithelium is acanthotic, and the rete pegs are elongated in an irregular pattern that *falsely* ("pseudo-") resembles squamous cell carcinoma.

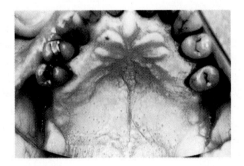

FIGURE 6-23
Nicotine stomatitis. The palate is whiter than normal and exhibits multiple small raised nodules with red umbilicated centers, particularly on the soft palate.

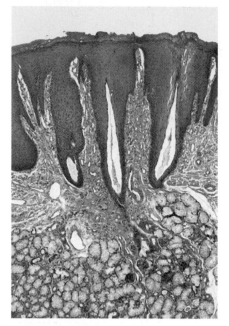

FIGURE 6-24

Nicotine stomatitis. The microscopic features of the small nodules reveal widened excretory ducts of minor salivary glands in which there is extensive squamous metaplasia of the normal cuboidal cells.

surface and may be fissured or wrinkled. Lesions may also occur on the buccal mucosa, particularly on the side of the mouth where the pipe or cigar is held.

HISTOPATHOLOGY

A biopsy of one of the umbilicated papules reveals a dilated salivary gland duct exhibiting squamous metaplasia of the ductal lining with hyperkeratosis and acanthosis of the adjacent surface epithelium. The connective tissue adjacent to the salivary gland duct exhibits variable degrees of chronic inflammation (Figure 6-24).

TREATMENT

Nicotine stomatitis does not appear to predispose the hard palate to malignancy. However, some authors suggest that the degree of smoking that causes nicotine stomatitis in the more anterior oral tissues also increases the risk of developing squamous cell carcinoma of the faucial and retromolar regions of the mouth and of the upper and lower respiratory tract. Nicotine stomatitis is rapidly resolved when the smoking habit stops.

PROLIFERATIVE VERRUCOUS LEUKOPLAKIA

■ PROLIFERATIVE VERRUCOUS LEUKOPLAKIA: diffuse white and/or papillary ("warty") area of the mucosa caused by varying degrees of epithelial hyperplasia; it has the potential to develop into verrucous carcinoma or well-differentiated squamous cell carcinoma.

Proliferative verrucous leukoplakia (PVL) is a recently delineated entity that occurs primarily in elderly patients. It is described as a diffuse leukoplakic area with varying degrees of whiteness and a surface texture consisting of both smooth and "warty" areas (Figure 6-25). The clinical course of PVL is exceedingly slow but relentless. There are often no identifiable causative factors.

The term *verrucous hyperplasia* is sometimes used to define a similar benign, largely exophytic type of undulating epithelial hyperplasia that if left untreated may or may not progress to a verrucous carcinoma. Its relationship to PVL is not completely understood but is believed to represent part of the spectrum of change found it that entity.

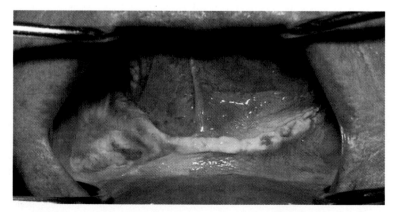

FIGURE 6-25

Proliferative verrucous leukoplakia. Both quadrants of the mandibular alveolar ridge are covered with a diffuse white lesion with some areas extensively thickened with a warty, friable surface. Fainter white areas extend into the buccal vestibule.

HISTOPATHOLOGY

The microscopic appearance of PVL exhibits a wide spectrum of the changes within the realm of epithelial hyperplasia. The changes range from mild forms of hyperorthokeratosis to verrucous carcinoma. Some cases that were followed for long periods have eventually developed focal areas of well-differentiated squamous cell carcinoma (Figure 6-26).

TREATMENT

During the early stages when lesions are small, treatment of PVL consists of local surgical excision. During later stages when lesions can extend over the entire arch(es), treatment becomes more difficult. In the maxilla, involvement of the soft palate, uvula, and tonsillar pillars can be problematic. In these areas the difficulty of surgical excision is due to the diffuse nature of the lesions and their proximity to structures that need to remain intact to enable mastication and speech. Recent refinements in the use of laser therapy have been helpful in arresting the progression of the disease process while preserving the vital anatomic structures.

EPITHELIAL ATROPHY

◼ EPITHELIAL ATROPHY: reduction in the normal thickness of epithelium.

Although hyperkeratosis usually occurs on the surface of normal or hyperplastic epithelium, it can also occur in association with atrophic epithelium. When a leukoplakia exhibits hyperkeratosis on the surface of atrophic epithelium, it is generally considered to be at greater risk of progressing to premalignancy (epithelial dysplasia) or malignancy than hyperkeratosis on the surface of normal or hyperplastic epithelium. Such an event commonly occurs on the lower lip of patients with prolonged actinic (solar) cheilitis before the development of squamous cell carcinoma.

ORAL SUBMUCOUS FIBROSIS

◼ ORAL SUBMUCOUS FIBROSIS: diffuse firm whitish areas of submucosal scarring usually caused by frequent and prolonged contact with betel nut quids, tobacco, or hot peppers; lesions have a higher than normal risk of developing squamous cell carcinoma.

Oral submucous fibrosis is a disorder that resembles scleroderma, except that it is limited to the oral cavity. The disease occurs primarily in India, Pakistan, and Burma, but cases also occur in China, Thailand, Nepal, and Vietnam. Although the exact cause of the disease remains unknown, it has been suggested that it probably results from a hypersensitivity to eating hot peppers (chilies), from betel nut chewing, or from protracted tobacco use. The epithelial atrophy in oral submucous fibrosis is at greater risk of progressing to premalignancy and malignancy than normal epithelium.

CLINICAL

Oral submucous fibrosis affects the oral tissue of the buccal mucosa, lips, soft palate, and occasionally the pharynx. The tissue is symmetrically affected and becomes progressively firm and pale. A common complaint is a progressive stiff-

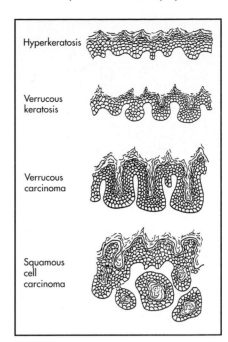

FIGURE 6-26

Proliferative verrucous leukoplakia. Diagram of the spectrum of histologic changes. Lesions slowly enlarge while progressing from the mildest form of hyperkeratosis through a stage of verrucous keratosis to verrucous carcinoma, with some lesions eventually becoming well-differentiated squamous cell carcinoma.

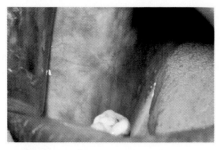

FIGURE 6-27

Oral submucous fibrosis. The buccal mucosa is pale and firm caused by the underlying fibrosis of the normally loose and soft connective tissue.

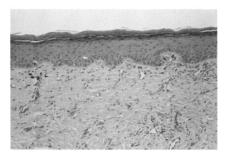

FIGURE 6-28

Oral submucous fibrosis. The overlying epithelium is thinned (atrophic), and the submucosa is composed of a dense fibrous connective tissue with a reduced vascularity.

ness of the cheeks, which inhibits the ability to open the mouth. The oral mucosa appears pale and atrophic (Figure 6-27).

HISTOPATHOLOGY

The earliest stage of the disease is characterized by chronic inflammation of the submucosal connective tissue. This stage is followed by a diffuse progressive fibrosis and atrophy of the overlying epithelium (Figure 6-28). The atrophic epithelium has a greater tendency to develop hyperkeratosis and epithelial dysplasia, which can progress to squamous cell carcinoma. For these reasons oral submucous fibrosis is considered a precancerous condition.

TREATMENT

Oral submucous fibrosis is usually diagnosed when the disease is at an advanced stage and lesions are widespread. At this stage surgical treatment is usually not possible, but systemic and intralesional injections of corticosteroids have been used with some success.

EPITHELIAL DYSPLASIA

■ EPITHELIAL DYSPLASIA: a premalignant change in epithelium characterized by a combination of individual cell and architectural alterations.

The development of a malignancy in stratified squamous epithelium occurs spontaneously or as a gradual process in which multiple minor individual cellular and tissue alterations eventually culminate in frank malignancy. The combination of tissue changes observed in the gradual transition to malignancy (premalignancy) is termed epithelial dysplasia.

Individul cell alterations (Figure 6-29) found in epithelial dysplasia include the following:

1. Prominent nucleoli
2. Hyperchromatic nuclei (hyperchromasia)
3. Nuclear pleomorphism
4. Altered nuclear/cytoplasmic ratio
5. Increased mitotic activity
6. Abnormal mitotic figures
7. Multinucleation of cells

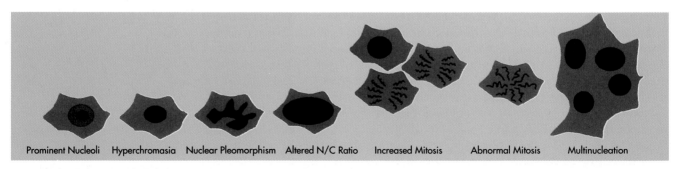

Prominent Nucleoli Hyperchromasia Nuclear Pleomorphism Altered N/C Ratio Increased Mitosis Abnormal Mitosis Multinucleation

FIGURE 6-29

Diagram of the individual cell alterations found in epithelial dysplasia. The degree of severity of an epithelial dysplasia is determined, in part, by the frequency and combination of these alterations.

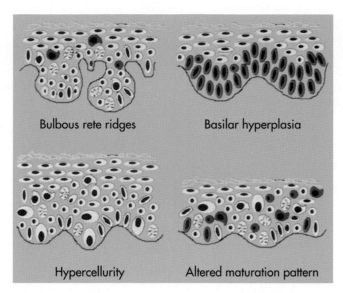

Bulbous rete ridges

Basilar hyperplasia

Hypercellurity

Altered maturation pattern

FIGURE 6-30

Diagram of the architectural alterations of the epithelium found in epithelial dysplasia. The degree of severity of the epithelial dysplasia is determined by the extent of these alterations combined with the individual cell abnormalities.

Architectural alterations (Figure 6-30) include combinations of the following:

1. Formation of bulbous rete pegs
2. Basilar hyperplasia
3. Hypercellularity
4. Altered maturation pattern of keratinocytes

The clinical appearance of epithelial dysplasia is most frequently observed as an area of leukoplakia (Figure 6-31) that is similar to other more innocuous appearing white lesions.

The degree of severity of an epithelial dysplasia is conveyed by assigning a grade of **mild, moderate,** or **severe/carcinoma in situ** based on its microscopic appearance (Figures 6-32, 6-33, and 6-34). It is important to note that the grade of an epithelial dysplasia can increase (become worse) with time. An epithelial dysplasia of the floor of the mouth or lateral border of the tongue in a cigarette smoker will, with time and continued smoking, increase its grade from mild to more severe. The time factor will vary extensively among individuals, from months to years. Equally important is that when a promoting factor is removed, some mild and incipient forms of epithelial dysplasia will regress (reverse), and the epithelium will revert to normal. In other forms of epithelial dysplasia, even with alteration of a contributing factor, reversal may not be possible, although the rate of progression to a more severe form is usually slowed. It appears doubtful that the *moderate* and *severe* forms of epithelial dysplasia can regress by simply removing the cause. In some forms the reversal of the moderate and severe forms of epithelial dysplasia may not be possible because the epithelial basement membrane may already be focally invaded. When the adjacent connective tissue is invaded with dysplastic epithelium, it is considered a squamous cell carcinoma.

Areas of epithelial dysplasia often exhibit a chronic lymphocytic infiltrate in the adjacent connective tissue, and lymphocytes extend upward into the deeper layers of the dysplastic epithelium. If the dysplasia is mild and the lymphocytic infiltrate is intense, the potential exists for an erroneous diagnosis. An epithelial dysplasia with an associated dense infiltrate of lymphocytes bears a striking re-

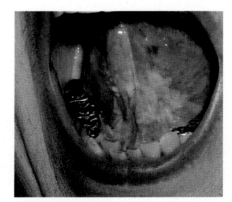

FIGURE 6-31

Epithelial dysplasia. The leukoplakic area on the ventral surface of the tongue is a common presentation of epithelial dysplasia in the oral cavity.

FIGURE 6-32

A, Diagram of *mild* epithelial dysplasia. **B,** Microscopic appearance of mild epithelial dysplasia.

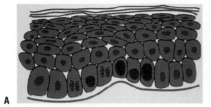
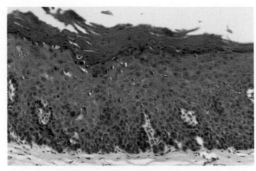

FIGURE 6-33

A, Diagram of *moderate* epithelial dysplasia. **B,** Microscopic appearance of moderate epithelial dysplasia.

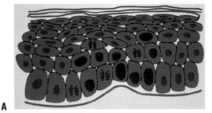
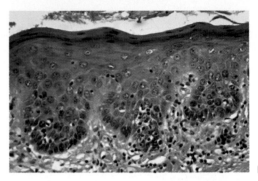

FIGURE 6-34

A, Diagram of *severe* epithelial dysplasia. **B,** Microscopic appearance of severe epithelial dysplasia.

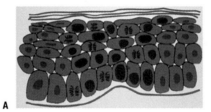
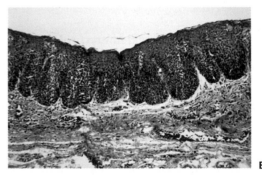

semblance to the dermatologic/mucosal condition of lichen planus. When an epithelial dysplasia has multiple histologic features in common with lichen planus, it has been term **"lichenoid dysplasia."** Because there have been many documented cases in which an intraoral squamous cell carcinoma has developed in the same location as lesions that have repeatedly been diagnosed as lichen planus, the question remains whether the initial lesion was in fact a lichenoid dysplasia rather than a lichen planus. Until more is known about these two conditions, the question remains unanswered. (See Chapter 8 for additional discussion.)

CARCINOMA IN SITU

■ CARCINOMA IN SITU: the most severe stage of epithelial dysplasia, involving the entire thickness of the epithelium, with the epithelial basement membrane remaining intact.

Carcinoma in situ, also referred to as *ca in situ* or *CIS*, is the most severe form of epithelial dysplasia and involves the entire thickness of the epithelium ("top-to-bottom change"). It is cytologically similar to squamous cell carcinoma except that architecturally the epithelial basement membrane remains intact and no invasion into the connective tissue has occurred. When dysplastic epithelial cells breach the basement membrane and spread (invade) into the connective tissue, allowing for the possibility of distant metastasis to occur, CIS becomes squamous cell carcinoma.

ERYTHROPLAKIA

■ ERYTHROPLAKIA: a red patch of the oral mucosa frequently caused by epithelial dysplasia, ca in situ, or squamous cell carcinoma.

Erythroplakia, also termed *"erythroplasia,"* was first used by Queyrat to describe a red, velvety lesion on the glans penis of elderly males. Literally, the term means "a red patch or plaque." The term is used to describe red mucosal lesions of the oral cavity that have no apparent cause.

CLINICAL
Erythroplakia of the mouth is usually an asymptomatic lesion that occurs primarily in older males who smoke cigarettes. It can be found on the floor of the mouth (Figure 6-35), lateral and ventral surfaces of the tongue, soft palate, and buccal mucosa.

The term **"speckled erythroplakia"** is often used to describe a lesion that is primarily red but exhibits interspersed focal white plaques (Figure 6-36). This lesion should be viewed with a high degree of suspicion because it has a high incidence of premalignant or malignant change. When obtaining a biopsy of this lesion, both red and white areas should be sampled.

HISTOPATHOLOGY
The microscopic evaluation of erythroplakias reveal that 60% to 90% are either epithelial dysplasias, carcinomas in situ, or squamous cell carcinomas. Consequently, oral erythroplakias should be viewed with a high degee of suspicion and routinely biopsied for histopathologic evaluation.

Three microscopic features of erythroplakias explain the deep red coloration of the lesions. First, erythroplakias lack the normal amount of surface layer keratin that normally diffuses the redness emanating from the underlying vasculature. Second, the remaining epithelial layers that normally cover the connective tissue papillae between the rete pegs are frequently reduced in thickness; therefore, the blood vessels normally present in the papillae are more visible from the surface than in normal mucosa. Third, in most erythroplakias, the size and number of vascular structures increase in response to the inflammation associated with the thinned and neoplastic epithelium (Figure 6-37).

TREATMENT
It is important that all erythroplakic lesions be biopsied to determine their exact nature. The treatment of erythroplakias depends on the specific histopathologic diagnosis of each case. Dysplasia and CIS are treated by local excision. Squamous cell carcinoma is treated more aggressively, depending on the clinical staging of the lesion.

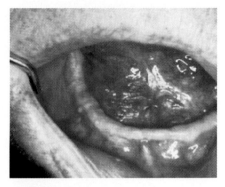

FIGURE 6-35
Erythroplakia. The red, slightly nodular area of the right anterior floor of the mouth is a common presentation of this clinical entity.

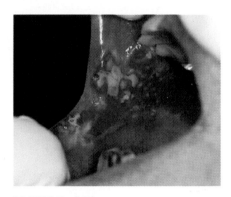

FIGURE 6-36
Speckled erythroplakia. The lesion in the right commissural area of the buccal mucosa exhibiting scattered white plaques against an erythematous background is a common presentation of dysplasia or early squamous cell carcinoma.

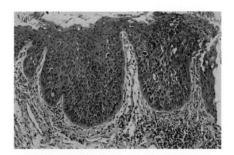

FIGURE 6-37
Carcinoma in situ. The microscopic alterations of the epithelium are severe. Areas of thickened epithelium that are adjacent to atrophic areas have inflamed connective tissue containing large vascular spaces. These microscopic features are responsible for the clinical appearance observed in erythroplakia or speckled erythroplakia.

MALIGNANT EPITHELIAL NEOPLASMS

SQUAMOUS CELL CARCINOMA

> ■ SQUAMOUS CELL CARCINOMA: malignant neoplasm of stratified squamous epithelium that is capable of locally destructive growth and distant metastasis.

Squamous cell carcinoma, sometimes termed *epidermoid carcinoma*, is defined as a malignant neoplasm derived from or exhibiting the morphologic features of squamous epithelium. As discussed earlier, squamous cell carcinoma is often the end stage of alteration in stratified squamous epithelium, beginning as an epithelial dysplasia and progressing until the dysplastic epithelial cells breach the basement membrane and invade the connective tissue. It also may arise de novo from the overlying stratified squamous epithelium and not have a prolonged premalignant phase.

Oral malignancies represent 3% of all cancer in males and 2% in females. The overall survival rate of patients with oral malignancies is 50%. They are responsible for 2% of the annual deaths in males and 1% in females. Each year approximately 30,000 new cases of oral cancer are diagnosed in the United States. The incidence of oral cancer differs extensively, depending on the tobacco habits prevalent in the various countries throughout the world. The incidence of oral cancer greatly increases in societies where extensive tobacco use begins early in life and is continuous.

Squamous cell carcinoma is by far the most common malignant neoplasm of the oral cavity, representing approximately 90% of all oral cancers. Although it occurs in various oral sites, it is most common on the lower lip, lateral borders of the tongue, and the floor of the mouth. The incidence of squamous cell carcinoma increases with age; most cases occur after 40 years of age.

A number of etiologic factors have been implicated in the development of oral squamous cell carcinoma. These include tobacco habits, alcohol consumption, viruses, actinic radiation, immunosuppression, nutritional deficiencies, preexisting diseases, and chronic irritation (Box 6-2).

Because the basal cells of oral epithelium have a higher than normal rate of mitotic activity, any factor that causes a disturbance in the quality or quantity of the cell-regulating proteins can induce unregulated (neoplastic) growth (Figure 6-38). Some of these proteins *("kinases")* interact with the proteins that coordinate cell replication *("cyclins")*. Others are regulatory proteins that influence the events associated with mitosis. These proteins are produced under the direction

---

■ **BOX 6-2**
Etiologic Factors Associated With Oral Squamous Cell Carcinoma

Smoked Tobacco
 Cigarettes
 Cigars
 Pipe

Smokeless Tobacco
 Snuff
 Chewing tobacco
 Quid (Pan)

Actinic Radiation

Infections
 Human papilloma virus
 Epstein-Barr virus
 Human immunodeficiency
  virus
 Candida albicans
 Treponema pallidum

Chronic Irritation
 Alcohol Consumption

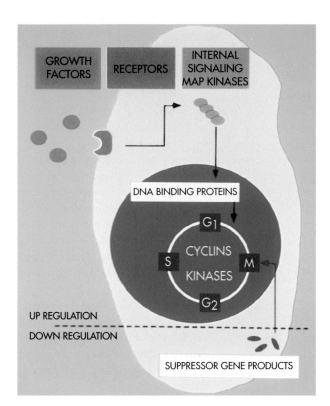

FIGURE 6-38
Common factors associated with regulation of cell growth.

of specific genes on specific chromosomes. The specific gene loci responsible for producing proteins that can upset the replication cycle of cells are termed *oncogenes*. When oncogenes are stimulated to overproduce proteins that stimulate mitosis (up regulation), the result is neoplastic growth. Alteration in the oncogene activity has been associated with one or more of the environmental factors (cofactors) mentioned in the following section. Some oncogenes prominently involved include the genomic loci that govern the epidermal growth factor (EGF) and transforming growth factor (TGF) and their receptors on the cell membrane (EGF-R and c-erb B); the internal signalling proteins (H-ras, G proteins, and kinases); and the nuclear DNA-binding transcription activator proteins (C-myc, C-fos, and C-myb). Neoplasia may also occur when the *suppressor genes* (antioncogenes) that normally function to shut down or control unnecessary cell cycling become deactivated. The most notable suppressor genes are those responsible for the p53 and the RB proteins.

Although the exact manner in which the following environmental factors or cofactors interact and interfere with the cell signaling and cycling mechanisms is unknown, they have been associated with an increase of oral squamous cell carcinoma.

Carcinogenic Factors

Tobacco

The habitual use of tobacco in its various forms, which consists primarily of cigarettes, cigars, pipe tobacco, snuff, chewing tobacco (Figure 6-39), and "quid," has been reported to be the most important factor associated with the transformation of normal mucosal epithelial cells to squamous cell carcinoma. Research indicates that 8 of every 10 patients with oral cancer had been long-term heavy smokers. As a carcinogen, smoked tobacco seems to be more potent than smokeless tobacco. The association between tobacco and cancer is further evidenced in patients who have received treatment for oral squamous cell carcinoma. Re-

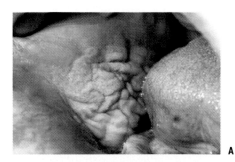

A

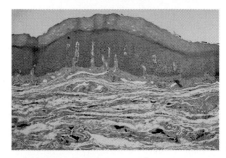

B

FIGURE 6-39
Tobacco chewer's pouch. A, Lesion of posterior vestibule and buccal mucosa with characteristic wrinkles and leukoplakic appearance. **B,** Microscopic appearance reveals a thickened layer of orthokeratin, acanthosis, and an undulating surface.

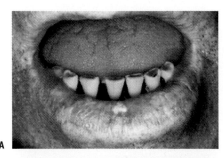

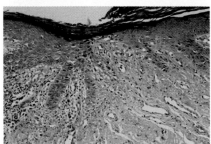

FIGURE 6-40

Actinic cheilitis. A, The lower lip is puffy with loss of the distinct vermilion border and is mottled with leukoplakic and atrophic areas. **B,** Microscopic features include hyperorthokeratosis, epithelial atrophy, dysplasia, basophilic degeneration of collagen, and telangiectasia.

search indicates that 30% to 37% of patients who continue to smoke after treatment develop a new lesion in another oropharyngeal site, whereas only 6% to 13% of those who quit develop new lesions.

Actinic radiation

Light-skinned individuals whose skin does not tan well and who sustain prolonged occupational or recreational exposure to direct sunlight are at greater risk of developing squamous cell carcinoma of the lower lip. Usually the lip goes through a series of preneoplastic changes that become progressively worse as the dose of actinic radiation accumulates and the patient ages. The sharp ridge or line of demarcation on the vermilion border is replaced by a puffy, rounded margin, and the skin develops multiple vertical creases. The exposed mucosal surface becomes mottled, consisting of red (atrophy) and white (hyperorthokeratosis) patches, and displays prominent superficial vascular structures (telangiectasia). This accumulation of changes is termed **actinic cheilitis** (also *solar cheilosis, solar keratosis,* or *solar elastosis*) (Figure 6-40). As time and exposure continue, recurring chronic ulcers frequently develop on the lip, lateral to the midline. Eventually, the ulcers stop healing, at which point biopsy usually reveals that a superficial well-differentiated squamous cell carcinoma has formed. Treatment of the altered tissue before the development of malignancy usually consists of superficial surgical removal of the damaged tissue ("lip stripping" or "lip shave"). When biopsy reveals the presence of invasion, surgical wedge resection is usually adequate unless metastasis has occurred.

Infections

Various infectious agents such as bacteria (syphilis) and fungi (chronic candidiasis) have been implicated as predisposing factors for oral squamous cell carcinoma. Convincing evidence firmly linking these agents to the development of squamous cell carcinoma has not been found. More substantial evidence of a link with an infectious agent has occurred with some viral agents. The most convincing is the association of the various genotypes of human papilloma virus (HPV) to anogenital squamous cell carcinoma. Although the mechanism is not completely elucidated, it is reported that the HPV early gene products E6 and E7 bind the host keratinocyte suppressor gene proteins p53 and/or RB, thus allowing uncontrolled cell cycling. Another possibility is that viral E6 and E7 oncoproteins induce overexpression of the epidermal growth factor receptor (EGF-R). Because of the difficulty isolating the HPV (usually HPV 16 and HPV 18) in squamous cell carcinoma of the head and neck compared with the cervical carcinoma, research has yet to produce the convincing link between oral lesions and the HPV that is present in lesions of the anogenital region.

Immunosuppression

Acquired immunodeficiency syndrome (AIDS) predisposes relatively young individuals to various oral and nonoral malignancies. Intraoral squamous cell carcinoma is among the number of malignant lesions that occur at a much younger age than normal for this condition and without the usual associated etiologic factors. Oral Kaposi sarcoma and lymphoma, which also occur at a younger age in AIDS patients, are much more common than squamous cell carcinoma.

Nutritional deficiencies

Patients with chronic iron deficiency anemia such as Plummer-Vinson syndrome develop gastrointestinal mucosal atrophy, including that of the oral cavity and have a higher susceptibility to esophageal and oral carcinomas. A direct causal relationship between low serum iron levels or other mineral deficiencies and cancer development has not been established.

Preexisting oral diseases

Oral submucous fibrosis (discussed earlier in this chapter) predisposes the oral mucosa to develop squamous cell carcinoma. Although there is some indication that chronic forms of oral lichen planus also predispose the oral mucosa to develop squamous cell carcinoma, this factor is still being debated (see Chapter 8).

Cofactors

Although not considered direct causes, several cofactors, such as alcohol consumption and chronic irritants caused by ill-fitting dentures, have been implicated in the progression of oral squamous cell carcinoma. The evidence for a direct topical effect by orally ingested alcohol is lacking because most chronic drinkers are also smokers. Most believe that the effect of alcohol on the induction of oral cancer is indirect and possibly a result of liver damage (cirrhosis) and an inability to detoxify the blood constituents. The association between cirrhosis of the liver and squamous cell carcinoma of the floor of the mouth and the tongue is especially high. When high alcohol intake is combined with heavy smoking, there is thought to be a synergistic effect, greatly increasing the incidence of oropharyngeal carcinoma.

CLINICAL

Oral squamous cell carcinoma has a number of different clinical presentations. The most common early presentations of intraoral squamous cell carcinoma are leukoplakias and erythroplakias. The more advanced lesions may first appear as a painless ulcer, a tumorous mass, or a verrucous (papillary) growth. Squamous cell carcinoma that has infiltrated deep into the connective tissue may have few surface changes but appears as a firm indurated area with associated loss of tissue mobility. On the floor of the mouth this commonly causes fixation of the tongue or inability to fully open the mouth. Carcinoma that invades from the gingiva into the underlying bone of the mandible or maxilla can result in loosening or loss of teeth, whereas those that penetrate deeply into the mandible with involvement of the inferior alveolar nerve can cause paraesthesia of the teeth and lower lip.

HISTOPATHOLOGY

Squamous cell carcinoma is diagnosed by histopathologically examining a representative biopsy of the neoplastic tissue. Common to all lesions is the presence of invasion into the underlying connective tissue and the inherent potential of malignant cells to erode the lymphatic and blood vessel walls, allowing them to be transported to distant sites (metastasis) (Figure 6-41).

Although all carcinomas have some capacity for metastasis, there is considerable variation in the potential of individual squamous cell carcinomas to metastasize. This potential is correlated to some extent with the histologic variation found in oral squamous cell carcinoma. The histologic variation is related to the degree of differentiation (grade) exhibited by the tumor cells and how closely the tissue architecture resembles normal stratified squamous epithelium. Tumors that produce significant amounts of keratin and exhibit some features of maturation from basal cells to keratin are considered as **well differentiated** (Figure 6-42). Tumors that produce little or no keratin but in which the epithelium still is recognizable as stratified squamous, despite its significant deviation from normal, are regarded as **moderately differentiated** (Figure 6-43). The tumors that produce no keratin, bear little resemblance to stratified squamous epithelium, exhibit a significant lack of normal architectural pattern and cohesiveness of cells, and exhibit extensive cellular abnormalities are designated as **poorly differentiated** (Figure 6-44).

As a general rule, squamous cell carcinomas of the lower lip tend to be well

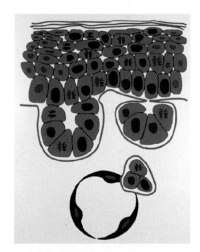

FIGURE 6-41

Diagram of the transition of epithelial dysplasia to invasive squamous cell carcinoma. Malignant cells have penetrated through the basement membrane into the underlying connective tissue, where they are capable of eroding into lymphatic vessels.

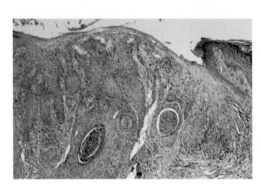

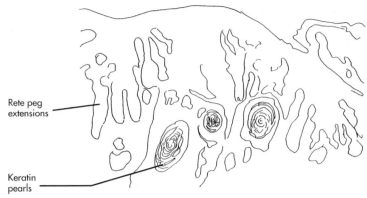

FIGURE 6-42

Well-differentiated squamous cell carcinoma. Microscopic features reveal irregularly elongated rete pegs invading the connective tissue and containing aberrant accumulations of keratin (keratin pearls).

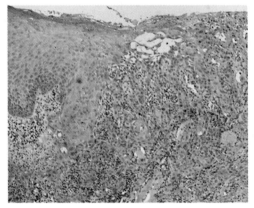

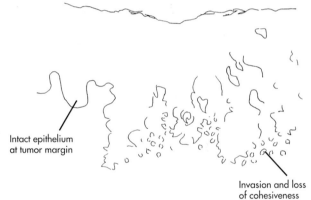

FIGURE 6-43

Moderately differentiated squamous cell carcinoma. The photomicrograph illustrates an abrupt line of demarcation between the normal epithelium *(left)* and the invasive neoplastic squamous epithelium that is *nonkeratinized* and exhibits loss of cellular cohesiveness.

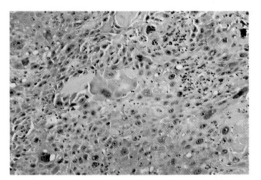

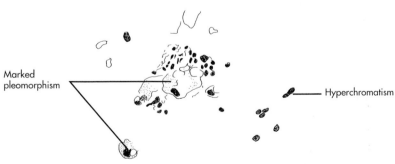

FIGURE 6-44

Poorly differentiated squamous cell carcinoma. The photomicrograph exhibits sheets of cells *lacking an architectural pattern* and exhibiting severe cellular abnormalities of hyperchromatism and pleomorphism.

differentiated; those that occur on the lateral borders of the tongue are often moderately differentiated, and those that involve the tonsillar region tend to be poorly differentiated. Although a number of different factors influence the biologic behavior of a tumor, such as anatomic structures and lymphatic drainage patterns, the degree of differentiation appears to be most important in determining its growth rate and ultimately its tendency to metastasize.

Sites and Incidence

The incidence of squamous cell carcinoma in various anatomic locations is significantly different; some areas appear to be relatively immune, whereas others appear to be particularly prone (Table 6-2). When all anatomic locations are considered, the lower lip is the most prone site. Within the oral cavity only, the lateral/ventral aspects of the tongue and the adjacent floor of the mouth are the most prone sites, followed by the posterior soft palate, particularly in the areas adjacent to the tonsillar pillars (Figure 6-45). Less frequently, the gingiva/alveolar ridge area is the site of origin, and the buccal mucosa, especially above the occlusal line, is seldom involved. Compared with other intraoral sites, carcinomas arising on the hard palate and dorsum of the tongue are relatively rare.

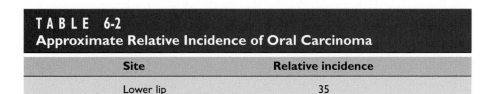

FIGURE 6-45

Diagram of the "horseshoe-shaped" intraoral area that is most prone to the development of squamous cell carcinoma. It consists of the anterior floor of the mouth, lateral borders of the tongue, tonsillar pillars, and lateral soft palate.

TABLE 6-2
Approximate Relative Incidence of Oral Carcinoma

Site	Relative incidence
Lower lip	35
Lateral/ventral tongue	25
Floor of mouth	20
Soft palate	15
Gingival/alveolar ridge	4
Buccal mucosa	1

Lower lip

Squamous cell carcinoma of the lower lip accounts for 30% to 40% of all oral carcinomas. It is much more common in males than females, occurring most commonly in patients who are in the fifth to eighth decade. Most lesions occur on the right or left vermilion borders (Figure 6-46) and seldom on the midline. In nearly all cases lesions are preceded by a prolonged period of actinic cheilitis, followed by an interval of recurring ulceration and encrustation. Eventually the ulcer fails to heal and develops a rolled border with indurated surrounding tissue. Squamous cell carcinomas of the lower lip are usually well differentiated and slow to metastasize. When metastases have not occurred, lesions are nearly 100% curable. Lesions present for prolonged periods usually metastasize first to the regional submental lymph nodes and then to the digastric and cervical nodes.

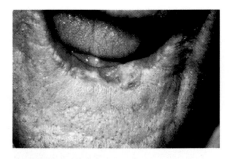

FIGURE 6-46

Squamous cell carcinoma of the lower lip.

Tongue

The lateral borders of the tongue (including the adjacent ventral surfaces) are the site of 25% of all oral squamous cell carcinomas and 50% of intraoral lesions. The lateral borders of the tongue are part of the U-shaped zone within the oral cavity and are high-risk anatomic sites for squamous cell carcinoma. The other sites comprising this zone are the anterior, right, and left floor of the mouth and the retromolar pad and adjacent areas of the soft palate. The dorsum of the tongue and hard palate appear to be relatively resistant to the initiation of new lesions, although extension from adjacent locations frequently occurs.

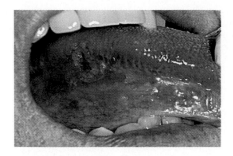

FIGURE 6-47

Squamous cell carcinoma of the lateral tongue.

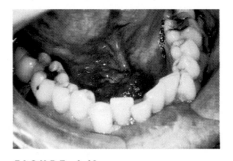

FIGURE 6-48

Squamous cell carcinoma of the anterior floor of the mouth.

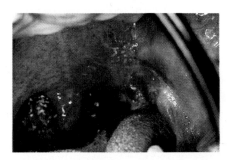

FIGURE 6-49

Squamous cell carcinoma of the left soft palate arising in an area of speckled erythroplakia.

Early lesions of the lateral surface of the tongue are usually located in the middle and posterior thirds (Figure 6-47). Commonly, lesions initially appear as an area of leukoplakia that in time ulcerates and develops raised or rolled borders. Other lesions may begin as focal areas of erythema or nodularity. Advanced lesions of all clinical types eventually ulcerate and produce extensive induration of the surrounding tissue, often resulting in immobility and altered speech. The initial appearance of some lesions often makes it impossible to clinically separate from chronic traumatic ulcers and require a biopsy to determine their true nature. Most lesions of the lateral border of the tongue are moderately differentiated squamous cell carcinomas. Metastasis commonly occurs early in the course of the disease and extends to the submandibular and deep cervical lymph nodes. Hemiglossectomy followed by radiotherapy are the treatments of choice. In general, the 5-year survival rate of patients with more advanced lesions is less than 30%.

Floor of the mouth

The floor of the mouth is the site of approximately 20% of all oral carcinomas and the third most common location of all intraoral squamous cell carcinomas. Most lesions are located in the anterior areas adjacent to the caruncles containing the orifices of Wharton ducts. Patients commonly are long-time smokers and/or heavy drinkers.

The clinical appearance of the early or initial lesions of the floor of the mouth commonly begins as an area of erythroplakia or speckled erythroplakia that gradually develops into an irregularly shaped central ulceration. As lesions progress the area becomes nodular and indurated and invades the deeper tissues (Figure 6-48). In advanced lesions fixation of the tongue and extension onto the gingiva are common. Most lesions in this area are moderately differentiated, metastasizing relatively early to the submandibular triangle and upper jugular chain lymph nodes. Treatment consists of surgery, often including the adjacent lymph nodes, followed by radiotherapy.

Soft palate

Squamous cell carcinoma of the soft palate occurs most commonly in its lateral posterior regions adjacent to the anterior faucial pillars. Lesions in this location represent approximately 15% of intraoral carcinoma. Patients commonly are heavy smokers with a high alcohol intake. Lesions are usually erythroplakic or a mixture of red and white plaquelike areas (Figure 6-49). Invasion often occurs before surface ulceration is evident. Most lesions are moderately to poorly differentiated, often invading the deeper structures and metastasizing to the cervical and jugular lymph nodes before large ulcerative or nodular lesions are present.

Gingiva/Alveolar ridge

Lesions of the gingiva and alveolar ridges represent 4% to 6% of intraoral carcinoma and commonly have the initial appearance of a verrucous leukoplakia or an ulceration with rolled borders (Figure 6-50). The mandible is affected more often than the maxilla; most lesions are present in the posterior areas. Lesions are usually well differentiated and invade the underlying bone, often by means of the periodontal membrane when teeth are present. Common presenting signs are extensive mobility and early tooth loss in the absence of advanced periodontal disease and sockets that fail to heal after extraction. In the mandible, metastasis is usually to the submandibular and cervical lymph nodes. Treatment consists of surgical excision; segmental resection may be necessary when bone invasion occurs.

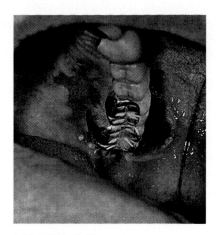

FIGURE 6-50

Squamous cell carcinoma of the gingiva and alveolar ridges.

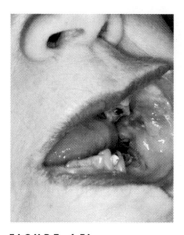

FIGURE 6-51

Squamous cell carcinoma of the buccal mucosa.

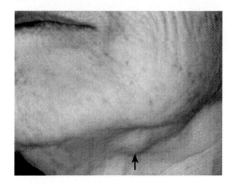

FIGURE 6-52

Enlarged firm fixed submandibular lymph node *(arrow)* caused by metastasis from an intraoral squamous cell carcinoma.

Buccal mucosa

The buccal mucosa is infrequently the site of squamous cell carcinoma, accounting for approximately 1% to 2% of intraoral carcinoma. Lesions usually occur as ulcers along the occlusal line (Figure 6-51) and are associated with surrounding induration caused by relatively rapid invasion of the deeper structures. Most lesions are moderately differentiated and metastasize to the submandibular lymph nodes. Treatment consists of surgical excision and/or radiotherapy.

Metastasis

Squamous cell carcinoma of the oral cavity spreads by invading the lymphatic vessels. Once inside these vessels, the tumor cells are carried to the regional lymph nodes, where they lodge and continue to proliferate. The proliferating tumors cells enlarge the lymph nodes and extend beyond their capsules into the surrounding tissue. These lymph nodes become easily palpable, appearing firm and fixed to the adjacent tissue. Enlarged, firm, and fixed lymph nodes are an ominous clinical sign (Figure 6-52).

The lymph nodes most commonly containing metastatic intraoral squamous cell carcinoma are the submandibular and the superficial and deep cervical nodes. Squamous cell carcinomas of the lower lip that become large enough to metastasize initially involve the submental nodes before spreading to the submandibular and cervical lymph nodes (Figure 6-53). Lesions that spread beyond the regional lymph nodes of the head and neck often metastasize to the lungs and liver.

Clinical staging of carcinomas of the head and neck (TNM system)

Clinical staging of carcinoma patients is used to designate the extent of disease in patients and to match it with what has been determined to be the most appropriate treatment for patients with comparable stages. The use of a uniform staging system provides meaningful comparisons of the results of specific types of treatments. The designations used in the TNM system (*T*, primary tumor; *N*, regional lymph node; *M*, distant metastasis) differ somewhat according to the anatomic site. For the oral cavity the TNM definitions and staging groups are outlined in Boxes 6-3 and 6-4.

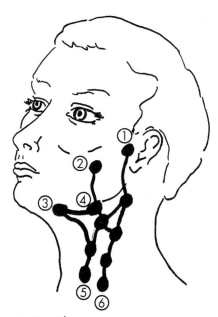

1. Parotid
2. Buccal
3. Submental
4. Submandibular
5. Deep cervical
6. Superficial cervical

FIGURE 6-53

Diagram of lymphatic drainage pathways and major lymph node clusters of the head and neck.

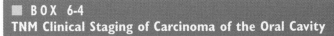

TREATMENT

Squamous cell carcinoma of the oral cavity is usually treated by surgical excision, radiation therapy, or both. Depending on the size, site, and stage of the lesion, surgical treatment may consist of local excision or a combination of local excision and regional lymph node dissection. For example, squamous cell carcinoma of the vermilion border of the lower lip is usually well differentiated, often diagnosed at an early stage, and can usually be cured by local excision. By contrast, squamous cell carcinomas of the lateral border of the tongue or floor of the mouth are usually less differentiated, often diagnosed at later stages, and quicker to metastasize. These lesions usually require extensive treatment (usually a combination of surgery, radiation, and possibly chemotherapy) and have a much poorer prognosis.

Less Common Forms

The overwhelming majority of squamous cell carcinomas of the oral cavity are the common generic morphologic types described in the previous section. The remaining oral squamous cell carcinomas consist of several morphologically distinct subtypes. The most common subtypes are verrucous carcinoma, spindle cell carcinoma, and nasopharyngeal carcinoma. On very rare occasions three other subtypes have been identified and will be discussed briefly. These are adenoid squamous cell carcinoma, adenosquamous carcinoma, and basaloid squamous carcinoma.

Verrucous carcinoma

■ **VERRUCOUS CARCINOMA:** distinct, diffuse, papillary, superficial, nonmetastasizing form of well-differentiated squamous cell carcinoma.

Ackerman first recognized verrucous carcinoma as a distinct entity in 1948. Although it also occurs in other anatomic sites, it most commonly occurs in the oral cavity.

CLINICAL

The tumor commonly occurs in males and tends to affect individuals over 60 years of age. Most intraoral cases involve the gingiva, alveolar mucosa, and buccal mucosa; however, the hard palate and floor of the mouth can also be involved. The tumor grows slowly, exhibits an exophytic papillary (warty) pattern (Figure 6-54), and tends to be diffusely distributed.

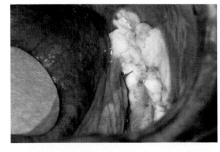

FIGURE 6-54

Verrucous carcinoma. Lesions commonly are diffuse, white, exophytic, and papillary.

HISTOPATHOLOGY

The surface of the tumor is usually papillary and covered by a thick layer of parakeratin. Deep crypts containing "plugs" of parakeratin usually occur between the elongated surface projections. The epithelium seldom exhibits severe dysplastic features. The basement membrane remains intact, and an intense chronic inflammatory cell infiltrate is often present in the underlying connective tissue. The interface between the tumor and the adjacent normal epithelium is usually well defined with minimal if any penetration of epithelial cells along a broad, blunt "pushing margin" of the bulb-shaped rete ridges (Figure 6-55). Compression of underlying superficial muscle bundles and saucerization of cortical bone are sometimes observed in long-standing lesions.

TREATMENT

Because of its superficial and cohesive growth pattern and sharply demarcated margins, verrucous carcinoma is ideally suited to treatment by either surgical excision or laser therapy. The prognosis is good because local excision is usually curative. New lesions in adjacent sites may occur.

Spindle cell carcinoma

> ■ SPINDLE CELL CARCINOMA: rare, unusal form of poorly differentiated squamous cell carcinoma consisting of elongated (spindled) epithelial cells that resemble a sarcoma.

Spindle cell carcinoma is an uncommon variant of squamous cell carcinoma in which the epithelial cells lose their cohesive character and rounded shape and resemble malignant fibroblasts (spindle cells). These lesions can be mistaken for fibrosarcoma.

CLINICAL

Spindle cell carcinoma occurs primarily in males and most often affects the lower lip and tongue. Occasionally, the alveolar mucosa or gingiva is involved.

HISTOPATHOLOGY

The lesion is usually ulcerated with malignant cells streaming from the tips of pointed and elongated epithelial rete pegs adjacent to the ulcerated zone. Curiously, the other layers of the epithelium exhibit a minimal degree of dysplasia. In some lesions, in addition to the spindle cell component, areas of recognizable squamous cell carcinoma with foci of keratin formation are sometimes observed. An inflammatory cell infiltrate consisting of lymphocytes and neutrophils or eosinophils is often present. Despite its apparent lack of differentiation, spindle cell carcinoma exhibits few mitotic figures and is often less aggressive than other forms of poorly differentiated carcinoma (Figure 6-56).

TREATMENT

Spindle cell carcinoma metastasizes and needs to be treated aggressively. Surgical excision appears to be the most effective mode of treatment.

Nasopharyngeal carcinoma

> ■ NASOPHARYNGEAL CARCINOMA: aggressive form of squamous cell carcinoma located in the nasopharynx and having varying levels of differentiation; often first discovered as a metastatic lesion in a lateral neck lymph node.

Of the anatomic locations immediately adjacent to the oral cavity, the nasopharynx is most commonly afflicted with squamous cell carcinoma. The lesions in

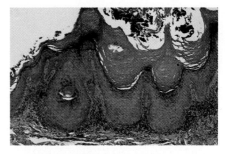

FIGURE 6-55

Verrucous carcinoma. The microscopic features exhibit extensive keratin production, forming fingerlike projections and filling deep crypts; acanthosis with broad blunt bulbous rete ridges compressing the underlying connective tissue; absent or minimal dysplasia, and an intact basement membrane.

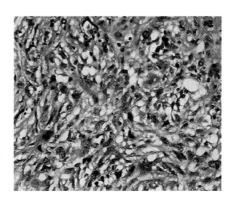

FIGURE 6-56

Spindle cell carcinoma. The microscopic features demonstrate a poorly differentiated lesion containing randomly oriented spindled epithelial cells resembling fibroblasts. The cells exhibit pleomorphism, hyperchromatism, and a lack of keratin production.

this site are usually less differentiated than those found in the oral cavity. In 1978 the WHO proposed that the various forms of squamous cell carcinoma found in the nasopharynx be divided into three categories based on their degree of histologic differentiation. The categories proposed were *keratinizing carcinoma, nonkeratinizing carcinoma,* and *undifferentiated carcinoma.* This has been widely accepted and useful in standardizing the histology and treatment of lesions in this anatomic location.

Patients with nasopharyngeal carcinoma do not fit the usual profile of those with oral squamous cell carcinoma, so a different etiologic factor has long been suspected. Although there is some evidence of an association with the Epstein-Barr virus (EBV) in the nonkeratinizing and undifferentiated types, the evidence is weaker for an association between the virus and the keratinizing type. No strong direct evidence has been established that supports a causal relationship between EBV and nasopharyngeal carcinoma.

CLINICAL

In the United States nasopharyngeal carcinoma accounts for 0.25% of all cancers and occurs in all age groups but more commonly in males by a 3:1 ratio. For unknown reasons nasopharyngeal carcinoma is one of the more common forms of cancer in China and accounts for 18% of all human malignancies. It is particularly prevalent in China's southern and northern provinces and on the island of Taiwan. Nasopharyngeal carcinoma is usually found during an investigation of an asymptomatic lateral neck mass because the lymph nodes of the lateral neck are the usual sites of initial metastases. Other presentations are nasal obstruction, unilateral otitis media, epistaxis, and otalgia.

HISTOPATHOLOGY

Keratinizing carcinoma of the nasopharynx represents 25% of nasopharyngeal carcinomas and exhibits all the features of the usual well or moderately differentiated squamous cell carcinoma found elsewhere in the oropharynx. Microscopic examination reveals distinct intercellular bridges (desmosomes), intracellular keratin production, and keratin pearl formation within islands of epithelial cells (Figure 6-57). **Nonkeratinizing carcinoma** also constitutes 25% of nasopharyngeal carcinomas. It exhibits the clumping features characteristic of squamous epithelium; individual cells exhibit distinct cytoplasm and visible desmosomes, but there is little or no evidence of keratin production (Figure 6-58). These cells clumps are like those of the transitional cell carcinoma of the urinary bladder. In the past, lesions with this histologic pattern were referred to as *transitional cell carcinoma.* **Undifferentiated carcinoma** is the most common form, representing 50% of these carcinomas. It differs from other carcinomas by having

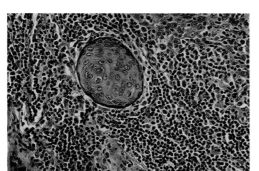
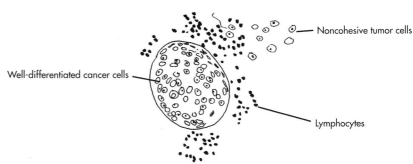

FIGURE 6-57

Nasopharyngeal carcinoma — *keratinizating type.* Microscopic features of the lesion exhibit a central island of well-differentiated squamous cell carcinoma.

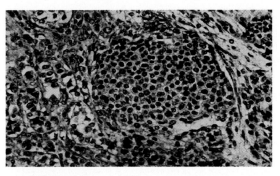
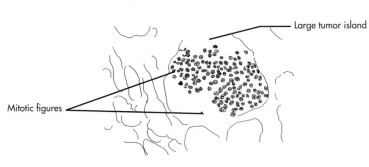

FIGURE 6-58

Nasopharyngeal carcinoma — *nonkeratinizing type.* Microscopic features of the lesion demonstrate sheets of randomly oriented poorly differentiated epithelial cells with no keratin production evident.

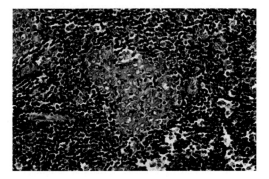
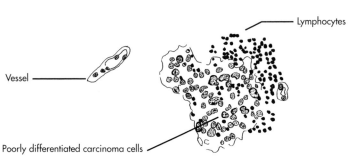

FIGURE 6-59

Nasopharyngeal carcinoma — *undifferentiated type.* Microscopic features of the lesion exhibit small islands and individual cells that are poorly differentiated against a background of densely packed normal lymphocytes.

neoplastic cells that are often difficult to recognize as being of epithelial origin. The cells have scant and indistinct cytoplasm surrounding a rounded vesicular nucleus with large prominent nucleoli. The cells may be in a syncytial arrangement rather than in the "sheets" that are common to squamous cell neoplasms. They are also distinguished by the presence of large aggregrates of nonneoplastic lymphocytes surrounding the epithelial component (Figure 6-59). Because of the intermingling of the two types of tissues, this form of the nasophyngeal carcinoma was previously designated as *lymphoepithelioma*. It is not uncommon for an individual lesion to have more than one of the three aforementioned histologic patterns.

TREATMENT

Because of the generally inaccessible anatomic location of a carcinoma in the nasopharynx, the immediate adjacency of vital structures, and the radiosensitivity of the two nonkeratinizing lesions, surgical treatment is usually not undertaken. The keratinizing type of carcinoma is not very radioresponsive; thus the 5-year survival rate of patients with these lesions is only 10% to 20%. Patients with nonkeratinizing lesions have variable responses to radiotherapy and have a 5-year survival rate of 35% to 50%. The undifferentiated lesions are most responsive to radiation and have a 5-year survival rate of 60%.

Adenoid squamous cell carcinoma

> ■ ADENOID SQUAMOUS CELL CARCINOMA: rare, low grade epithelial malignancy of the sun-exposed skin of the face and lower lip.

The adenoid squamous cell carcinoma is a well-differentiated neoplasm that occurs primarily on the face, including the vermilion border of the lower lip. It does not occur within the oral cavity. This tumor is referred to by a number of names including *adenoacanthoma, acantholytic squamous cell carcinoma,* and *pseudoglandular squamous cell carcinoma.*

CLINICAL
Lesions arise on sun-damaged skin, specifically in areas of actinic (solar) keratosis of the acantholytic type.

HISTOPATHOLOGY
The tumor tends to be well circumscribed at its lateral and deep margins and resembles the profile of keratoacanthoma. The peripheral cells of the tumor exhibit the features of a well-differentiated squamous cell carcinoma and one or more irregular, slitlike, or cystic areas containing acantholytic and dysplastic cells.

Surgical excision of an adenoid squamous cell carcinoma is the treatment of choice and is usually curative. If the tumor is incompletely excised, it can recur locally; however, metastasis is rare.

Adenosquamous carcinoma

> ■ ADENOSQUAMOUS CARCINOMA: rare, aggressive carcinoma of the mucosa consisting of a mixture of malignant squamous and glandular cells.

CLINICAL
Adenosquamous carcinoma is a rare, aggressive carcinoma that occurs within the oral and nasal cavities and in the larynx. Within the oral cavity it occurs primarily on the floor of the mouth and the hard palate.

HISTOPATHOLOGY
Adenosquamous carcinoma appears to be simultaneously derived from the surface mucosa and the adjacent minor salivary gland ducts. The histologic appearance resembles a high-grade mucoepidermoid carcinoma.

TREATMENT
The tumor has a marked tendency to metastasize to regional lymph nodes and distant sites. Because of its metastatic potential, the tumor has a poor prognosis.

Basaloid squamous cell carcinoma

> ■ BASALOID SQUAMOUS CELL CARCINOMA: rare, aggressive form of poorly differentiated squamous cell carcinoma consisting of medullary patterns of cells with central areas of necrosis.

The basaloid squamous cell carcinoma (BSCC) is a relatively new entity first described in 1986. Before it was defined as a separate entity, the basaloid squamous cell carcinoma was often diagnosed as an adenoid cystic carcinoma or an adenoid type of basal cell carcinoma.

CLINICAL

It is an aggressive malignancy that occurs primarily at the base of the tongue, larynx, pyriform sinus, and tonsil. Males are affected far more often than females; the gender ratio is approximately 7:1. Most of the reported cases have been in habitual smokers, many of whom also consumed significant amounts of alcohol. The average age of the patients affected by this tumor is approximately 60 years.

HISTOPATHOLOGY

Lesions are composed of closely packed, moderately pleomorphic, basaloid cells that form variable-sized islands and cords. The larger islands of tumor cells often exhibit a central focus of comedo type (doughnutlike) necrosis. The smaller islands of tumor cells often exhibit prominent individual cell necrosis (apoptosis). Cells at the periphery of the tumor islands tend to exhibit nuclear palisading. A cribriform growth pattern similar to that seen in adenoid cystic carcinoma is frequently present. Many cases exhibit a zone of stromal hyalinization around the neoplastic islands. Mitotic figures, including atypical forms, are often numerous. Foci of squamous differentiation are always present. This most commonly consists of cells with abundant eosinophilic cytoplasm or collections of keratinized cells within the basaloid cell islands. Keratin pearl formation may or may not be present. The junction between the squamous cells and the adjacent basaloid tumor cells is usually abrupt, with little or no transition. In most cases the overlying surface epithelium exhibits severe dysplasia or carcinoma in situ, which is in continuity with the basaloid squamous cell carcinoma.

TREATMENT

At the time of initial diagnosis, the majority of patients with basaloid squamous cell carcinoma exhibit metastases to regional lymph nodes or distant metastases (stage III or IV diseases). Like the adenosquamous carcinoma, the basaloid squamous cell carcinoma tends to metastasize widely and has a poor prognosis.

Basal cell carcinoma

> ■ BASAL CELL CARCINOMA: common, locally destructive, nonmetastasizing malignancy of the skin composed of medullary patterns of basaloid cells.

Basal cell carcinoma is a malignant tumor of hair-bearing areas of the skin. It does not arise on mucous membranes; however, it can involve mucous membranes by directly spreading from adjacent skin. The majority of basal cell carcinomas arise on the sun-exposed skin of the upper part of the face, including the forehead and ears, in individuals with fair skin. Individuals with dark skin are rarely affected. Chronic occupational or recreational exposure to direct sunlight (actinic radiation) is a known etiologic factor for this tumor. Males are more commonly affected than females. The incidence of basal cell carcinoma is particularly high in regions with high temperatures and low humidity. Notable examples are Queensland in Australia and Arizona in the United States. Basal cell carcinoma can develop in patients who are in the fourth decade of life, but it usually develops in older patients. An exception is seen in patients with the nevoid basal cell carcinoma syndrome (Gorlin-Goltz syndrome), in which the tumors develop in patients in the second and third decades of life.

CLINICAL

The basal cell carcinoma starts as a slightly elevated papule that slowly enlarges and eventually develops a central, crusted ulcer with an elevated smooth-rolled border (Figure 6-60). If untreated, the tumor enlarges and invades adjacent tissues and structures by direct extension (Figure 6-61) but rarely metastasizes. Al-

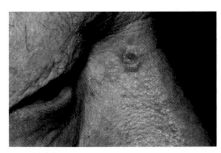

FIGURE 6-60

Basal cell carcinoma. Early incipient lesion on the bridge of the nose that exhibits the raised smooth borders with the depressed center.

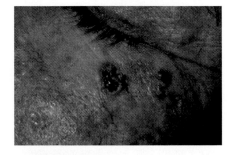

FIGURE 6-61

Basal cell carcinoma. Advanced lesion with characteristic irregular shape and central nonhealing ulcer. An adjacent satellite lesion is present.

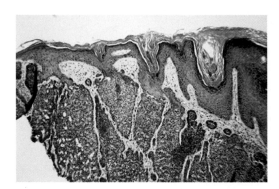

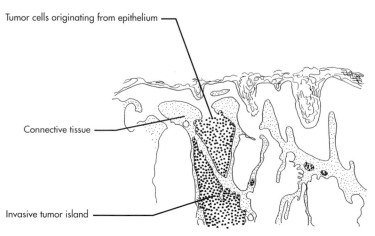

Tumor cells originating from epithelium

Connective tissue

Invasive tumor island

FIGURE 6-62

Basal cell carcinoma. Microscopic features of raised margin illustrate a proliferation of cells from the basal cell layer and extension of the tumor cells laterally beneath the overlying normal skin.

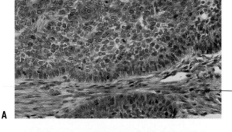

A

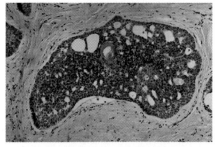

B

FIGURE 6-63

Basal cell carcinoma. A, High-power microscopy of islands of basal cell carcinoma with a peripheral layer of palisaded cells and a central area composed of uniform basal and parabasal cells. **B,** Medium-power microscopy of an island of basal cell carcinoma exhibiting the less common microcystic (adenoid) pattern. Included is a focal area of keratinization.

though most basal cell carcinomas are solitary tumors, those occurring in the Gorlin-Goltz syndrome are multiple.

HISTOPATHOLOGY

The basal cell carcinoma is characterized by a proliferation of basaloid epithelial cells (Figure 6-62) exhibiting a spectrum of growth patterns ranging from solid (Figure 6-63, *A*) to adenoid or cystic (Figure 6-63, *B*). The cells at the periphery of the tumor islands are usually palisaded and hyperchromatic. The central cells may be polyhedral, oval, round, or spindle shaped. Intercellular bridges are seldom seen in routine tissue sections. Mitotic figures can vary from few to numerous. Apoptosis (individual cell death) of tumor cells is commonly seen. The fibrous stroma around the tumor islands is variably cellular and often exhibits large amounts of acid mucopolysaccharides. During tissue processing, dehydration causes the mucopolysaccharides to shrink, resulting in the formation of retraction spaces (clefts) that separate the stroma from the tumor islands. This is a common but not a constant histologic artifact seen in tissue sections of basal cell carcinoma. Another frequently seen feature in the stroma of basal cell carcinoma is an increase in the elastic tissue content.

TREATMENT

Basal cell carcinoma can be treated by a number of modalities. The most common are excisional surgery, radiation, and electrocautery. In an individual case the modality of treatment is dictated by a variety of factors. The most common are size and site of the lesion and the age of the patient. Although basal cell carcinoma has a distinct tendency to recur after conservative treatment, the cure rate using the previously mentioned modalities is approximately 95%.

MELANOMA

■ MELANOMA: malignant neoplasm of melanocytes occurring on skin and mucosal surfaces that commonly has a radial and superficial initial growth period before it extends into the deeper underlying tissues and metastasizes.

Melanoma, also termed "malignant melanoma," most commonly occurs on the skin, where it is divided into four main types: (1) *superficial spreading*, (2) *lentigo maligna*, (3) *acral-lentiginous*, and (4) *nodular*.

Melanomas also occur on the mucous membranes, including the oral mucosa. On the skin melanomas tend to develop on the sun-exposed areas in fair-skinned individuals who have had prolonged exposure to strong direct sunlight. Recent data from Scandinavia, Australia (Queensland), and the United States indicate that the incidence of cutaneous melanoma is increasing, having tripled in the last 40 years. Although the median age of patients with the initial diagnosis of skin lesions is 53, it is the most common malignancy of young, white adults, occurring more commonly in males than in females. Sunshine (actinic radiation) is the only factor that is strongly implicated in the etiology of skin melanoma. Since melanoma also occurs on surfaces not exposed to the sun, other unknown factors most likely exist.

Oral melanoma is considered rare when compared to the incidence of skin melanoma. Oral melanoma, like skin melanoma, occurs in patients who are in the 40- to 60-year age group. Most cases of oral melanoma arise on the hard palate and maxillary gingiva.

ORAL MELANOMA

Oral melanoma can be dark brown, bluish-black, or black. Occasionally, a non-pigmented melanoma ("amelanotic melanoma") is found that is reddish rather than brown or black. Most lesions have an early macular pattern and become papular and/or nodular in later stages. A nodular melanoma occurs that does not have a significant macular stage.

Most melanomas within the oral cavity tend to grow in two phases: an initial **radial-growth phase** followed by a **vertical-growth phase.** During the radial-growth phase the neoplastic cells spread laterally in all directions but remain confined to the surface epithelium. The vertical-growth phase begins when the neoplastic cells invade and populate the connective tissue. The duration of the radial-growth phase can differ significantly among different types of melanoma.

SUPERFICIAL SPREADING MELANOMA

■ **SUPERFICIAL SPREADING MELANOMA:** most common form of malignant melanoma, initially appearing as an irregularly shaped brown-black macular area with jagged borders and satellite lesions in which areas of nodular melanoma eventually develop.

CLINICAL
Superficial spreading melanoma is the most common type of melanoma on skin and on mucous membranes, accounting for approximately 80% of all lesions. Superficial spreading melanoma is most commonly found in middle-age patients. The radial-growth phase consists of a tan, brown, or black variegated macule or plaque that exhibits an irregular outline (Figure 6-64). Frequently, one or more nearby satellite lesions are present. The radial-growth phase may last from several months to several years. During this phase the lesion becomes larger, more intensely pigmented, and eventually nodular and ulcerated.

HISTOPATHOLOGY
The radial-growth phase is characterized by the presence of large atypical melanocytes within the epithelial layer that exhibit abundant pale cytoplasm and are arranged in small round clusters at the epithelial connective tissue interface

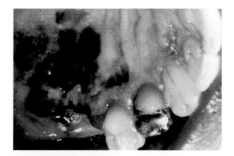

FIGURE 6-64
Superficial spreading melanoma. The lesion is brown-black with irregular margins and multiple satellite lesions. The location on the anterior palate is common. (Courtesy Dr. A.M. Rees.)

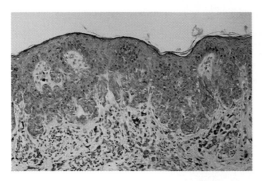
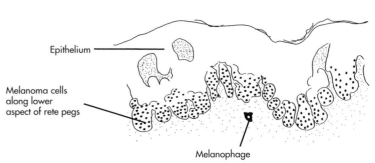

Epithelium

Melanoma cells
along lower
aspect of rete pegs

Melanophage

FIGURE 6-65

Superficial spreading melanoma. Microscopic features of a lesion before the vertical-growth stage (invasion) reveal the proliferation of abnormal melanocytes within the basal cell layer, producing a nodular pattern of the tips of the rete pegs. The dark coloration of most lesions is due to the greatly increased numbers of atypical melanocytes and the resulting excess melanin production. The melanin is usually contained within melanophages located in both the upper layers of the epithelium and underlying connective tissue.

(Figure 6-65). Focal microinvasion is usually evident. The term "pagetoid" is usually used to describe the clear cells in the unique intraepithelial growth pattern in superficial spreading melanoma. The nodular and ulceration stage is characterized by frank invasion of the connective tissue by tumor cells, which are usually arranged in an alveolar pattern. The individual tumor cell exhibits abundant pale cytoplasm containing variable amounts of fine, powdery melanin that imparts a "dusty" appearance to the cytoplasm. Mitotic figures may or may not be conspicuous. Significant pseudoepitheliomatous hyperplasia of the overlying epithelium may accompany the invading tumor cells. The diagnosis of melanoma can be confirmed with positive immunohistochemical stains for S-100, HMB-45, and vimentin.

LENTIGO MALIGNA MELANOMA

> ■ LENTIGO MALIGNA MELANOMA: slowly evolving melanoma that developes within a preexisting pigmented macular lesion on the *sun-exposed* skin of elderly patients.

CLINICAL

Lentigo maligna melanoma occurs only on sunexposed areas of the skin, primarily on the cheeks and temples of elderly white men and women. It is an uncommon form of melanoma, representing 5% of lesions. It usually arises in a preexisting pigmented lesion known as *Hutchinson melanotic freckle* and evolves slowly over a period of 15 or more years. The lentigo maligna presents as a relatively large, irregular and asymmetric, variegated macular lesion. The color varies extensively from a light tan to black, the latter usually indicative of malignancy. Some lesions exhibit a central area of pale scarring, a sign that some regression has occurred.

HISTOPATHOLOGY

In lentigo maligna melanoma the epithelium is atrophic; the basal layer exhibits increased numbers of cytologically atypical melanocytes with variable amounts of coarse melanin granules. Although in most instances the atypical melanocytes are singularly scattered throughout the basal layer, some small nests of cells may also be present. Intraepithelial spreading of tumor cells may be present. As the lesion progresses, the intensity of the pigmentation increases and individual atypical melanocytes begin appearing in the superficial connective tissue. This early invasive or vertical-growth phase is usually accompanied by a fibroblastic and lymphohistiocytic host response. During the advanced invasive phase the neoplastic melanocytes are often spindle shaped and may exhibit desmoplasia or neurotropism.

ACRAL LENTIGINOUS MELANOMA

■ ACRAL LENTIGINOUS MELANOMA: brown, irregularly shaped macular lesion of the *unexposed* skin of the hands and feet that undergoes progression to nodular melanoma.

Acral lentiginous melanoma occurs on the palms of the hands, soles of the feet, and nails beds (especially the thumb and great toe). It is purported to have a mucosal counterpart that is found on the mucocutaneous junction and the oral mucous membranes. This type of melanoma is clinically and histologically similar to the lentigo maligna melanoma; however, its biologic behavior is much more aggressive.

CLINICAL
Acral lentiginous melanomas occur in all races and appear to be unrelated to exposure to sunlight. They represent 8% of all melanomas. This type of melanoma starts as a *brown* variegated macule with irregular borders. As the tumor enlarges it becomes ulcerated, papular, or nodular, which is indicative of its transition to the vertical-growth phase. In the mouth the diagnosis of oral acral lentiginous melanoma is seldom made because in this location it is clinically and microscopically indistinguishable from superficially spreading melanoma.

HISTOPATHOLOGY
The macular phase of skin lesions exhibits a basilar proliferation of individual large atypical melanocytes that impart a vacuolated appearance to the basal region of the epithelium. Mitotic figures may or may not be seen during the radial growth phase. The basal arrangement of the palisaded melanoma cells constitutes the lentiginous pattern. As the tumor assumes a papular and nodular appearance, confluent masses of neoplastic melanocytes, which are frequently spindle shaped, extend into the connective tissue. Many of these lesions exhibit a marked infiltrate of lymphocytes that may assume a lichenoid pattern at the epithelial-mesenchymal junction. In these cases a lymphocytic infiltrate can obscure the presence of the neoplastic melanocytes. Detailed microscopic examination supplemented with immunohistochemical staining is required in these cases.

NODULAR MELANOMA

■ NODULAR MELANOMA: a form of melanoma of the skin, and occasionally the mucosa, that arises as a raised mass with a limited macular radial-growth phase, quickly invades and metastasizes, and consists of a wide variety of cell shapes and sizes.

Nodular melanoma is the second most common form of melanomas, accounting for 15% of these lesions. It primarily occurs on skin but is also found on oral

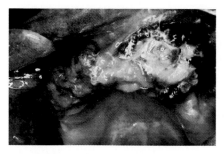

FIGURE 6-66

Nodular melanoma. The lesion is large with a nodular surface containing ulceration and areas of dark and partial pigmentation intermingled with nonpigmented areas.

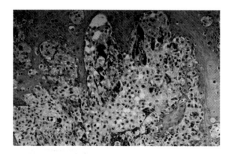

FIGURE 6-67

Nodular melanoma. Microscopic features reveal a variety of cell types. The most common is a large epithelioid cell with either a clear or pink cytoplasm. Other cells are spindled and some are small, round, and dense, resembling lymphocytes. Melanin deposits are sporadically distributed.

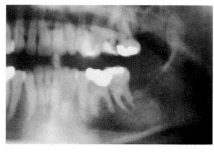

FIGURE 6-68

Metastatic adenocarcinoma from breast. The radiograph reveals a large mixed radiolucent-radiopaque area in the posterior mandible.

mucous membranes. It differs significantly from the other types by having little or no radial-growth phase but exhibiting a prominent vertical-growth phase almost from its inception. Occasionally, lesions do not contain clinically or even microscopically detectable melanin-induced pigmentation.

CLINICAL

The lesion consists of combinations of pink, red, brown, and black nodules, many of which are ulcerated (Figure 6-66). Evidence of metastasis is found early in the disease process.

HISTOPATHOLOGY

In most cases by the time a tissue sample is secured, the connective tissue is usually densely packed with tumor cells. The cells exhibit a variety of morphology types, the most common being epithelioid with lightly pink or clear cytoplasms; others are spindle-shaped and lymphocyte-like (Figure 6-67). Different parts of the tumor may have different mixtures of the cell types. Normal and abnormal mitotic figures and pleomorphic cells are frequent. Melanin deposition is usually sporadic with large areas devoid of such deposits. In other areas heavy deposits of melanin granules are commonly present and usually obscure the features of the individual cells. The surface epithelium at the margins of the tumor is usually free of the malignant cells, indicating the absence of a radial-growth phase.

TREATMENT

The key to the treatment of melanoma is early diagnosis while it is still in its radial-growth phase, followed by prompt surgical excision of the lesion. During the radial-growth phase melanomas are "thin"; that is, most of the tumor cells are located in or immediately adjacent to the epithelium and can therefore be excised with relative ease. When measuring the thickness of melanoma, it has been shown that melanomas that are less than 0.76 mm thick rarely metastasize; most are cureable. Such tumor thickness is determined during microscopic evaluation by the pathologists, who use a micrometer to measure from the top of the granular layer of the epithelium to the level of the deepest tumor cell.

In addition to tumor thickness, the rate of mitotic activity within the vertically growing neoplastic cells has also proven to be a valuable prognostic indicator for melanoma. Other factors that have some effect on the prognosis of melanoma include gender of the patient, anatomic site of the lesion, and the presence or absence of tumor-infiltrating lymphocytes.

Because of its prominant vertical-growth pattern, nodular melanoma tends to invade deeply and metastasize early. Melanomas that have metastasized to regional lymph nodes or distant sites have a relatively poor prognosis. Chemotherapy and immunotherapy for metastatic melanomas are presently at the experimental and clinical stages of development. Regardless of treatment, nodular melanoma that has entered the vertical-growth phase exhibits a relatively poor prognosis.

METASTASES TO THE JAWS

Metastasis to the oral region from a malignant tumor elsewhere in the body is an uncommon but clinically important finding because it may be the first indication that the patient has a distant primary tumor. The vast majority of metastases from distant primary lesions to the oral region occur in the mandible, although the maxilla can also be affected. Although metastatic lesions within the mandible can be asymptomatic, most patients experience some degree of discomfort or pain, which is often followed by loosening of teeth or unilateral paresthesia or anesthesia of the lower lip or chin. The development of these symptoms should alert the clinician to the potential presence of metastatic disease. Some degree of swelling or expansion of the mandible, primarily in the molar region, is also often present. The pathway for the metastatic spread of tumor cells to the mandible from a distant primary, such as the kidney, has usually been ascribed to the paravertebral plexus of veins (Batson plexus).

The radiologic appearance of the mandible at the site of a metastatic tumor deposit can range from an ill-defined radiolucency to an ill-defined radiopacity, or it may appear as a mixed radiolucent/radiopaque lesion (Figure 6-68). The microscopic appearance usually suggests that a lesion is metastatic because the cells will often be present in clusters of various sizes that are separated by normal resident tissue or fibrous connective tissue replacement (Figure 6-69).

The majority of tumors that metastasize to the jaw are adenocarcinomas. The site of origin of the most common primary tumors and the approximate relative frequency of metastasis to the jaws are as follows: breast (30%), lung (20%), kidney (15%), thyroid (5%), prostate (5%), colon (5%), stomach (5%), and cutaneous melanoma (5%).

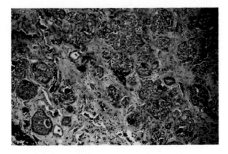

FIGURE 6-69

Metastasis to the jaws. The microscopic features of soft tissue removed from within the mandible suggest a metastatic lesion because the cells are in small clusters separated by relatively normal connective tissue. Some cell nests contain pools of eosinophilic coagulum that suggests the lesion is an adenocarcinoma.

ADDITIONAL READING

KERATOACANTHOMA

Eversole LR, Leider AS, Alexander G. Intraoral and labial keratoacanthoma. *Oral Surg Oral Med Oral Pathol.* 1982; 54:663-667.

Goodwin RE, Fisher GH. Keratoacanthoma of the head and neck. *Ann Otol Rhinol Laryngol.* 1980; 89:72.

LABIAL MELANOTIC MACULE

Ho KK, Dervan P, O'Loughlin S, Powell FC. Labial melanotic macule: a clinical, histopathologic, and ultrastructural study. *J Am Acad Dermatol.* 1993; 28:33-9.

Weathers DR, Corio RL, Crawford BE, Giansanti JS and others. The labial melanotic macule. *Oral Surg.* 1976; 42:196-205.

ORAL MELANOTIC MACULE

Page LR, Corio RL, Crawford BE, Giansanti JS and others. The oral melanotic macule. *Oral Surg.* 1977; 44:219-226.

MELANOACANTHOMA

Goode RK, Crawford BE, Callihan MD, Neville BW. Oral melanoacanthoma. *Oral Surg Oral Med Oral Pathol.* 1983; 56: 622-628.

Lambert WC, Lambert MW, Mesa ML, Schnieder LC and others. Melanoacanthoma and related disorders: simulants of acral-lentiginous (P-P-S-M) melanoma. *Int J Dermatol.* 1987; 26:508-10.

Tomich CE, Zunt SL. Melanoacanthosis (melanoacanthoma) of the oral mucosa. *J Dermatol Surg Oncol.* 1990; 16:231-6.

Wright JW, Binnie WH, Byrd DL, Dunsworth AR. Intraoral melanoacanthoma. *J Periodontol.* 1982; 54:107-111.

NEVUS

Barker GR, Sloan P. An intraoral combined blue naevus. *Br J Oral Maxillofac Surg.* 1988; 26:165-168.

Buchner A, Hanson LS. Pigmented nevi of the oral mucosa: a clinicopathologic study of 36 new cases and review of 15 cases from the literature: part 2: analysis of 191 cases. *Oral Surg Oral Med Oral Pathol.* 1987; 63:676-682.

SMOKER'S MELANOSIS

Axell T, Hedin A. Epidemiologic studies of excessive oral melanin pigmentation with special reference to the influence of tobacco habits. *Scand J Dent Res.* 1982; 90:434-442.

Brown FH, Houston GD. Smoker's melanosis: a case report. *J Periodontol.* 1991; 62:524-7.

Merchant HW, Haynes LE, Ellison LT. Soft-palate pigmentation in lung disease, including cancer. *Oral Surg Oral Med Oral Pathol.* 1976; 41:726-733.

LEUKOPLAKIA

Abbey LM. Precancerous lesions of the mouth. *Curr Opin Dent.* 1991; 1:773-6.

Albrecht M, Banoczy J, Dinya E, Tamas G. Occurrence of oral leukoplakia and lichen planus in diabetes mellitus. *J Oral Pathol Med.* 1992; 21:364-6.

Banoczy J. Oral leukoplakia and other white lesions of the oral mucosa related to dermatological disorders. *J Cutan Pathol.* 1983; 10:238-56.

Bouquot JE. Reviewing oral leukoplakia: clinical concepts for the 1990s. *J Am Dent Assoc.* 1991; 122:80-2.

Bouquot JE, Gnepp DR. Laryngeal precancer: a review of the literature, commentary, and comparison with oral leukoplakia. *Head Neck.* 1991; 13:488-97.

Silverman S, Gorsky M, Lozada F. Oral leukoplakia and malignant transformation: a followup study of 257 patients. *Cancer*. 1984; 53: 563-568.

Waldron CA, Shafer WG. Leukoplakia revisited: a clinicopathologic study of 3256 oral leukoplakias. *Cancer*. 1975; 36:1386-1392.

WHO Collaborating Centre for Oral Precancerous Lesions. Definition of leukoplakia and related lesions: an aid to studies on oral precancer. *Oral Surg Oral Med Oral Pathol*. 1978; 46:518-539.

LEUKOEDEMA

Archard HO, Carlson KP, Stanley HR. Leukoedema of the human oral mucosa. *Oral Surg Oral Med Oral Pathol*. 1968; 25: 717-728.

Martin JL. Leukoedema: a review of the literature. *J Natl Med Assoc*. 1992; 84:938-40.

van Wyk CW, Ambrosio SC. Leukoedema: ultrastructural and histochemical observations. *J Oral Pathol*. 1983; 12:319-329.

NICOTINE STOMATITIS

Reddy CR, Kameswari VR, Ramulu PG. Histopathological study of stomatitis nicotina. *Br J Cancer*. 1971; 25:403.

Thoma KH. Stomatitis nicotina and its effect on the palate. *Am J Orthod Oral Surg*. 1941; 27:38.

PROLIFERATIVE VERRUCOUS LEUKOPLAKIA

Hall JM, Cohen MA, Moreland AA. Multiple and confluent lesions of oral leukoplakia: proliferative verrucous leukoplakia. *Arch Dermatol*. 1991; 127:887-890.

Hansen LS, Olson JA, Silverman S. Proliferative verrucous leukoplakia: a long-term study of thirty patients. *Oral Surg Oral Med Oral Pathol*. 1985; 60:285-98.

EPITHELIAL DYSPLASIA

Abdelsayed RA. Study of human papillomavirus in oral epithelial dysplasia and epidermoid carcinoma in the absence of tobacco and alcohol use. *Oral Surg Oral Med Oral Pathol*. 1991; 71:730-2.

De Jong WF, Albrecht M, Banoczy J, van der Waal I. Epithelial dysplasia in oral lichen planus: a preliminary report of a Dutch-Hungarian study of 100 cases. *Int J Oral Surg*. 1984; 13:221-5.

Gregg TA, Cowan CG, Kee F. Trends in the relative frequency of histologically diagnosed epithelial dysplasia and intra-oral carcinoma in Northern Ireland, 1975-1989. *Br Dent J*. 1992; 173:234-6.

Kaugars GE, Burns JC, Gunsolley JC. Epithelial dysplasia of the oral cavity and lips. *Cancer*. 1988; 62:2166-70.

Kaugars GE, Mehailescu WL, Gunsolley JC. Smokeless tobacco use and oral epithelial dysplasia. *Cancer*. 1989; 64:1527-30.

Odukoya O, Gallagher G, Shklar G. A histologic study of epithelial dysplasia in oral lichen planus. *Arch Dermatol*. 1985; 121:1132-6.

Pindborg JJ, Reibel J, Holmstrup P. Subjectivity in evaluating oral epithelial dysplasia, carcinoma in situ and initial carcinoma. *J Oral Pathol*. 1985; 14:698-708.

ERYTHROPLAKIA

Crissman JD, Visscher DW, Sakr W. Premalignant lesions of the upper aerodigestive tract: pathologic classification. *J Cell Biochem Suppl*. 1993; 17F:49-56.

Mashberg A. Erythroplasia: the earliest sign of asymptomatic oral cancer. *J Am Dent Assoc*. 1978; 96:615-620.

Shafer WG, Waldron CA. Erythroplakia of the oral cavity. *Cancer*. 1975; 36:1021-1028.

Shear M. Erythroplakia of the mouth. *Int Dent J*. 1972; 22:460.

SQUAMOUS CELL CARCINOMA

Cowan JM, Beckett MA, Ahmed-Swan S, Weichselbaum RR. Cytogenetic evidence of the multistep origin of head and neck squamous cell carcinoma. *J Natl Cancer Inst*. 1992; 84:793-797.

Gupta PC, Pindborg JJ, Mehta FS. Comparison of carcinogenicity of betel quid with and without tobacco: an epidemiological review. *Ecol Dis*. 1982; 1:213-9.

Krolls SO, Hoffman S. Squamous cell carcinoma of the oral soft tissues: a statistical analysis of 14,253 cases by age, sex and race of patients. *J Am Dent Assoc*. 1976; 92:571-574.

Krutchkoff DJ, Chen J, Katz RV. Oral cancer: a survey of 566 cases from the University of Connecticut oral pathology biopsy service, 1975-1986. *Oral Surg Oral Med Oral Pathol*. 1990; 70:192-198.

Mashberg A, Morrisey JB, Garfinkel L. A study of the appearance of early asymptomatic squamous cell carcinoma. *Cancer*. 1973; 32:1436-1445.

Murphy GF, Elder DE. *Non-melanocytic Tumors of the Skin: Atlas of Tumor Pathology, AFIP Fascicle 1*. Washington, DC: Armed Forces Institute of Pathology: 1991. Third Series.

Pindborg JJ. *Oral Cancer and Precancer*. Bristol, England: John Wright & Sons Ltd; 1980.

Vokes EE, Weichselbaum RR, Lippman SM, Hong WK. Head and neck cancer. *N Engl J Med*. 1993; 1894-194.

Wright BA, Binnie WH, Wright JM. *Oral Cancer: Clinical and Pathological Considerations*. Boca Raton, Florida: CRC-Press; 1988.

ADENOID SQUAMOUS CELL CARCINOMA

Johnson WC, Helwig EB. Adenoid squamous cell carcinoma (adenoacanthoma): a clinicopathologic study of 155 patients. *Cancer*. 1966; 19:1639-1650.

Jones AC, Freedman PD, Kerpel SM. Oral adenoid squamous cell carcinoma: a report of three cases and review of the literature. *J Oral Maxillofac Surg*. 1993; 51:676-81.

ADENOSQUAMOUS CARCINOMA

Gerughty RM, Hennigar GR, Brown FM. Adenosquamous carcinoma of the nasal, oral and laryngeal cavities: a clinicopathologic survey of ten cases. *Cancer.* 1968; 22:1140-1155.

Lam KY, Loke SL, Ma LT. Histochemistry of mucin secreting components in mucoepidermoid and adenosquamous carcinoma of the oesophagus. *J Clin Pathol.* 1993; 46:1011-5.

BASALOID SQUAMOUS CARCINOMA

Banks ER, Frierson HF, Mills SE, George E and others. Basaloid squamous cell carcinoma of the head and neck: a clinicopathologic and immunohistochemical study of 40 cases. *Am J Surg Pathol.* 1992; 16:939-946.

Klijanienko J, el-Naggar A, Ponzio-Prion A, Marandas P and others. Basaloid squamous carcinoma of the head and neck: immunohistochemical comparison with adenoid cystic carcinoma and squamous cell carcinoma. *Arch Otolaryngol Head Neck Surg.* 1993; 119:887-90.

Wain SL, Kier R, Vollmer RT, Bossen EH. Basaloid-squamous cell carcinoma of the tongue, hypopharynx and larynx: report of 10 cases. *Hum Pathol.* 1986; 7:1158-1166.

MELANOMA

Breslow A. Thickness, cross-sectional areas and depth of invasion in the prognosis of cutaneous melanoma. *Ann Surg.* 1970; 172:902-908.

Eisen D, Voorhees JJ. Oral melanoma and other pigmented lesions of the oral cavity. *J Am Acad Dermatol.* 1991; 24:527-537.

Elder DE, Murphy GF. *Melanocytic Tumors of the Skin: Atlas of Tumor Pathology, AFIP-Fascicle 2.* Washington, DC: Armed Forces Institute of Pathology: 1991. Third Series.

Guzzo M, Grandi C, Licitra L, Podrecca S and others. Mucosal malignant melanoma of head and neck: forty-eight cases treated at Istituto Nazionale Tumori of Milan. *Eur J Surg Oncol.* 1993; 19:316-9.

Joughin K, Antonyshyn O, Myrden JA. Mucosal malignant melanoma of the paranasal sinuses. *Ann Plast Surg.* 1992; 29:353-6.

Lombardi T, Haskell R, Morgan PR, Odell EW. An unusual intraosseous melanoma in the maxillary alveolus. *Oral Surg Oral Med Oral Pathol Oral Radiol Endod.* 1995; 80:677-82.

Manganaro AM, Hammond HL, Dalton MJ, Williams TP. Oral melanoma. *Oral Surg Oral Med Oral Pathol Oral Radiol Endod.* 1995; 80:670-6.

Rapini RP, Golitz LE, Greer RO, Krekorian EA and others. Primary malignant melanoma of the oral cavity. *Cancer.* 1985; 55:1543-1551.

Regezi J, Hayward J, Pickens T. Superficial melanomas of the oral mucous membranes. *Oral Surg Oral Med Oral Pathol.* 1978; 45:730-740.

Snow GW, van der Waal I. Mucosal melanomas of the head and neck. *Otolaryngol Clin North Am.* 1986; 19:537-547.

Stern SJ, Guillamondegui OM. Mucosal melanoma of the head and neck. *Head Neck.* 1991; 13:22-7.

Trotti A, Peters LJ. Role of radiotherapy in the primary management of mucosal melanoma of the head and neck. *Semin Surg Oncol.* 1993; 9:246-50.

METASTASIS

Batson OV. The function of the vertebral veins and their role in the spread of metastasis. *Ann Surg.* 1940; 112:138.

Clausen F, Poulsen H. Metastatic carcinoma to the jaws. *Acta Pathol Microbiol Scand.* 1963; 57:361.

Friedman M, Roberts N, Kirshenbaum GL, Colombo J. Nodal size of metastatic squamous cell carcinoma of the neck. *Laryngoscope.* 1993; 103:854-6.

Wanamaker JR, Kraus DH, Eliachar I, Lavertu P. Manifestations of metastatic breast carcinoma to the head and neck. *Head Neck.* 1993; 15:257-62.

Watkinson JC, Todd CE, Paskin L, Rankin S and others. Metastatic carcinoma in the neck: a clinical, radiological, scintigraphic and pathological study. *Clin Otolaryngol.* 1991; 16:187-92.

ORAL INFECTIONS

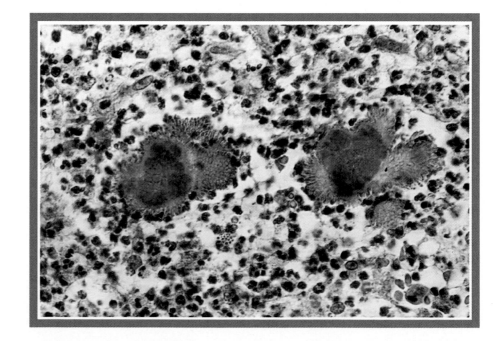

VIRAL INFECTIONS

Viruses are among the simplest and smallest microorganisms that infect humans. They consist of a single or double strand of either DNA or RNA surrounded by a protein coat termed a *capsid*. These two structures constitute the nucleocapsid or *core* of the virus. The core of the virus *(virion)* is responsible for infection. Because a virion lacks the necessary cytoplasmic constituents of higher life forms, it is unable to perform metabolic or protein synthesis functions. A virus is an obligate parasite because it must enter a host cell of a higher life form to replicate and undertake macromolecular synthesis. Viruses are not able to enter all of the cells they encounter, only those cells that possess a surface receptor specific for that virus. The matching of a virus with a specific cell type is termed *tropism*. Viruses are tissue and species specific; they infect some species of the animal kingdom and not others. There are some viruses that only infect humans.

Before most viruses can infect cells and replicate, they must bind specific molecules ("ligands") located on their outermost protein coat ("envelope") to a receptor on the wall of a tropic cell (Figure 7-1). When the match occurs, the virion penetrates the cell wall and enters the cell's cytoplasm. Upon entry into a cell some viruses shed their envelope by integrating it into the host's cell surface. Once inside the cell the virion undergoes sufficient disintegration to allow segments of its nucleic acids to integrate into the host's genome. DNA viruses can immediately enter the nucleus and fuse with the host cell's DNA, whereas the RNA viruses remain in the cytoplasm during their intracellular cycle. The exception to this usual mechanism is the RNA *retroviruses* that utilize the host cell's DNA to replicate their RNA genome. Although each family of viruses uses a cell's replication mechanism in a different way, all viruses alter the usual metabolic and protein synthesis pathways of the host in some way to serve their own needs. This process often results in the death of the host cell, allowing the dispersed replicated viruses to infect the cells of adjacent tissue.

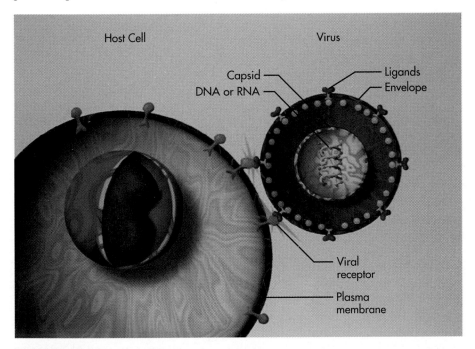

FIGURE 7-1

Diagram of the basic structure of a virus *(right)* that consists of an outer envelope containing specific binding ligand molecules and an inner capsid containing DNA or RNA chromatin. The virus is achieving "tropism," matching its ligand molecules with compatible surface viral receptors of a host cell.

■ LATENCY: a prolonged stage of some viral infections in which the viral core is integrated within cellular components, but its presence is not detectable clinically or with the use of laboratory methods.

Some virions remain harmlessly integrated within the genome of the host cell for prolonged periods. This occurs if the body's immune system attenuates the activity of the virus or if the infection is sufficiently nontoxic that cell death does not occur. This state of attenuated activity has been termed *viral latency*. During this stage there are usually no apparent clinical lesions or detectable viral antigens expressed on the surface of the infected cell. This unique ability of a virus to avoid detection and destruction by the immune system and therapeutic agents is particularly common in some members of the herpes family of viruses but also occurs in other viruses. Viral latency is considered to play an important role in carcinogenesis, acting as a predisposing cofactor necessary for the development of a large array of neoplasms. Latency is considered the reason for long delays in the onset of symptoms of patients infected with the HIV-1 virus.

At present, there are not many therapeutic agents available that are effective in curtailing viral infections. Consequently, viral infections usually continue until the host's own immune system is capable of dealing with them.

The three most commonly encountered families of viruses within the oral cavity are the herpes, coxsackie, and papovaviruses. In each viral family one member commonly predominates in occurrence and clinical significance, whereas the rest are less frequently encountered.

HERPES VIRUSES

The herpes family of viruses consists of the following:

Herpes simplex 1 (HSV-1)
Herpes simplex 2 (HSV-2)
Varicella-zoster virus (VZV)
Epstein-Barr virus (EBV)
Cytomegalovirus (CMV)
Human herpesvirus 6 (HH6)

Three members of the herpes virus family are **neurotropic** (HSV-1, HSV-2, and VZV) and three are **lymphotropic** (EBV, CMV, and HH6); all herpes viruses are capable of entering and replicating in **epithelial cells.** HSV-1 and HSV-2 are closely related and share many common antigens but still have some detectable glycoprotein surface receptors that differ. There are also some important differences in their biologic activity because HSV-2 possesses oncogenic potential. EBV is associated with epithelial and lymphoid malignancies. At this time little is known of the biologic activity of the HH6 virus except that it is secreted in the saliva of nearly all children and is found in the lymphocytes of lymphoproliferative diseases in adults.

Herpes Simplex Virus

The core of the herpes simplex virus (HSV) consists of a single strand of DNA. The chromatid contains more than 80 genes that are divided into three groups according to their function during replication. The large genome of this virus allows it to encode numerous proteins of replication and cellular metabolism, making it able to survive and become ubiquitous in the population. The virus is lytic to human epithelial cells and latent in neural tissue (Figure 7-2). Replication occurs primarily in epithelial cells, resulting in cell death and the release of

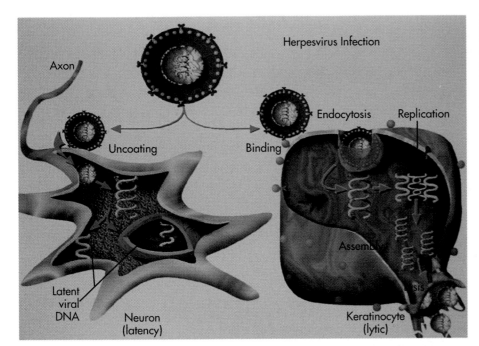

FIGURE 7-2

Diagram of the two basic types of herpes simplex infection. Lytic infections *(right)* commonly occur after endocytosis of the herpes virus into the keratinocyte. Replication and reassembly ensues that overwhelms the host cell and causes it to burst, which releases large numbers of viruses. Latent infections *(left)* commonly occur in the cell body of neurons where the viral DNA remains dormant within the cytoplasm or nucleus until it is activated to replicate and migrate along a neural axis to an epithelial surface.

up to 200,000 virions. During release not all of the virions acquire an envelope from the cell's cytoplasmic membrane; the survival time of these virions is therefore very short.

CLINICAL

HSV usually enters the body through breaks in the skin, although there is considerable evidence that it can penetrate intact mucous membranes. HSV-1 occurs primarily in lesions located above the waist, and HSV-2 occurs in lesions below the waist. In approximately 10% of the cases HSV-2 can be found in oral lesions and HSV-1 can be found in genital lesions.

Patients infected with HSV-1 or HSV-2 experience an initial primary infection followed by a state of latency. In some patients there are repeated recurrences of the infection. Most cases of initial (primary) herpes infection do not produce clinical lesions and have minimal clinical symptoms. Thus most patients are unaware that the virus has entered their body. The virus pentrates the mucosal barrier without visible lesions or symptoms. Because the virus is neurotropic, it infects the peripheral nerves and migrates to a regional ganglion where it remains dormant (latent). In this location it is undected by the immune system, protected from therapeutic agents, and not diagnosed until activated. Activation results in migration along the nerve axon to surface epithelial cells. This migration can be triggered by a number of factors that may include emotional stress, trauma, cold, sunlight, gastric upset, fever, the menstrual cycle, and any number of other factors that result in suppression of the immune system.

Whether patients have primary or secondary occurrences, the incubation period before the emergence of visible lesions ranges between 1 and 26 days but is most commonly 7 to 8 days. Patients usually notice altered sensation in the affected tissue, usually characterized by fullness or a lack of tactile or sensory perception. At this stage and during the vesicular stage that follows, the patient's saliva and genital secretions are highly contagious. It is important to note that the virus may continue to shed into the saliva and other mucosal secretions without active lesions on the epithelial surfaces.

Acute primary herpetic gingivostomatitis

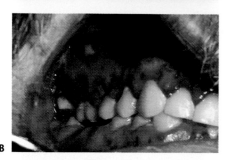

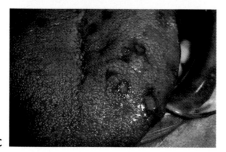

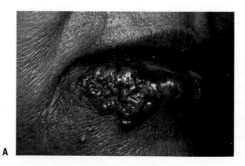

FIGURE 7-3

Acute primary herpetic gingivostomatitis. Multiple shallow punctate lesions on both keratinizing and gland-bearing mucosa. **A,** Lower lip; **B,** gingiva; and **C,** tongue.

> ■ ACUTE PRIMARY HERPETIC GINGIVOSTOMATITIS: an uncommon clinical presentation of an initial herpes simplex infection in which multiple shallow ulcers are present throughout both the keratinized and gland-bearing intraoral surfaces; accompanied by systemic symptoms of fever, lymphadenopathy, and myalgia.

Approximately 1% of initial oral infections with HSV-1 or HSV-2 occur as a highly visible and acutely symptomatic primary infection. These infections usually occur in young children, although they also occur in adults. The initial oral infection can vary and is termed *acute primary herpetic gingivostomatitis.*

Mild forms exhibit multiple small punctate shallow ulcers involving both keratinizing and nonkeratinizing oral mucosal surfaces. The ulcers may be confined to the gingiva, or they may involve various sites from the lips and perioral skin to the nasopharynx (Figure 7-3).

Severe forms may present as large diffuse whitish ulcers that exhibit scalloped borders and erythematous halos. These lesions lack the characteristic distinct individual punctate appearance of lesions seen in the milder form. The different appearance results from the coalescence of many small ulcers into single, large superficial ulcers.

In both the mild and severe forms of primary herpetic gingivostomatitis, the patient experiences fever and lymphadenopathy that last from 2 to 10 days. Muscle soreness (myalgia) and inability to masticate and swallow food are common problems. If patients are healthy, the signs and symptoms may only last from 2 to 4 days.

In immunocompromised patients a prolonged form of acute primary herpetic gingivostomatitis may develop. Commonly, these patients are receiving chemotherapy for a malignancy, are organ transplant recipients, or have a congenital or acquired immunodeficiency syndrome (AIDS). Surface lesions in these patients are often larger and deeper than those found in relatively healthy patients. In patients with the most severe forms of immunocompetency, such as those with late stage AIDS, lesions are even deeper with friable and necrotic centers and are accompanied by severe pain.

Secondary oral herpes simplex

Recurrent oral herpes simplex. The two main clinical types of recurrent oral herpes simplex infections based on the location of the lesions are **recurrent herpes labialis** and **recurrent intraoral herpes.** Recurrent herpes labialis affects the lips, whereas recurrent intraoral herpes involves the slope of the hard palate or maxillary gingiva. Both are commonly associated with recent dental treatment and present as a cluster of small vesicular lesions. The clinical appearance of the lesions found in the two types differs. Because the labial lesions often involve the skin, they will form identifiable fluid-filled vesicles that rupture, ulcerate, and resolve as crusted brownish lesions (Figure 7-4). Intraoral lesions are

FIGURE 7-4

Recurrent herpes labialis. A, Early stages consisting of fluid-filled viral vesicles. **B,** Late stage demonstrating brownish crusted lesions.

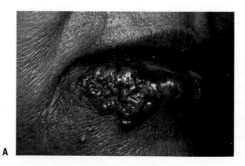

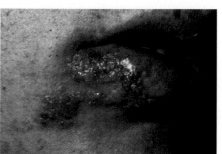

found on mucous membranes and seldom form a clinically visible vesicle. Lesions are punctate with red or white bases that slowly disappear (Figure 7-5).

Recurrent herpes labialis

■ **RECURRENT HERPES LABIALIS:** episodic occurrences of a cluster of vesicles and shallow ulcers localized to the lateral aspects of the lips in patients with latent herpes simplex infections dormant in ganglia that innervates the lips; lesions are triggered by a variety of internal and external factors.

Herpes labialis is by far the most common form of recurrent herpes simplex infections. It affects the lips and occurs in 15% to 20% of those who have had a primary infection. It is commonly termed a "cold sore" because it often occurs after an upper respiratory viral infection. Reactivation of a latent herpes simplex virus residing in the trigeminal ganglion can be triggered by prolonged exposure to sunlight, trauma and manipulation of the lips, fever, immunosuppression, menstruation, and periods of stress and anxiety. Unfortunately, there are presently few definitive treatments for herpes labialis. Empiric treatments include keeping the lesions soft and covered with an ointment to prevent further spreading and secondary bacterial infection. At present, the use of antiviral agents such as acyclovir has been beneficial. Although patients experience significant discomfort in the area, they do not exhibit elevated temperatures and seldom exhibit lymphadenopathy.

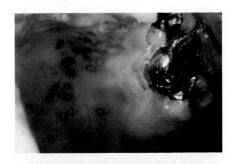
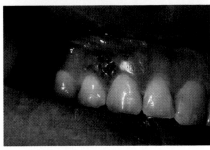

FIGURE 7-5

Recurrent intraoral herpes. A, Common intraoral site on posterior palate over greater palatine foramina. **B,** Occasionally encountered gingival lesions.

Recurrent intraoral herpes

■ **RECURRENT INTRAORAL HERPES:** episodic occurrences of an intraoral cluster of symptomatic shallow punctate ulcers, commonly but not exclusively, on the mucosa overlying the greater palatine foramina typically appearing after dental procedures in the area.

Recurrent intraoral herpes is relatively uncommon and often occurs after dental treatment or injection of a local anesthetic into the area. Some intraoral locations seem to be more prone to recurrent lesions than others. The most common site is the hard palate over the greater palatine foramina. Other intraoral sites include the free and attached gingiva, especially the maxillary gingiva, and the lateral aspects of the tongue. Although the diagnosis of a recurrent intraoral herpes simplex is primarily a clinical one, when lesions occur in the less common sites, they frequently remain undiagnosed until confirmed with a biopsy that includes an incipient vesicle. In patients who are immunosuppressed, the intraoral recurrent lesions are often substantially larger and deeper and accompanied by fever and lymphadenopathy, resembling a prolonged acute primary form of the disease. There is no known treatment for recurrent intraoral herpes simplex. Establishing the diagnosis and alleviating the patient's concerns about a more serious disease are usually sufficient.

Herpetic whitlow

■ **HERPETIC WHITLOW:** a primary or secondary herpes simplex infection localized to the hands or fingers and acquired by direct contact with an active lesion.

Before the time when gloves were required for all clinical procedures, herpetic whitlow was a common occurrence on the hands of health care workers. In addition to infection by direct contact with oral lesions, herpetic whitlow can occur

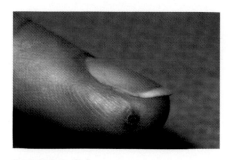

FIGURE 7-6

Herpetic whitlow. Painful, inflamed herpetic lesion on finger.

by autoinoculation from oral or genital lesions. Lesions are usually vesicular or pustular and surrounded by a wide zone of erythema (Figure 7-6). Throbbing pain, high fever, and regional lymphadenopathy of the arm or axilla are common. The symptoms are often of sufficient severity to incapacitate the patient for 1 or more weeks. Restricting contact with others is usually advisable because lesions on the fingers are highly contagious.

HISTOPATHOLOGY

During the prodromic stage before vesicle formation, the infected epithelial cells accumulate fluid and swell. This gives the cytoplasm a vacuolated appearance termed *ballooning degeneration*. Some cells exhibit nuclear changes consisting of margination of the chromatin and the presence of large eosinophilic *intranuclear inclusion bodies*. Papules and vesicles develop when the accumulation of intracellular and intercellular edema results in cell lysis. At this stage occasional *multinucleated epithelial giant cells* are present. Papules develop on the skin when exudate is present, and vesicles develop when the lesions are primarily composed of clear transudate. On mucosal surfaces pustules or vesicles seldom occur because the epithelium is fragile and ruptures readily, leaving a punctate shallow ulcer. Microscopic examination of an intact vesicle reveals a fluid-filled intraepithelial vesicle (blister) containing fibrin, ballooning degenerated and multinucleated epithelial cells, and some acute inflammatory cells (Figure 7-7, *A*). The large number of liberated viruses is not visible with light microscopy. The base of the lesion may exhibit an intact basal cell layer or, more commonly, an inflamed zone of connective and/or granulation tissue.

DIAGNOSIS

Diagnosis of a herpes simplex infection is usually based on the clinical findings. When the diagnosis is not readily apparent, one or more of the following laboratory procedures may be useful.

Biopsy. Ideally, an excisional biopsy of an intact vesicle is obtained. The viral cytopathic effects, including cellular ballooning degeneration, multinucleated epithelial cells, and nuclear inclusions, can be observed in routine hematoxylin and eosin (H&E) stained tissue slides. Immunostains utilizing monoclonal antibodies applied to the fixed tissue sections can be used to identify specific types and subtypes of the herpes virus.

Cytologic smear. The specimen is obtained by puncturing an intact vesicle and expressing the vesicular (blister) fluid onto a glass slide or by mechanically removing cells from the base or edges of an ulcerated lesion and smearing them onto microscopic slides. The smears are stained and examined for the cytopathic effects (CPE) of the virus on the epithelial cells. The CPE observed include the presence of inclusion bodies, ballooning degeneration, and multinucleation of epithelial cells (Figure 7-7, *B*). The test is not specific for HSV because similar CPE are found in the epithelium of VZV lesions.

Culture. The culture specimen is best obtained from intact vesicles or pustules. Contents of a needle aspiration are optimal, but a cotton swab may also be used to directly inoculate a tissue culture. The cultured cells are examined for CPE on epithelial cells. High concentrations of the virus will produce changes in the cultured cells after 24 hours; the mean time for a positive test is 1 to 3 days.

Fluorescent antibody. The specimen consists of smears or suspensions of cells stained with antibodies against HSV-1 and HSV-2 antigens. Antibodies are

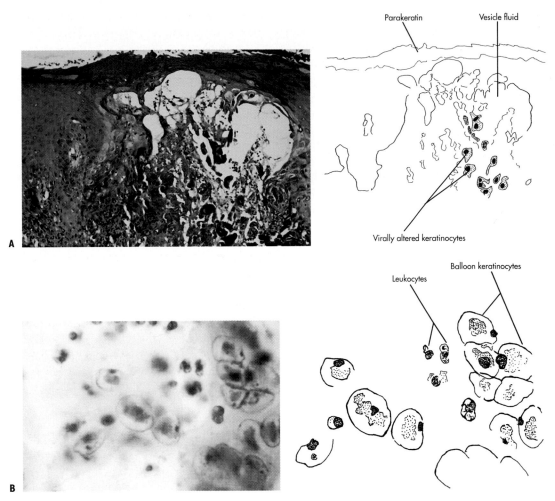

FIGURE 7-7

Herpes simplex. A, Photomicrograph of an intact intraepithelial viral vesicle that exhibits fluid, virally altered cells, and necrotic debris. **B,** Cytologic smear of viral vesicle contents that reveals enlarged and ballooned keratinocytes and associated leukocytes.

labeled with a fluorescent dye that is visible microscopically or with spectroscopic instruments. This method is not as sensitive as the culture method.

Serology. This is an indirect test in which blood samples are tested to detect antibody levels in the serum against specific viral antigens. Serology is sensitive only for primary infections because levels of circulating antibody in recurrent disease are usually too low to be detected.

TREATMENT

Treatment of HSV infections varies with the type and location of the infection and the systemic condition of the patient. In general, resolution of viral lesions depends on the competency of the patient's immune system. Therapeutic agents are of little help except in immunocompromised patients. Of the antiviral agents available for HSV, only *acyclovir* is effective. Acyclovir is most effective in the treatment of primary genital lesions and only marginally effective for recurrent genital or primary and recurrent oral infections. Treatment of primary oral lesions is palliative when oral rinses and analgesics are used. Antibiotics are often prescribed for the prevention of secondary infections. Treatment of the recurrent labial and intraoral lesions has been previously discussed.

Varicella-Zoster Virus

The varicella-zoster virus (VZV) is a member of the herpes family of viruses and shares many features with the herpes simplex virus. The primary infection of VZV is known as *varicella* or "chicken pox"; the recurrent disease is termed *herpes zoster* or "shingles". Primary infections are followed by a period of latency during which the neurotropic virus resides in the regional ganglia. Later, if the host's immune system is overwhelmed or suppressed, the virus may emerge to produce recurrent disease along a specific dermatome. Like HSV, the epithelial lesions are intraepithelial fluid-filled vesicles on the skin or mucosal surfaces. The VZV differs in that its initial mode of contact is by inhalation of droplets that enter the body through the respiratory system. In this location replication occurs before systemic spreading via the blood stream as a viremia, after which skin and mucosal eruptions appear. The VZV is structurally similar to other members of the herpes family, differing by having only minor variations in the ratio of guanine-cytosine amino acids in its genome.

CLINICAL

Varicella (chicken pox)

■ VARICELLA: primary infection of the varicella-zoster virus acquired during childhood that produces a generalized symptomatic maculopapular rash of the skin, malaise, fever, and minor lesions throughout the oral cavity.

Varicella is the initial infection of VZV and is usually acquired in childhood. Unlike HSV infections the primary infection is usually symptomatic and includes fever, headache, malaise, sore throat, and lung congestion. In the Western world 90% of the adult population will contact the virus and harbor it in its latent form. After an incubation period of approximately 2 weeks, patients develop a cutaneous hemorrhagic maculopapular rash accompanied by malaise and a low-grade fever. Lesions quickly progress to vesicles and pustules that rupture and become crusted (Figure 7-8). For approximately 1 week new lesions will continue to appear so that a mixture of lesions at various stages of development and resolution is always present. Small numbers of vesicular lesions are usually present on the oral mucosa, including the tongue, buccal mucosa, gingiva, palate, and oropharynx. The oral vesicles rupture early and are usually seen as small ulcers that closely resemble aphthous ulcerations. The oral lesions are not particularly painful. Occasional pustular skin lesions become secondarily infected and may heal as a small depressed scar ("pock"). When acquired in adulthood the disease may be severe and progress to interstitial pneumonia. If patients are immunocompromised, widespread dissemination can result in death.

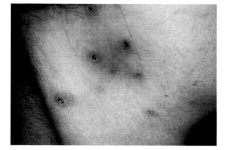

FIGURE 7-8

Varicella (chicken pox). Crusted lesions (pox) of skin of the late stage of a primary infection of the varicella-zoster virus in a young patient.

Herpes zoster (shingles)

■ HERPES ZOSTER: a regional occurrence of the varicella-zoster virus that appears as vesicular eruptions of the skin or mucosa in a distinctive unilateral pattern; pain persists for prolonged periods after lesions heal.

Herpes zoster is the recurrent form of a varicella infection. It affects 10% to 20% of the population and can occur at any age but is more common in the elderly and the immunocompromised. On the skin the predominant clinical feature is a *unilateral* linear vesicular rash outlining the cutaneous distribution (dermatome) of the affected peripheral nerve. Coalescence of the vesicles, followed by crusting, occurs quickly. When herpes zoster involves the trigeminal nerve, unilateral facial and oral lesions may develop along the ophthalmic, maxillary, and mandibular distribution of the nerve (Figure 7-9, *A*). Lesions on the intra-oral mucosal surfaces are sharply and distinctively unilateral along the nerve distribution (Figure 7-9, *B*). The mucosal lesions develop as fragile vesicles that rupture easily and are usually seen as crateriform ulcers that may persist from 2 to 3 weeks, usually healing within a month.

Lesions produce pain on both skin and mucous membranes. During the few days before the eruption of the vesicles, the patient experiences pain, paresthesia, and dysesthesia in the affected dermatome. When lesions appear, patients usually experience a stinging pain. In older patients the pain may persist for a month or more after the lesions have healed. This condition is termed *postherpetic neuralgia* and is characterized by burning and severe pain. The healed area may remain hypersensitive for months or years.

In the immunocompromised patient, besides developing deeper and more widespread lesions, the condition may become chronic with persistent pain and occasional central nervous system (CNS) involvement and death.

HISTOPATHOLOGY

The tissue changes in lesions of varicella and herpes zoster are essentially the same as in those of HSV. During the prodromal period epithelial cells containing replicating viruses exhibit cytoplasmic swelling due to intracellular edema (ballooning degeneration), margination of nuclear chromatin, and the formation of intranuclear inclusion bodies. Multinucleation of epithelial cells will also be seen when intraepithelial vesicles have formed. The postvesicular ulcer is similar to any other shallow ulcer characterized by a fibrinopurulent exudate covering a zone of granulation tissue.

DIAGNOSIS

The presence of unilateral lesions along dermatomes of the peripheral nerves is pathognomonic for herpes zoster. In varicella or herpes zoster when the classic distribution of lesions is not present, as often occurs in immunocompromised patients, and when involvement is more diffuse, one or more of the following laboratory techniques may be diagnostically helpful.

Cytologic smear

The specimen consists of fluid obtained from vesicles and smeared on slides. The presence of epithelial cells that exhibit cytopathic changes including ballooning degeneration, intranuclear inclusions, and multinucleation shows a positive finding of a viral infection. Unfortunately, HSV infection will give a similar result.

Culture

Swabs of vesicle fluid or lesional tissue are cultured in the same manner as for HSV.

Fluorescent antibody

Microscopic examination of a sample of lesional tissue is reacted with an antibody to the VZV, labeled with fluorscein dye, and viewed with ultraviolet light.

Serology

This indirect test measures the level of the circulating VZV antibody and is mainly used to document the presence of the virus and the severity of the infection. It is most effective in primary infections of varicella when antibody levels are high. Recurrent lesions of herpes zoster will only have detectable antibodies several weeks after the appearance of lesions and in only 50% of the cases.

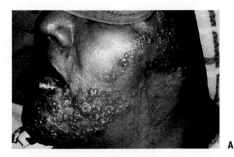
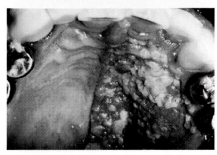

FIGURE 7-9

Herpes zoster (shingles). A, Multiple unilateral painful vesicles following the mandibular branch of the trigeminal nerve. **B,** Multiple vesicles on an erythematous base with a unilateral, sharp line of demarcation that corresponds to the nerve distribution of the palate.

Epstein-Barr Virus

The Epstein-Barr virus (EBV) is a member of the herpes virus group and exhibits tropism for human B lymphocytes. By means of the lymphocytes the virus can gain passage to the epithelial cells of the oropharynx and nasopharynx. The mechanism for infection of epithelial cells of the lateral borders of the tongue in HIV-positive patients is unknown. EBV is known to be a causative factor in infectious mononucleosis, Burkitt lymphoma, and nasopharyngeal carcinoma. In patients with acquired and congenital immunodeficiency conditions, EBV is found in B-cell lymphomas and in white lesions ("hairy leukoplakia") on the lateral borders of the tongue.

The structure of EBV is similar to that of HSV and VZV and has an array of detectable antigens specific for the virus and some that are differentially expressed during an infectious process. The target cell receptors are located on the surface of the B lymphocytes, which after binding with EBV, undergo rapid mitosis that in turn activates T lymphocytes. The *heterophile antibody* is a by-product of the rapid increase in B lymphocytes. It is an IgM class antibody that recognizes and binds the Paul-Bunnell antigen of sheep and bovine red blood cells. This is a particularly useful test for the diagnosis of infectious mononucleosis. Antibodies to the other EBV antigens are also used diagnostically. These include the Epstein-Barr virus nuclear antigen (EBNA), which is a late antigen found in infections; early antigens (EA-R) found in Burkitt lymphoma, and ER-D, found in infectious mononucleosis; and the viral capsid antigen (VCA), which is a late antigen found in all cells actively producing a virus. The B lymphocyte stimulation of T lymphocytes is considered part of how the body controls infection by the virus. Patients with transient or permanently impaired T-cell function have difficulty coping with EBV, resulting in chronic states of EBV infection. Alteration of this mechanism may be responsible for the development of some manifestations of the acquired immunodeficiency syndrome.

CLINICAL

EBV is transmitted through saliva containing the virus, which was shed from the epithelial cells of the oropharynx of infected patients. Since nearly 70% of the adult population harbors the EBV virus and since it is periodically shed in the saliva, opportunities for contact are frequent.

> ■ INFECTIOUS MONONUCLEOSIS: a debilitating initial infection of Epstein-Barr virus characterized by fatigue, malaise, lymphadenopathy, fever, and other symptoms that persist for prolonged periods; occurs primarily in young adults.

When the initial infection is acquired during early childhood, it is mild and usually subclinical. In contrast, when acquired in adolescence or young adulthood, it frequently leads to the development of **infectious mononucleosis (IM).** IM can be a severe, debilitating condition characterized by lymphadenopathy, malaise, pharyngitis, fatigue, fever, hyperplastic tonsils, thrombocytopenia, and splenomegaly. Intraorally, patients often exhibit multiple petechiae of the soft palate (Figure 7-10). The condition generally persists for 4 to 6 weeks; however, lymphadenopathy and the minor degrees of fatigue and malaise persist for several months.

HISTOPATHOLOGY

Tissue from either the tonsils or enlarged lymph nodes exhibit germinal hyperplasia and large, abnormal, nonneoplastic T lymphocytes. The aberrant lymphocytes are basophilic with a vacuolated cytoplasm and large, kidney-shaped nuclei.

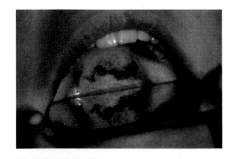

FIGURE 7-10

Infectious mononucleosis. Multiple coalesced petechiae of the soft palate in a young patient.

Diagnosis is based on a combination of clinical findings, a positive heterophilic antibody test, and/or EBV antigens. Cultures for EBV are not available on a routine diagnostic basis.

TREATMENT
Acyclovir is of little help in relieving symptoms and in controlling the course of diseases caused by EBV. Rest and restricting periods of exertion are of most value.

Cytomegalovirus
The cytomegalovirus (CMV) is similar in structure to the other members of the herpes family of viruses. It is primarily acquired as an infection in early childhood. If contracted during fetal development from an infected mother, stillbirth is a possible outcome. Up to 1% of newborns have been found to carry the virus. CMV is found in saliva, breast milk, urine, and semen. It is transmitted through blood-to-blood and intimate contacts and organ transplants. CMV has a latency period during which it may reside or replicate in the epithelial cells of the kidney or oropharynx.

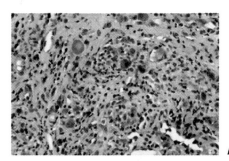

CLINICAL
In children and young adults the virus is usually transmitted through the saliva of infants. In these patients the symptoms are mild and consist of pharyngitis, malaise, fever, and lymphadenopathy. Blood smears may exhibit the same atypical lymphocytes as those observed in infectious mononucleosis. During periods of reduced immunocompetence or immunosuppression, the virus is reactivated and produces symptoms similar to infectious mononucleosis. Severe infections can result in hepatitis, pneumonia, thrombocytopenia, or encephalitis. In patients with acquired immunodeficiency syndrome, it can be fatal.

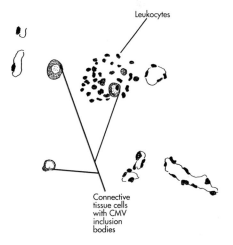

HISTOPATHOLOGY
Characteristic tissue changes are found primarily after reactivation in immunosuppressed patients or in patients who have died of lymphoma or leukemia. In these patients parenchymal and individual cells within the surrounding connective tissue are greatly enlarged (cytomegaly) and contain large intranuclear inclusion bodies (Figure 7-11, *A*). The presence of CMV can be revealed using DNA in situ hybridization (Figure 7-11, *B*).

TREATMENT
No reliable treatment or vaccine is available at present.

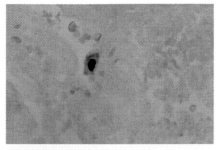

COXSACKIE VIRUSES
The coxsackie viruses are part of the picornavirus family, one of the largest and most prevalent of the RNA viruses. This family also includes the rhinoviruses of the common cold. Because the coxsackie virus has a portal of entry through the oropharynx and gastrointestinal tract, it is part of the subgroup of enteroviruses that also includes the polioviruses and the echoviruses. Coxsackie viruses have a wide range of tissues for which they exhibit tropism. Included among the tissues is the epithelium of the oropharynx. There are two types, coxsackie A and coxsackie B, each with multiple subtypes (A1 to A23 and B1 to B6). The diseases affecting the oral region are of the coxsackie A group. The major ones are herpangina (most subtypes); hand, foot, and mouth disease (A9, A16); and lymphonodular pharyngitis (A10).

FIGURE 7-11

Cytomegalovirus ulcer. A, Photomicrograph of a zone of granulation tissue at the base of an ulcer containing enlarged cells with intranuclear inclusion bodies in routine H&E stained tissue. **B,** Tissue with an immunoprobe for cytomegalovirus using DNA in situ hybridization *(red-stained cell).*

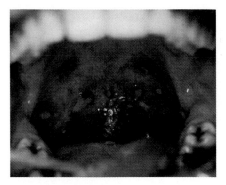

FIGURE 7-12

Herpangina. Multiple, small vesicular and punctate lesions of the posterior soft palate and nasopharynx.

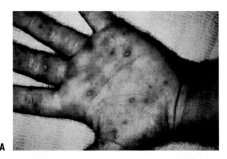

A

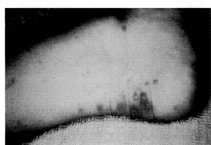

B

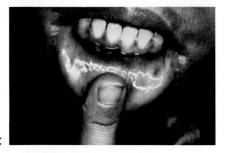

C

FIGURE 7-13

Hand, foot, and mouth disease. Eruption of small vesicles on the palms of the hands (**A**), feet (**B**), and lower lip of a young patient (**C**). (Courtesy Dr. W. Goebel.)

Herpangina

> ■ HERPANGINA: a nontreatable mild infection caused by a mixture of coxsackie A viruses localized to the posterior soft palate and nasopharynx that consist of multiple small shallow ulcers resembling a herpetic infection that lasts for approximately 1 week.

Herpangina is a misnomer because it is not caused by a herpes virus, as its name implies. It is transmitted by inhalation of airborne droplets or by contact with saliva containing the coxsackie A virus. The virus can survive outside the body for 2 to 4 hours. Herpangina frequently occurs in outbreaks, particularly among schoolchildren. Nearly all of the subtypes can be isolated from oral lesions. Patients usually develop a permanent immunity to a particular member of a subgroup but not to other members.

CLINICAL

Symptoms are usually mild and of short duration, lasting no more than 1 week. Patients complain of a sore throat and difficulty when swallowing. There may be a mild fever and some malaise. Small vesicular or punctate lesions with a white base will be present on the posterior soft palate near the uvula and anterior fauces of the tonsils (Figure 7-12). The lesions rarely appear anterior to this region. This is of particular help in distinguishing this entity from other viral diseases and herpetiform aphthous ulcers.

TREATMENT

Because the symptoms are mild and of short duration, no specific treatment is necessary.

Hand, Foot, and Mouth Disease

> ■ HAND, FOOT, AND MOUTH DISEASE: a highly contagious systemic infection of coxsackie A viruses (usually subtypes 9 and 16) of limited duration in which vesicular eruptions occur on the palms of hands, soles of feet, and mucosa of the anterior part of the mouth.

Hand, foot, and mouth disease is usually caused by subtypes A9 and A16 of coxsackie virus A, but others have also been isolated. It is highly contagious and occurs in local outbreaks, mostly among children in the 1-to 5-year-age group.

CLINICAL

During the short incubation period the patient experiences malaise, low-grade fever, nausea, and an eruption of small vesicles on an erythematous base on the palms of the hands and the feet (Figure 7-13, *A* and *B*). Within 1 to 2 days oral vesicles and ulcers appear on the mucous membranes and are usually confined to the anterior part of the mouth (Figure 7-13, *C*). Lesions are uncommon in the oropharyngeal area, which differs from herpangina.

HISTOPATHOLOGY

The tissue contains intraepithelial vesicles and epithelial cells exhibiting ballooning degeneration. Because coxsackie viruses are RNA types, infected cells usually contain microscopically visible eosinophilic intracytoplasmic inclusion bodies.

TREATMENT

Hand, foot, and mouth disease is self-limiting and lasts from 1 to 2 weeks with only mild symptoms. No specific treatment is necessary.

Acute Lymphonodular Pharyngitis

■ ACUTE LYMPHONODULAR PHARYNGITIS: a localized infection of coxsackie A virus (subtype 10) consisting of yellow or white papules surrounded by an erythematous zone confined to the lymphoid tissues of the posterior soft palate and nasopharynx that lasts from 1 to 2 weeks.

Acute lymphonodular pharyngitis is caused by the coxsackie A10 virus. It occurs as an endemic outbreak among schoolchildren. The condition does not produce the usual vesicles and superficial ulcers seen in other viral lesions and is therefore often misdiagnosed or overlooked.

CLINICAL
The characteristic lesions are located in the same anatomic region of the mouth as herpangina. They appear as raised white or yellow papules or nodules that do not ulcerate. Usually multiple lesions are present that are surrounded by an erythematous zone. Typical locations include the uvula, soft palate, anterior fauces, and posterior oropharynx. Lesions are preceded by a 2-to 10-day incubation period accompanied by a mild headache, fever, and sore throat. The duration of the symptoms and lesions varies from 1 to 2 weeks.

HISTOPATHOLOGY
The lesions consist of raised epithelium due to underlying, densely packed lymphocytes, which in some areas may still have identifiable lymphoid germinal centers. The overlying epithelium may contain intracytoplasmic inclusion bodies.

TREATMENT
The disease is self-limiting and mild in nature; no specific treatment is required.

TOGAVIRUS

The togavirus is an enveloped, single-stranded RNA virus consisting of four major groups. The Rubivirus group is the only important member of this family because it has the rubella virus as its only member. The disease caused by this virus is also referred to as **rubella** or commonly as *German measles*. Most members of the togavirus family do not infect humans. Although the rubella virus causes only a mild exanthematous skin rash in children, it can cause serious developmental defects in a developing fetus during the first trimester of pregnancy.

Rubella

■ RUBELLA: a systemic viral infection beginning in the respiratory tract and extending to the circulatory system; produces a papular skin rash, fever, and malaise that last from 1 to 2 weeks; capable of producing congenital defects during pregnancy.

CLINICAL
Rubella is a respiratory virus, differing from the other members of the togaviruses. It infects by entering the upper respiratory system and lungs, spreading to the local lymph nodes and eventually into the blood stream as a viremia. This stage represents the prodromal period, which lasts approximately 2 weeks. At this point, even before the emergence of a rash, the virus is shed and can be spread through the inhalation of respiratory droplets. During the prodromal period and subsquent viremia, fever, malaise, and headache are common. When the disseminated virus reaches the skin, a papular rash develops and lasts for another 1 to 2 weeks. No specific oral lesions are noted on the mucosa. The

spreading of the rubella virus to pregnant women during endemic outbreaks is of major concern. When pregnant women contract rubella, particularly when their immunity is less than adequate, the virus is allowed to enter the fetal circulatory system, producing defects in the developing tissues and organs. Major risk of a developmental defect is present until the twentieth week of gestation. Common congenital defects include deafness, degrees of blindness, and cardiovascular alterations. In severe cases miscarriage or stillbirths can occur.

TREATMENT
Rubella that occurs during childhood, when symptoms are mild, requires no specific treatment. At present, prevention is the main thrust in the management of outbreaks of rubella. Dependable vaccines have recently been developed and are being made widely available in an attempt to eradicate the virus from the human population. Eradication is thought to be an attainable goal because the virus has one subtype and infects humans only. Expectant mothers who are not sure of their immune status to the rubella virus should be vaccinated as a preventive measure.

PARAMYXOVIRUSES

The paramyxoviruses are large RNA viruses; the measles and mumps viruses are the two most prominent members. Both viruses are transmitted through saliva and therefore have implication to health care workers who must recognize the presence of these diseases in their patients to prevent transmission. The viruses are easily transmitted; 85% to 90% of the population contracts the virus before they are 15 years of age.

Measles

■ MEASLES: a highly contagious systemic viral infection contracted through the respiratory system and spread through the circulatory system with a predilection for skin blood vessels that produce a skin rash and sometimes pneumonia and encephalitis.

Measles is one of the most severe and widespread of the childhood exanthematous diseases. It is also one of the most common. The virus enters the body through the respiratory system and undergoes rapid replication within the respiratory epithelium before spreading to the regional lymph nodes and throughout the body via the circulatory system. The virus has a predilection for blood vessel walls, particularly those of the skin, and produces the characteristic erythematous rash.

CLINICAL
Excruciating headaches, a rash, photophobia, high fever, and a cough are the hallmarks of a measles infection. After an incubation period of 8 to 10 days, the virus spreads to the brain, superficial blood vessels, conjunctiva, urinary tract, gastrointestinal tract, and oral mucosa. Symptoms emanate from all sites during the next week. Lesions referred to as *Koplik spots* infrequently occur on the oral mucous membranes. They are usually asymptomatic, transient in nature, and often overlooked, appearing as small white papules on an erythematous base on the buccal mucosa. Palatal petechia and generally inflamed mucous membranes and gingiva are also present during the peak of the infection. The possible complication of fatal forms of encephalitis or viral pneumonia is of concern. Patients become contagious approximately 4 days before they feel ill, making intervention to prevent spread of the virus difficult. A skin rash eventually appears, indicating the presence of the disease.

TREATMENT

Measles is treated symptomatically with analgesics, fluids, and rest. Immuno-compromised patients are administered immune serum globulin, which is most effective if administered within 6 days of the initial exposure. Most of the treatment strategy is aimed at preventing measles from spreading because local epidemics occur easily. Since 1977 the United States has had a mass vaccination program against measles. The measles, mumps, and rubella vaccines are administered after a baby is 15 months old.

Mumps (Epidemic Parotitis)

■ MUMPS: a localized viral infection contracted through the respiratory system that primarily affects one or more major salivary glands with swelling and pain; occasionally affects other organs; and produces fever and malaise.

The mumps virus is a paramyxovirus that has only one subtype. It is worldwide in distribution and, where no vaccination programs exist, occurs throughout the year. Evidence of infection is present in 85% to 90% of individuals by the age of 15, although not all will have obvious symptoms. The virus is spread through saliva and nasal droplets and is communicable during the prodromic period and up to 1 week before the onset of clinical signs and symptoms. It infects and replicates in the respiratory mucosa before disseminating to the salivary glands, CNS, testes, ovaries, pancreas, and occasionally, the eyes and middle ear. Usually, involvement of tissues other than the parotid glands is not severe.

CLINICAL

Patients with classic mumps manifest swelling of one or both parotid glands in addition to the usual signs and symptoms of viral infections such as headache, fever, and malaise. In some patients the submandibular glands will also be involved. The enlarged glands are very painful, especially at meal time. A noteworthy clinical sign is the elevation of the earlobe on one or both of the affected sides when it is viewed from behind the patient. This is indicative of involvement of the tail of the parotid gland. This sign helps to differentiate mumps from nonparotid causes of facial swelling such as a dental abcess and associated cellulitis. Intraorally, the papilla over the opening of Stensen duct on the buccal mucosa may be enlarged. Symptoms may last as long as 4 to 5 weeks. In some patients involvement of the major salivary glands does not occur, making diagnosis more difficult. In these cases the diagnosis is made by detecting viral-specific antibodies in the blood or by recovering the mumps virus from the urine.

TREATMENT

There are no antiviral agents available for the treatment of mumps. Patients are treated symptomatically with analgesics, bedrest, and a bland diet. As with measles and rubella, mumps is managed through aggressive vaccination programs for young children in an attempt to reduce the presence of the virus in the population.

HUMAN PAPILLOMA VIRUSES

The human papilloma viruses (HPV) are part of the papovavirus family. They are DNA (double-stranded) viruses with a spherical virion measuring 50 nm in diameter. Structurally, they consist of a nucleocapsid without an outer envelope. Based on analysis by DNA sequencing, more than 50 HPV subtypes have been identified to date. These have been grouped according to the specific diseases in which the clusters of subtypes are found. HPV exhibits tropism for epithelial cells and is found in normal oral mucosa, presumably in a latent stage, and in many other benign, premalignant, and malignant lesions. Within the oral cavity the clinical entities that contain one or more of the HPV subtypes are squamous papilloma (HPV-6 and HPV-11); verruca vulgaris (HPV-2 and HPV-6); and condyloma acuminatum (HPV-6, HPV-11, and HPV-45).

Certain HPV subtypes have been associated with some hyperplastic, dysplastic, and neoplastic epithelial lesions.

Mucosal lesions containing one or more HPV subtypes appear clinically as single or multiple areas of thickened epithelium, often with a papillary surface. The presence of fine hairlike surface projections (papillary) is common in some lesions. Lesions may be raised and exhibit a thin stalk (pedunculated) or flat and diffuse on a broad base (sessile). Most are whitish, but the flatter, broad-based lesions may be reddish or exhibit the pinkish color of normal oral mucosa.

Squamous Papilloma

> ■ SQUAMOUS PAPILLOMA: a papillary focal epithelial hyperplasia common in the posterior aspect of the mouth, containing koilocytic cells and HPV-6 and HPV-11.

Squamous papillomas are the most common benign neoplasms of oral epithelium. They are present throughout the mouth in patients of all ages. There is a higher incidence on the soft palate, faucial pillars, and uvular areas. They are usually solitary lesions; however, multiple lesions can occasionally occur in young patients. Koilocytes may or may not be evident in the epithelium. Although these lesions do not appear to contain HPV genomic material, in situ DNA hybridization research indicates that HPV subtypes 6 and 11 are usually detectable.

Verruca Vulgaris

> ■ VERRUCA VULGARIS: a papillary focal epithelial hyperplasia commonly containing koilocytic cells of HPV-2 or HPV-6; commonly occurs on the hands and in the anterior aspect of the mouths of children.

Verruca vulgaris is generally known as a *wart* when it occurs on skin. It is commonly found on the hands and fingers of children. The virus contained within the epithelial cells can be spread by autoinoculation; lesions spread from the fingers to other sites, particularly the lips, hard palate, and gingiva. HPV subtypes 2 and 6 are present in nearly all of these lesions.

CLINICAL

The lesions are exophytic, keratinized, sessile papules or nodules with "warty" (cauliflower) surfaces (Figure 7-14, *A*). Lesions measure 2 to 5 mm in diameter, although much larger lesions occasionally occur. The skin and oral mucosal lesions are similar in appearance except that the oral lesions are usually white, whereas the skin lesions are usually grayish-brown. This difference in coloration between skin and mucosal lesions is primarily related to the moist environment of the mouth as compared with the dry environment on the skin surface.

HISTOPATHOLOGY

Lesions consist of papillary epithelial proliferations that contain multiple fingerlike projections exhibiting hyperkeratosis and a prominent granular cell layer. Mild degrees of basilar hyperplasia and radially oriented rete pegs are present (Figure 7-14, *B*). Variable numbers of superficial epithelial cells with shrunken nuclei and perinuclear clearing (koilocytosis), which indicates HPV infection, are seen. The connective tissue exhibits dilated vascular channels and some vari-

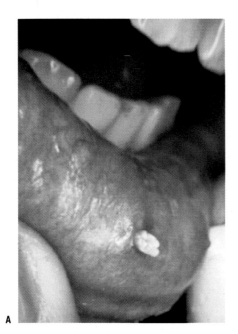

A

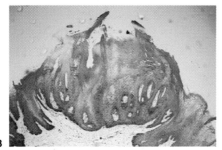

B

FIGURE 7-14

Verruca vulgaris. **A,** Clinical appearance of mucosal lesions are white, solitary, and exophytic, with a stalk and a papillary (warty) surface. **B,** Low-power photomicrograph reveals extensive keratin production, acanthosis, and radially oriented rete pegs.

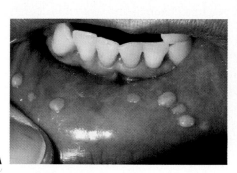
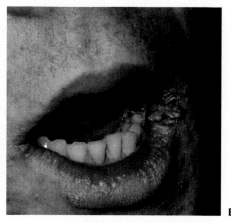

FIGURE 7-15

Condyloma acuminatum. **A,** Multiple sessile flat lesions with pebbly surfaces. **B,** Papillary lesions present in the left corner of lower lip.

able numbers of chronic inflammatory cells. Lesions display viral particles, both ultrastructurally and immunohistochemically.

TREATMENT
Some lesions will regress spontaneously. Those that persist should be excised surgically. Recurrence of intraoral lesions may occur but is uncommon.

Condyloma Acuminatum

> ■ CONDYLOMA ACUMINATUM: multiple papillary or sessile focal areas of epithelial hyperplasia of the genital and oral mucosas that contain koilocytes and HPV-6 or HPV-11 and are difficult to eradicate.

Condyloma acuminatum, commonly termed *genital or venereal wart,* occurs most commonly on the genitalia; however, oral lesions are common. The lesions are caused by the human papilloma virus (usually HPV-6 and HPV-11). Although many oral lesions are acquired through oral-genital sexual contact, some cases are transmitted though nonsexual contact or autoinoculation from genital lesions. Oral lesions in young children can be particularly problematic because sexual abuse may be involved.

CLINICAL
Condyloma acuminatum presents as solitary or multiple, pinkish, sessile papules or plaques with a pebbled surface (Figure 7-15, *A*) or as pedunculated papillary lesions (Fig 7-15, *B*). Oral lesions occur predominantly on the nonkeratinized mucosa of the lips, floor of the mouth, lateral and ventral surfaces of the tongue, buccal mucosa, and soft palate. Gingival lesions do occur; however, they are uncommon.

HISTOPATHOLOGY
Lesions are characterized by an epithelial proliferation exhibiting broad, blunt, or rounded surfaces. The epithelium may be either nonkeratinized or parakeratinized. Often lesions will exhibit a marked degree of acanthosis and/or pseudoepitheliomatous hyperplasia with a moderate to marked degree of basilar hyperplasia (Figure 7-16, *A*). Increased numbers of mitotic figures are usually present in the basilar region. The spinous layer of the epithelium is generally hypercellular with a variable degree of nuclear pleomorphism. A characteristic fea-

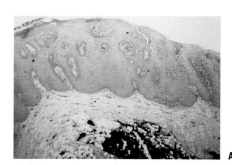
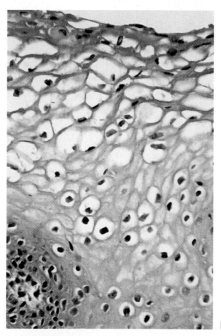

FIGURE 7-16

Condyloma acuminatum. **A,** Low-power photomicrograph of a common flat lesion exhibiting extensive epithelial hyperplasia with acanthosis and fusion and blunting of rete pegs. **B,** Medium-power photomicrograph of spinous cell layer containing clear cells with shrunken nuclei and perinuclear clear zones (koilocytes).

ture of condyloma acuminatum is the presence of variable numbers of superficial spinous cells exhibiting shrunken nuclei with perinuclear clear zones (koilocytes), indicative of an HPV infection (Figure 7-16, *B*). The connective tissue is usually edematous, exhibiting prominent vascular channels and a variable degree of chronic inflammation.

TREATMENT

A solitary, small condyloma is best treated by a simple excision that includes a narrow border of clinically normal mucosa around the base of the stalk. Multiple small isolated lesions are similarly treated. Large fleshy lesions are more difficult to treat. Surgery or removal by laser is the preferred treatment modality for these lesions. Although topical podophyllin is used for treating genital lesions, it is hazardous for treating oral lesions and therefore contraindicated. Recurrence of treated lesions is common.

Focal Epithelial Hyperplasia

■ FOCAL EPITHELIAL HYPERPLASIA: multiple papillary or sessile areas of epithelial hyperplasia of the oral mucosa in young patients of specific population isolates that frequently regress spontaneously; the epithelium is extensively acanthotic and contains koilocytes and HPV-13 and HPV-32.

Focal epithelial hyperplasia, commonly known as *Heck disease*, is a condition found primarily in isolated groups of native Indians of North and Central America and Brazil, northern native peoples, and other groups in Europe and Africa. The lesions are usually multiple and often involve the buccal and labial mucosa of the mouth. Lesions are sessile and may be pink or white. Although most lesions occur in children, they can also be found in older age groups. Most regress spontaneously. If lesions persist, they can be surgically excised. The lesions contain abundant HPV-13 and HPV-32.

HISTOPATHOLOGY

The surface of lesions of focal epithelial hyperplasia is characterized by greatly thickened layers of parakeratin and extensive acanthosis. Epithelial cells of the upper spinous layer display enlarged nuclei and vacuolated clear cytoplasm (koilocytes) indicative of an HPV infection. The basal cell layer exhibits increased mitotic activity. The associated connective tissue is usually loose and well vascularized, exhibiting a variable infiltrate of lymphocytes.

TREATMENT

Those lesions that do not regress spontaneously can be surgically excised. Until the diagnosis has been firmly established for individual patients, lesions should be surgically excised and submitted to a laboratory for a definitive diagnosis.

RETROVIRUSES

The members of the retrovirus family have been extensively studied for some time because of their known oncogenic potential in animals. The first retrovirus that exhibited this potential was the Rous sarcoma virus. Once injected into chickens, it rapidly produced sarcomas. In 1981 during the search for the causative agent of the acquired immunodeficiency syndrome (AIDS), another retrovirus, the T-cell lymphotropic virus 1 (HTLV-1), was found to be the causative agent of T-cell leukemia in humans. Shortly thereafter, a retrovirus was isolated from a patient with AIDS and named the human immunodeficiency virus (HIV). The virus became known as **HIV-1;** a less common variant of the virus **(HIV-2)** has been isolated from patients with a similar disorder in regions of West Africa.

Human Immunodeficiency Virus (HIV)

The human immunodeficiency virus (HIV) exhibits tropism for T lymphocytes, macrophages, and certain nerve cells. The viral envelope contains specific surface glycoproteins, notably gp120 and gp41, that bind with the CD4 receptors on the surface of the T lymphocyte helper cells and macrophages (Figure 7-17, *A*). Successful binding allows the contents of the viral core to enter the cytoplasm of the host cell, leaving the viral envelope behind. The core contains enzymatic proteins p24, p9, and p7 that are necessary for the virus to use the constituents of the host cell for replication. Once within the cell the RNA of the viral

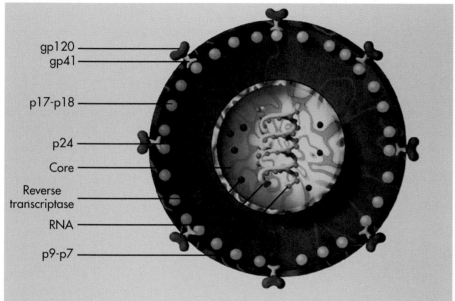

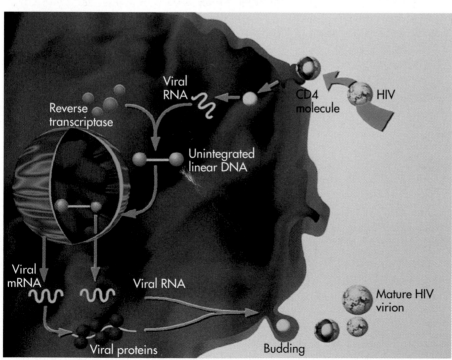

FIGURE 7-17

Human immunodeficiency virus. A, Diagram of a retrovirus with essential envelope glycoproteins, core enzymatic proteins, and RNA chromatin. **B,** Process of replication of an HIV retrovirus within a target cell with CD4 receptors on surface.

nucleocapsid uses the viral enzyme **reverse transcriptase** to synthesize strands of viral DNA, using the viral RNA as the template. The newly formed viral DNA enters the host nucleus and becomes spliced into the genome of the host cell. The integrated viral genome is now able to maintain a dormant or latent state. Periodically, this integrated proviral DNA is transcribed to RNA where it directs the metabolic activity of the host cell to synthesize more HIV RNA genome; the retroviral structural proteins *gag*, *pol*, and *env*; and the replication regulatory proteins *nef*, *tat*, and *rev* (Figure 7-17, *B*). The level of metabolic and mitotic activity of the host CD4 cell is believed to be a factor in the rate in which the disease progresses in an individual patient. In patients with lower levels of CD4 cell stimulation, there may be a prolonged period of latency before the devastating clinical effects of an HIV infection are apparent. In patients with active or chronic infections that heightened the activity level of the CD4 cells, there is a noticeable increase in the rate in which the disease progresses. This is believed to result from the infectious agents acting as mitogenic stimulators of the CD4 cells that have been previously genetically altered by the retrovirus. This results in the production of overwhelming amounts of viral protein that leads to the rapid and premature death of the stimulated CD4 immune cell. To sustain adequate immune function, a helper/suppressor T-cell ratio of 2:1 is required. During the latency-like state, which may last for 3 to 8 years, a slow but progressive functional deterioration of the T4:T8 cell ratio occurs until the immune system can no longer prevent normal commensal or latent organisms from becoming potent infective agents. Normal patients harbor 800 to 1200 such T-cells per cubic millimeter. With progressive CD4 lymphocyte depletion, immunosuppression becomes increasely more severe with the emergence of pre-AIDS opportunistic infection. Once the CD4 lymphocyte count falls below 200 cells per cm and the ratio of helper/suppressor cells is reversed, a diagnosis of AIDS is made.

The drastic reduction in total lymphocytes, particularly the CD4 lymphocytes, results in the loss of production of the noncellular components of the defense system of the body. These include the essential lymphokine factors such as interleukin 2 (IL2), interferon (IF), the macrophage activating factor (MAF), and the factors that stimulate the production of natural killer (NK) cells. Additionally, a gammaglobulinemia, which is often associated with a compensatory increase in the number of B-cells, may occur.

CLINICAL

Systemic

After initial contact with HIV, there is a 2- to 6-week delay before antibodies to the virus are detectable in the blood. Most patients are unaware of their status during this time. Some patients will experience a noticeable initial period of malaise, lethargy, mild temperature elevation, headache, arthralgia, myalgia, chronic cough, and possibly a skin rash. These symptoms are similar to those of flu or a mild form of infectious mononucleosis. This is usually followed by a period of latency that may last for 6 months in infants and 1 or more years in adults. During this period some patients have no symptoms other than the gradual development of chronic lymphadenopathy.

Over the next 3 to 5 years, some or all of the following insidious symptoms of pre-AIDS gradually appear:

Night sweats/malaise/fever
Weight loss
Memory loss/mild dementia
Chronic infections

Generalized lymphadenopathy

Diarrhea

Once the CD4 lymphocyte count approaches or falls below 200, one or more of the following severe and disabling symptoms appears, heralding the onset of AIDS:

Pneumocystis carinii pneumonia

Bacterial pneumonia

Cryptosporidiosis

Toxoplasmosis

Cerebral meningitis

Kaposi sarcoma

Non-Hodgkin lymphoma

Generalized herpes simplex/varicella-zoster infections

Cytomegalovirus retinitis/pneumonia/colitis

Candidiasis/cryptococcosis/coccidioidosis/histoplasmosis or other deep mycotic infections

Mycobacterium avium-intracellulare infections

■ **BOX 7-1**
Oral Lesions of HIV-Positive Pre-AIDS Patients

"Hairy" leukoplakia
Acute pseudomembraneous candidiasis
Diffuse herpes simplex
 gingivostomatitis
Gingivitis/periodontitis
Acute nonspecific ulcers
Diffuse varicella-zoster lesions

■ **BOX 7-2**
Common Oral Lesions in Patients With AIDS

Candidiasis	HIV gingivitis/periodontitis
Intraoral	Acute nonspecific ulcers
Esophageal	Chronic ulcers
"Hairy" leukoplakia	*Cryptococcus neoformans*
Diffuse herpes simplex gingivostomatitis	*Histoplasma capsulatum*
Diffuse varicella-zoster lesions	Cytomegalovirus
Kaposi sarcoma	Herpes simplex
Non-Hodgkin lymphoma	

Oral manifestation

The oral manifestations of HIV-infected patients are multiple and varied and are occasionally the first sign that the patients harbor the virus. The lesions that develop are due to an inadequate immune surveillance system and consist of either opportunistic infections or neoplasms. Box 7-1 lists the oral lesions found in pre-AIDS patients when CD4 lymphocyte counts are reduced and range from 800 to 200 cells per cubic millimeter.

Whether patients are symptomatic, when their blood CD4 lymphocyte count becomes less than 200 per cc or constitutes less that 14% of the total normal lymphocyte count they are determined to have progressed to AIDS. The oral conditions that may occur in patients with AIDS are listed in Box 7-2.

Occurring less frequently within the oral cavity of AIDS patients are one or more of the lesions listed in Box 7-3.

■ **BOX 7-3**
Infrequent Oral Conditions Found in AIDS Patients

Atypical tuberculosis
Coccidiodomycosis
Molluscum contagiosum infection
Toxoplasmosis
Bacillary angiomatosis
Condyloma acuminatum
Enlarged parotid glands
Xerostomia
Squamous cell carcinoma

■ "HAIRY" LEUKOPLAKIA: white patches of the lateral borders of the tongue with a tendency for vertical linear folds found in latency stages of HIV infected patients, with the thickened epithelium containing an upper zone of clear cells (koilocytes), most of which contain Epstein-Barr virus.

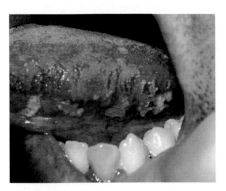

FIGURE 7-18

"Hairy" leukoplakia. White lesions with vertical striations on the lateral surface of the tongue; common in HIV-positive patients but occasionally found in patients with other causes of immunosuppression.

"Hairy" leukoplakia

"Hairy" leukoplakia is a white lesion located primarily on the lateral borders of the tongue and occasionally on the adjacent buccal mucosa. The lesion has a linear, folded appearance that was originally described as "hairlike" (Figure 7-18). It appears during the late latency stages of HIV infections and is considered a precusor of AIDS. Because other conditions can mimic "hairy" leukoplakia, it is important to remember that its clinical presence alone is not indicative of an HIV-positive status. Histologic features of "hairy" leukoplakia include hyperparakeratosis and acanthosis with a zone of enlarged cells (koilocyte-like cells) in the upper region of the stratum spinosum (Figure 7-19, *A*). The koilocytotic cells usually contain the EBV as evidenced by immunohistochemistry or in situ hybridization (Figure 7-19, *B*). Because other causes of immunosuppression will also have these findings, the presence of the HIV antibody in the serum is necessary for a diagnosis of an HIV-positive status. Many of these lesions will also show superficial colonization by *Candida albicans*. The underlying connective tissue is usually free of an inflammatory reaction to the organisms, which is indicative of a diminished level of immunoreactivity.

Candidiasis. Persistent and refractory acute or chronic forms of *C. albicans* infection of the oral mucous membranes, in an otherwise healthy patient, is an important early indicator of impending deterioration of the immune system in HIV-positive patients. It is often associated with nasopharyngeal, esophageal, epiglottic, and larnygeal candidiasis (Figure 7-20). Other species of *Candida* including *C. tropicalis*, *C. glabrata*, and *C. parapsilosis* are commonly found in HIV-positive patients and may account for differences in their responses to treatment.

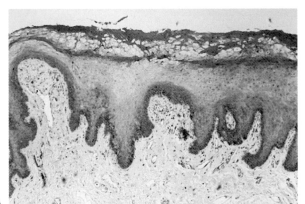

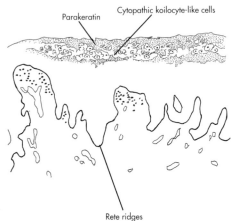

Parakeratin

Cytopathic koilocyte-like cells

Rete ridges

A

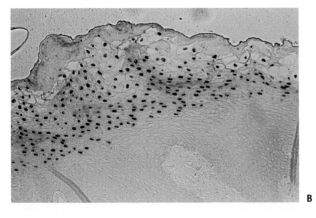

B

FIGURE 7-19

"Hairy" leukoplakia. A, Low-power photomicrograph of a lesion from the lateral surface of the tongue that exhibits characteristic hyperparakeratosis and acanthosis with a zone of vaculolated koilocyte-like cells. **B,** Presence of EBV in the upper layers of the epithelium as revealed by in situ hybridization.

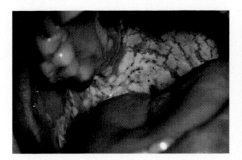

FIGURE 7-20

HIV candidiasis. Persistent acute pseudomembraneous candidiasis on the palate.

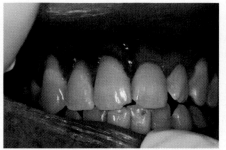

FIGURE 7-21

HIV gingivitis. Atypical, intensely erythematous gingival inflammation involving several teeth with uninvolved adjacent gingiva.

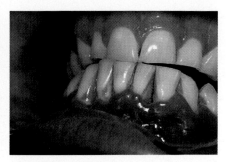

FIGURE 7-22

HIV periodontitis. Focal areas of an advanced gingival recession and an erythematous gingiva with features suggestive of a superimposed ANUG.

Deep (invasive) fungal infections. Although candidiasis is the most common infection in HIV-positive patients, infections by mycotic organisms capable of penetrating into the underlying connective tissue are occasionally encountered. The most common of these infections is histoplasmosis. It is characterized by mucosal ulceration or red granular swellings. The organisms are easily detectable in a biopsy specimen. Oral lesions are usually only a manifestation of a more widespread systemic infection.

Gingivitis/periodontitis associated with HIV infection. Some HIV-positive patients will develop a form of atypical gingivitis/periodontitis. The involved gingiva in these patients has an unusual intensity consisting of a wide zone of erythema that affects both the free and attached gingiva (Figure 7-21). The distribution of the lesions is unique in that some teeth are spared, whereas others are severely affected (so-called "skip lesions"). The condition is rapidly progressive, moving quickly from a gingivitis to a periodontitis (Figure 7-22), and is unresponsive to the usual treatments. In many cases the gingivitis occurs as an atypical form of acute necrotizing ulcerative gingivitis (ANUG) often superimposed on a rapidly progressive periodontitis. The periodontitis differs significantly from the usual type in that there is commonly a rapid denuding of the gingival tissue with resultant exposure of the alveolar bone. The condition is accompanied by severe pain and spontaneous bleeding, which is uncommon in periodontal disease in non-HIV patients.

Acute nonspecific ulcers. The oral ulcers in HIV-positive patients resemble larger and deeper versions of aphthous ulcers (Figure 7-23). They are crateriform with a large erythematous halo. The edges are often sharp or thickened. The center will quickly expose bone or penetrate muscle unless it is treated. Treatment involves tissue examination to determine if the lesion is the result of a specific infection such as herpes, CMV, or an invasive fungus. If no specific infectious organism is identified, as is often the case, steroid therapy is usually effective.

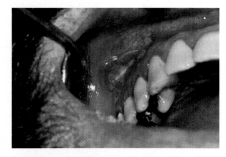

FIGURE 7-23

Acute nonspecific ulcer. Deep crateriform ulcer with rolled borders and no identifiable causative factor that is penetrating the underlying muscle in an HIV-positive patient.

Kaposi sarcoma

■ KAPOSI SARCOMA: macular or nodular vascular lesions occurring singularly or in multiples on the mucosa and skin of HIV-infected patients; lesions consist of proliferating atypical endothelial cells and are indicative that the patient has AIDS.

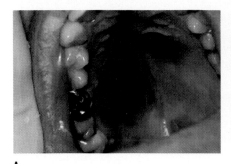
A

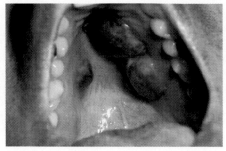
B

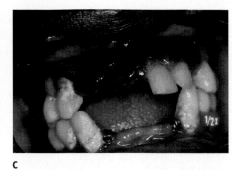
C

FIGURE 7-24

Kaposi sarcoma. A, Diffuse, purplish macular lesion on the right side of the hard palate.
B, Nodular form of Kaposi sarcoma involving both the right and left sides of the palate. **C,** Combined macular and nodular lesions of the anterior maxillary gingiva.

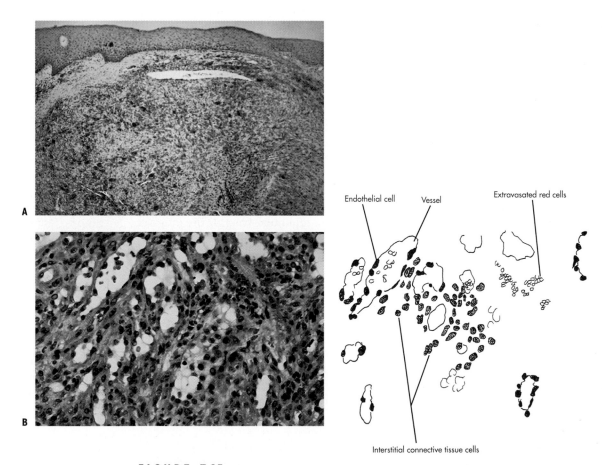

FIGURE 7-25

Kaposi sarcoma. A, Low-power photomicrograph reveals a circumscribed submucosal nodule of highly vascular tissue with abundant extravasated red blood cells. **B,** High-power photomicrograph revealing abnormally shaped and incompletely formed blood vessels composed of rounded, plump endothelial cells.

Oral lesions of Kaposi sarcoma eventually occur in 10% to 20% of HIV-positive male patients and are more common in those patients who acquire the virus through sexual transmission rather than intravenous drug abuse. The lesions are reddish to deep purple and may be macular or nodular (Figure 7-24, *A* and *B*). The predominant locations within the oral cavity are the hard and soft palates, followed by the maxillary gingiva (Figure 7-24, *C*). The early macular lesions are difficult to differentiate from a persistent hematoma, whereas the early nodular lesions resemble pyogenic granuloma. On the gingiva, large lesions will often interfere with mastication. Large palatal lesions interfere with speech and may undergo spontaneous bleeding. Oral lesions may or may not be accompanied by skin lesions.

The histopathology of Kaposi sarcoma is not always distinctive in the early lesions because the tissue may resemble other benign vascular lesions such as capillary hemangioma or pyogenic granuloma. The more mature lesions exhibit a proliferation of hyperchromatic spindle-shaped or oval endothelial cells arranged in an irregular vascular pattern (Figure 7-25, *A*). In some lesions distinct vascular spaces are present that have plump and rounded endothelial cells projecting into the vascular lumina (Figure 7-25, *B*), whereas in others there are only occasional slitlike spaces with a few distinct vessels. Extravasated red blood cells and hemosiderin deposits are characteristically present.

Patients with lesions and few other outward signs of their HIV status are often anxious to have them removed. Diagnosis should be confirmed by biopsy because hematomas, pyogenic granulomas, and other vascular lesions may have similar clinical appearances. Lesions have been treated by radiotherapy; surgery; and intralesional injections of Adriamycin, vinblastine, vincristine, bleomycin, and other antimetabolites. Small lesions have been eliminated with sclerosing agents. Some preliminary research suggests that removing small, early lesions may prevent the development of additional ones.

Non-Hodgkin lymphoma. The lymphomas seen in HIV-positive patients are primarily the B-cell type of lesions. Although the lesions are not common within the oral cavity, they have been reported in nearly all anatomic locations. They are characterized by their rapid appearance and growth, which quickly undergoes ulceration. The borders are raised, rolled, and indurated (Figure 7-26). The histopathology reveals a uniform distribution of a single cell type, usually consisting of the less mature forms of B-cells and immunoblasts (Figure 7-27). Many cells exhibit features in common with Burkitt lymphoma. The presence of lymphoma in HIV-positive patients is a sign of a poor prognosis.

Viral infections. The viral infections in HIV positive patients are usually exacerbations of previous latent infections. In these patients the reactivated form does not remain localized and transient as occurs in non-immunocompromised individuals. The recurrences more closely resemble primary infections, except that the viral infections are of an *indefinite* duration and capable of causing the death of the patient if they are not promptly and adequately treated. The viral infections usually found are herpes simplex and varicella, which appear as multiple diffuse ulcers that are larger and deeper than usual. CMV also occurs and is believed to be responsible for the bilateral swelling of the parotid glands and the reduction in salivary flow, which results in xerostomia. CMV is also found in deep focal ulcers and is thought to be responsible, along with EBV, for the generalized lymphadenopathy. EBV has been found in "hairy" leukoplakia and is thought to be the causative agent for that lesion. HPV infections are common in HIV-positive patients and are responsible for condyloma acuminatum and multifocal papular lesions resembling those seen in focal epithelial hyperplasia (Heck disease).

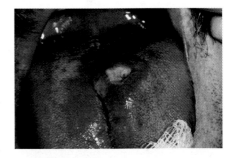

FIGURE 7-26

Non-Hodgkin lymphoma. Rapidly enlarging lesion with central ulceration on the dorsal side of the tongue.

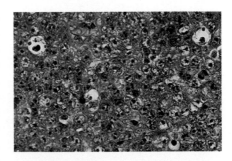

FIGURE 7-27

Non-Hodgkin lymphoma. High-power photomicrograph demonstrating densely packed large immature lymphocytes and immunoblasts in a lymphoma in an HIV-positive patient.

BACTERIAL INFECTIONS

Streptococcus

The streptococci are a large group of gram-positive organisms, mostly facultative anaerobes, that grow in pairs or short chains. They are classified according to the clinical diseases that they cause, their serologic properties, hemolytic potential, and metabolic/biochemical properties. Two members of streptococci are of particular importance within the oral cavity. They are *Streptococcus pyogenes*, a beta hemolytic streptococcus that is responsible for pharyngitis, tonsillitis, and some atypical forms of mucositis and gingivitis; and *Streptococcus viridens*, an alpha nonhemolytic streptococcus that is a normal inhabitant of the oral cavity and is of importance in the pathogenesis of dental caries and bacterial endocarditis.

Pharyngitis/Tonsillitis

Pharyngitis/tonsillitis, also referred to as "strept throat," is an acute condition caused by a beta hemolytic streptococcus. It occurs primarily in young patients who are 5 to 15 years of age. It is spread by the inhalation of infected droplets present in crowded conditions. Symptoms of infection occur 2 to 4 days after contact and may include a sudden onset of elevated temperature, throat soreness, chills, malaise, cervical lymphadenopathy, and headache. Within a few days petechiae may occur on the soft palate. All the oral mucous membranes may be erythematous and uncomfortable. Differentiation from the more common viral pharyngitis is required before treatment.

Scarlet Fever

Scarlet fever is a complication of a streptococcal oropharyngeal infection. It occurs when the beta hemolytic streptococci become systemically disseminated. The injury caused by the bacterial toxins to the walls of the small, superficial vessels results in a skin rash that is particularly noticeable on the face. The oral cavity is often affected and exhibits generalized edema, elongation of the uvula, and diffuse petechiae. The dorsal surface of the tongue becomes whitened and the fungiform papillae become erythematous and enlarged, appearing as small, red papules against a white background. This appearance of the tongue has been referred to as "strawberry tongue." The skin rash lasts about 1 week and is followed by a period of desquamation. The development of acute glomerulonephritis and rheumatic fever is of greatest concern. Most patients recover from glomerulonephritis, but rheumatic fever may permanently damage the heart valves. This predisposes the damaged valves to recurring infections during subsequent transit bacteremias. The chronic condition of recurring infections of the heart valves, primarily the mitral valve, is termed *subacute bacterial endocarditis* and is of great concern in the practice of dentistry. Patients with this condition are required to have prophylactic premedication with antibiotics before receiving invasive dental treatments.

Staphylococcus

The members of the genus *Staphylococcus* are potent human pathogens that produce purulent exudate (pus) and cause a large array of diseases. The staphylococcus microorganism is a round, gram-negative, facultative anaerobic bacterium that grows in clusters. It is found on the skin and oronasopharyngeal surfaces of all humans. Members of this genus are the cause of most acute infections that occur after trauma and surgical procedures when aseptic technique is not rigidly followed. Staphylococci are capable of survival on nonhuman, dry surfaces for prolonged periods and are easily transferrable. *S. aureus* is the best known strain of this genus; it is responsible for most common acute skin infections such as folliculitis, furuncles, and carbuncles ("boils"). Fortunately, the organisms are very susceptible to heat and chemical sterilization and can be controlled when proper aseptic protocols are followed.

Impetigo

■ IMPETIGO: acute pustular eruptions of the perioral skin of children with neglected oral hygiene in which S. *aureus* is the most common pathogen.

Impetigo is the common name given to an acute pustular eruption of the perioral skin (Figure 7-28) in which *S. aureus* is the most commonly found pathogen. It occurs in children with neglected personal hygiene who often scratch the lesions, spreading the bacteria to other parts of the face in a linear or excoriated pattern. In some instances the fingernail beds also become infected. The clinical similarity between impetigo and perioral primary or recurrent herpes infections and allergic stomatitis can sometimes pose a diagnostic problem. Cultures from smears of lesional exudate are used to identify the causative organisms before treatment. Treatment consists of using both topical and systemic antibiotics. *S. aureus* is very sensitive to systemically administered penicillin.

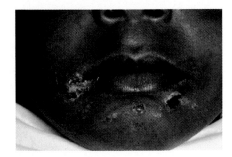

FIGURE 7-28

Impetigo. Pustular and crusted perioral lesions commonly harboring S. *aureus* pathogens in a young patient.   (Courtesy Dr. S. Rovin and Dr. W. Sabes.)

Osteomyelitis

S. aureus is most commonly found in the acute forms of osteomyelitis, which occurs as a result of direct invasion through a break in the overlying skin or through hematologic spread from an adjacent or remote focus of infection. Acute suppurative osteomyelitis is commonly found in younger patients whose long bones possess highly vascularized metaphyseal areas. Within the oral cavity, osteomyelitis is more common in the mandible than in the maxilla. It usually occurs after dental caries and pulpitis progress to an intraosseous periapical infection. In these infections *S. aureus* is the organism most commonly cultured from the exudate. Treatment of deep infections of bone are often more difficult than soft tissue lesions and require prolonged high doses of penicillin or intravenous therapy.

Mycobacterium

Strains of the genus *Mycobacterium* are among the oldest and most treatment-resistant infections known to man. They are aerobic bacilli with a cell wall containing a high lipid component. This feature makes them resistant to medications that are in an aqueous solution. As aerobes they are able to survive and flourish in oxygenated environments such as the lungs. Their lipid cell wall also presents difficulty in detection with common histologic screening stains such as gram, Giemsa, and hematoxylin/eosin (H&E) stains. Special acid-fast staining techniques are required for their detection in tissue sections. The common human infections by this genus include tuberculosis (*M. tuberculosis*) and leprosy (*M. leprae*), both of which have been the source of numerous worldwide epidemics. With an increase in immunodeficiency syndromes there has been a resurgence of cases of tuberculosis. The resurgence is complicated because of the emergence of new atypical strains, the most prevalent being *M. avium-intracellulare* that is particularly common in patients with AIDS.

Tuberculosis

■ TUBERCULOSIS: chronic granulomatous infection of the lungs caused by M. *tuberculosis*, which is spread by aerosols; can occasionally have associated chronic oral ulcers and/or enlarged nasopharyngeal and cervical lymph nodes.

Tuberculosis is spread by aerosols that usually enter the body through the lungs and lodge in the terminal alveoli. The bacilli are phagocytized and spread throughout the adjacent tissue by means of the motile macrophages present in the lungs. Within macrophages the microorganisms are protected by their lipid outer coat and are able to undergo rapid replication that eventually destroys the host cell, liberating large numbers of bacilli to invade new peripheral sites. These phagocytic cells spread the organisms to the regional lymph nodes and, if not halted by the immune system, to other organs such as the kidneys, bone marrow, and brain. Pivotal to the ability of the body to restrict the spread of the tuberculosis bacilli is its development of ample numbers of antibodies. The presence of an antibody response in an infected patient can be detected by a positive skin reaction when challenged with fragments of the protein structure of the bacteria. This is referred to as the purified protein derivative (**PPD**) test and is widely used to identify those individuals who have contracted the organism, either recently or in the past.

CLINICAL

Oral lesions have been found in 3.5% of patients with systemic tuberculosis. They are rarely seen unless the patient also has lung and possibly other systemic involvement. Patients who are immunocompromised have a much higher incidence of oral lesions. The lesions are commonly infected with atypical forms of the organisms such as *M. avium-intracellulare.*

The clinical appearance of an oral lesion is as a chronic ulcer with indurated borders (Figure 7-29) or as a swelling in the tonsils, other lymphoid-rich areas of the posterior aspect of the mouth and the nasopharynx, and regional cervical lymph nodes. Lesions may also be found intraosseously and may appear as chronic osteomyelitis that eventually drain and produce bony sequestra.

HISTOPATHOLOGY

The microscopic appearance of the lesions within the oral cavity is the same as in the lungs, consisting of granulomas exhibiting a central necrotic focus surrounded by mononuclear cells and multinucleated Langhans giant cells. The granuloma is usually surrounded by a mantle of lymphocytes and fibrous tissue. Arrested lesions may show areas of dystrophic calcifications.

TREATMENT

Treatment of *M. tuberculosis* infections is difficult because the lesions are resistant to common antibiotics. To avoid resistant strain development, two antimycobacterial agents are combined—isoniazid and rifampin. Treatment extends over a period of 18 to 24 months.

Treponema pallidum

■ SYPHILIS: a sexually transmitted local and systemic infection caused by *Treponema pallidum* with three progressive clinical stages—a primary chancre at the point of contact, a secondary skin rash and mucous patches, and tertiary (late) systemically disseminated lesions; all are effectively treated with penicillin.

The microorganism *T. pallidum* is part of the order Spirochaetales, in which all members are thin, elongated, coiled, or helical structures that are gram-negative. The bacteria of this order are commonly referred to as "spirochetes." *T. pallidum* is the most common and is responsible for **syphilis,** the sexually transmitted disease that has been a major health problem for centuries. It occurs as a communicable disease in humans because it does not survive well outside of

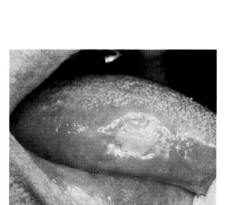

FIGURE 7-29

Tuberculosis. Chronic shallow nonhealing ulcer of the lateral surface of the tongue with associated induration.   (Courtesy Dr. F.M. Lucatorto.)

the human body. Adequate research to completely understand its pathogenesis and the defense of the body against it is still lacking. Diagnosis is often difficult because the clinical manifestations are widely varied and often imitate many other conditions during each of its many stages of progression. To add to the diagnostic problems, *T. pallidum* is difficult to visualize microscopically because it does not absorb the routine screening stains available clinically. Instead, more complex laboratory procedures are required such as the application of a Warthin-Starry stain (Figure 7-30), a dark-field illumination and detection of the antibodies to the spirochetes tagged with fluorscein dyes and illuminated with ultraviolet light.

Syphilis

CLINICAL

Untreated syphilis progresses through three clinical stages of infection: (1) primary syphilis, (2) secondary syphilis, and (3) tertiary (late) syphilis. The primary and secondary stages are closely associated in time and may even overlap, whereas tertiary or late syphilis may be separated by a period of latency that lasts from several to many years and varies extensively between individuals.

Primary syphilis occurs as a localized lesion at the site of contact and is termed a *chancre*. Chancres occur primarily on the genitals and less commonly within and around the oral cavity (Figure 7-31). In these locations spirochetes undergo rapid replication and enter the lymphatics and blood stream. There is an asymptomatic incubation period that averages 21 days, which is followed by an open wound that teems with spirochetes. At this stage the serologic tests will be negative, but a diagnosis can be made using dark-field or immunofluorescent staining and by microscopically viewing lesional tissue or exudate. Without treatment primary lesions heal in 3 to 6 weeks; with treatment, healing occurs in 10 to 14 days.

Secondary syphilis develops 2 to 6 months after the initial infection if the primary stage is not treated. Some unhealed chancres may still be present. The secondary lesions occur on the skin and mucous membranes and are morphologically diverse. They can occur as macular, papular, follicular, lenticular, papulosquamous, flat papillary (condyloma lata), pustular, nodular, or mucous membrane patches. The lesions may simultaneously appear in many anatomic areas, or they may be localized to one area such as the mucous membranes (Figure 7-32). The lymph nodes are almost always involved at this stage, and needle aspirates will contain the organisms. The skin and mucous membrane lesions exhibit large numbers of spirochetes; serology tests will be positive. With or without treatment, secondary lesions heal in 2 to 4 weeks. Patients will not be noticeably ill during the secondary stage of the disease.

Tertiary syphilis is also referred to as late syphilis. It may occur in some patients despite the apparent, successful treatment of the earlier disease. It involves primarily the CNS and cardiovascular system. This stage has recently been well documented in patients with AIDS. This stage follows a prolonged period of latency in which the patient periodically experiences some minor exacerbations of the condition. The most serious complication occurs during pregnancy and results in the birth of a fetus with congenital syphilis. In patients with tertiary syphilis, nearly every organ of the body is affected. Lesions termed *gummas* can destroy the nose, palate, and tongue. In bones the tertiary lesions produce osteomyelitis and destroy joints. The most serious complication of late syphilis is the destruction of the walls of the large blood vessels, resulting in aneurysms and cardiac insufficiency. Neural involvement leads to dementia and strokes.

Congenital syphilis is due to a transplacental infection with *Treponema pallidum* during fetal development. The extent of involvement varies from an over-

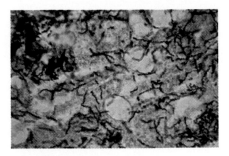

FIGURE 7-30

Syphilis. High-power photomicrograph of tissue from the secondary lesion illustrated in Figure 7-32; the Warthin-Starry stain reveals numerous coiled spirochetes.

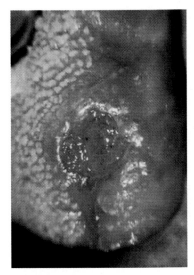

FIGURE 7-31

Syphilis. Primary lesion (chancre) of the anterior dorsal tongue at the point of initial contact with a *T. pallidum* pathogen. (Courtesy Dr. F.M. Lucatorto.)

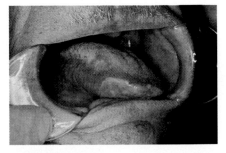

FIGURE 7-32

Syphilis. Secondary lesion on the ventral surface of the tongue (mucous patch).

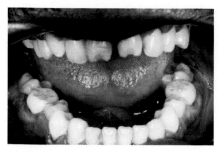

FIGURE 7-33

Congenital syphilis. The patient exhibits anomalously shaped teeth consisting of incisors with screwdriver-shaped crowns and notched incisal edges and molars with constricted crowns and a lack of cuspal development (mulberry molars).

whelming infection leading to infant death to an infection with a period of latency in which the disease is not suspected until 12 or more months after birth. In these patients a rash will eventually appear and the destruction of bones, nerves, and some organs will occur. The classic descriptions of saber (pointed) shins, rhagades (perioral vertical creases), frontal bossing, and saddle nose (destruction of the nasal spine) are commonly used to describe the primary manifestations of the infection. **Hutchinson triad** (which consists of blindness, deafness, and dental anomalies) is also used to describe the findings of congenital syphilis. The dental anomalies are due to failure of some incisal and cuspal growth centers to form. This results in anterior teeth that are narrower at the incisal edge than at the middle third ("screwdriver teeth") and/or are notched ("Hutchinson incisors"), pegged-shaped laterals, and molars with constricted and atrophic cusps ("mulberry molars") (Figure 7-33).

DIAGNOSIS

Since primary and secondary manifestations of syphilis have exudative lesions, dark-field examination and direct immunofluorescent staining can be used to facilitate the detection of the organisms. The culture of lesional tissue cannot be used for diagnostic purposes. Screening tests such as the VDRL (Venereal Disease Research Laboratory) test and the RPR (rapid plasma reagin) test are frequently used. These tests are not specific for *T. pallidum* and have a risk of false-positive results. More dependable tests are those using antibodies specific for antigenic markers of *T. pallidum*. The most commonly used are the fluorescent treponemal antibody absorption (FTA-ABS) test, the microhemagglutination assay—*T. pallidum* (MHA-TP), and the enzyme-linked immunosorbent assay (ELISA).

TREATMENT

The long-acting penicillins are the antibiotics of choice and are very effective in the treatment of all stages of syphilis.

Actinomyces

Cervicofacial Actinomycosis

■ **CERVICOFACIAL ACTINOMYCOSIS:** an acute deep suppurative abcess of the upper neck, perioral area, and jaws with an associated draining sinus tract that contains "sulfur granules" and purulent exudate caused by the filamentous anaerobic gram-positive bacteria—*Actinomyces israelii*.

Cervicofacial actinomycosis is caused by an infection by normal commensal (endogenous) organisms of humans and does not require contact with an infected individual. The pathogen is a filamentous bacteria of the genus *Actinomyces*, usually the anaerobic, gram-positive, *Actinomyces israelii*. This family of bacteria includes other members that normally inhabit the oral cavity but are seldom pathogenic. These include *A. naeslundii*, *A. odontolyticus*, and *A. viscosus*. All members of the genus are constituents of dental calculus, the calcified encrustation on teeth. Infections by *A. israelii* are classified according to the anatomic area involved. In most cases evidence exists of a previous injury or surgical procedure, which allows the organisms to invade an anaerobic environment within the tissue. In the oral, head, and neck areas the infection is referred to as **cervicofacial actinomycosis.**

CLINICAL

The deep infections of cervicofacial actinomycosis are caused by *A. israelii*, normally present in tonsillar crypts, carious teeth, and calculus deposits. Traumatic

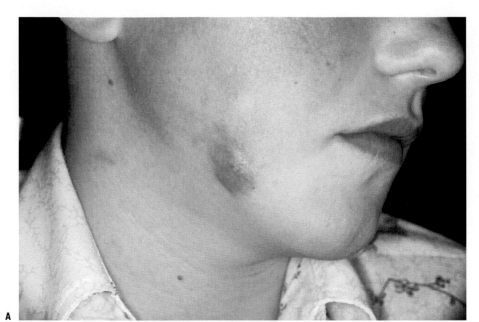

FIGURE 7-34

Cervicofacial actinomycosis. A, A young patient with a sinus tract on facial skin due to an infection of actinomyces following a traumatic injury to the teeth and maxilla 3 months earlier. **B,** Photomicrograph of purulent exudate from a deep abscess composed of neutrophils and containing calcified bacterial colonies with a periphery of filamentous organisms radiating in a sunburst or "ray" pattern (sulfur granules).

A

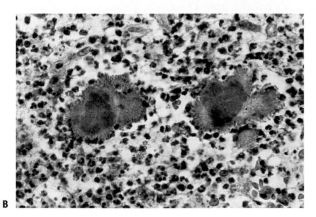

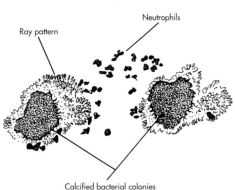

Ray pattern   Neutrophils

Calcified bacterial colonies

B

incidents such as a dental extraction, a periapical infection following an open pulpitis, or a pericoronitis around a partially impacted tooth are potential opportunities for the organisms to become infective. Once infection occurs, an acute inflammatory reaction ensues. In soft tissue, swelling and intense pain are frequent. Bacterial invasion into bone initiates a localized osteomyelitis that can cause a great deal of bone destruction, nodular reactive periosteitis, and soft tissue abscesses that give rise to a regional nodularity with draining sinus tracts on the surface of the skin (Figure 7-34, *A*) and mucosa. The clinical presentation of the soft tissue has led to the term "lumpy jaw" disease. The exudate emanating from the draining sinus tracts will often contain small, clinically visible yellowish-green calcified structures referred to as **"sulfur granules."** These represent calcified colonies of *A. israelii* and are indicative of actinomycosis.

HISTOPATHOLOGY

The tissue changes in actinomycosis are those of an acute abscess, consisting of a central cavity containing purulent exudate that surrounds multiple calcified colonies of filamentous bacteria. The central area of a colony stains hematoxylin positive and appears somewhat amorphous, whereas the periphery consists of filamentous organisms arranged in a sunburst or "ray" pattern. The filaments stain positively with both eosin and periodic acid-Schiff (PAS). The surrounding purulent exudate is composed primarily of neutrophils (Figure 7- 34, *B*). The presence of the calcified filamentous bacterial colonies located deep in the tissue is diagnostic for actinomycosis.

TREATMENT

Treatment of actinomycosis consists of surgical drainage and debridement followed by a high daily dosage of penicillin for at least 10 days. Large lesions require an extended course of intravenously administered penicillin to achieve a complete cure.

MYCOSES

Candida albicans

The genus *Candida* includes eight species of fungi of which *Candida albicans* is by far the most prevalent. *C. albicans* can be present as a yeast (spore), a yeast with pseudohyphae, or as long, branching septate hyphae. The hyphal form is usually present when organisms are isolated from an infectious process.

Candidiasis

Candidiasis is now widely accepted as an encompassing term for the many clinical forms of infection by members of the genus *Candida*. Other synonyms used are "candidosis" and "moniliasis." All of the genus are present as commensals that become infective when an alteration in the immunity of the host occurs. Among opportunistic infectious agents, they are usually the first to take advantage of any reduction in the defense system of the host cell.

CLINICAL

Within the oral cavity infections by *C. albicans* occur on the surface of the mucosa where they assume several clinical forms. Some are white and may rub off easily, whereas others do not. Some appear bright red, which is due to atrophy and erosion of the epithelium and an intense inflammation of the underlying connective tissue. A classification of the basic types of oral candidiasis is presented in Box 7-4. Other entities associated with infections of *Candida albicans* are listed in Box 7-5.

Candidiasis is the classic prototype of an opportunistic infection. It is a commensal organism within the oral cavity that becomes pathogenic when appropriate predisposing factors exist. A large number of factors may predispose the oral tissue to the development of candidiasis (Box 7-6).

■ BOX 7-4
Classification of Basic Types of Oral Candidiasis

Acute
  Pseudomembraneous ("thrush")
  Atrophic ("erythematous")

Chronic
  Hyperplastic ("candidal leukoplakia")

■ BOX 7-5
Oral Lesions Associated With Candida albicans

Angular cheilitis ("perlèche")
Median rhomboid glossitis
Chronic mucocutaneous candidiasis

■ BOX 7-6
Factors Predisposing Oral Tissues to Candidiasis

Acidic saliva	Malnutrition/gastrointestinal malabsorption
Xerostomia	Carbohydrate-rich diets
Nocturnal denture wearing	Diabetes mellitus
Heavy smoking	HIV infection
Blood group O individuals	Endocrine abnormalities
Immunologic disorders	Epithelial dysplasia
Antibiotic therapy	Blood dyscrasia and malignancy
Steroid therapy	Radiation/chemotherapy
Iron, folic acid, and vitamin deficiencies	Old age/infancy

Acute Pseudomembraneous Candidiasis (Thrush)

■ ACUTE PSEUDOMEMBRANEOUS CANDIDIASIS: a clinical form of *C. albicans* infection that consists of creamy, loose patches of desquamative epithelium containing numerous matted mycelia over an erythematous mucosa that is easily removed; common in patients with more severe predisposing factors.

Acute pseudomembranous candidiasis is characterized by the presence of white "curds" or creamy, loose patches in various intraoral sites. The white patches can be easily removed with a tongue depressor or gauze (Figure 7-35). The underlying mucosa is erythematous and may bleed slightly. The pseudomembrane consists of desquamative and necrotic epithelial cells and numerous matted and tangled mycelia (hyphae) of *C. albicans*. The lesions are commonly found in newborns before they acquire a competent immune system. Some common causes of this form of candidiasis include the prolonged use of antibiotics, which disrupts the balance in the oral flora; the use of systemic steroids, which induces immunosuppression; HIV infection; chronic xerostomia due to radiation therapy, chemotherapy, or medications; Sjögren syndrome; and diabetes mellitus. The diagnosis of candidiasis can be confirmed with PAS stained cytology smears of the pseudomembrane (Figure 7-36). The matted hyphae will be preferentially stained, allowing the diagnosis to be made rapidly and accurately. To differentiate between the various strains of *Candida* requires the use of immunohistochemical techniques. Cultures are a much slower method and usually unnecessary in view of the clinical findings and cytologic smear results. Treatment with antifungal medication is effective in relieving symptoms and most infections within 1 to 2 weeks. If lesions do not undergo immediate regression, the patient may be severely immunosuppressed and/or harboring other species of *Candida*. These patients may require more potent medications than the usual azole derivatives such as amphotericin B, which is usually administered intravenously and requires hospitalization.

Atrophic (Erythematous) Candidiasis

■ ATROPHIC (ERYTHEMATOUS) CANDIDIASIS: a clinical form of *C. albicans* infection in which the mucosa is thinned, smooth, and bright red with symptoms of burning and increased sensitivity; commonly found on the palate under a denture but also on the tongue and other mucosal surfaces.

In non-immunosuppressed patients, atrophic (erythematous) candidiasis is most commonly found in patients with ill-fitting dentures or in those who wear their dentures continuously. It has also been referred to as "denture sore mouth" and appears as a generalized red area of atrophic tissue, commonly on the palate (Figure 7-37, *A*). It is found primarily under maxillary dentures in older patients and more commonly in those patients who do not adequately clean or remove their dentures at night. In the early stages areas of superficial erosion and petechiae may be present. The chief complaint is of a continuous burning sensation of the affected area. Atrophic candidiasis can also affect the tongue, in which case the tongue exhibits a smooth and "beefy" red appearance (Figure 7-37, *B*). This appearance is due to the loss of the filiform papilla, a generalized thinning of the epithelium, and excessive inflammation of the connective tissue. Patients complain of intense sensitivity and pain on exposure to hot and cold liquids, spicy foods, and alcoholic beverages. Cytologic smears usually fail to reveal hyphal forms of the fungal organisms, although careful scrutiny may reveal occasional fungal spore forms. In these cases cultures may be useful in confirming that a fungal infection is actually present. Because of its distinctive clinical ap-

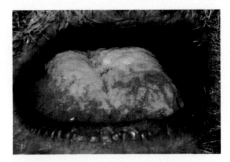

FIGURE 7-35

Acute pseudomembranous candidiasis (thrush). Tongue exhibits a superficial layer of loose, cream-colored deposit with raised curdlike patches that can be removed, revealing an erythematous base.

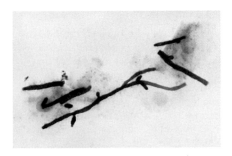

FIGURE 7-36

Acute pseudomembranous candidiasis. Cytologic smear of whitish pseudomembrane stained with PAS demonstrating the branching hyphae and budding yeasts superimposed on desquamated superficial squames.

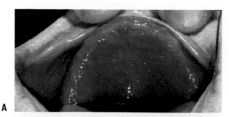

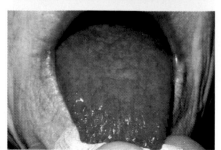

FIGURE 7-37

Atrophic (erythematous) candidiasis. A, Intensely erythematous and atrophic mucosa under a maxillary denture that is highly sensitive and periodically painful. **B,** A smooth, "beefy" red, sensitive tongue due to the loss of papillae resulting from a long-term persistent candidasis. Also present is a mild form of *C. albicans*–induced angular cheilitis (perlèche).

pearance, particularly in a susceptible patient, empirical treatment with antifungal agents in an ointment base applied to the tissue surface of the denture can be instituted. Resolution of the condition over a period of 1 to 2 weeks confirms the diagnosis. To achieve a long-term cure, the predisposing factors need to be identified and corrected and the existing infection needs to be topically or systemically treated.

Chronic Hyperplastic Candidiasis

> ■ **CHRONIC HYPERPLASTIC CANDIDIASIS:** a clinical form of *C. albicans* infection consisting of white plaques or papules against an erythematous background containing hyphae in the parakeratin layer of the thickened epithelium.

Chronic hyperplastic candidiasis usually presents as a white mucosal plaque. It is most commonly found on the buccal mucosa along the occlusal line, widening as it approaches the commissure (Figure 7-38), and also on the laterodorsal surfaces of tongue and the alveolar ridges. Since it presents a mucosal white patch or plaque, it is frequently termed "candidal leukoplakia." The lesion is often discovered during the microscopic evaluation of a routine biopsy of a leukoplakic lesion when the hyphal forms of the organism are observed. At times chronic hyperplastic candidiasis presents as white papules against an erythematous background and resemble a "speckled leukoplakia" or "speckled erythroplasia," conditions that commonly exhibit microscopic features of epithelial dysplasia. Because of its close clinical resemblance to a premalignant lesion, biopsy is necessary.

Tissue specimens usually exhibit hyperparakeratosis containing variable numbers of hyphae that vertically invade the parakeratin. Although the hyphae can often be seen with routine H&E stains, most cases require PAS or silver stains to demonstrate their presence. Variable numbers of neutrophils, sometimes occurring as microabscesses (Munro abscesses) within the parakeratin layer, are commonly seen. The spinous layer of the epithelium usually thickens (acanthosis) and the rete pegs become longer. The underlying connective tissue exhibits an inflammatory infiltrate consisting of plasma cells and lymphocytes.

Because the fungal organisms are found on or near the epithelial surface, topical antifungal medication is more effective than medication administered for systemic effect. Since candidiasis is an opportunistic infection, attempts should be made to identify and correct predisposing factors to prevent recurrence.

Angular Cheilitis (Perlèche)

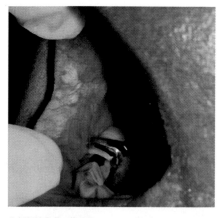

FIGURE 7-38

Chronic hyperplastic candidiasis (candidal leukoplakia). Localized white mucosal patch that is asymptomatic and does not rub off on the mucosa adjacent to the commissure.

> ■ **ANGULAR CHEILITIS (PERLÈCHE):** symptomatic bilateral fissures of the corners of the mouth that are common in patients with *C. albicans* infection in other parts of the mouth and often intensified with mouth overclosure; requires treatment with antifungal medication.

Angular cheilitis is a bilateral chronic inflammation of the corners ("angles") of the mouth, characterized by atrophy and linear fissures (Figure 7-39). Although the lesions may occur alone, they are often associated with intraoral acute pseudomembranous or atrophic lesions in other parts of the mouth. Angular cheilitis is common in patients with a loss of vertical dimension due to tooth loss, attrition of teeth, or old dentures. Secondary infections with bacteria sometimes occur, complicating treatment. In the past this lesion was considered to be a sign of vitamin B deficiency and treatment efforts were often erroneously directed toward correcting only that condition. Although jaw overclosure may mechanically intensify angular cheilitis and provide a favorable environment for growth, it is not the sole cause. Treatment consisting only of increasing the vertical dimension is insufficient to correct the problem. As with all lesions of candidiasis, treatment is a twofold process that consists of identifying the predisposing factors and eradicating local infection. Antifungal ointments alone or in combination with antibiotics, if a bacterial infection is present, are usually effective in treating angular cheilitis.

Median Rhomboid Glossitis

■ MEDIAN RHOMBOID GLOSSITIS: an asymptomatic, elongated, erythematous patch of atrophic mucosa of the middorsal surface of the tongue due to a chronic *C. albicans* infection.

Median rhomboid glossitis represents an area of chronic candidiasis located on the middorsum of the tongue. In the past it was thought to represent a developmental defect and was therefore not treated. The lesion starts as a narrow, mildly erythematous area located along the median fissure of the tongue (Figure 7-40). The lesion is asymptomatic and enlarges slowly, often remaining unnoticed by the patient for many years. If undiagnosed and untreated, the lesion gradually enlarges and exhibits the erythematous nodular hyperplasia characteristic of chronic hyperplastic candidiasis. In some patients a lesion develops on the midline of the palate opposite the tongue lesion. Because median rhomboid glossitis can be clinically suspicious, it is occasionally biopsied. Treatment consists of identifying and managing predisposing factors and the application of topical antifungal agents for prolonged periods.

For convenience, the clinical term *chronic multifocal oral candidiasis* is sometimes used to describe patients exhibiting more than one of the above chronic forms of candidiasis. Lesions may persist for many years but do not usually involve other anatomic sites. The reason for the site specificity of these low-grade infections is not known. The intervening mucosa is unaffected. Many of the patients are smokers and/or denture wearers. Unless the predisposing factors are identified and corrected, treatment with an antifungal medication is effective only as a temporary measure.

Chronic Mucocutaneous Candidiasis

Chronic mucocutaneous candidiasis (CMC) is a term used to describe a condition in which persistent and refractory candidiasis occurs on the mucous membranes, skin, and nails of the affected patients (Figure 7-41). Most of these patients exhibit endocrinopathies or defects of the immune system.

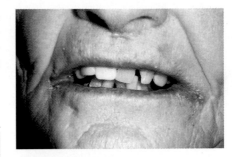

FIGURE 7-39

Angular cheilitis (perlèche). Severe fissures in the corners (angles) of the mouth in a patient with adult onset diabetes mellitus.

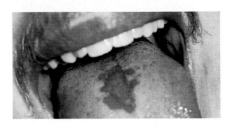

FIGURE 7-40

Median rhomboid glossitis. The localized midline area of atrophy and erythema is usually asymptomatic, present for prolonged periods, and gradually increases in size with the surface becoming increasingly pebbly or nodular. Hyphae of *C. albicans* are commonly found in the parakeratin layer.

A 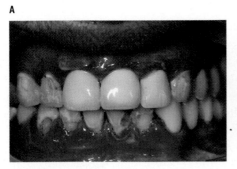 B C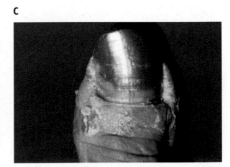

FIGURE 7-41

Chronic mucocutaneous candidiasis. A patient with refactory candidiasis of the oral mucous membranes **(A)**, eye lids **(B)**, and skin surrounding the nail bed **(C)**.

Histoplasma capsulatum

Histoplasmosis

■ HISTOPLASMOSIS: a chronic lung infection common in the Mississippi Valley due to inhalation of spores of *Histoplasma capsulatum;* may have associated intraoral lesions consisting of a chronic ulcer resembling a malignancy and is best treated with amphotericin B.

Histoplasmosis is a **deep mycotic infection** in which the organism *H. capsulatum* infects the lungs through inhalation of airborne spores (conidia). Fortunately, most cases are asymptomatic, and only 1% of the infected hosts develop a clinically detectable pneumonia. In even fewer cases the disease disseminates to other organs and tissues. Histoplasmosis occurs throughout the temperate zones of the world. In North America endemic areas are located in the Mississippi and Ohio River Valleys of the United States. Endemic areas are also found in various locations in Central and South America. The organisms are present as saprophytic spores found in soil contaminated by bat and bird droppings. Inhalation of spores occurs when the dust and soil of attics, caves, and other roosting areas of birds and bats are disturbed. In some endemic areas 70% of the inhabitants will have positive skin tests, yet few will recall having acquired the infection.

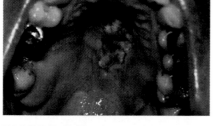

FIGURE 7-42

Histoplasmosis. A lesion of the palate in a patient with AIDS that exhibits an irregularly shaped deep ulcer with central necrosis over granulation tissue.

CLINICAL

Patients with symptoms of infection exhibit a short, transient period of fever, malaise, cough, and dyspnea. Immunity develops rapidly in nearly all patients. In the rare instances in which the immunity of the patient does not arrest or otherwise contain the disease, granulomas and cavitation of lung tissue occurs, often followed by dissemination of the disease to the regional lymph nodes and adjacent anatomic structures. In chronic forms of the disease, dissemination to the skin and oral mucous membranes may be the first signs of infection.

Oral lesions of histoplasmosis occur primarily on the gingiva, tongue, palate, and buccal mucosa. The lesions are granulomatous and appear initially as a nodule and later as a chronic ulcer with raised, rolled borders and induration of the surrounding tissue (Figure 7-42). The clinical appearance closely resembles that of carcinoma or tuberculosis. On the gingiva it may appear as a diffuse granulomatous process with underlying alveolar bone loss and loosening of teeth. Because lesions can resemble many other conditions, histoplasmosis is seldom suspected initially. The diagnosis is usually determined after laboratory examination of an incisional biopsy. In patients with immunodeficiencies, lesions of histoplasmosis may be multiple and widely disseminated. Cervical lymphadenopathy is common, and brain involvement may occur.

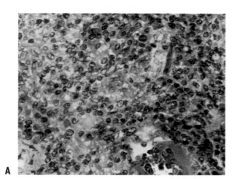

A

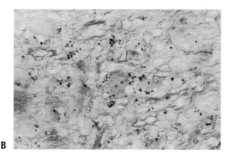

B

FIGURE 7-43

Histoplasmosis. A, Photomicrograph of H&E stained granulomatous tissue composed of histiocytes and occasional multinucleated giant cells. **B,** Same tissue with PAS stain reveals numerous small spores of *H. capsulatum* (small red dots).

HISTOPATHOLOGY

Histoplasmosis is a granulomatous infection characterized by the formation of multiple, small, often inconspicuous granulomas composed of histiocytes, many of which contain variable numbers of organisms. The granulomas are often obscured by a generalized background of histiocytes, lymphocytes, and plasma cells. Scattered multinucleated giant cells may be present (Figure 7-43, *A*). The organism is usually present in its spore form, measures 2 to 5μm in diameter, and is located within the histiocytes and multinucleated cells and interspersed among the other inflammatory cells. With routine H&E tissue stains, spores can only be seen when present in large numbers. However, they are more easily visualized with PAS (Figure 7-43, *B*) and methenamine silver stains, which selectively stain the small spores.

DIAGNOSIS

Histoplasmosis is diagnosed by combining data obtained from clinical evaluation, microscopic examination, culture, serologic findings, and the histoplasmin skin test. The histoplasmin skin test uses *inactivated* mycelia or yeast of the organism but is not an effective test in endemic areas of the world where a large proportion of the population has had subclinical contact with the spores and has antibodies to the organisms. The most sensitive and reliable test for histoplasmosis is the immunodiffusion test, which detects the patient serum antibody to the **H** and **M** antigen of *H. capsulatum*. DNA probes are also available.

TREATMENT

For disseminated histoplasmosis, administration of amphotericin B remains the therapy of choice, whereas the azoles are used as adjuncts. In patients with immunodeficient disorders such as AIDS, recurrence of the infection is a continuing problem.

Coccidioides immitis

Coccidioidomycosis

> ■ **COCCIDIOIDOMYCOSIS**: a chronic lung infection due to inhalation of spores of *Coccidioides immitis* common in the San Joaquin Valley of California that may have associated chronic ulcers in the mouth resembling a malignancy; best treated with amphotericin B.

Coccidioidomycosis is a deep fungal infection of lungs that is common in patients in the arid parts of North and South America and caused by inhaled spores of *C. immitis* that are present in dust. One of the largest endemic areas for this disease is in the central valley of California, where it is known as **"San Joaquin Valley Fever"** or simply **"Valley Fever."** Other endemic areas in North America include the Maricopa and Pima counties of Arizona, parts of southwest Texas, and northern Mexico.

CLINICAL

Approximately 40% of individuals exposed to *C. immitis* will develop significant lung and respiratory symptoms, fever, cough, chest discomfort, and arthralgia at the time of initial exposure. A small percentage of these patients will develop disseminated disease. Fatal outcomes are rare unless the patient is severely immunocompromised. Disseminated organisms may involve the skin and oral mucous membranes. Intraorally, the mucosal lesions usually resemble other granulomatous diseases, with ulceration and induration as prominent features. As with other deep fungal infections, clinical distinction from carcinoma is not possible, and microscopic examination of a tissue sample and testing for seroimmunoreactivity is therefore essential.

HISTOPATHOLOGY

Coccidioidomycosis is characterized by multiple focal granulomas containing large macrophages, lymphocytes, plasma cells, and multinucleated giant cells. Liquefactive necrosis and exudate may be seen in the center of the granulomas. PAS and methenamine silver stains reveal large spherules (10 to 60 µm in diameter) filled with endospores measuring 2 to 5 µm in diameter.

DIAGNOSIS

The diagnosis of a *C. immitis* infection utilizes fractions of the organism in the mycelial phase **(coccidioidin)** and the spherule phase **(spherulin)** as antigens to test for the presence of the antibody. A positive skin reaction can be observed 2 to 4 weeks after the patient has had contact with the organism. Serum antibody levels can be monitored by immunodiffusion and latex particle agglutination tests.

TREATMENT

Ketoconazole is effective in mild infections. Recurrence is often a problem after cessation of azole therapy. Permanent cures usually require amphotericin B therapy, particularly in the more serious infections.

Cryptococcus neoformans

Cryptococcosis

■ CRYPTOCOCCOSIS: a chronic infection of the lungs due to the inhalation of spores of *Cryptococcus neoformans* carried in bird droppings, with a predilection for spread to the CNS; oral chronic ulcers primarily occur in immunocompromised patients and are best treated with amphotericin B.

C. neoformans, the causative organism of cyrptococcosis, is a universally distributed fungus that is present in the droppings of pigeons. As in most deep fungal infections, the spores are transmitted as aerosols through the respiratory passages into the lungs, where primary lesions occur. Of particular concern with infections of *C. neoformans* is the predilection for spreading to the CNS.

CLINICAL

Most patients are not aware of initial contact with *C. neoformans*, whereas others may experience mild flulike symptoms. In some patients the primary lung infection results in a residual nodule that can be mistaken for a carcinoma. CNS involvement is usually in the form of a severe meningitis, but on occasion granulomas that produce neurologic defects are located within the brain. Oral lesions usually occur in patients who are severely immunosuppressed or suffering from leukemia or lymphoma. The lesions present as ulcers and granulomas that penetrate into bone or perforate the palate.

HISTOPATHOLOGY

Tissue contains multiple focal granulomas exhibiting numerous lymphocytes and plasma cells. Macrophages and multinucleated giant cells containing fungal organisms are present in clusters or singly throughout the lesion. The infective form of the fungus is a budding yeast that measures 5 to 20 μm in diameter and exhibits a thick mucicarmine-positive capsule that resembles a halo.

TREATMENT

The treatment of choice for cryptococcosis is amphotericin B, which must be supplemented with 5-fluorocytosine when neurologic involvement is present. In many cases, particularly in the immunosuppressed patient, relapse is a problem after therapy stops.

Blastomyces dermatitidis

North American Blastomycosis

■ NORTH AMERICAN BLASTOMYCOSIS: an uncommon, rarely symptomatic, chronic lung infection due to inhalation of spores of *Blastomyces dermatitides;* has associated skin lesions and occasional chronic mouth ulcers that resemble malignancy and are best treated with amphotericin B.

Blastomycosis is caused by *B. dermatitidis* and occurs predominantly in patients in North America and parts of Africa. As with other deep mycotic infections, a primary infection of the lungs results from the inhalation of spores. The exact reservoir of the organisms is still unknown. Attempts to culture organisms from the soil in endemic areas has been unsuccessful.

CLINICAL

Similar to many other deep mycoses, most of the primary infections of blastomyces are asymptomatic. When symptoms do occur, they are usually flulike in nature unless a disseminated infection occurs. Skin involvement is common, beginning as a rash or papular eruptions that become pustular and eventually ulcerative. Intraoral lesions are crateriform and indurated, simulating a squamous cell carcinoma.

HISTOPATHOLOGY

Cutaneous or mucosal lesions are characterized by a central ulcer, and the adjacent epithelium exhibits a pseudoepitheliomatous hyperplasia, which may lead to an erroneous suspicion of malignancy. The connective tissue is granulomatous, consisting of histiocytes, lymphocytes, plasma cells, and multinucleated giant cells. Budding spores measuring 8 to 15 μm in diameter are found in areas of inflammation, particularly within the cytoplasm of multinucleated giant cells (Figure 7-44).

DIAGNOSIS

Although not entirely specific, two antigenic tests based on the use of fractions of *B. dermatitidis* in the mycelial (blastomycin) and yeast phases are available. Immunodiffusion tests are more reliable but are technically difficult to perform. The microscopic and culture appearances of the organism are important in making the diagnosis.

TREATMENT

Except for uncomplicated lung infections that can be treated with ketoconazole, the treatment of choice for blastomycosis is amphotericin B.

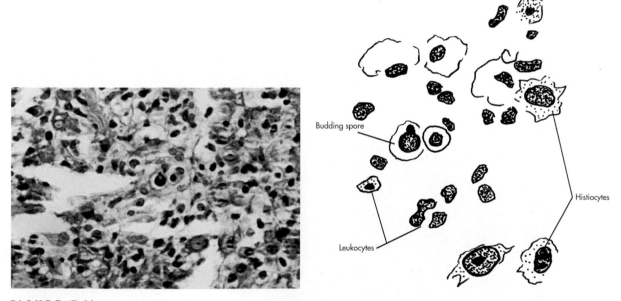

FIGURE 7-44

Blastomycosis. A photomicrograph of granulation tissue from the base of a chronic ulcer with PAS stain revealing the presence of a budding spore *(center area)* typical of *B. dermatitidis* with surrounding histiocytes, multinucleated giant cells, and leukocytes.

Aspergillus

Aspergillosis

> ■ ASPERGILLOSIS: an infection commonly located in the lungs of immunocompromised patients and occasionally occurring as a destructive lesion of the maxillary sinuses, anterior palate, and nasal passages due to the inhalation of spores of *Aspergillus fumigatus* and *A. flavus*; best treated in the oral area with surgical debridement followed by amphotericin B and azole fungicides and with management of the predisposing condition.

Aspergillosis is caused by the *Aspergillus* species of fungi. The species most frequently found in opportunistic infections are *A. fumigatus* and *A. flavus*. Usually, healthy individuals are not susceptible to infection with this organism. Although the fungal spores are widespread in the environment, they are not part of the human flora. *Aspergillus* is a major cause of mycotic infections in domestic farm animals and birds, in which it remains as a large reservoir. Acquisition of an infection with this organism by humans requires a severely compromised or debilitated host such as occurs in AIDS and in immunosuppressed organ transplant recipients.

CLINICAL
Human infections by *A. fumigatus* are increasing as a result of the growing number of patients who take immunosuppressive drugs for organ transplantation and the growing population of immunodeficient patients. In these patients infection usually occurs in the lungs and is manifested by the formation of a **"fungus ball."** In the oral area nearly all cases involve the anterior palate, nasal spine and passages, and maxillary sinuses. In these areas swelling is a common presenting symptom that has a radiographic appearance characterized by dense radiopacities within an area of bone destruction. Lesions may extend to the floor of the orbit, resulting in visual disturbances.

HISTOPATHOLOGY
The organisms are usually present in the center of an area of necrosis and exudate, which is surrounded by a typical granulomatous reaction with dense infiltrates of histiocytes, lymphocytes, and plasma cells. The presence of the fungus is demonstrated with PAS or methenamine silver stains, which reveal large branching septate hyphae, conidiophores, and conidiospores (Figure 7-45).

FIGURE 7-45

Aspergillosis. Photomicrograph of tissue from a "fungus ball" of maxillary sinus stained with PAS revealing the septate hyphae with conidiospores.

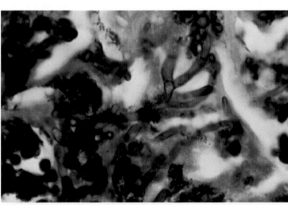

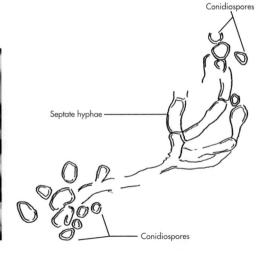

Conidiospores

Septate hyphae

Conidiospores

DIAGNOSIS

The diagnosis of aspergillosis in humans relies heavily on the clinical circumstances of the infection, the anatomic site of the infection, and the microscopic findings. Culture is difficult and is often negative. No skin sensitivity or serum reactivity tests are useful because most of the affected patients are immunodeficient.

TREATMENT

A major component of the treatment of aspergillosis is the surgical debridement of the sequestered bone and necrotic tissue in which the organisms reside. To be effective, aggressive treatment with amphotericin B and azole systemic fungicides is necessary. Until the underlying predisposing factors are corrected, the prognosis is not favorable.

ZYGOMYCOTA MUCOR/RHIZOPUS

Rhinocerebral Zygomycosis

■ RHINOCEREBRAL ZYGOMYCOSIS: a chronic destructive infection of the mid-face and nasal passages, occurring in patients with uncontrolled diabetes mellitus and in severely immunocompromised patients; due to members of Mucor or Rhizopus of the phylum Zygomycota; best treated with surgical debridement, followed by amphotericin B and management of the predisposing condition.

Zygomycosis is caused by fungal organisms of the phylum Zygomycota that contains the genera Mucor and Rhizopus, which is the same order of fungi that constitutes the mold on bread and fruit. Collectively, human infections by these organisms are termed **zygomycosis** because any one of a large number of the members of this phylum may be involved. In the past they were termed **"phycomycosis,"** reflecting an older term for one of the genera. More recently they were referred to as **"mucormycosis,"** the name of one of the orders of Mucorales.

The most common human disease process produced by these organisms is **rhinocerebral zygomycosis,** so named because it primarily affects the nose, maxillary sinus, and midface, with frequent extension to the brain.

CLINICAL

The fungi responsible for zygomycosis flourish in an acidic environment, usually in patients with severe ketoacidosis due to uncontrolled diabetes mellitus. Other severely immunosuppressed and debilitated patients are also susceptible to infection by this organism. The fungus tends to invade and block major blood vessels, resulting in ischemic necrosis, gangrene, and large tissue defects.

HISTOPATHOLOGY

The typical microscopic features of zygomycosis include extensive tissue necrosis and the presence of numerous large fungal hyphae. The hyphae are coenocytic (nonseptate) and can be seen with routine H&E stains. They exhibit a ribbonlike appearance, with budding and dichotomous branching (Figure 7-46). Numerous sporangiospores are also present.

TREATMENT

Treatment of zygomycosis is similar to that of aspergillosis, consisting of surgical curettage, aggressive therapy with amphotericin B, and management of the underlying predisposing condition.

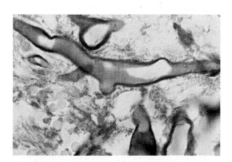

FIGURE 7-46

Zygomycosis. Photomicrograph of H&E stained tissue from an immunosuppressed patient with a destructive lesion of the anterior maxilla revealing large ribbonlike tubular nonseptate structures budding at right angles against a background of necrotic debris.

ADDITIONAL READING

VIRAL INFECTIONS

HERPES INFECTIONS

Herpes Simplex

Ashley R, Wald A, Corey L. Cervical antibodies in patients with oral herpes simplex virus type 1 (HSV-1) infection: local anamnestic responses after genital HSV-2 infection. *J Virol.* 1994; 68:5284-6.

Burke EM, Karp DL, Wu TC, Corio RL. Atypical oral presentation of herpes simplex virus infection in a patient after orthotopic liver transplantation. *Eur Arch Otorhinolaryngol.* 1994; 251:301-3.

Carrega G, Castagnola E, Canessa A, Argenta P and others. Herpes simplex virus and oral mucositis in children with cancer. *Support Care Cancer.* 1994; 2:266-9.

Detjen PF, Patterson R, Noskin GA, Phair JP and others. Herpes simplex virus associated with recurrent Stevens-Johnson syndrome: a management strategy. *Arch Intern Med.* 1992; 152:1513-6.

Dohvoma CN. Primary herpetic gingivostomatitis with multiple herpetic whitlows. *Br Dent J.* 1994; 177:251-2.

Glick M, Muzyka BC, Lurie D, Salkin LM. Oral manifestations associated with HIV-related disease as markers for immune suppression and AIDS. *Oral Surg Oral Med Oral Pathol.* 1994; 77:344-9.

Jones AC, Freedman PD, Phelan JA, Baughman RA and others. Cytomegalovirus infections of the oral cavity: a report of six cases and review of the literature. *Oral Surg Oral Med Oral Pathol.* 1993; 75:76-85.

Jones AC, Migliorati CA, Baughman RA. The simultaneous occurrence of oral herpes simplex virus, cytomegalovirus, and histoplasmosis in an HIV-infected patient. *Oral Surg Oral Med Oral Pathol.* 1992; 74:334-9.

King DL, Steinhauer W, Garcia-Godoy F, Elkins CJ. Herpetic gingivostomatitis and teething difficulty in infants. *Pediatr Dent.* 1992; 14:82-5.

Lavelle CL. Acyclovir: is it an effective virostatic agent for orofacial infections? *J Oral Pathol Med.* 1993; 22:391-401.

MacPhail LA, Hilton JF, Heinic GS, Greenspan D. Direct immunofluorescence vs. culture for detecting HSV in oral ulcers: a comparison. *J Am Dent Assoc.* 1995; 126:74-8.

Miller CS. Herpes simplex virus and human papillomavirus infections of the oral cavity. *Semin Dermatol.* 1994; 13:108-17.

Miller CS, Redding SW. Diagnosis and management of orofacial herpes simplex virus infections. *Dent Clin North Am.* 1992; 36:879-95.

Robinson PA, High AS, Hume WJ. Rapid detection of human herpes simplex virus type 1 in saliva. *Arch Oral Biol.* 1992; 37:797-806.

Rodu B. New approaches to the diagnosis of oral soft-tissue disease of viral origin. *Adv Dent Res.* 1993; 7:207-12.

Spruance SL. The natural history of recurrent oral-facial herpes simplex virus infection. *Semin Dermatol.* 1992; 11:200-6.

Yamamoto T, Osaki T, Yoneda K, Ueta E. Immunological investigation of adult patients with primary herpes simplex virus-1 infection. *J Oral Pathol Med.* 1993; 22:263-7.

Varicella-Zoster

Balfour HH. Current management of varicella zoster virus infections. *J Med Virol.* 1993; 1(suppl):74-81.

Cohen PR. Tests for detecting herpes simplex virus and varicella-zoster virus infections. *Dermatol Clin.* 1994; 12:51-68.

Gershon AA. Varicella-zoster virus: prospects for control. *Adv Pediatr Infect Dis.* 1995, 10:93-124.

Gnann JW. New antivirals with activity against varicella-zoster virus. *Ann Neurol.* 1994; 35(suppl):S69-72.

Liesegang TJ. Biology and molecular aspects of herpes simplex and varicella-zoster virus infections. *Ophthalmology.* 1992; 99:781-99.

Liesegang TJ. The biology of herpes simplex and varicella zoster virus infections. *Int Ophthalmol Clin.* 1993; 33:81-93.

Meier JL, Straus SE. Comparative biology of latent varicella-zoster virus and herpes simplex virus infections. *J Infect Dis.* 1992; 166(suppl 1):S13-23.

Plotkin SA. Vaccines for varicella-zoster virus and cytomegalovirus: recent progress. *Science.* 1994; 265:1383-5.

Rockley PF, Tyring SK. Pathophysiology and clinical manifestations of varicella zoster virus infections. *Int J Dermatol.* 1994; 33:227-32.

Straus SE. Overview: the biology of varicella-zoster virus infection. *Ann Neurol.* 1994; 35(suppl):S4-8.

Tyring SK. Natural history of varicella zoster virus. *Semin Dermatol.* 1992; 11:211-7.

Whitley RJ. Therapeutic approaches to varicella-zoster virus infections. *J Infect Dis.* 1992; 166(suppl 1):S51-7.

Epstein-Barr

Chow VT. Cancer and viruses. *Ann Acad Med Singapore.* 1993; 22:163-9.

Iezzoni JC, Gaffey MJ, Weiss LM. The role of Epstein-Barr virus in lymphoepithelioma-like carcinomas. *Am J Clin Pathol.* 1995; 103:308-15.

Kadin ME. Pathology of Hodgkin's disease. *Curr Opin Oncol.* 1994; 6:456-63.

Khan G, Coates PJ. The role of Epstein-Barr virus in the pathogenesis of Hodgkin's disease. *J Pathol.* 1994; 174:141-9.

Klein G. Role of EBV and Ig/myc translocation in Burkitt lymphoma. *Antibiot Chemother.* 1994; 46:110-6.

Lee JH, Lee SS, Park JH, Kim YW and others. Prevalence of EBV RNA in sinonasal and Waldeyer's ring lymphomas. *J Korean Med Sci.* 1994; 9:281-8.

Nalesnik MA, Starzl TE. Epstein-Barr virus, infectious mononucleosis, and posttransplant lymphoproliferative disorders. *Transplant Sci.* 1994; 4:61-79.

Raab-Traub N. Epstein-Barr virus infection in nasopharyngeal carcinoma. *Infect Agents Dis.* 1992; 1:173-84.

Vousden KH, Farrell PJ. Viruses and human cancer. *Br Med Bull.* 1994; 50:560-81.

Cytomegalovirus

Hanshaw JB. Cytomegalovirus infections. *Pediatr Rev.* 1995; 16:43-8.

Ho M. Advances in understanding cytomegalovirus infection after transplantation. *Transplant Proc.* 1994; 26(5 suppl 1): 7-11.

Markham A, Faulds D. Ganciclovir: an update of its therapeutic use in cytomegalovirus infection. *Drugs.* 1994; 48:455-84.

Nardiello S, Digilio L, Pizzella T, Galanti B. Cytomegalovirus as a co-factor of disease progression in human immunodeficiency virus type 1 infection. *Int J Clin Lab Res.* 1994; 24: 86-9.

Spaete RR, Gehrz RC, Landini MP. Human cytomegalovirus structural proteins. *J Gen Virol.* 1994; 75(pt 12):3287-308.

Starr SE. Cytomegalovirus vaccines: current status. *Infect Agents Dis.* 1992; 1:146-8.

Wagstaff AJ, Bryson HM. Foscarnet: a reappraisal of its antiviral activity, pharmacokinetic properties and therapeutic use in immunocompromised patients with viral infections. *Drugs.* 1994; 48:199-226.

Human Herpesvirus 6

Borysiewicz LK, Sissons JG. Cytotoxic T cells and human herpes virus infections. *Curr Top Microbiol Immunol.* 1994; 189:123-50.

Cantin E, Chen J, Gaidulis L, Valo Z and others. Detection of herpes simplex virus DNA sequences in human blood and bone marrow cells. *J Med Virol.* 1994; 42:279-86.

Golden MP, Kim S, Hammer SM, Ladd EA and others. Activation of human immunodeficiency virus by herpes simplex virus. *J Infect Dis.* 1992; 166:494-9.

Hill AE, Hicks EM, Coyle PV. Human herpes virus 6 and central nervous system complications. *Dev Med Child Neurol.* 1994; 36:651-2.

Oda Y, Katsuda S, Okada Y, Kawahara EI and others. Detection of human cytomegalovirus, Epstein-Barr virus, and herpes simplex virus in diffuse interstitial pneumonia by polymerase chain reaction and immunohistochemistry. *Am J Clin Pathol.* 1994; 102:495-502.

Sumiyoshi Y, Akashi K, Kikuchi M. Detection of human herpes virus 6 (HHV 6) in the skin of a patient with primary HHV 6 infection and erythroderma. *J Clin Pathol.* 1994; 47:762-3.

COXSACKIE A VIRUSES

Hyypia T, Stanway G. Biology of coxsackie A viruses. *Adv Virus Res.* 1993; 42:343-73.

Nakayama T, Urano T, Osano M, Hayashi Y and others. Outbreak of herpangina associated with Coxsackie virus B3 infection. *Pediatr Infect Dis J.* 1989; 8:495-8.

TOGAVIRUSES

Rubivirus

Broor S, Kapil A, Kishore J, Seth P. Prevalence of rubella virus and cytomegalovirus infections in suspected cases of congenital infections. *Indian J Pediatr.* 1991; 58:75-8.

Forng RY, Frey TK. Identification of the rubella virus nonstructural proteins. *Virology.* 1995; 206:843-53.

Frey TK. Molecular biology of rubella virus. *Adv Virus Res.* 1994; 44:69-160.

Mumps and Rubella Consensus Conference. *Can Commun Dis Rep.* 1994; 20:165-76.

Robinson J, Lemay M, Vaudry WL. Congenital rubella after anticipated maternal immunity: two cases and a review of the literature. *Pediatr Infect Dis J.* 1994; 13:812-5.

PARAMYXOVIRUSES

Bakshi SS, Cooper LZ. Rubella and mumps vaccines. *Pediatr Clin North Am.* 1990; 37:651-68.

Breuer J, Jeffries DJ. Control of viral infections in hospitals. *J Hosp Infect.* 1990; 16:191-221.

Glick M, Goldman HS. Viral infections in the dental setting: potential effects on pregnant HCWs. *J Am Dent Assoc.* 1993; 124:79-86.

Smith H. Mumps. *Practitioner.* 1990; 234:903-4.

Weber DJ, Rutala WA, Orenstein WA. Prevention of mumps, measles, and rubella among hospital personnel. *J Pediatr.* 1991; 119:322-6.

Wharton M, Cochi SL, Williams WW. Measles, mumps, and rubella vaccines. *Infect Dis Clin North Am.* 1990; 4:47-73.

HUMAN PAPILLOMA VIRUSES

Baum BJ, O'Connell BC. The impact of gene therapy on dentistry. *J Am Dent Assoc.* 1995; 126:179-89.

Costa LJ, Silveira FR, Batista JM, Birman EG. Human papilloma virus: its association with epithelial proliferative lesions. *Braz Dent J.* 1994; 5:5-10.

Ferenczy A. Epidemiology and clinical pathophysiology of condylomata acuminata. *Am J Obstet Gynecol.* 1995; 172(4 pt 2):1331-9.

Gall SA. Human papillomavirus infection and therapy with interferon. *Am J Obstet Gynecol.* 1995; 172(4 Pt 2):1354-9.

Herrington CS. Human papillomaviruses and cervical neoplasia: I: classification, virology, pathology, and epidemiology. *J Clin Pathol.* 1994; 47:1066-72.

Herrington CS. Human papillomaviruses and cervical neoplasia: II: interaction of HPV with other factors. *J Clin Pathol.* 1995; 48:1-6.

McCance DJ. Human papillomaviruses. *Infect Dis Clin North Am.* 1994; 8:751-67.

McLachlin CM. Pathology of human papillomavirus in the female genital tract. *Curr Opin Obstet Gynecol.* 1995; 7:24-9.

Wu TC. Immunology of the human papilloma virus in relation to cancer. *Curr Opin Immunol.* 1994; 6:746-54.

HECK DISEASE

Carlos R, Sedano HO. Multifocal papilloma virus epithelial hyperplasia. *Oral Surg Oral Med Oral Pathol.* 1994; 77:631-5.

Chindia ML, Awange DO, Guthua SW, Mwaniki DL. Focal epithelial hyperplasia (Heck's disease) in three Kenyan girls: case reports. *East Afr Med J.* 1993; 70:595-6.

Cohen PR, Hebert AA, Adler-Storthz K. Focal epithelial hyperplasia: Heck disease. *Pediatr Dermatol.* 1993; 10:245-51.

Costa LJ, Silveira FR, Batista JM, Birman EG. Human papilloma virus—its association with epithelial proliferative lesions. *Braz Dent J.* 1994; 5:5-10.

Landells ID, Prendiville JS. Oral mucosal lesions in a Somali boy. *Pediatr Dermatol.* 1994; 11:274-6.

Obalek S, Janniger C, Jablonska S, Favre M and others. Sporadic cases of Heck disease in two Polish girls: association with human papillomavirus type 13. *Pediatr Dermatol.* 1993; 10:240-4.

Tan AK, Tewfik TL, Moroz B, Thibault MJ and others. Focal epithelial hyperplasia. *Otolaryngol Head Neck Surg.* 1995; 112:316-20.

Vilmer C, Cavelier-Balloy B, Pinquier L, Blanc F and others. Focal epithelial hyperplasia and multifocal human papillomavirus infection in an HIV-seropositive man. *J Am Acad Dermatol.* 1994; 30:497-8.

RETROVIRUSES

Human Immunodeficiency Virus

Andris JS, Capra JD. The molecular structure of human antibodies specific for the human immunodeficiency virus. *J Clin Immunol.* 1995; 15:17-26.

Beard WA, Wilson SH. Site-directed mutagenesis of HIV reverse transcriptase to probe enzyme processivity and drug binding. *Curr Opin Biotechnol.* 1994; 5:414-21.

Bolognesi DP. Approaches to HIV vaccine design. *Trends Biotechnol.* 1990; 8:40-5.

Bour S, Geleziunas R, Wainberg MA. The human immunodeficiency virus type 1 (HIV-1) CD4 receptor and its central role in promotion of HIV-1 infection. *Microbiol Rev.* 1995; 59:63-93.

Centers for Disease Control. Update: HIV-2 infection—United States. *JAMA.* 1989; 262:1579, 1583.

Coleman DC, Bennett DE, Sullivan DJ, Gallagher PJ and others. Oral Candida in HIV infection and AIDS: new perspectives/new approaches. *Crit Rev Microbiol.* 1993; 19:61-82.

del Guercio P. AIDS and immune dysfunction: alternative etiologic mechanisms. *Contrib Microbiol Immunol.* 1989; 11: 289-304.

Flaitz CM, Nichols CM, Hicks MJ. An overview of the oral manifestations of AIDS-related Kaposi's sarcoma. *Compendium.* 1995; 16:136-8, 140, 142.

Fox PC. Saliva and salivary gland alterations in HIV infection. *J Am Dent Assoc.* 1991; 122:46-8.

Garfunkel AA, Glick M. Common oral findings in two different diseases—leukemia and AIDS: part 2. *Compendium.* 1992; 13:550, 552-3, 556.

Glick M, Garfunkel AA. Common oral findings in two different diseases—leukemia and AIDS: part 1. *Compendium.* 1992; 13:432, 434, 436.

Greenspan JS, Greenspan D, Winkler JR. Diagnosis and management of the oral manifestations of HIV infection and AIDS. *Infect Dis Clin North Am.* 1988; 2:373-85.

Hellen CU, Wimmer E. Viral proteases as targets for chemotherapeutic intervention. *Curr Opin Biotechnol.* 1992; 3:643-9.

Jindal JR, Campbell BH, Ward TO, Almagro US. Kaposi's sarcoma of the oral cavity in a non-AIDS patient: case report and review of the literature. *Head Neck.* 1995; 17:64-8.

Kanki PJ. Clinical significance of HIV-2 infection in West Africa. *AIDS Clin Rev.* 1989; 95-108.

Kaplan M. Human retroviruses: a common virology. *Transfus Med Rev.* 1989; 3(1 suppl 1):4-8.

Khoo SH, Wilkins EG. Controversies in anti-retroviral therapy of adults. *J Antimicrob Chemother.* 1995; 35:245-62.

Levy JA. Viral and cellular factors influencing HIV tropism. *Adv Exp Med Biol.* 1991; 300:1-15.

McGrath MS, Ng VL. Human retrovirus-associated malignancy. *Cancer Treat Res.* 1989; 47:267-84.

Reichart PA. Oral manifestations of recently described viral infections, including AIDS. *Curr Opin Dent.* 1991; 1:377-83.

Reichart PA, Gelderblom HR, Becker J, Kuntz A. AIDS and the oral cavity: the HIV-infection: virology, etiology, origin, immunology, precautions and clinical observations in 110 patients. *Int J Oral Maxillofac Surg.* 1987; 16:129-53.

Roberts MW, Brahim JS, Rinne NF. Oral manifestations of AIDS: a study of 84 patients. *J Am Dent Assoc.* 1988; 116:863-6.

Schiodt M, Pindborg JJ. AIDS and the oral cavity: epidemiology and clinical oral manifestations of human immune deficiency virus infection: a review. *Int J Oral Maxillofac Surg.* 1987; 16:1-14.

Sciubba JJ. Recognizing the oral manifestations of AIDS. *Oncology.* 1992; 6:64-70, 75.

Silverman S. AIDS update: oral manifestations and management. *Dent Clin North Am.* 1991; 35:259-67.

Silverman S, Wara D. Oral manifestations of pediatric AIDS. *Pediatrician.* 1989; 16:185-7.

Stewart GT. The epidemiology and transmission of AIDS: a hypothesis linking behavioural and biological determinants to time, person and place. *Genetica.* 1995; 95:173-93.

Swanstrom R. Characterization of HIV-1 protease mutants: random, directed, selected. *Curr Opin Biotechnol.* 1994; 5:409-13.

Update: HIV-2 infection—United States. *MMWR.* 1989; 38:572-4, 579-80.

van der Waal I, Schulten EA, Pindborg JJ. Oral manifestations of AIDS: an overview. *Int Dent J.* 1991; 41:3-8.

Weber J. The biology and epidemiology of HIV infections. *J Antimicrob Chemother.* 1989; 23(suppl A):1-7.

BACTERIAL INFECTIONS

STREPTOCOCCUS

Barnett BO, Frieden IJ. Streptococcal skin diseases in children. *Semin Dermatol.* 1992; 11:3-10.

Bernard P. Dermo-hypodermal bacterial infections: current concepts. *Eur J Med.* 1992; 1:97-104.

Bialecki C, Feder HM, Grant-Kels JM. The six classic childhood exanthems: a review and update. *J Am Acad Dermatol.* 1989; 21(5 pt 1):891-903.

Bratton RL, Nesse RE. St. Anthony's fire: diagnosis and management of erysipelas. *Am Fam Physician.* 1995; 51:401-4.

Cherry JD. Contemporary infectious exanthems. *Clin Infect Dis.* 1993; 16:199-205.

Friedman AD. Superficial bacterial and fungal infections of the skin. *Adv Pediatr Infect Dis.* 1990; 5:205-19.

Hartley AH, Rasmussen JE. Infectious exanthems. *Pediatr Rev.* 1988; 9:321-9.

Kahn RM, Goldstein EJ. Common bacterial skin infections. Diagnostic clues and therapeutic options. *Postgrad Med.* 1993; 93:175-82.

Quinn RW. Comprehensive review of morbidity and mortality trends for rheumatic fever, streptococcal disease, and scarlet fever: the decline of rheumatic fever. *Rev Infect Dis.* 1989; 11:928-53.

Stevens DL. Invasive group A *streptococcus* infections. *Clin Infect Dis.* 1992; 14:2-11.

Stevens DL. Invasive group A streptococcal infections: the past, present and future. *Pediatr Infect Dis J.* 1994; 13:561-6.

Tomiyama J, Hasegawa Y, Kumagai Y, Adachi Y and others. Acute febrile mucocutaneous lymph node syndrome (Kawasaki disease) in adults: case report and review of the literature. *Jpn J Med.* 1991; 30:285-9.

Wickboldt LG, Fenske NA. Streptococcal and staphylococcal infections of the skin. *Hosp Pract.* 1986; 21:41-7.

STAPHYLOCOCCUS

Aly R. The pathogenic staphylococci. *Semin Dermatol.* 1990; 9:292-9.

Bass JW. Treatment of skin and skin structure infections. *Pediatr Infect Dis J.* 1992; 11:152-5.

Marples RR, Richardson JF, Newton FE. Staphylococci as part of the normal flora of human skin. *Soc Appl Bacteriol Symp Ser.* 1990; 19:93S-99S.

Sippe JR. Common skin infections. *Aust Fam Physician.* 1991; 20:783-4, 787, 790-4.

MYCOBACTERIUM

Bloom BR, Flynn J, McDonough K, Kress Y, Chan J. Experimental approaches to mechanisms of protection and pathogenesis in *M. tuberculosis* infection. *Immunobiology.* 1994; 191:526-36.

Crawford JT. New technologies in the diagnosis of tuberculosis. *Semin Respir Infect.* 1994; 9:62-70.

Dannenberg AM. Roles of cytotoxic delayed-type hypersensitivity and macrophage-activating cell-mediated immunity in the pathogenesis of tuberculosis. *Immunobiology.* 1994; 191:461-73.

Drobniewski FA, Kent RJ, Stoker NG, Uttley AH. Molecular biology in the diagnosis and epidemiology of tuberculosis. *J Hosp Infect.* 1994; 28:249-63.

Dunlap NE, Kimerling ME. Drug-resistant tuberculosis in adults: implications for the health care worker. *Infect Agents Dis.* 1994; 3:245-55.

Ford JG, Felton CP. Tuberculosis: pathogenesis and laboratory diagnosis. *Occup Med.* 1994; 9:561-74.

Grange JM. Diagnostic tests for tuberculosis and their evaluation. *Semin Respir Infect.* 1994; 9:71-7.

Lowrie DB, Tascon RE, Colston MJ, Silva CL. Towards a DNA vaccine against tuberculosis. *Vaccine.* 1994; 12:1537-40.

O'Brien RJ. Drug-resistant tuberculosis: etiology, management and prevention. *Semin Respir Infect.* 1994; 9:104-12.

Rook GA, al Attiyah R, Filley E. New insights into the immunopathology of tuberculosis. *Pathobiology.* 1991; 59: 148-52.

Rook GA, Hernandez-Pando R. T cell helper types and endocrines in the regulation of tissue-damaging mechanisms in tuberculosis. *Immunobiology.* 1994; 191:478-92.

Shinnick TM, King CH, Quinn FD. Molecular biology, virulence, and pathogenicity of mycobacteria. *Am J Med Sci.* 1995; 309:92-8.

Swanson DS, Starke JR. Drug-resistant tuberculosis in pediatrics. *Pediatr Clin North Am.* 1995; 42:553-81.

Waxman S, Gang M, Goldfrank L. Tuberculosis in the HIV-infected patient. *Emerg Med Clin North Am.* 1995; 13:179-98.

TREPONEMA PALLIDUM

Goens JL, Janniger CK, De Wolf K. Dermatologic and systemic manifestations of syphilis. *Am Fam Physician.* 1994; 50:1013-20.

Larsen SA, Steiner BM, Rudolph AH. Laboratory diagnosis and interpretation of tests for syphilis. *Clin Microbiol Rev.* 1995; 8:1-21.

Sanchez MR. Infectious syphilis. *Semin Dermatol.* 1994; 13: 234-42.

Starling SP. Syphilis in infants and young children. *Pediatr Ann.* 1994; 23:334-40.

Stoll BJ. Congenital syphilis: evaluation and management of neonates born to mothers with reactive serologic tests for syphilis. *Pediatr Infect Dis J.* 1994; 13:845-52.

ACTINOMYCES

Bhatti SA. Cervicofacial actinomycosis in pregnancy. *Br Dent J.* 1989; 166:83-5.

Foster SV, Demmler GJ, Hawkins EP, Tillman JP. Pediatric cervicofacial actinomycosis. *South Med J.* 1993; 86:1147-50.

Friduss ME, Maceri DR. Cervicofacial actinomycosis in children. *Henry Ford Hosp Med J.* 1990; 38:28-32.

Happonen RP. Immunocytochemical diagnosis of cervicofacial actinomycosis with special emphasis on periapical inflammatory lesions. *Proc Finn Dent Soc.* 1986; 82(suppl 7-8):1-50.

Lerner PI. The lumpy jaw: cervicofacial actinomycosis. *Infect Dis Clin North Am.* 1988; 2:203-20.

Martin MV. Antibiotic treatment of cervicofacial actinomycosis for patients allergic to penicillin: a clinical and in vitro study. *Br J Oral Maxillofac Surg.* 1985; 23:428-34.

MYCOSES

CANDIDA ALBICANS

Allen CM. Animal models of oral candidiasis: a review. *Oral Surg Oral Med Oral Pathol.* 1994; 78:216-21.

British Society for Antimicrobial Chemotherapy Working Party. Antifungal chemotherapy in patients with acquired immunodeficiency syndrome. *Lancet*. 1992; 340:648-51.

Challacombe SJ. Immunologic aspects of oral candidiasis. *Oral Surg Oral Med Oral Pathol*. 1994; 78:202-10.

Epstein JB, Stevenson-Moore P, Scully C. Management of xerostomia. *J Can Dent Assoc*. 1992; 58:140-3.

Fotos PG, Hellstein JW. *Candida* and candidosis: epidemiology, diagnosis and therapeutic management. *Dent Clin North Am*. 1992; 36:857-78.

Fotos PG, Ray TL. Oral and perioral candidosis. *Semin Dermatol*. 1994; 13:118-24.

Garber GE. Treatment of oral *Candida mucositis* infections. *Drugs*. 1994; 47:734-40.

Greenspan D. Treatment of oral candidiasis in HIV infection. *Oral Surg Oral Med Oral Pathol*. 1994; 78:211-5.

Iacopino AM, Wathen WF. Oral candidal infection and denture stomatitis: a comprehensive review. *J Am Dent Assoc*. 1992; 123:46-51.

Jeganathan S, Chan YC. Immunodiagnosis in oral candidiasis: a review. *Oral Surg Oral Med Oral Pathol*. 1992; 74:451-4.

Jeganathan S, Lin CC. Denture stomatitis: a review of the aetiology, diagnosis and management. *Aust Dent J*. 1992; 37:107-14.

Jones AC, Bentsen TY, Freedman PD. Mucormycosis of the oral cavity. *Oral Surg Oral Med Oral Pathol*. 1993; 75:455-60.

Korting HC. Clinical spectrum of oral candidosis and its role in HIV-infected patients. *Mycoses*. 1989; 32(suppl 2):23-9.

Langford A. Gingival and periodontal alterations associated with infection with human immunodeficiency virus. *Quintessence Int*. 1994; 25:375-87.

Lynch DP. Oral candidiasis: history, classification, and clinical presentation. *Oral Surg Oral Med Oral Pathol*. 1994; 78:189-93.

McCarthy GM. Host factors associated with HIV-related oral candidiasis: a review. *Oral Surg Oral Med Oral Pathol*. 1992; 73:181-6.

Odom RB. Common superficial fungal infections in immunosuppressed patients. *J Am Acad Dermatol*. 1994; 31(3 pt 2):S56-9.

Samaranayake LP. Oral mycoses in HIV infection. *Oral Surg Oral Med Oral Pathol*. 1992; 73:171-80.

Scully C, de Almeida OP. Orofacial manifestations of the systemic mycoses. *J Oral Pathol Med*. 1992; 21:289-94.

Scully C, el-Kabir M, Samaranayake LP. *Candida* and oral candidosis: a review. *Crit Rev Oral Biol Med*. 1994; 5:125-57.

HISTOPLASMA CAPSULATUM

Bullock WE. Interactions between human phagocytic cells and *Histoplasma capsulatum*. *Arch Med Res*. 1993; 24:219-23.

de Almeida OP, Scully C. Oral lesions in the systemic mycoses. *Curr Opin Dent*. 1991; 1:423-8.

Dijkstra JW. Histoplasmosis. *Dermatol Clin*. 1989; 7:251-8.

Dobleman TJ, Scher N, Goldman M, Doot S. Invasive histoplasmosis of the mandible. *Head Neck*. 1989; 11:81-4.

Kauffman CA. Newer developments in therapy for endemic mycoses. *Clin Infect Dis*. 1994; 19(suppl 1):S28-32.

Sarosi GA, Davies SF. Therapy for fungal infections. *Mayo Clin Proc*. 1994; 69:1111-7.

Stansell JD. Fungal disease in HIV-infected persons: cryptococcosis, histoplasmosis, and coccidioidomycosis. *J Thorac Imaging*. 1991; 6:28-35.

Tomecki KJ, Dijkstra JW, Hall GS, Steck WD. Systemic mycoses. *J Am Acad Dermatol*. 1989; 21:1285-93.

Wheat J. Endemic mycoses in AIDS: a clinical review. *Clin Microbiol Rev*. 1995; 8:146-59.

Wheat J. Histoplasmosis and coccidioidomycosis in individuals with AIDS: a clinical review. *Infect Dis Clin North Am*. 1994; 8:467-82.

Wheat J. Histoplasmosis: recognition and treatment. *Clin Infect Dis*. 1994; 19(suppl 1):S19-27.

Wheat LJ. Diagnosis and management of histoplasmosis. *Eur J Clin Microbiol Infect Dis*. 1989; 8:480-90.

Zuckerman JM, Tunkel AR. Itraconazole: a new triazole antifungal agent. *Infect Control Hosp Epidemiol*. 1994; 15:397-410.

COCCIDIOIDES IMMITIS

Bosso JA. Fungal infections in pediatric patients. *Pharmacotherapy*. 1990; 10(pt 3):150S-153S.

British Society for Antimicrobial Chemotherapy Working Party. Antifungal chemotherapy in patients with acquired immunodeficiency syndrome. *Lancet*. 1992; 340:648-51.

De Repentigny L, Kaufman L, Cole GT, Kruse D and others. Immunodiagnosis of invasive fungal infections. *J Med Vet Mycol*. 1994; 32(suppl 1):239-52.

Einstein HE, Johnson RH. Coccidioidomycosis: new aspects of epidemiology and therapy. *Clin Infect Dis*. 1993; 16:349-54.

Galgiani JN. Coccidioidomycosis: changes in clinical expression, serological diagnosis, and therapeutic options. *Clin Infect Dis*. 1992; 14(suppl 1):S100-5.

Graybill JR. Treatment of coccidioidomycosis. *Ann N Y Acad Sci*. 1988; 544:481-7.

Graybill JR. Treatment of coccidioidomycosis. *Curr Top Med Mycol*. 1993; 5:151-79.

Harley WB, Blaser MJ. Disseminated coccidioidomycosis associated with extreme eosinophilia. *Clin Infect Dis*. 1994; 18:627-9.

Hobbs ER. Coccidioidomycosis. *Dermatol Clin*. 1989; 7:227-39.

Kappe R, Seeliger HP. Serodiagnosis of deep-seated fungal infections. *Curr Top Med Mycol*. 1993; 5:247-80.

Kaufman L. Laboratory methods for the diagnosis and confirmation of systemic mycoses. *Clin Infect Dis*. 1992; 14(suppl 1):S23-9.

Knoper SR, Galgiani JN. Systemic fungal infections: diagnosis and treatment: I: coccidioidomycosis. *Infect Dis Clin North Am*. 1988; 2:861-75.

Pappagianis D. Coccidioidomycosis. *Semin Dermatol*. 1993; 12:301-9.

Pappagianis D, Zimmer BL. Serology of coccidioidomycosis. *Clin Microbiol Rev*. 1990; 3:247-68.

Sarosi GA, Davies SF. Therapy for fungal infections. *Mayo Clin Proc*. 1994; 69:1111-7.

Stevens DA. Coccidioidomycosis. *N Engl J Med.* 1995; 332:1077-82.

CRYPTOCOCCUS NEOFORMANS

Almeida OP, Scully C. Oral lesions in the systemic mycoses. *Curr Opin Dent.* 1991; 1:423-8.

Kozel TR. Antigenic structure of *Cryptococcus neoformans* capsular polysaccharides. *Immunol Ser.* 1989; 47:63-86.

Levitz SM. The ecology of *Cryptococcus neoformans* and the epidemiology of cryptococcosis. *Rev Infect Dis.* 1991; 13: 1163-9.

Lucatorto FM, Eversole LR. Deep mycosis and palatal perforation with granulomatous pansinusitis in acquired immunodeficiency syndrome: case reports. *Quintessence Int.* 1993; 24:743-48.

Patterson TF, Andriole VT. Current concepts in cryptococcosis. *Eur J Clin Microbiol Infect Dis.* 1989; 8:457-65.

Treseler CB, Sugar AM. Fungal meningitis. *Infect Dis Clin North Am.* 1990; 4:789-808.

White MH, Armstrong D. Cryptococcosis. *Infect Dis Clin North Am.* 1994; 8:383-98.

Zuckerman JM, Tunkel AR. Itraconazole: a new triazole antifungal agent. *Infect Control Hosp Epidemiol.* 1994; 15:397-410.

BLASTOMYCES DERMATITIDIS

Baily GG, Robertson VJ, Neill P, Garrido P and others. Blastomycosis in Africa: clinical features, diagnosis, and treatment. *Rev Infect Dis.* 1991; 13:1005-8.

Bradsher RW. A clinician's view of blastomycosis. *Curr Top Med Mycol.* 1993; 5:181-200.

Bradsher RW. Blastomycosis. *Clin Infect Dis.* 1992; 14(suppl 1):S82-90.

Bradsher RW. Macrophages and *Blastomyces dermatitidis.* *Immunol Ser.* 1994; 60:553-65.

Kaufman L. Laboratory methods for the diagnosis and confirmation of systemic mycoses. *Clin Infect Dis.* 1992; 14(suppl 1):S23-9.

Maxson S, Miller SF, Tryka AF, Schutze GE. Perinatal blastomycosis: a review. *Pediatr Infect Dis J.* 1992; 11:760-3.

Medoff G, Kobayashi GS. Systemic fungal infections: an overview. *Hosp Pract.* 1991; 26:41-52.

Mikaelian AJ, Varkey B, Grossman TW, Blatnik DS. Blastomycosis of the head and neck. *Otolaryngol Head Neck Surg.* 1989; 101:489-95.

Steck WD. Blastomycosis. *Dermatol Clin.* 1989; 7:241-50.

ASPERGILLUS

De Foer C, Fossion E, Vaillant JM. Sinus aspergillosis. *J Craniomaxillofac Surg.* 1990; 18:33-40.

Fraser RS. Pulmonary aspergillosis: pathologic and pathogenetic features. *Pathol Annu.* 1993; 28(pt 1):231-77.

Hartwick RW, Batsakis JG. Sinus aspergillosis and allergic fungal sinusitis. *Ann Otol Rhinol Laryngol.* 1991; 100(5 pt 1): 427-30.

Hearn VM, Mackenzie DW. Antigenic structure of *Aspergillus* species. *Immunol Ser.* 1989; 47:87-111.

Kauffman HF, Beaumont F. Serological diagnosis of *Aspergillus* infections. *Mycoses.* 1988; 31(suppl 2):21-6.

Rhodes JC, Jensen HE, Nilius AM, Chitambar CR and others. *Aspergillus* and aspergillosis. *J Med Vet Mycol.* 1992; 30 (suppl 1):51-7.

ZYGOMYCOTA MUCOR/RHIZOPUS

Adam RD, Hunter G, DiTomasso J, Comerci G. Mucormycosis: emerging prominence of cutaneous infections. *Clin Infect Dis.* 1994; 19:67-76.

Armstrong D. Problems in management of opportunistic fungal diseases. *Rev Infect Dis.* 1989; 11(suppl 7):S1591-9.

de Almeida OP, Scully C. Oral lesions in the systemic mycoses. *Curr Opin Dent.* 1991; 1:423-8.

de Biscop J, Mondie JM, Venries de la Guillaumie B, Peri G. Mucormycosis in an apparently normal host: case study and literature review. *J Craniomaxillofac Surg.* 1991; 19:275-8.

Forteza G, Burgeno M, Martorell V, Sierra I. Rhinocerebral mucormycosis: presentation of two cases and review of the literature. *J Craniomaxillofac Surg.* 1988; 16:80-4.

Ingram CW, Sennesh J, Cooper JN, Perfect JR. Disseminated zygomycosis: report of four cases and review. *Rev Infect Dis.* 1989; 11:741-54.

Rinaldi MG. Zygomycosis. *Infect Dis Clin North Am.* 1989; 3:19-41.

Van der Westhuijzen AJ, Grotepass FW, Wyma G, Padayachee A. A rapidly fatal palatal ulcer: rhinocerebral mucormycosis. *Oral Surg Oral Med Oral Pathol.* 1989; 68:32-6.

IMMUNE-MEDIATED DISORDERS

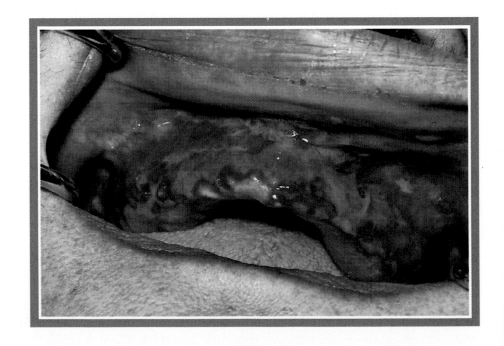

A t present, the diseases discussed in this chapter are considered to be of immune origin, although in the future, specific infectious etiologic agents may be identified for some or all. Regardless of the initiating agents, it is the interactions of the immune system, which protects and heals the body, that contribute substantially to the magnitude of the disease process. Common to most of the inflammatory reactions in the diseases discussed in this chapter is the dominance of T lymphocytes, chiefly the CD4 and CD8 subtypes. When disease mainly targets the surface epithelium, it is characterized by a substantial increase in the number of *Langerhans cells.* The Langerhans cell, an integral part of the cellular component of the intraepithelial immune system, is an antigen-processing cell with a role equivalent to that of the macrophage of connective tissue. Its role is to initiate a cascade of cellular and humoral immune responses. In many of the diseases to be discussed, antibodies against normal mucosal and skin epithelium can also be found in the circulation, further evidence of an autoimmune type of disease. These findings have prompted continuing research for exogenous agents that are capable of penetrating the skin and mucosal barrier, stimulating Langerhans cells and altering normal antigenic determinants to the extent that antibodies are produced against the body's own tissue.

RECURRENT APHTHOUS STOMATITIS

Recurrent aphthous stomatitis (RAS) is a common disease in humans. Within the oral cavity RAS is the most common condition affecting the mucosal soft tissue. Approximately 15% to 20% of the world population is afflicted by this condition. It appears to be more common in North America where specific socio-ecomonic and age groups reveal incidences of nearly 40%. In the English speaking world the lesions are commonly known as **"canker sores"** and are often confused with recurrent herpes simplex infections. RAS is an enigma to researchers because clinical lesions that occur in association with a large number of disparate local and systemic conditions are found to have a single pattern of histopathologic features. This has lead many researchers to view the lesions of RAS as a common mucosal manifestation of many different disease processes, each of which is mediated through the immune system. In some conditions, similar lesions can be found on the mucosal surfaces of the anogenitalia. Within the oral cavity RAS occurs in three distinct clinical forms: *aphthous minor, aphthous major,* and *herpetiform ulcers.* RAS also occurs in association with chronic gastrointestinal disturbances and other systemic conditions, the most notable of which is *Behçet syndrome.*

Aphthous ulcers are usually diagnosed on the basis of their clinical signs and symptoms because there are no reliable laboratory tests. During a brief preulcerative phase a subtle, specific microscopic change is present that is sometimes helpful. Once ulceration occurs the tissue changes are nonspecific, resembling an ulcer due to many other causes.

ASSOCIATED SYSTEMIC CONDITIONS

The majority of patients with recurrent aphthous ulcers are otherwise healthy. In a minority the presence of chronic RAS lesions is associated with a systemic condition. The systemic conditions most consistently associated with chronic and recurring aphthous lesions are Behçet syndrome and the chronic gastrointestinal malabsorption disturbances, particularly Crohn disease and gluten-sensitive enteropathy (celiac disease). Often, the malabsorption syndromes are mild or even symptomless but still appear capable of producing nutritional deficiencies of folic acid, vitamin B_{12}, and iron, all of which have been implicated in patients with chronic recurrent aphthous ulcers. Many patients can correlate ulcerative episodes with the ingestion of certain foods, most notably nuts and chocolate, whereas others have chronic asthma and/or multiple allergies. Correlation has been found with the menstrual cycle, periods of stress and anxiety, and a family history of lesions. It has recently been discovered that patients who are immunodeficient, particularly those that are HIV positive, become prone to prolonged, severe attacks of aphthouslike lesions. Because of the wide variety of associated conditions, no unifying theory of pathogenesis has yet evolved other than the lesions appear to be related to the immune system.

APHTHOUS MINOR

> ■ APHTHOUS MINOR: commonly encountered, painful, small superficial ulcers of the oral gland-bearing mucosa that occur episodically in clusters of one to five lesions.

Aphthous minor is the clinical form of virtually all RAS lesions. The other forms, major and herpetiform, together are estimated to occur less than 5% of the time.

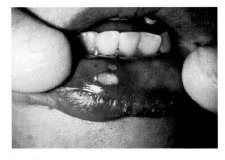

FIGURE 8-1

Recurrent aphthous minor. Lesions are shallow crateriform ulcers with a whitish-yellow base and an erythematous halo.

CLINICAL

Oral lesions of RAS minor occur episodically, with less than five ulcers present at any one time. During an attack new lesions may continually appear for a 3- to 4-week period, with each lesion lasting 10 to 14 days. The ulcers are located on the gland-bearing mucosa, usually sparing the attached gingiva, hard palate, and dorsum of the tongue. Individual lesions are round but may be elliptical if they are located in a crease or fold of the tissue. Individual lesions are small, 0.5 mm to 1 cm in diameter, shallow with sharp crateriform edges, and have a whitish yellow base and an erythematous halo or flare on the surrounding mucosa (Figure 8-1). Patients complain of pain that is out of proportion to the size of the lesion. The most common locations for lesions are the mucosal surfaces of the lips, posterior soft palate, and anterior fauces. Other less common locations are the ventral and lateral borders of the tongue and the anterior floor of the mouth.

When lesions occur on the labial mucosa, a history of a minor traumatic incidence can often be elicited. In some lesions multiple malaligned teeth with sharp incisal edges, particularly cuspids that are labially displaced, are present in the area in which patients usually experience lesions. Although mechanical irritants are not known to be the cause of aphthous ulcers, they often seem to precipitate the appearance of individual aphthous ulcers during an episodic period. Lesions of the soft palate and ventral tongue usually appear spontaneously without known precipitating traumatic incidents.

The clinical course of minor aphthous ulcers differs significantly from minor lacerations of the mucosa of non–aphthous-prone individuals. Traumatic breaks in the mucosa of non–aphthous patients will exhibit some tenderness for 1 or 2 days and heal uneventfully in 5 or 6 days. When slight and superficial mucosal lacerations occur in patients with a predisposition for aphthous ulcers, tenderness intensifies to pain in a few days and continues to intensify for 7 to 10 more days before finally healing in 10 to 14 days. Between episodes patients subject to RAS have normal reactions and healing times for minor lacerations. Oddly, surgical procedures on the mucosa during an aphthous attack heal normally.

HISTOPATHOLOGY

Mild tissue changes can be found during the preulcerative or prodromal stage. They consist of a mild T4 lymphocyte (helper/inducer) infiltrate concentrated in perivascular locations of the submucosal tissue. Later, T-cells are observed within the epithelium with vacuolization and necrosis of individual epithelial cells that eventuates in epithelium disintegration and ulceration. During this second phase the underlying connective tissue contains dense infiltrates of lymphocytes of the T8 (suppressor/cytotoxic) subset. The perivascular infiltrates are found more deeply in the submucosal tissue than normally occurs during the inflammatory cellular response from minor lacerations in non-aphthous patients. The ulcer surface is covered by a fibrinopurulent exudate overlying a zone of granulation tissue in which neutrophils, macrophages, and plasma cells are prominent, but mast cells and eosinophils are found in scant amounts (Figure 8-2). During the healing phase there is normal transformation of granulation tissue to fibrous tissue with epithelial migration over the surface. During this final phase the predominant lymphocyte subset reverts back to a T4 population.

TREATMENT

The treatment of recurrent aphthous ulcers is varied with proponents for each of a wide variety of remedies. Because there is no treatment to prevent a predisposition for future attacks, treatments are directed toward reducing the intensity and length of each episode. The most successful treatment is the application of gel- or cream-based topical steroids, particularly those on the higher end of the potentcy scale. In severe and persistent cases the administration of systemic steroids for 1 week has been shown to be effective. When only a few lesions are present in the parts of the mouth accessible to the patient, self-administered chemical cautery or styptic agents such as powdered alum and powdered boric acid have been used to reduce the duration of lesions. In addition to sterilizing the wound, these agents produce a layer of the patient's own devitalized tissue that acts as an occlusive "bandage" over the lesion, separating the oral environment from the immune response of the tissue. Although this does not prevent new lesions from occurring, reducing their duration is of great help to the patient. Oral rinses containing the antimicrobials chlorhexidine and tetracycline provide short-term relief in some patients, and when used on a daily basis during recurring bouts, they serve to lengthen the period between episodes. If patients are found to be deficient in folic acid, vitamin B_{12}, or iron, dietary supplementation is sometimes useful. Patients found to be gluten-sensitive require long-term dietary modification. Reduction of oral lesions often coincides with the improvements to the gastrointestinal tract.

APHTHOUS MAJOR

■ APHTHOUS MAJOR: one or two uncommon, large, superficial painful ulcers usually present on the labial mucosa and soft palate.

Aphthous major is uncommon but is still the second most common form of RAS. It was previously referred to as *periadenitis mucosa necrotica recurrens*, reflecting the propensity of the lesions to occur over areas of mucosa containing a large number of minor salivary glands.

CLINICAL

Lesions are large, compared with aphthous minor, ranging from 5 to 20 mm or more in size. They occur in fewer numbers, usually only one or two at a time and primarily in two locations—the mucosa of the lips (Figure 8-3, *A*) and the poste-

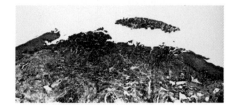

FIGURE 8-2

Recurrent aphthous minor. Microscopic appearance of the ulceration exhibiting a fibrinopurulent exudate over granulation tissue containing an infiltrate of mixed acute and chronic inflammatory cells.

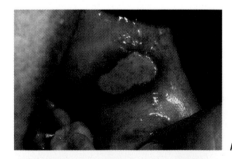

A

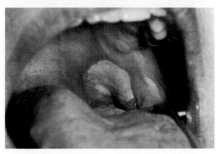

B

FIGURE 8-3

Recurrent aphthous major. Large shallow ulcers of labial mucosa (**A**) and lateral soft palate (**B**). Lesions are painful and exhibit characteristic erythematous halo.

rior soft palate/anterior fauces area (Figure 8-3, *B*). Lesions are crateriform and deeper than aphthous minor lesions and last for much longer periods, often up to 6 weeks. Pain is severe, making eating difficult, particularly when lesions are located in the posterior aspect of mouth. Aphthous major ulcers usually do not occur until after puberty, and in some patients they may be a problem for as long as 20 years. Deep and persistent lesions may become secondarily infected with bacterial and fungal organisms. When healing occurs, scar with tissue contracture often results. This is an unusual occurrence on oral mucosal surfaces because most minor injuries heal without noticeable scar formation.

HISTOPATHOLOGY

The tissue changes are similar to those in aphthous minor. The inflammation extends deep into the underlying connective tissue, and perivascular infiltrates of lymphocytes are a prominent finding. The surface of the ulcer is covered with a fibrinopurulent exudate over granulation tissue. The healing period for prolonged lesions differs from aphthous minor because the connective tissue destruction is often more extensive, requiring replacement of large amounts of normal structures with scar tissue before complete healing.

TREATMENT

The management of aphthous major usually requires an emphasis on the combined use of short term systemic and topical steroids. Antimicrobial rinses may be required as an adjunct to reduce or prevent secondary infection. Use of topical anesthetic is sometimes necessary to allow adequate nutritional intake. If lesions are in the posterior aspect of the mouth, topical anesthetics must be judiciously administered because extension of the anesthetic effect to the epiglottis could result in serious consequences to the patient while eating.

HERPETIFORM ULCERS

> ■ HERPETIFORM ULCERS: rare, multiple, small, painful, superficial ulcers with episodes of long duration that occur on gland-bearing and keratinizing mucosas.

Herpetiform ulcers are the least common form of RAS and the form most often misdiagnosed. They are frequently mistaken for primary herpes simplex infections, which they closely resemble clinically, hence their name.

CLINICAL

Patients with herpetiform ulcers have prolonged episodes of widely distributed intraoral lesions of small (3 to 6 mm in diameter), shallow, and crateriform ulcers (Figure 8-4). An episode may last for weeks to months, and some patients may experience lesions nearly continously for several years. During prolonged attacks individual lesions heal while new ones continually reappear. They are seldom found in patients who are in their late teens, as is common with aphthous minor, or in childhood, as is common with primary herpetic stomatitis, the condition that the ulcers clinically resemble. Although most lesions are found almost exclusively on the gland-bearing mucosa, these lesions may also occur on some keratinizing surfaces. Since the presence of lesions on the keratinizing mucosal surfaces is common in primary herpes infection, herpetiform ulcers are often misdiagnosed as a herpes infection. Pain that is more excessive than is warranted by the size of the lesions is a prominent feature of this condition.

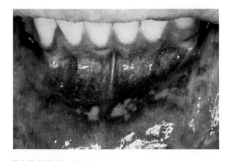

FIGURE 8-4

Herpetiform (aphthous) ulcers. Clusters of small shallow aphthous ulcers of the labial mucosa resembling lesions of a herpes simplex infection.

Due to the ease of confusing herpetiform aphthous lesions with primary herpetic stomatitis, laboratory tests are often necessary to rule out a viral etiology. Cytology smears do not show the cytopathic effects of a viral infection, and the multinucleated epithelial cells found in viral infections are not present. Viral cultures, immunofluorescence for the herpes antigen, and ultrastructural examination for the presence of the virus are negative.

HISTOPATHOLOGY

The microscopic features of individual lesions are identical to lesions of aphthous minor. Lesions tend to be shallow with little connective tissue destruction; thus scarring does not occur.

TREATMENT

The use of systemic steroids is often the only effective method of managing herpetiform ulcers. It may require the prolonged use of low-dose steroid treatment to prevent rapid recurrence of lesions during a prolonged attack. Because of the large number of widely dispersed lesions, treatment with topical steroids or chemical cauterizations is often not practical or effective. Some patients have obtained temporary relief with oral rinses of tetracyclines. In other patients, this form of management is of little value.

BEHÇET SYNDROME

> ■ BEHÇET SYNDROME: a systemic condition of uncertain origin consisting of multiple oral, anogenital, and ocular aphthouslike lesions; frequently has central nervous system (CNS) involvement and arthralgia.

Behçet syndrome is an uncommon condition that is systemic in nature but has multiple superficial painful ulcers of the oral mucosa identical to recurrent aphthous minor ulcers as one of its consistent symptoms. At present, the etiology of Behçet syndrome is unknown. It has been shown that many patients with Behçet syndrome have circulating antibodies specific for a herpes virus; however, evidence is insufficient to draw a conclusion of a viral etiology.

CLINICAL

A prominent and consistent feature of Behçet syndrome is the presence of intraoral ulcers identical to aphthous minor ulcers with similar lesions present in the anogenital area. Patients consistently have ocular lesions of varying degrees of severity, ranging from photophobia to uveitis. The presence of oral, anogenital, and ocular aphthouslike lesions is usually sufficient to make the diagnosis of Behçet syndrome. Other common features of the syndrome include arthralagia, thrombophlebitis, CNS involvement, and macular and pustular skin lesions.

HISTOPATHOLOGY

The tissue changes of ulcerative lesions are similar to that of aphthous minor except that the vascular component is more prominent. Blood vessel walls exhibit infiltrates of inflammatory cells, resulting in a severe vasculitis that appears to destroy the vessel walls.

TREATMENT

Although the condition may undergo spontaneous remission for prolonged periods, in most patients the use of systemic steroids is necessary to achieve relief of symptoms and to prevent serious ocular damage during an episode.

MUCOSAL AND SKIN CONDITIONS

LICHEN PLANUS

> ■ L I C H E N P L A N U S : a skin disease common within the oral cavity, where it appears as either white reticular, plaque, or erosive lesions with a prominent T lymphocyte response in the immediate underlying connective tissue.

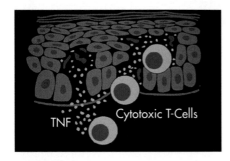

FIGURE 8-5

Lichen planus. Diagram of the cytotoxic T lymphocytes stimulated by intraepithelial Langerhans cells emitting tumor necrosis factor (TNF) that contributes to the degeneration of the epithelium.

Lichen planus (LP) is a common skin disease that affects approximately 1% of the population. Lesions occur on cutaneous and oral surfaces (40%); on cutaneous alone (35%), and on mucosal only (25%).

At present, the etiologic agent initiating LP is unknown. Research exploring the pathogenesis of LP has become focused on the role of the epithelial antigenic processing macrophage, the Langerhans cell, and its interaction with the abundant T lymphocytes that accumulate in the immediate underlying connective tissue. Some investigators believe that the Langerhans cell recognizes an antigen that is similar to antigens on the keratinocytes of patients with certain classes of major histocompatibility antigens. Thus during the processing of antigens and stimulation of T lymphocytes by the Langerhans cell, lymphocytes cytotoxic to epithelial cells are produced (Figure 8-5). The identity of the initial stimulating antigen is still unknown.

There have been reports in the literature that LP may be responsible for the subsequent development of squamous cell carcinoma. Although the documentation of many of the reported cases is not always complete, malignancy is estimated to occur in 0.4% to 2% of LP patients when lesions persist for 5 or more years. Because many dysplasias have a dense infiltrate of lymphocytes in the same location as is found in LP, it is possible that some cases thought to be LP preceding a malignancy on a histologic basis were really cases of epithelial dysplasia. At present, cases of epithelial dysplasia with an LP-like infiltrate of lymphocytes have been designated as *lichenoid dysplasia*. Another consideration when evaluating cases of transformed LP is that reports indicate many lesions are located on the lateral borders of the tongue, areas that are highly susceptible to the development of carcinoma regardless of prior disease processes. Some researchers believe that mucosa that is subjected to prolonged LP becomes more susceptible to a secondary initiating carcinogen than adjacent areas. Regardless, there are still well-documented cases of malignant lesions arising in locations uncommon for carcinoma and where there has been long-term presence of LP.

CLINICAL

LP has a wide range of clinical appearances that correlate closely with the severity of the disease process. There are three distinct clinical presentations: **reticular, erosive,** and **plaque.** It is common for patients to have a combination of the reticular and erosive forms. Plaque LP usually occurs alone and resembles most other forms of leukoplakia. Oral LP occurs in men and women between the ages of 30 and 70, and children and adolescents are rarely affected.

Reticular LP of the mucous membranes is easily diagnosed due to its unique and distinctive pattern. It consists of raised, thin, white lines that connect in arcuate patterns, producing a lacework or reticular appearance against an erythematous background (Figure 8-6). The white lines are referred to as *striae of Wickham*. Patients with reticular LP seldom have symptoms and are usually unaware of their condition unless it is noticed by their dentist or dental hygienist. A lesion may become sensitive if an area becomes atrophic or erosive due to an intensification of the condition. Reticular LP most commonly occurs on the buccal mucosa and the buccal vestibule, and the tongue and gingiva are the next

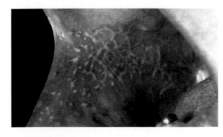

FIGURE 8-6

Lichen planus. Clinical appearance of the lacework pattern of the reticular form of the disease.

most common locations. It is unusual for lesions to occur only on the hard or soft palates without involving most of the other oral mucosal surfaces. A feature of reticular LP is that it is usually bilateral.

Erosive LP appears as a mixture of erythematous and white pseudomembranous areas (Figure 8-7). Frequently, the junction between the erosive areas and the normal mucosa exhibits a faint whitish tinge that resembles radiating striae. The whitish peripheral zone is most often present on the buccal mucosa and vestibule areas. Patients with this form of LP complain of a sore mouth that is sensitive to cold and hot, spicy foods, and alcoholic beverages. When erosive LP is severe, most patients seek a bland liquid diet. During examination, touching the areas produces pain and bleeding. In most cases it is not possible to make the correct diagnosis without a biopsy of the perilesional tissue. The clinical appearance of the erosive LP is difficult to differentiate from candidiasis, mucous membrane pemphigoid, pemphigus vulgaris, and discoid lupus erythematosus. After prolonged involvement with erosive LP, areas of hyperpigmentation (melanosis) will occasionally occur on the mucosa in the healed areas.

Plaque LP appears as a white raised or flattened area on the oral mucous membranes and is indistinguishable from other focal leukoplakias (Figure 8-8). The most common location is on the tongue, where it produces irregular white smooth areas and raised plaques. Often more than one area is involved, particularly on the dorsal surface of the tongue.

Other clinical forms of LP have been occasionally described that appear to be either a variant of plaque LP or are transient in nature. One of these is **atrophic LP.** The clinical appearance of atrophic LP is identical to the erythematous background of the reticular form and may be part of the transitional stage from reticular to erosive LP. Atrophic LP is most common on the gingiva and buccal mucosa. A rare form of LP consisting of large bullae ranging in size from 4 mm to 2 cm is **bullous LP.** The bullae are of brief duration and rupture almost immediately; with the loss of the separated epithelium, the underlying connective tissue is exposed and the lesion becomes an erosive LP. Reports indicate that bullous lesions occur primarily on the posterior buccal mucosa.

Patients with a depletion of immunocompetent cells and who require infusion of competent cells in the form of bone marrow transplants or transfusions often develop a condition referred to as **graft-versus-host disease (GVHD).** This condition develops when the acquired immunocompetent T lymphocytes attack the host cells of patients who are not sufficiently histocompatible. This is the opposite of what occurs when a healthy patient receives an incompatible graft and his immune system attempts to reject the graft. Part of the host cell response to GVHD is a skin and mucous membrane reaction that is histologically identical to LP. The oral changes may be the first indication that a serious problem exists that can be fatal if not treated. Death frequently follows if the immunodeficient patient has received a large transfusion of improperly prepared blood in which the lymphocytes have not been removed.

LP of the skin assumes a very different appearance than lesions of the mucous membranes. **Cutaneous lichen planus** is purported to occur in 35% to 44% of patients who seek medical attention for oral lesions. On the skin lesions appear as clusters or diffuse areas of raised purplish papules with a white keratotic "cap." Since lesions are usually itchy, patients commonly produce linear excoriations that result in the development of a linear pattern of additional lesions along the scratch marks (Figure 8-9). The development of skin lesions extending along areas of injury or irritation is referred to as the **Koebner phenomenon.** This characteristic feature of LP may explain the increased size and intensity of oral lesions in areas prone to chronic irritation from teeth and toothbrushing. These areas are commonly the buccal mucosa along the occlusal line and commissure, the lateral borders of the tongue, and the marginal gingiva.

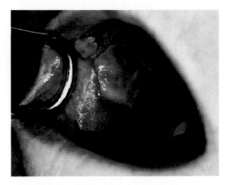

FIGURE 8-7

Lichen planus. Clinical appearance of the symptomatic erosive form of the disease on the buccal mucosa, exhibiting a large area of erosion against an erythematous background.

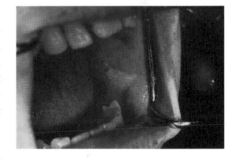

FIGURE 8-8

Lichen planus. Plaque form of lichen planus on the buccal mucosa.

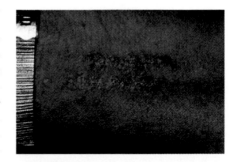

FIGURE 8-9

Lichen planus. Papular skin lesions distributed in a linear pattern on the flexor surface of the wrist.

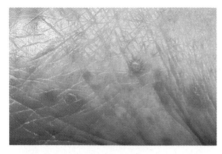

FIGURE 8-10

Lichen planus. Papular lesions on the skin of the sole of the foot.

Cutaneous lesions can occur on almost any part of the body (Figure 8-10) including the scalp and nail beds but are most prevalent on the upper trunk, the flexor surfaces of the arms and legs, and the genitalia.

DIAGNOSIS

LP is often diagnosed based on clinical information only, especially when reticular LP is present with its characteristic striae of Wickham in a lacework or annular pattern against an erythematous background. The erosive and plaque variants of LP always require laboratory evaluation because they can clinically resemble a number of other mucosal lesions including malignancy. Incisional biopsy is required for histologic and direct immunofluorescent examinations.

HISTOPATHOLOGY

The histologic features vary with the clinical types of LP. Reticular LP consists of focal areas of epithelial hyperplasia in which the surface contains a thick layer of orthokeratin or parakeratin. The spinous cell layer may be thickened (acanthosis) with shortened and pointed ("sawtooth") rete pegs. The thickened areas are seen clinically as striae of Wickham. Between these areas the epithelium is thinned (atrophic) with loss of rete peg formation. The adjacent underlying connective tissue contains a narrow dense accumulation of T lymphocytes that transgresses the basement membrane and is observed in the basilar and parabasilar cell layers of the epithelium (Figure 8-11, *A*). Within the epithelium, rounded or ovoid amorphous eosinophilic bodies referred to as *Civatte bodies* are sometimes present. They are thought to represent apoptotic (dead) keratinocytes or other necrotic epithelial components that are transported to the connective tissue for phagocytosis. Immunofluorescent examination demonstrates a deposit of fibrinogen along the basement membrane with vertical extensions into the immediate underlying connective tissue. Immunohistochemistry using the antibody to the S-100 protein indicates an increase in the Langer-

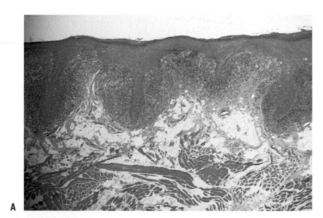

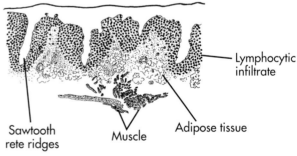

Lymphocytic infiltrate

Sawtooth rete ridges

Muscle

Adipose tissue

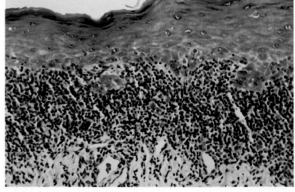

FIGURE 8-11

Lichen planus. Microscopic features demonstrating the characteristic narrow dense band of T lymphocytes in the immediately adjacent connective tissue of reticular LP **(A)** and atrophic/erosive LP **(B)**.

hans cells in the midlayers of the epithelium. Occasionally, lymphoid follicles will be found deeper in the connective tissue in patients with long-term disease.

Erosive LP exhibits an extensively thinned epithelium in which there are areas of complete loss of rete peg formation and a dense infiltrate of T lymphocytes obscuring the basement membrane and extending well into the middle and upper levels of the epithelium. Liquefaction of the basement membrane and vacuolization and destruction of the basal cells is present in most areas (Figure 8-11, *B*). Occasionally, subepithelial separation will be present. Often, the epithelium is lost, exposing the underlying connective tissue. The lymphocytes are confined to a narrow zone in the upper layers of the connective tissue.

Plaque LP resembles the histology of the striae of reticular LP but without the intermittent atrophic areas of the epithelium. It consists of generalized hyperorthokeratosis or hyperparakeratosis combined with acanthosis. There may be loss of rete pegs at the epithelial-connective tissue interface or alteration of their shape into a "sawtooth" pattern. The basement membrane is noticeably thickened. The band of T lymphocytes present in the superficial connective tissue is less dense than in reticular LP, with only occasional cells found in the lower levels of the epithelium.

The tissue diagnosis of LP can often be difficult but may be greatly aided by the use of immunofluorescence (Figure 8-12). All forms of LP will be negative for IgG, IgM, and IgA antibodies but positive for fibrinogen (Figure 8-13).

TREATMENT

After diagnosis most clinicians do not think it is necessary to treat small areas of the reticular or plaque type of LP unless they become symptomatic, persistent, or widespread. Erosive LP is commonly treated and responds well to topical steroids such as fluocinonide. In more resistant cases systemically administered methylprednisolone is effective when used either alone or in combination with topical steroids. Intralesional injections of corticosteroids have been used with degrees of success but are not well accepted by patients, particularly if there are multiple lesions. The application of retinoic acid derivatives has been tried but is clinically unproven and has undesirable side effects.

LICHENOID DRUG REACTIONS

■ LICHENOID DRUG REACTIONS: the presence of lesions resembling erosive lichen planus mainly on the buccal mucosa; associated with the ingestion of some categories of medications.

The prevalence of oral lichenoid drug reactions is increasing due to the recognition that the entity has an etiology that is distinct from the traditional forms of LP. The increased occurrence may be due to the introduction of new categories of medications that have a greater tendency for lichenoid reactions as a side effect in individuals who are prone to this condition. The antibiotics, antihypertensives, gold compounds, diuretics, antimalarials, and nonsteroidal antiinflammatory medications are noteworthy (Box 8-1).

■ BOX 8-1
Major Categories of Medications Associated With Lichenoid Drug Reactions

Antibiotics	Diuretics
Antihypertensives	Gold compounds
Antimalarials	Nonsteroidal antiinflammatories

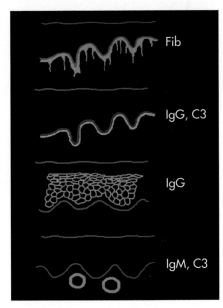

FIGURE 8-12

Lichen planus. Diagram of immunofluorescent patterns and antibodies of the common autoimmune conditions found within the oral cavity. From top to bottom: lichen planus, *fibrinogen* in a shaggy pattern at the basement membrane; mucous membrane pemphigoid, *IgG* and *C3* in a smooth pattern at the basement membrane; pemphigus vulgaris, *IgG* in a "fishnet" pattern outlining cells of the epithelium; erythema multiforme, *IgM* and *C3* in a perivascular pattern within the deeper connective tissue.

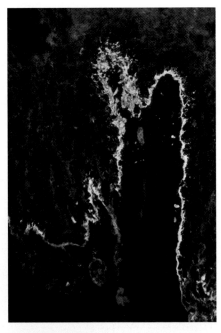

FIGURE 8-13

Lichen planus. Photomicrograph of immunofluorescent pattern of linear deposit of fibrinogen at the basement membrane.

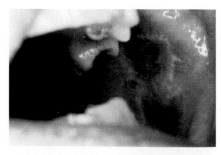

FIGURE 8-14

Lichenoid drug reaction. Clinical lesion on the buccal mucosa with central erythematous area and surrounding radiating white striae.

CLINICAL

Within the oral cavity, lesions are primarily located on the posterior buccal mucosa. Lesions are usually painful and exhibit a central erythematous area of erosion with a surrounding zone of radiating striae that gradually fade ("sunburst" appearance) (Figure 8-14).

HISTOPATHOLOGY

Histologically the tissue exhibits changes that are identical to erosive LP. The diagnosis of lichenoid drug reaction is usually made when the tissue report indicates that the lesion is consistent with LP and disappears after the offending medication is withdrawn.

TREATMENT

Treatment with the usual topical steroids must be combined with cessation or reduction in the dose of the offending medication to provide more than temporary relief.

MUCOUS MEMBRANE PEMPHIGOID

> ■ MUCOUS MEMBRANE PEMPHIGOID: a desquamating condition of mucous membranes in which the autoimmune reaction occurs at the level of the basement membrane and commonly affects the gingiva before extending to other mucosal locations.

The term **mucous membrane pemphigoid (MMP)** is often used synonymously with **cicatricial pemphigoid (CP),** particularly among dermatologists. The patients seen by dermatologists occasionally have involvement of the eye mucous membranes that results in scar formation (cicatrix) and nasal mucosal lesions in addition to those found within the oral cavity. On rare occasions patients with CP may also have one or more associated lesions on the skin, usually in the head and neck areas. In all locations there is atrophy of the epithelium followed by separation from the connective tissue at the level of the basement membrane, leaving painful, irregular erosive areas. When this basic disease process occurs *exclusively* on the oral mucous membranes, it is now thought to be a slightly different than when other tissues are involved, hence the name mucous membrane pemphigoid. When it is restricted to the gingiva only, it is the most common disease entity of a diagnostic grouping of clinical lesions collectively referred to as *desquamative gingivitis.* A disease with a similar pathogenesis that primarily involves the skin and produces large, fluid-filled blisters is referred to as **bullous pemphigoid** (BP). In 10% to 20% of the cases of BP, oral lesions can also be found.

The pathogeneses of MMP, CP, and BP are similar, which is revealed by immunologic and biochemical studies. The principal target of the autoantibodies is the BP-1 antigen, a 230 kD protein that is located in the hemidesmosome apparatus located at the base of the basal cell adjacent to the basement membrane (Figure 8-15). The autoantibody that combines with the BP-1 antigen is an IgG class antibody, which precipitates a complement (C3) reaction that produces the disease process leading to the breakdown of the adhesive factors that anchor the epithelium to the basement membrane and the connective tissue. Immunofluorescence stains reveal the autoantibody-antigen reaction and C3 to be present in a linear deposit along the basement membrane. This is sufficiently specific to be used routinely for diagnostic purposes to differentiate MMP, CP, and BP from pemphigus vulgaris and erosive LP, the other two oral lesions with similar clinical features.

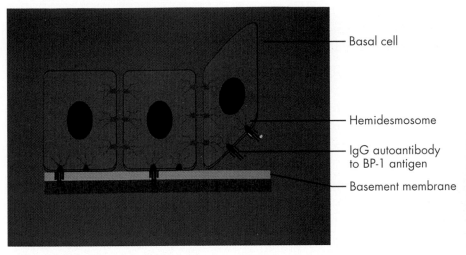

FIGURE 8-15

Mucous membrane pemphigoid. Diagram of the separation of the epithelium from the connective tissue at the level of the basement membrane as a result of IgG type autoantibody combining BP-1 antigen of the hemidesmosome.

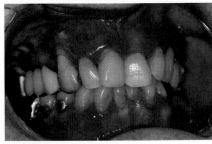

FIGURE 8-16

Mucous membrane pemphigoid. Gingiva containing patchy areas of erythema and atrophy with loss of normal stippling.

CLINICAL

Within the oral cavity, lesions first appear on the attached and free gingiva as irregular patches of erythema with associated loss of visible stippling (Figure 8-16). If they are not diagnosed and treated, they may remain confined to the gingiva for long periods before extending to adjacent tissue. While lesions are on the gingiva, minor irritation such as routine brushing results in the separation of the epithelium from the connective tissue and a blood-filled blister or exposed connective tissue (desquamation) (Figure 8-17). Under a denture the tissue will appear as a generalized area of erythema and erosion (Figure 8-18). A clinical test that can be performed in this case consists of rubbing or pushing on the tissue with a blunt instrument or gauze to determine if a blister forms in the next 1 to 2 minutes. The production of a blister or bulla indicates a positive **Nikolsky sign.** A positive Nikolsky sign is not specific for MMP because it may be present in other conditions that have defects in cell cohesion or basement membrane attachment. Often, patients will exhibit linear erosions along the free margins of the gingiva. These are the result of toothbrushing and flossing on the affected tissue.

If untreated, lesions will progressively involve the buccal mucosa, palate, and floor of the mouth. Extension into the nasopharynx, larynx, and esophagus has been observed. Genital lesions are present in 25% of the cases. Far more common and of greater concern is involvement of the eye conjunctiva. In this location bullae, erosions, and generalized erythema can occur that result in scarring and the formation of adhesive tissue bands extending from the lid to the sclera, referred to as *symblepharon.* Untreated eye lesions can lead to serious loss of visual acuity.

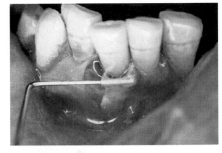

FIGURE 8-17

Mucous membrane pemphigoid. Gingiva exhibits loss of adhesion of epithelium to connective tissue.

DIAGNOSIS

Evaluation of tissue specimens with light microscopy and direct immunofluorescence is necessary to distinguish the various diseases with a positive Nikolsky sign. Of importance is the localization of the histologic site of tissue separation and the identification of the specific immunoglobulin profile at the site of the

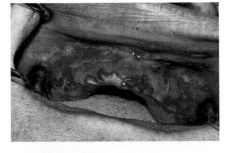

FIGURE 8-18

Mucous membrane pemphigoid. Multiple diffuse areas of superficial erosions *(white)* against an erythematous background due to mechanical forces of a denture on the fragile atrophic epithelium.

TABLE 8-1
Tissue Diagnosis of Erosive Diseases of the Mucosa

Disease	Location of defect	Target antigen	Immunofluorescence
Erosive lichen planus	Basement membrane	Unknown	Fibrinogen
Mucous membrane pemphigoid	Hemidesmosome	BP-1	IgG, C3; linear pattern
Pemphigus vulgaris	Desmosomes	Desmoglein II	IgG; fishnet pattern
Erythema multiforme	Basement membrane	Immune complexes	IgM, C3; perivascular pattern

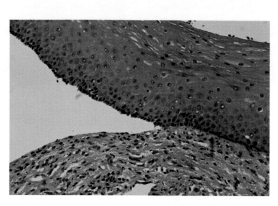 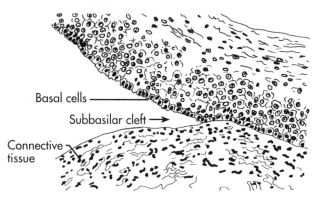

Basal cells

Subbasilar cleft →

Connective tissue

FIGURE 8-19

Mucous membrane pemphigoid. Photomicrograph of mucosa demonstrating lack of rete pegs and loss of adhesion of the epithelium with cleavage at the level of basement membrane.

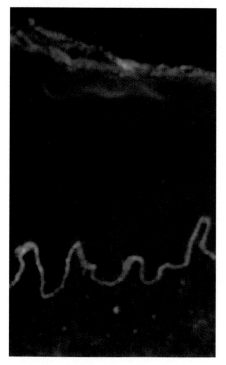

FIGURE 8-20

Mucous membrane pemphigoid. Immunofluorescence reveals a solid yellow-green line, indicating the presence of IgG antibody complexed to the antigen at the basement membrane.

antigen-antibody reaction (Table 8-1). In MMP the splitting occurs at the level of the basement membrane because the targeted antigen is located in the lamina lucida zone of the basment membrane.

HISTOPATHOLOGY
The microscopic findings consist of a thinned epithelium that exhibits some attenuation of the rete pegs. A separation occurs at the basement membrane and leaves a connective tissue that is diffusely infiltrated with lymphocytes with some plasma cells and occasional eosinophils (Figure 8-19). Vasodilatation is prominent in the underlying connective tissue. Immunofluorescence stains reveal a deposit of the IgG antibody and C3 that follows the basement membrane in a linear pattern (Figure 8-20).

TREATMENT
Patients are managed with a combination of systemic and topical steroids. Treatment of early lesions, particularly when confined to a few areas of the gingiva, will prevent progression of the disease and the necessity to treat serious eye afflictions with prolonged steroid therapy.

PEMPHIGUS VULGARIS

> ■ PEMPHIGUS VULGARIS: a desquamating condition of the oral mucosa and skin in which autoantibodies react and destroy antigenic components of the desmosomes of the intermediate cells, producing epithelial separation above the basal cell layer.

Pemphigus vulgaris (PV) and its less common variants are part of a group of dermatologic diseases in which there is epithelial desquamation due to autoantibod-

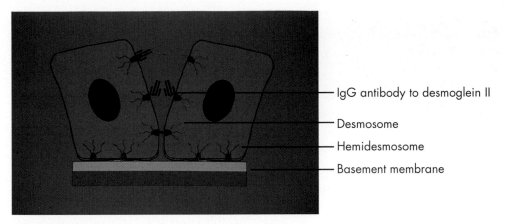

IgG antibody to desmoglein II

Desmosome

Hemidesmosome

Basement membrane

FIGURE 8-21

Pemphigus vulgaris. Diagram of destruction of intraepithelial adhesion resulting from binding of the IgG antibody to the desmoglein II protein of the desmosome.

ies that attack the desmosome of the *intercellular* cohesive system. The loss of adhesion occurs between the cells located in the zone above the basal cell layer and results in **suprabasilar bullous formation.** Other members of this disease group *(pemphigus vegetans, pemphigus foliaceus,* and *pemphigus erythematosus)* represent milder forms and do not involve the oral cavity as extensively as PV. If untreated, PV can be a serious life-threatening disease with a mortality rate of over 70%. With aggressive treatment patient death rate is greatly reduced.

Destruction of the adhesive factors of the suprabasilar spinous cells is referred to as **acantholysis.** Although this process is still not completely understood, some progress has been made. It is established that intercellular adhesion of oral keratinocytes is accomplished by desmosomes and extracellular proteins. Within the desmosomes there is a group of intracellular proteins referred to as **desmoplakin,** whereas the extracellular proteins that surround the cell, providing the intercellular "glue," are collectively called **cadherins.** In PV the target antigen is thought to be one of the cadherins, desmoglein II—the 130 kD protein (Figure 8-21); in the variant pemphigus foliaceus, the target antigen is desmoglein I—the 165 kD cadherin protein.

Autoantibodies to the desmoglein I protein of PV can be detected circulating in the patient's serum and have been found to fluctuate with the intensity of the disease process. Experimentally, these same antibodies have been isolated and transferred to animals where they were found to attack normal skin, producing lesions similar to PV in humans. The initial causative factors leading to the production of these autoantibodies in selected individuals is still unknown. The fact that certain ethnic groups are more prone to develop PV has lead to the theory that a genetic predisposition exists. The development of PV is thought to predispose patients having specific major histocompatibility antigens on their skin and mucosal keratinocytes.

CLINICAL

PV is most prevalent in patients in the 40- to 60-year-old age group. It has a higher incidence in individuals of Mediterranean and Ashkenazic Jewish decent and those with specific histocompatibility antigens. Drugs such as penicillamine and the presence of a preexisting malignancy *(paraneoplastic PV)* appear to cause lesions in patients that are identical to those of the common form of PV.

PV mainly affects the skin of the torso. In nearly 50% of the patients with cutaneous PV, the oral lesions precede the presence of skin lesions, often by as

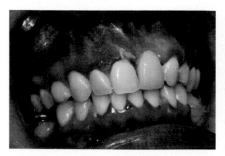

FIGURE 8-22

Pemphigus vulgaris. Gingiva demonstrating erosive lesion of the free margin of gingiva in an area commonly irritated during toothbrushing.

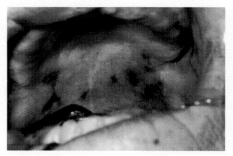

FIGURE 8-23

Pemphigus vulgaris. Multiple erosive lesions of the soft palate.

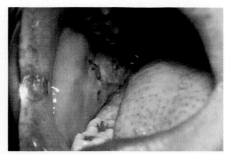

FIGURE 8-24

Pemphigus vulgaris. Erosive lesions of the posterior buccal mucosa.

much as a year. Other mucous membranes such as the nasopharynx, esophagus, vagina, and cervix can also be involved. Bullae are commonly present on skin but are rare on the oral mucosa. Intraoral lesions are common on the soft palate where they have a brief, usually undetected bullous stage. In this and most other intraoral locations the delicate surface layers are quickly lost, leaving the commonly observed erythematous area that is sensitive to hot, cold, spicy foods, and alcoholic liquids. The free margin of the gingiva (Figure 8-22), where chronic abrasion during toothbrushing is common, and the lateral borders of the tongue, where constant frictional activity occurs, will have larger and more intensely symptomatic erosive lesions. Lesions are commonly found on the other mucosal surfaces of the mouth, particularly the soft palate (Figure 8-23) and buccal mucosa (Figure 8-24). Both skin and mucosal tissue will have a positive Nikolsky sign (Figure 8-25). On the skin the individual lesions are produced by briefly appearing blisters that collapse with the formation of a brittle reddish crust (scab) (Figure 8-26).

HISTOPATHOLOGY

The microscopic appearance of PV exhibits epithelium of normal thickness and normal rete peg formation. Mild inflammation is found in the underlying connective tissue. The basal cell layer is intact, but the cells of the suprabasilar layer are separated (acantholysis) and float freely in a fluid-filled intraepithelial space (Figure 8-27). The cells lose their polygonal shape and become rounded with less cytoplasm visible around the nucleus. This gives the cells a malignant appearance when viewed on a cytology slide. These cells have been given the name

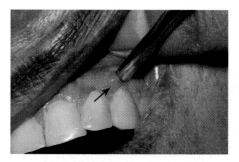

FIGURE 8-25

Pemphigus vulgaris. Blister formation (*arrow*) on normal-appearing gingiva after the movement of mirror handle under pressure indicative of positive Nikolsky sign.

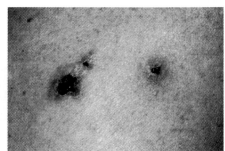

FIGURE 8-26

Pemphigus vulgaris. Dry, crusted lesions on the skin.

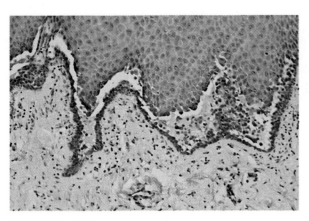

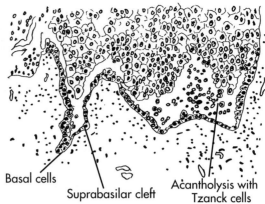

Basal cells
Suprabasilar cleft
Acantholysis with
Tzanck cells

FIGURE 8-27

Pemphigus vulgaris. Photomicrograph of epithelium exhibiting rete pegs and a zone of acantholysis above the basal cell layer. Spinous cells (Tzanck cells) are present floating freely in the fluid-filled intraepithelial space.

of **Tzanck cells** and are a characteristic finding in the fluid in the area of epithelial separation in PV.

Immunofluorescence is a most valuable aid in the diagnosis of this condition. In the early stages of the disease before the development of superbasalar separation and the presence of Tzanck cells, it may be the only means of diagnosis. It is also most helpful in detecting the disease on tissue biopsied from a perilesional location. The test reveals the presence of the IgG antibody in a "fishnet" pattern due to its attachment to the periphery of the cells in the spinous layers of the epithelium (Figure 8-28).

TREATMENT

Treatment of PV is aggressive and requires a prolonged high dosage of prednisolone in the range of 150 to 360 mg daily for 6 to 10 weeks. Since the side effects of prolonged high doses of steroids can be severe, doses are often reduced after an initial period and are used in combination with other nonsteroid immunosuppressant drugs such as azathioprine. In most cases the condition eventually goes into remission and doses are greatly reduced or even withdrawn for a time. With modern combinations of medications, mortality rates have been drastically reduced; 10% of the patients surcome to the complications of prolonged steroid therapy and the associated secondary infection and even fewer to PV itself.

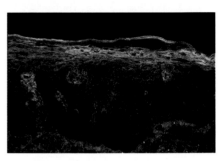

FIGURE 8-28

Pemphigus vulgaris. Immunofluorescent pattern of the IgG antibody adherence to the desmosomal protein (desmoglein) located on the periphery of epithelial intermediate cells, producing a "fishnet" pattern of binding sites.

EPIDERMOLYSIS BULLOSA

■ EPIDERMOLYSIS BULLOSA: a generalized desquamating condition of the skin and mucosa with associated scarring, contractures, and dental defects that occur in three main hereditary forms in children and one acquired form in adults.

Epidermolysis bullosa (EB) is an encompassing term for a large group of clinically similar disease processes that have in common the separation of the epithelium from the underlying connective tissue and the formation of large blisters that frequently result in extensive and often immobilizing scar formation. There are four basic types, each with multiple subtypes; three of the types have hereditary patterns, and one is acquired in later life. The acquired form is the only one

TABLE 8-2
Major Categories of Epidermolysis Bullosa

Type	Genetic pattern	Level of separation	Defective structure
HEREDITARY			
Simplex	Autosomal dominant	Intraepithelial	Linking proteins
Junctional	Autosomal recessive	Lamina lucida	Anchoring filaments
Dystrophic	Autosomal dominant/recessive	Sublamina densa	Type VII collagen
ACQUIRED			
Acquisita	None	Sublamina densa	Type VII collagen

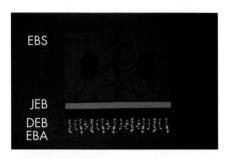

FIGURE 8-29

Epidermolysis bullosa. Diagram of the various target sites where destruction of the components of epithelial adhesion occurs in the three major hereditary forms of epidermolysis bullosa: simplex *(EBS);* junctional *(JEB);* dystrophic *(DEB);* and the acquired form, acquisita *(EBA).*

thought to be solely of autoimmune origin. This simplified classification is based on a mixture of clinical and morphologic criteria.

The three major hereditary types of EB are (1) **epidermolysis bullosa simplex (EBS),** in which there is intraepithelial cleavage due to cytolysis of the basal or intermediate cell layer (*epidermolytic type*); (2) **junctional epidermolysis bullosa (JEB),** in which the cleavage is within the basement membrane at the level of the anchoring filaments contained within the lamina lucida (*lamina lucidolytic type*); and (3) **dystrophic epidermolysis bullosa (DEB),** in which the cleavage takes place at the level of the type VII collagen-anchoring fibrils located beneath the lamina densa of the basement membrane where they extend into the dermis (*dermolytic type*). The diagnosis of the hereditary forms is best made with ultrastructural analysis because the break in adhesion is not a result of an antigen-antibody reaction that can be detected with the usual immunofluorescent methods. Rather, the defect in epithelial adhesion is due to congenitally absent or greatly reduced specific molecular factors (Figure 8-29). When electron microscopy is not available, panels of complex immunohistochemical research using monoclonal antibodies against various constituents of the adhesive mechanism (*immunofluorescence mapping*) have been used to detect the absent factors (Table 8-2).

In the acquired type of EB, **epidermolysis bullosa acquisita (EBA),** there are detectable IgG (and sometimes IgA) autoantibodies to type VII collagen. In skin and mucosa, anchoring fibrils composed of type VII collagen are important constituents of the complex adherence system of epithelium to dermis. They attach the lamina densa portion of the basement membrane to the underlying dermis. The attachment of autoantibodies to type VII collagen triggers a complement-mediated inflammatory reaction that can result in severe damage to the anchoring fibrils.

CLINICAL

Epidermolysis bullosa simplex is a mild form of EB with an autosomal dominant hereditary pattern. Lesions occur over sites of friction or trauma and usually involve the hands, feet, and neck and occasionally the knees and elbows. Teeth are not affected, but mild intraoral blisters are found. EBS appears during infancy, improving significantly by puberty.

Junctional epidermolysis bullosa is a severe form of EB inherited as an autosomal recessive trait. It has previously been referred to as *EB letalis* because some infants died within the first few months of life. Hemorrhagic blisters and loss of nails; large blisters of the face, trunk, and extremities; and generalized scarring and atrophy are common. Intraorally, large, fragile, hemorrhagic blisters of the palate and crusted granular hemorrhagic lesions are present in perioral and perinasal locations. Erupted teeth exhibit hypoplastic and severely pitted enamel that rapidly develops caries.

Dystrophic epidermolysis bullosa occurs in both an autosomal dominant and a recessive form with the recessive phenotype exhibiting the most severe forms of the disease. Lesions are apparent at birth and arise at sites of pressure such as the occiput, back, elbows, buttocks, and fingers. The bullae rupture, leaving painful ulcers that heal with large and deep scars that undergo contracture leading to loss of mobility and clawlike hands (Figure 8-30). Fingernails and toenails are seldom present in adolescents and adults. There may be marked skin depigmentation and deficient hair. The teeth exhibit delayed eruption and enamel hypoplasia with rapid caries development. Blistering and scarring around the oral cavity result in a diminished opening, ankyloglossia, and loss of vestibular sulci with resultant difficulty in providing dental treatment. Attempts at maintaining normal oral hygiene generate more blister formation.

Epidermolysis bullosa acquisita is a nonhereditary form of EB that is manifested in adulthood. It has been associated with multiple myeloma; diabetes mellitus; amyloidosis; tuberculosis; and inflammatory bowel disease, particularly Crohn disease. The clinical findings closely resemble those of the less severe (autosomal dominant) forms of JEB, which is also a disease of the type VII anchoring fibrils. There are trauma- or friction-induced blisters of the knees, elbows, and the dorsal side of the hands and feet that heal with scars and milia. In some cases loss of nails and alopecia are common. Intraorally, blisters are rare but when present produce scarring and a diminished oral opening, leading to the deterioration of oral hygiene; caries; and periodontal disease.

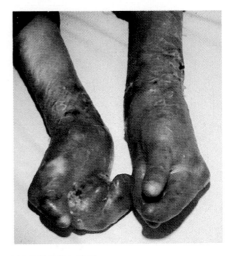

FIGURE 8-30

Epidermolysis bullosa. Clawlike hands due to deep scars and contractures of the soft tissue in a young patient with the recessive dystrophic form of epidermolysis bullosa.

HISTOPATHOLOGY

The tissue of EBS exhibits a zone of cleavage above the basal cell layer. In the remaining types of EB the separation is subepithelial (Figure 8-31).

TREATMENT

Since the hereditary forms of EB are not immune- or inflammatory-mediated conditions but represent adhesive factors to that form, no specific treatment is available. Meticulous wound healing techniques, the prevention of infections, and the systemic use of phenytoin (Dilantin), the anticonvulsant also known to inhibit collagenase activity, have been helpful in ameliorating the morbidity of the disease. Although the acquired form (EBA) has an autoimmune basis, treatment with high doses of corticosteroids and immunosuppressant medications has not been substantially beneficial. Maintenance of the patient's nutritional status is required in cases of restricted oral opening and esophageal strictures.

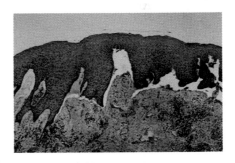

FIGURE 8-31

Epidermolysis bullosa. Photomicrograph of the acquisita form demonstrating the separation of the epithelium from the connective tissue at the level of the basement membrane.

ERYTHEMA MULTIFORME

> ■ ERYTHEMA MULTIFORME: a widespread hypersensitivity reaction that occurs in mild and severe forms that has tissue reactions centered around the superficial vessels of the skin and mucous membranes; usually occurs in patients as the result of an inciting agent.

Erythema multiforme (EM) is an inflammatory disease of immune origin that affects the skin and mucous membranes with a wide spectrum of manifestations and varying degrees of severity. In most patients, an inciting agent can be identified. Common precipitating factors are (1) infections such as herpes simplex, mycoplasma pneumonia, and histoplasmosis; (2) drugs—most commonly sulfas, penicillin, Dilantin, barbiturates, iodines, and salicylates; (3) some gastrointestinal conditions—noteably Crohn disease and ulcerative colitis; and (4) other con-

■ BOX 8-2
Common Precipitating Factors of Erythema Multiforme

Infections
   Herpes simplex
   Mycoplasma pneumonia
   Histoplasmosis

Drugs
   Sulfas
   Penicillin
   Dilantin
   Barbiturates
   Iodines
   Salicylates

Gastrointestinal
   Crohn disease
   Ulcerative colitis

Others
   Malignancies
   Radiation therapy
   Vaccination

FIGURE 8-32

Erythema multiforme. Diagram of perivascular inflammation and associated mixed inflammatory cells due to the immune complex binding to the vessel walls and the liberation of lytic enzymes toxic to epithelial cells.

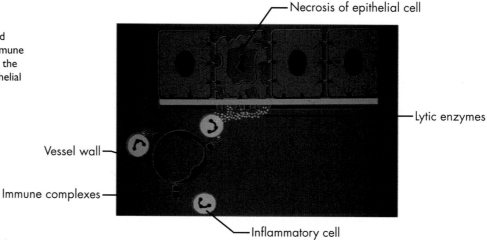

Necrosis of epithelial cell

Lytic enzymes

Vessel wall

Immune complexes

Inflammatory cell

ditions such as malignancy, radiation therapy, and recent vaccination (Box 8-2). There are still many cases in which a precipitating factor cannot be identified.

The pathogenesis of EM is mostly unknown. Research has identified circulating immune-related complexes that appear after patients have encountered some infections, particularly herpes and mycoplasma, and after allergic reactions to medications. The surface epithelium and the walls of blood vessels in the lamina propria appear to be targeted, with the resulting skin and mucosal reactions ranging from a mild erythema to widespread necrosis with sloughing of the epithelial layer (Figure 8-32).

CLINICAL

EM appears in three clinical forms: (1) **EM minor,** (2) **chronic EM minor,** and (3) **EM major.** Another condition, **toxic epidermal necrolysis (TEN),** is considered by some researchers to be a severe form of EM major that is associated with a high mortality rate.

EM minor is a disease that primarily involves the skin; the oral mucosa is involved in 25% of cases. Lesions occur on the skin or mucosa. Before the appearance of lesions there is a 3- to 7-day prodromic period in which patients experience severe headache, fever, and malaise. The prodromic period is followed by an emergence of the classic skin lesion that is variously referred to as a *target,*

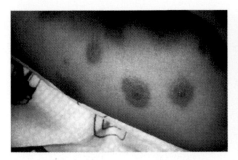

FIGURE 8-33

Erythema multiforme. Skin of a young patient exhibiting characteristic "target" lesions.

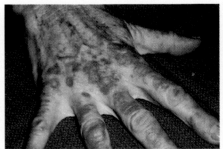

FIGURE 8-34

Erythema multiforme. Skin lesions of the chronic form of EM minor demonstrating long-standing multiple small "target" lesions.

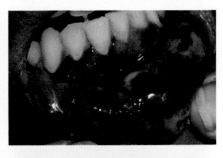

A

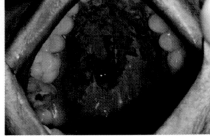

B

FIGURE 8-35

Erythema multiforme. A, Erosive lesions of the labial mucosa and gingiva. **B,** Diffuse area of superficial sloughing and focal erosions of the palate.

bullseye, or *iris* lesion (Figure 8-33). Each of the descriptive terms denotes the common appearance of a concentric erythematous patch with a peripheral thin zone of pallor followed by one or more additional thin erythematous rings. In the early stages the center of the ring develops a raised papule or small bulla that collapses, producing a transient central erosion that quickly heals and returns to normal, which then produces the "center of the bullseye." Individual target lesions range from a few millimeters to many centimeters and are distributed mostly on the flexor surfaces of the extremities; the trunk and facial surfaces are less frequently involved. Although the condition can occur in individuals of any age, young adults are most commonly involved. The condition is self-limiting, usually resolving in 2 to 3 weeks. Treatment sometimes helps to shorten this period. Recurrent episodes of the disease are not uncommon.

Chronic EM minor is the mildest form of EM. Skin lesions are smaller in size and of shorter duration and distribution than in the other forms. In chronic EM minor the patient may have lesions continually for 1 or more years. In these patients the appearance of the lesions is similar to that of a disseminated viral eruption (Figure 8-34). Individual lesions will disappear rather than developing into large "target" lesions.

Oral lesions in both forms of EM minor are similar, varying from focal erosions resembling aphthous ulcers to more diffuse areas of erythema or erosions that are painful to the patient (Figure 8-35). In general, the lesions are very nonspecific and require the presence of associated cutaneous lesions and a compatible history to make the diagnosis. Tissue examination is of little help but may be useful in ruling out other more histologically specific diseases.

EM major is an acute form of the disease with severe involvement of both the skin and mucous membranes. Although the typical target lesions found in other forms of EM will be present, large bullae of both the mucous membranes and skin are characteristic of this severe form of the disease. The bullae quickly collapse, producing whitish pseudomembranes on the mucosa and dark red crusted lesions on the dry skin surfaces. These are particularly noteworthy on the lips (Figure 8-36) and eyes because after sleeping, patients are often unable to open their eyes or part their lips due to the encrustations. The very acute form of the disease is confined to young adults and is referred to as **Stevens-Johnson syndrome.** Mucosal lesions of Stevens-Johnson syndrome are usually extensive and involve the mouth, eyes, esophagus, and genitalia. The oral lesions are very painful, and eye lesions may lead to scarring and partial blindness.

Toxic epidermal necrolysis is considered an extremely severe form of EM major and is often fatal. Large sheets of skin become necrotic and slough, exposing denuded connective tissue that can result in massive loss of electrolytes and

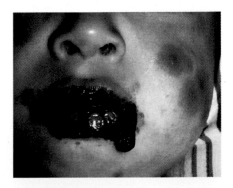

FIGURE 8-36

Erythema multiforme. Acute form of EM major (Stevens-Johnson syndrome) in 2-year-old male exhibiting characteristic target lesions of the skin and hemorrhagic encrustations of the lips.

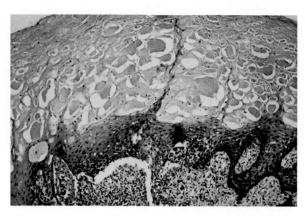

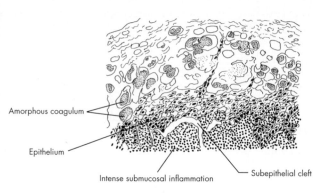

FIGURE 8-37

Erythema multiforme. Photomicrograph of mucosal tissue with extensive intraepithelial pooling of eosinophilic coagulum, separation of the epithelium from connective tissue (bulla formation), and intense chronic inflammatory cell infiltrates. (From Sklar G. Oral lesions of erythema muliforme: histologic and histochemical observations. *Arch Dermatol.* 1965; 92:495.)

widespread infection. The skin areas clinically resemble severe burns caused by scalding water. Oral lesions in these patients are similar to the sloughing lesions found in Stevens-Johnson syndrome but are even more diffuse and widespread.

HISTOPATHOLOGY

The tissue changes of EM are variable, reflecting the wide spectrum of clinical presentations. The tissue changes in the milder forms of the disease are often described as nonspecific, but some consistent features have been described. Intercellular and intracellular edema of the overlying epithelium with focal microvesicle formation is one of the more consistent findings. Sometimes the edema results in a pooling of an eosinophilic amorphous coagulum within the epithelium that has been described as "keratin mucopolysaccharide dystrophy" (Figure 8-37). Migration of both mononuclear and polymorphonuclear cells into all layers of the epithelium is common. In some cases, acanthosis and irregular elongation of rete pegs is present. A generalized diffuse infiltrate of mixed mononuclear cells of the upper portion of the lamina propria is common. Vasodilatation of blood vessels with marked connective tissue edema and a tendency for interstitial transudate pooling often results in large zones of separation at the basement membrane level. Immunofluorescent stains indicate that these zones are negative for antigen-antibody reactions. The perivascular infiltrate of mononuclear cells that is present around blood vessels that are deep in the lamina propria and within muscle layers is somewhat distinctive. The deep perivasculitis is positive with immunofluorescence for IgM and C3 (Figure 8-38). This finding, combined with the other tissue and clinical findings, is of considerable help in diagnosing EM.

TREATMENT

The success of the treatment depends on the clinician's ability to find and neutralize the initiating factor. If episodes follow herpes attacks, prophylactic management of the herpes with acylovir has been effective. In most chronic cases finding and treating the inciting agent is not always possible. The condition is generally self-limiting except in some chronic forms when, if left untreated, it could extend for years. Treatment in mild cases is symptomatic and consists of antihistamines, analgesics and antipyretics combined with oral rinses of antihistamine, or the use of a topical steroid. Systemic steroids are sometimes used, but

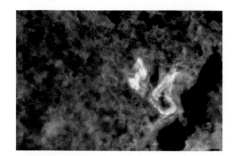

FIGURE 8-38

Erythema multiforme. Immunofluorescent pattern of the IgM antibody in a perivascular pattern deep within the connective tissue. A similar pattern occurs at the same site with C3.

research shows that there is little difference in the length of time in which lesions resolve with steroid administration when compared with other more conservative forms of treatment.

LUPUS ERYTHEMATOSUS

■ LUPUS ERYTHEMATOSUS: a chronic inflammatory condition of the skin, connective tissue, and specific internal organs that has associated circulating autoantibodies to DNA and other nuclear and RNA proteins and circular whitish buccal mucosal lesions and erythematous rashes of the sun-exposed skin.

Lupus erythematosus (LE) occurs in three clinical forms that represent the severity and distribution of involvment. The mildest form, **discoid lupus erythematosus (DLE),** is chronic and confined to the sun-exposed skin of the face, scalp, and ears but also involves the oral mucosa. The intermediate form, **subacute cutaneous lupus erythematosus (SCLE),** is more widespread and affects the head and neck, the upper trunk, and the extensor surfaces of the arms. The severest form, **systemic lupus erythematosus (SLE),** primarily involves the organs, especially the kidneys. Rashes occur periodically on the upper trunk and face.

The pathogenesis of LE is still not fully understood. There is ample evidence that the immune system becomes altered and is responsible for the deleterious changes that take place within the basal cells, collagen, and vascular tissue. Autoantibodies to DNA and other nuclear and ribonuclear protein antigens are present in the blood; there is an increase in B-cell function and a decrease in the number of suppressor T-cells; and circulating autoantibodies that exhibit cross-reactivity with antigenic determinants on multiple tissues are found. Recently it has become apparent that individuals may have a genetic predisposition to the development of some forms of the disease. Although there is some speculation that the disease is initiated by a viral agent, no scientific evidence has yet been found for this theory. The apparent role of UV light on the development of lesions on exposed cutaneous surfaces is still unknown.

Systemic Lupus Erythematosus
SLE is the most common form of the disease and the form with the highest morbidity. Most of the systemic problems are related to the kidneys, where damage to the glomeruli can be severe. Patients experience widespread arthritis and arthralgia; heart and lung involvement; anemia and bone marrow depression; and diffuse vasculitis and skin rashes, most notably the "butterfly rash" over the malar areas of the face (Figure 8-39). Fatigue, malaise, fever, and psychosis are commonly found in those affected. The disease primarily affects females, usually during the childbearing years. Oral lesions are found in 21% of patients with SLE.

Subacute Cutaneous Lupus Erythematosus
SCLE affects the skin of the upper parts of the body, with systemic and musculoskeletal components mildly involved. Chronic skin rashes are present for months but eventually heal. Symptoms of muscle and joint stiffness and malaise and fatigue are common. Circulating antinuclear antibodies (ANA) and antibodies to cytoplasmic constituents similar to those found in Sjögren syndrome are also found.

Discoid Lupus Erythematosus
DLE is the form of the disease in which the cutaneous and mucosal lesions of the face are the most prominent findings. Scalp involvment with hair loss (alopecia) is also common.

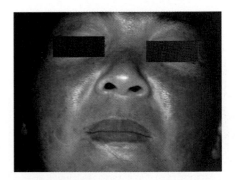

FIGURE 8-39

Lupus erythematosus. Vasculitis and skin rash over malar areas of face ("butterfly rash") that intensify with exposure to sunlight are common in most forms of the disease.

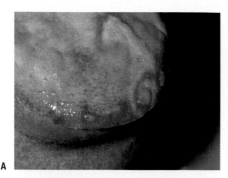

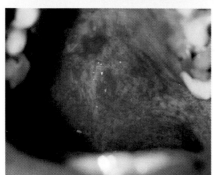

FIGURE 8-40

Lupus erythematosus. Patient with oral mucosal lesions of the tongue **(A)** and palate consisting of diffuse and annular leukoplakic lesions, erythematous areas, and chronic ulcerations **(B).** Intraoral lesions are most frequently found in patients with the discoid form of LE but may be present to a lesser degree in all forms of the disease.

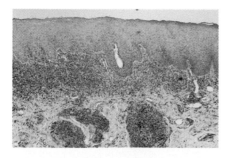

FIGURE 8-41

Lupus erythematosus. Microscopic appearance of mucosal lesions exhibiting a parakeratinizing surface with a dense infiltrate of lymphocytes in the immediate underlying connective tissue. In the deeper areas there are characteristic large focal and perivascular accumulations of lymphocytes.

CLINICAL

Oral lesions occur in approximately 24% of patients affected with DLE and are similar to the oral lesions found in other forms of LE. In SLE oral lesions are less common, present only in 21% of cases, but are often more symptomatic and involve more intraoral structures. Oral mucosal lesions can be found in all forms of LE appearing as annular leukoplakic areas and/or erythematous erosions or chronic ulcerations (Figure 8-40). This lesion is most commonly found in patients with DLE. In milder forms an ulcer may not develop, and lesions appear as an area of chronic erythema that is sensitive, often with a burning sensation. The long-standing chronic lesion may have few symptoms and be present as a leukoplakic patch that does not ulcerate. Although oral lesions are occasionally the first physical sign of LE, in most cases, oral and skin lesions appear simultaneously.

HISTOPATHOLOGY

The microscopic features of mucosal lesions of LE are remarkably similar to those found in LP and graft-versus-host disease. The target antigen appears to be in the basal and parabasal layers of the epithelium where large numbers of T lymphocytes accumulate and degeneration of cells occurs. An increase in the thickness of the basement membrane and epithelial atrophy with loss of rete peg formation are common. The presence of concentrations of lymphocytes in the immediate underlying lamina propria, deep focal accumulations of lymphocytes with germinal centers, and perivascular infiltrates of lymphocytes (Figure 8-41) is helpful in differentiating lesions of LE from LP. In the more chronic lesions the presence of hyperorthokeratosis and surface depressions containing keratin ("keratin plugging") suggest that a lesion is LE rather than LP. Direct immunofluorescence reveals a granular linear pattern to the IgA, IgM, and IgG immunoglobulins; fibrinogen; and C3. Such a pattern is not sufficiently specific to be diagnostic for LE but can be of help in distinguishing LE lesions from LP because LP is not usually reactive to any of the immunoglobulins. The most specific diagnostic test for SLE is the antinuclear antigen (ANA) and the LE cell tests. Unfortunately, these test are usually negative in patients with DLE.

TREATMENT

Cutaneous lesions of DLE are treated with topical steroids, antimalarials, and sulfones. The more severe forms of the disease requires steroids or combinations of steroids and immunosuppressive drugs such as cyclophosphamide and azathioprine. Oral lesions can be refractory to topical treatment, requiring systemic steroids to obtain relief of symptoms.

PROGRESSIVE SYSTEMIC SCLEROSIS

■ **PROGRESSIVE SYSTEMIC SCLEROSIS (SCLERODERMA):** a generalized condition characterized by replacement of the normal connective tissue with dense collagen bundles resulting in fibrosis, loss of mobility, and altered function of organs.

Progressive systemic sclerosis (PSS) is preferred to the older term, *scleroderma*. The disease has three main presentations: (1) the **diffuse** (classic) form, in which there is generalized involvment of both the body surfaces and the visceral organs; (2) as part of the **CREST syndrome;** and (3) **localized,** which may appear as one of three clinical subtypes referred to as *morphea, linear,* or *"en coup de sabre."* The basic disease process is a slow, continuous replacement of the usual vascular loose connective tissue with densely packed collagen bundles with few blood vessels evident. When the skin becomes involved, it loses its softness and elasticity and becomes tight and firmly adhered to the underlying muscle and bone, resulting in progressive loss of mobility of the hands, joints, or other moving internal or external anatomic structures. Because of this feature, at one time the condition was referred to as "hidebound disease." The disease primarily affects females and initially appears during middle-age.

The pathogenesis of the progressive fibrous replacement of the normal connective tissue is not completely known. Recent research has found circulating immune complexes that are toxic to capillary endothelial cells, which chronically damages these blood vessels and stimulates nearby fibroblasts to produce collagen. In severe diffuse forms of the disease, patients exhibit specific circulating and tissue antinuclear antibodies. Some CREST syndrome patients exhibit the antibody to the protein contained within the centromere of the cell. This is most common in patients who have Raynaud disease as a prominent feature of their disease process. In some cases defective fibroblast function is found to be the fundamental disease process.

In the diffuse form of PSS most of the skin is involved, as are the esophagus, intestines, lungs, kidneys, and heart. The skin becomes firm and immovable with loss of adnexal structures such as hair and the sebaceous and sweat glands. A restricted oral opening and sclerodactyly are prominent in the late stages of the disease (Figure 8-42). The CREST syndrome, of which PSS is a part, consists of calcinosis (C), Raynaud disease (R), esophageal strictures (E), sclerodactyly (S), and telangiectasia (T) of the skin.

The localized form of PSS is limited to regions of the skin and does not have visceral involvement. The clinical subtypes of localized PSS merely reflect the morphologic cutaneous surfaces affected by the disease.

CLINICAL

The oral and facial manifestations of PSS are found most often in patients with the diffuse form and those with CREST syndrome. The major oral problem is the progressive restriction of the oral opening and the loss of saliva production that leads to a xerostomia and its associated complications. These conditions combined with dysphagia due to esophageal strictures result in a diminished ability to eat and have the required dental care. Other findings include generalized induration of the mucosal tissue; altered tongue function; and alteration in the fibrous component of the gingiva, resulting in advanced periodontitis. Symptomatic alterations in the temporomandibular joint include clicking, crepitation, and pain that sometimes is associated with erosion of bone. Cortical erosion of the bone at the angle of the mandible and the coronoid process is occasionally observed. In less than a third of the patients, widening of the periodontal membrane will be found in the late stage of the disease.

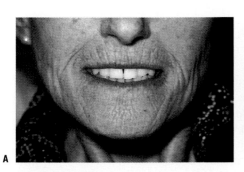
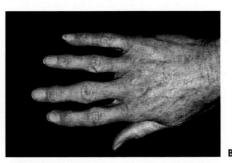

A   B

FIGURE 8-42

Progressive systemic sclerosis. Patients exhibit superficial tissue that becomes firm and immovable resulting in contracture of the lips and a limited mouth opening **(A)** and fingers with tightly bound skin (sclerodactyly) with reduced mobility **(B)**.

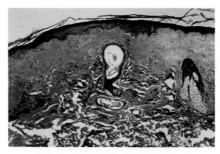

FIGURE 8-43

Progressive systemic sclerosis. Photomicrograph of the skin reveals a dense hyalinized collagen deposit immediately below the epithelium that is replacing most dermal appendages and other anatomic structures.

HISTOPATHOLOGY

The tissue reveals diffuse deposits of dense hyalinized collagen replacing the normal anatomic structures. In the skin the sweat glands, hair follicles, and sebaceous glands are lost and the overlying epithelium is thinned (Figure 8-43). Hyalinization occurs around blood vessels, and adipose tissue is lost. In the early stages perivascular infiltrates of mononuclear inflammatory cells are common, followed by a gradual decrease in the number of small blood vessels and a simultaneous increase in the density of the collagen.

TREATMENT

In some patients spontaneous remissions have occurred. Use of systemic steroids has been of some help in reducing the rate of progression of the disease. In general, no treatment is presently available to completely halt the disease process.

ALLERGIC REACTIONS

Allergic reactions, which occur after repeated contact with an external antigen **(allergin)** in previously sensitized individuals, are immune inflammatory responses mediated by the IgE immunoglobulin. After initial contact IgE is secreted by lymphoblasts into the circulatory system where it binds to specific receptors on basophils and mast cells, sensitizing the cells to the external agent for months or years. In 5% to 10% of the population, individuals are prone to developing large numbers of IgE sensitized mast cells; when reexposed to the allergin, they bind it in large amounts. Binding of the allergin to IgE antibodies attached to mast cells or basophils triggers the cell's cytoplasm to degranulate. For degranulation to occur two surface IgE antibodies must be bridged by the same binding allergin. The released cytoplasmic granules have high concentrations of the vasodilators—histamine and serotonin; heparin; eosinophil chemotactic factor; slow-reacting substance anaphylaxis (SRS-A); and bradykinin. The actions of these chemical mediators on the surrounding tissue accounts for the symptoms seen in allergic patients. The severity of the reactions is governed by the following: the patient's concentration of IgE, the susceptibility of the mast cells to degranulation, the sensitivity of the endothelial and other target cells to the released mediators, and the presence of sufficient neutralizing mediators. These factors are variable in each patient, and many are genetically determined. Thus some individuals are more prone to severe and recurring reactions than others.

CONTACT STOMATITIS

Hypersensitivity to allergins are commonly observed within the oral cavity. Since some of the most common allergins are foods, patients who are sensitive to specific foods will exhibit mucosal reactions soon after contact. Common foodstuff includes nuts, shellfish, fruits, and some vegatables. Other allergins are chemical in nature (haptens) and require conjugation with proteins to become effective allergins. This process occurs with the aid of the intraepithelial Langerhans cell where the hapten is converted into a competent antigen and is presented to the T lymphocytes for sensitization and production of IgE with specific receptors. These allergins are metals; dental materials; flavoring and other chemicals in toothpaste, mouthwash, and chewing gum; ingredients in rubberdam and latex gloves; and cosmetics such as lipstick. Drugs and other medications comprise a large category of allergins. Most notable are the penicillins and sulfa drugs. Many of these allergins are ingested, which allows for quick access into the blood stream. In the blood stream the allergins may sensitize immune cells in all parts of the body, resulting in life-threatening vasodilatation and edema in the airway and/or other organs. When such a reaction is severe, it is referred to as *anaphylactic shock*. Because of the large number of possible allergins, the sensitizing agent may remain undiscovered.

CLINICAL

The usual oral mucosal reactions to the presence of a sensitizing allergin is erythema and edema. When the gingiva is involved, the tissue is a uniform bright red in all quadrants (Figure 8-44, *A*). This is in contrast to the dental-plaque–related gingivitis that is usually present in some locations and usually is confined to an area close to the free gingival margin with the attached gingiva of relatively normal color. The buccal mucosa is generally puffy and dark red. Closer examination reveals that the superficial capillaries are engorged and ejected. The lips are frequently involved and appear swollen, erythematous, and subject to erosive areas and chronic ulceration (Figure 8-44, *B*). The patients complain of a burning sensation and sensitivity to hot, cold, alcohol, and spicy foods and liquids. An allergy to denture base material is unusual, occurring when the acrylic has been incompletely cured. In these cases, the distribution corresponds to all tissue surfaces that are in contact with the denture base. This distribution pattern distinguishes true allergic reactions to denture acrylic from similarly appearing acute atrophic (erythematous) candidiasis that occurs on the palate only.

HISTOPATHOLOGY

The epithelium usually exhibits intracellular and intercellular edema (spongiosis). Occasionally, vesicular formation occurs that may be located within the epithelium or at the basement membrane. The connective tissue exhibits engorged and dilated blood vessels against a background of edema and an infiltrate of lymphocytes and plasma cells. The infiltrates are often concentrated in perivascular locations, especially in the deeper areas. In some lesions the allergin elicits a heavy plasma cell response. Lesions containing dense infiltrates of plasma cells are commonly associated with allergies to flavoring in chewing gum and mouthwash and have been referred to as *plasma cell gingivitis*. Presence of increased numbers of eosinophils is a frequent tissue finding in allergic reactions.

ANGIOEDEMA

> ■ ANGIOEDEMA: a recurring rapid swelling of the lips and adjacent structures in susceptible patients that occurs after contact with an allergin, antiinflammatory medication, or exposure to the elements.

Angioedema is a common clinical presentation of a group of allergic conditions with different etiologic pathways. The previous term, *angioneurotic edema*, is no longer used because the condition is not thought to be related to psychologic problems or other nervous system stimulation as initially described by Quincke in 1882. Within the oral area angioedema usually develops rather quickly as a regional, painless swelling of the lips, anterior cheek, or tongue (Figure 8-45). It is of great concern when the more posterior anatomic structures are involved because the airway becomes subject to compromise, creating an emergency situation. Upon cessation of contact with the allergin, the swelling subsides rapidly on its own, usually within 24 to 48 hours. The two basic forms of angioedema are **acquired** and **hereditary.**

Acquired angioedema is the most common form and is frequently the result of recent ingestion of a medication. Most of the acquired types are IgE

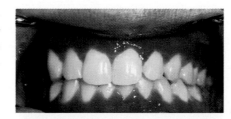
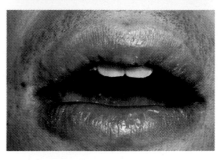

FIGURE 8-44

Contact stomatitis. Patient with generalized erythema and edema of the gingiva **(A)** and swollen lips with small fissures and erosive areas due to a hypersensitivity to an unidentified allergin **(B).**

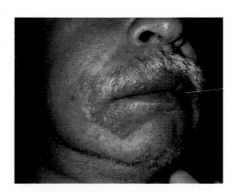

FIGURE 8-45

Acquired angioedema. Patient with swelling of the lips and right cheek with transepithelial oozing and crusting of transudate that began 3 days after receiving penicillin during root canal treatment.

immune-mediated, particularly those initiated by penicillin. Other types are of nonimmune origin such as occurs in patients receiving the nonsteroidal antiinflammatory drugs aspirin and indomethacin. These medications act directly on the mast cell, destabilizing the cell membrane and thereby facilitating degranulation and liberating chemical mediators of inflammation. In other types, the angiotensin-converting enzyme inhibitors such as captopril and enalaprilate cause a nonimmune-mediated angioedema by enhancing the activity of bradykinin, one of the inflammatory mediators liberated from mast cells during degranulation. In some patients ingestion of medication is not required with the angioedema occurring after exposure to cold, sun, or exercise.

Hereditary angioedema, a rare form of the disease, is inherited as an autosomal dominant trait. In these patients the swelling develops after mild trauma to the area. In the oral area lesions are frequently preceded by a tooth extraction. Unlike the acquired form, lesions of hereditary angioedema may involve the gastrointestinal and respiratory tracts. Involvement of these areas usually results in a medical emergency because intense pain and vomiting or laryngeal constriction often ensues. The hereditary form of angioedema is due to a hereditary deficiency of the C1 esterase inhibitor (C1INH) of the complement casade. Without the inhibitor very little provocation is required to precipitate activation of the complement system, leading to vascular dilatation and tissue edema.

POSSIBLE IMMUNE-MEDIATED REACTIONS

CHEILITIS GLANDULARIS

■ CHEILITIS GLANDULARIS: enlargement of the lower lip due to chronic inflammation of the minor salivary glands and distention of excretory ductal structures.

Cheilitis glandularis is an uncommon inflammatory condition of the minor salivary glands of the lower lip. Multiple etiologic factors have been attributed to the condition, but the basic initiating factors are still unknown. Because this condition clinically resembles cheilitis granulomatosa, a disease considered to have an immune-mediated component, it is discussed in this chapter to help differentiate the two conditions.

CLINICAL

Cheilitis glandularis is a condition of the lower lip that occurs primarily in middle-age and older men. The lip becomes greatly enlarged and everted, exposing the labial mucosa to the sun and atmospheric elements. The exposed surfaces become dry and pale and contain multiple small reddish nodules (Figure 8-46). The nodules represent openings of excretory ducts of minor salivary glands that have become congested with retained mucin. With bimanual palpation, mucin can be expressed from the nodules. This is a useful diagnostic test for this condition.

HISTOPATHOLOGY

The connective tissue of the lower lip contains multiple chronically inflamed minor salivary glands with distended and tortuous excretory ducts. The ducts generally contain inspissated mucin with fibrous tissue, lymphocytes, and plasma cells replacing the acini. The ducts exhibit focal areas of metaplasia to a stratified

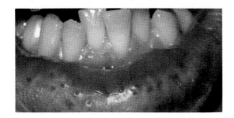

FIGURE 8-46

Cheilitis glandularis. A long-standing enlarged lower lip with a pale, dry surface containing multiple small raised papules (enlarged duct openings) is characteristic of this condition.

squamous epithelium. Bacteria commonly enter the ductal structures, causing the production of purulent exudate, which replaces the mucin. In this acute form of the disease there is often associated deep abscesses throughout the lip with frequent draining sinus tracts.

TREATMENT

Surgery is the preferred method of treatment, usually in the form of a vermilionectomy. In more severe and long-standing conditions, extensive surgical reduction of the lip may be required. Untreated affected lips are thought to have an increased risk of developing carcinoma.

CHEILITIS GRANULOMATOSA

> ■ CHEILITIS GRANULOMATOSA: a recurrent or persistent enlargement of the lip commonly associated with Melkersson-Rosenthal syndrome consisting of noncaseating granulomas, generalized edema, and vascular changes.

Cheilitis granulomatosa is a recurrent or persistent enlargement of the lip that is commonly associated with Melkersson-Rosenthal syndrome (MRS). The other features of MRS are generalized orofacial swelling, peripheral facial nerve paralysis, and a fissured tongue. The etiology of the condition is unknown but is thought to represent hypersentivity to the bacteria in a chronic focus of infection in another nearby location.

CLINICAL

Affected patients are found in all age groups, with a median age of 25 years. Exacerbation of the generally enlarged lower lip occurs on a regular basis and may be associated with other intraoral swellings, particularly of the palate and the floor of the mouth. In addition to the cosmetic problem the enlarged and disfigured lip often produces difficulties for the patient during eating, drinking, and speaking (Figure 8-47).

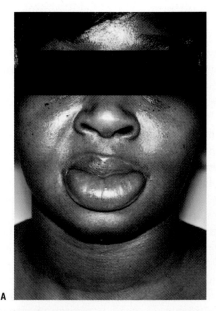 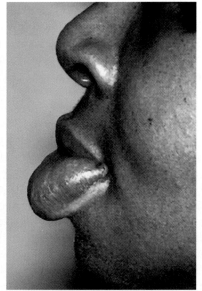

A   B

FIGURE 8-47
Cheilitis granulomatosa. Enlarged and disfigured lower lip, which is apparent in frontal **(A)** and lateral **(B)** views. The condition also produces difficulties in eating and speaking.

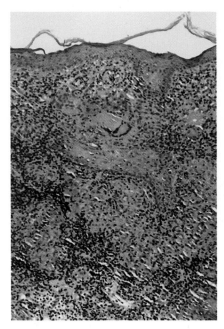

FIGURE 8-48

Cheilitis granulomatosa. Microscopic features reveal multiple focal granulomas composed of epithelioid cells and giant cells surrounded by lymphocytes, plasma cells, and edematous connective tissue.

HISTOPATHOLOGY

The characteristic feature of the tissue is the presence of multiple noncaseating granulomas that are located close to the vascular structures. The granulomas are composed of epithelioid cells and giant cells (Figure 8-48); occasionally there are nearby aggregates of lymphocytes and plasma cells. Generalized edema and dilated blood vessels are also present throughout the connective tissue.

TREATMENT

The most successful treatment has been the indentification and removal of coexisting infections, often of odontogenic origin. Surgical resection of the enlarged and usually everted lip is sometimes effective. Intralesional injection of steroid solutions has generally shown little effect.

SARCOIDOSIS

> ■ SARCOIDOSIS: a chronic disease affecting the skin, mucosa, salivary glands, lungs, and other organs; consists of multiple noncaseating epithelioid granulomas and fibrosis of adjacent tissue.

Sarcoidosis is a chronic disease consisting of multiple granulomas of the skin, mucosal surfaces, salivary glands, lungs, and occasionally other major organs. At present, the etiology of sarcoidosis is unknown. Research has revealed some features of the disease that may eventually be useful in identifying the causative factors: some ethnic groups are more susceptible than others; the hormonal status of the patients may play a role; the patients' major histocompatibility antigen status is important, particularly those having HLA-B5, -B7, -B8, HLA-A9, HLA-Cw7, and HLA-DR3 types; patients are allergic to antigens found in some infectious agents such as mumps, tuberculosis, and candida; often patients have reduced levels of circulating T lymphocytes; some patients have altered CD4/CD8 ratios; and some have elevated levels of serum lysozymes and serum angiotensin-converting enzymes.

CLINICAL

Sarcoidosis is common in black populations of the Caribbean, Peurto Rico, and Africa. African Americans have a higher incidence of the disease than the rest of the population. In America, the disease is usually contracted before the age of 40 and is significantly more frequent in women than men. In Europe the disease is found in a slightly older age group and is equally distributed among the sexes.

The patients' symptoms are generally nonspecific. Patients complain of a general lack of energy and difficulty in breathing. The lungs appear to be initially involved with extension through the lymphatics to the hilar and mediastinal lymph nodes. Many patients have multiple erythematous skin nodules and swelling of the parotids and/or the submandibular glands. Other involvement of the head and neck area is common, with lymph nodes exhibiting enlargement and lesions present in and around the nasal passages. Lesions have been known to develop in bone but are rare. Approximately 25% of patients will have eye involvement, particularly of the uveal tract. A combination of lesions of the uveal tract, parotid gland, and seventh cranial nerve has been described as **Heerfordt syndrome** (uveoparotid fever).

Oral lesions appear as diffuse submucosal enlargements or focal firm nodules. Ulceration is uncommon, and lesions are usually completely symptomless. Lesions have been reported on the lips, tongue, buccal mucosa, gingiva, hard and soft palate (Figure 8-49), and floor of the mouth.

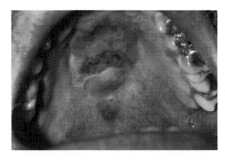

FIGURE 8-49

Sarcoidosis. The soft palate contains a firm raised diffuse nodular lesion with a focal area of ulceration.

HISTOPATHOLOGY

The tissue contains multiple granulomas in a nodular pattern, each consisting of an accumulation of epithelioid macrophages and multinucleated giant cells (Figure 8-50). The granulomas are similar to those found in tuberculosis but differ in that there is an absence of the central caseating necrosis and a reduced lymphocyte infiltrate. The periphery of each granuloma is composed of a cellular fibrous connective tissue. The multiple nuclei of the giant cells are often arranged in a ring around the periphery and may additionally contain some stellate-shaped structures that have been described as "asteroid bodies." Electron microscopy reveals that these structures are phagocytized cellular debris. Because the cellular features are similar to other infectious or foreign body granulomas, bacterial and fungal stains are usually applied and the tissue is viewed with polarized light to rule out these causative factors.

DIAGNOSIS

In disseminated cases urinalysis will reveal an increase in calcium levels and serum analysis will reveal an increase in calcium, immunoglobulins, lysozymes, and angiotensin-converting enzymes. The traditional test is the Kveim reaction, which is performed by injecting a suspension of human antigenic extract from the spleen tissue of patients with sarcoidosis into the forearm of patients who are suspected of having the disease. Positive patients will develop a sarcoid lesion in 4 to 6 weeks.

TREATMENT

Patients are generally treated with steroids, particularly if lung lesions are present. Immunosuppressant drugs are also used either alone or in combination with other modalities. Spontaneous resolution of lesions is also known to occur. Prognosis is good in nearly all treated cases.

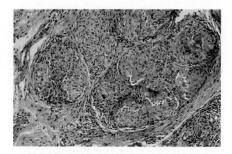

FIGURE 8-50

Sarcoidosis. Tissue exhibits multiple non-caseating granulomas consisting of epithelioid cells and multinucleated giant cells and surrounded by thin bands of fibrous tissue. Few lymphocytes are observed in the adjacent connective tissue.

ADDITIONAL READING

GENERAL

Eversole LR. Immunopathology of oral mucosal ulcerative, desquamative, and bullous diseases. *Oral Surg Oral Med Oral Pathol.* 1994; 77:555-71.

Fine J-D, ed. *Bullous Diseases: Topics in Clinical Dermatology Series.* New York: Igaku-Shoin Medical Publishers; 1993.

Provost TT, Weston WL. *Bullous Diseases.* St Louis: Mosby; 1993.

RECURRENT APHTHOUS STOMATITIS

Bagan JV, Sanchis JM, Milian MA, Penarrocha M and others. Recurrent aphthous stomatitis: a study of the clinical characteristics of lesions in 93 cases. *J Oral Pathol Med.* 1991; 20:395-7.

Endre L. Recurrent aphthous ulceration with zinc deficiency and cellular immune deficiency. *Oral Surg Oral Med Oral Pathol.* 1991; 72:559-61.

Field EA, Brookes V, Tyldesley WR. Recurrent aphthous ulceration in children: a review. *Int J Paediatr Dent.* 1992; 2:1-10.

Hunter IP, Ferguson MM, Scully C, Galloway AR and others. Effects of dietary gluten elimination in patients with recurrent minor aphthous stomatitis and no detectable gluten enteropathy. *Oral Surg Oral Med Oral Pathol.* 1993; 75:595-8.

McCartan BE, Sullivan A. The association of menstrual cycle, pregnancy, and menopause with recurrent oral aphthous stomatitis: a review and critique. *Obstet Gynecol.* 1992; 80:455-8.

Meiller TF, Kutcher MJ, Overholser CD, Niehaus C and others. Effect of an antimicrobial mouthrinse on recurrent aphthous ulcerations. *Oral Surg Oral Med Oral Pathol.* 1991; 72:425-9.

Nolan A, Lamey PJ, Milligan KA, Forsyth A. Recurrent aphthous ulceration and food sensitivity. *J Oral Pathol Med.* 1991; 20:473-5.

Nolan A, McIntosh WB, Allam BF, Lamey PJ. Recurrent aphthous ulceration: vitamin B_1, B_2 and B_6 status and response to replacement therapy. *J Oral Pathol Med.* 1991; 20:389-91.

Pedersen A. Recurrent aphthous ulceration: virological and immunological aspects. *APMIS Suppl.* 1993; 37:1-37.

Pedersen A, Hougen HP, Kenrad B. T-lymphocyte subsets in oral mucosa of patients with recurrent aphthous ulceration. *Oral Pathol Med.* 1992; 21:176-80.

Pedersen A, Madsen HO, Vestergaard BF, Ryder LP. Varicella-zoster virus DNA in recurrent aphthous ulcers. *Scand J Dent Res.* 1993; 101:311-3.

Pedersen A, Pedersen BK. Natural killer cell function and number in peripheral blood are not altered in recurrent aphthous ulceration. *Oral Surg Oral Med Oral Pathol.* 1993; 76:616-9.

Porter SR, Kingsmill V, Scully C. Audit of diagnosis and investigations in patients with recurrent aphthous stomatitis. *Oral Surg Oral Med Oral Pathol.* 1993; 76:449-52.

Regezi JA, Macphail LA, Richards DW, Greenspan JS. A study of macrophages, macrophage-related cells, and endothelial adhesion molecules in recurrent aphthous ulcers in HIV-positive patients. *J Dent Res.* 1993; 72:1549-53.

Savage NW, Seymour GJ. Specific lymphocytotoxic destruction of autologous epithelial cell targets in recurrent aphthous stomatitis. *Aust Dent J.* 1994; 39:98-104.

Wray D, Charon J. Polymorphonuclear neutrophil function in recurrent aphthous stomatitis. *J Oral Pathol Med.* 1991; 20:392-4.

BEHÇET SYNDROME

Bhatia V, Menon RK, Gupta AK, Band AH, Menon PS. Behçet syndrome. *Indian Pediatr.* 1984; 21:249-51.

de Merieux P, Spitler LE, Paulus HE. Treatment of Behçet's syndrome with levamisole. *Arthritis Rheum.* 1981; 24:64-70.

Kikuchi K, Suga T, Senoue I, Nomiyama T and others. Esophageal ulceration in a patient with Behçet's syndrome. *Tokai J Exp Clin Med.* 1982; 7:135-43.

Lehner T, Welsh KI, Batchelor JR. The relationship of HLA-B and DR phenotypes to Behçet's syndrome, recurrent oral ulceration and the class of immune complexes. *Immunology.* 1982; 47:581-7.

Wilkey D, Yocum DE, Oberley TD, Sundstrom WR and others. Budd-Chiari syndrome and renal failure in Behçet disease. *Am J Med.* 1983; 75:541-50.

LICHEN PLANUS

Bricker SL. Oral lichen planus: a review. *Semin Dermatol.* 1994; 13:87-90.

Eisen D. The therapy of oral lichen planus. *Crit Rev Oral Biol Med.* 1993; 4:141-58.

Eisenberg E. Lichen planus and oral cancer: is there a connection between the two? *J Am Dent Assoc.* 1992; 123:104-8.

Holmstrup P. The controversy of a premalignant potential of oral lichen planus is over. *Oral Surg Oral Med Oral Pathol.* 1992; 73:704-6.

Oliver GF, Winkelmann RK. Treatment of lichen planus. *Drugs.* 1993; 45:56-65.

Sigurgeirsson B, Lindelof B. Lichen planus and malignancy: an epidemiologic study of 2071 patients and a review of the literature. *Arch Dermatol.* 1991; 127:1684-8.

Silverman S. Lichen planus. *Curr Opin Dent.* 1991; 1:769-72.

Zegarelli DJ. The treatment of oral lichen planus. *Ann Dent.* 1993; 52:3-8.

LICHENOID DRUG REACTIONS

Halevy S, Sandbank M, Livni E. Macrophage migration inhibition factor release in lichenoid drug eruptions. *J Am Acad Dermatol.* 1993; 29:263-5.

Halevy S, Shai A. Lichenoid drug eruptions. *J Am Acad Dermatol.* 1993; 29:249-55.

Shiohara T, Moriya N, Nagashima M. Induction and control of lichenoid tissue reactions. *Springer Semin Immunopathol.* 1992; 13:369-85.

MUCOUS MEMBRANE PEMPHIGOID

Anhalt GJ, Morrison LH. Bullous and cicatricial pemphigoid. *J Autoimmun.* 1991; 4:17-35.

Chan LS, Yancy KB, Hammerberg C, Soong HK and others. Immune-mediated subepithelial blistering diseases of mucous membranes. *Arch Dermol.* 1993; 129:448-455.

Mutasim DF, Pelc NJ, Anhalt GJ. Cicatricial pemphigoid. *Dermatol Clin.* 1993; 11:499-510.

Van Joost T, Van't Veen AJ. Drug-induced cicatricial pemphigoid and acquired epidermolysis bullosa. *Clin Dermatol.* 1993; 11:521-7.

Vincent SD, Lilly GE, Baker KA. Clinical, historic, and therapeutic features of cicatricial pemphigoid: a literature review and open therapeutic trial with corticosteroids. *Oral Surg Oral Med Oral Pathol.* 1993; 76:453-9.

PEMPHIGUS VULGARIS

Amagai M, Klaus-Kovtun V, Stanley JR. Autoantibodies against a novel epithelial cadherin in pemphigus vulgaris, a disease of cell adhesion. *Cell.* 1991; 67:869-77.

Becker BA, Gaspari AA. Pemphigus vulgaris and vegetans. *Dermatol Clin.* 1993; 11:429-52.

Gorsky M, Raviv M, Raviv E. Pemphigus vulgaris in adolescence. *Oral Surg Oral Med Oral Pathol.* 1994; 77:620-2.

Karpati S, Amagai M, Prussick R, Cehrs K and others. Pemphigus vulgaris antigen: a desmoglein type of cadherin is localized within keratinocyte desmosomes. *J Cell Biol.* 1993; 122:409-15.

Mutasim DF, Pelc NJ, Anhalt GJ. Paraneoplastic pemphigus, pemphigus vulgaris, and pemphigus foliaceus. *Clin Dermatol.* 1993; 11:113-7.

Plott RT, Amagai M, Udey MC, Stanley JR. Pemphigus vulgaris antigen lacks biochemical properties characteristic of classical cadherins. *J Invest Dermatol.* 1994; 103:168-72.

Rook AH. Photophoresis in the treatment of autoimmune disease: experience with pemphigus vulgaris and systemic sclerosis. *Ann N Y Acad Sci.* 1991; 636:209-16.

Setoyama M, Hashimoto K, Tashiro M. Immunolocalization of desmoglein I (band 3 polypeptide) on acantholytic cells in pemphigus vulgaris, Darier's disease, and Hailey-Hailey's disease. *J Dermatol.* 1991; 18:500-5.

EPIDERMOLYSIS BULLOSA

Burgeson RE. Type VII collagen, anchoring fibrils, and epidermolysis bullosa. *J Invest Dermatol.* 1993; 101:252-5.

Crawford EG, Burkes EJ, Briggaman RA. Hereditary epidermolysis bullosa: oral manifestations and dental therapy. *Oral Surg Oral Med Oral Pathol.* 1976; 42:490-500.

Fine J-D. Epidermolysis bullosa: clinical aspects, pathology, and recent advances in research. *J Dermatol.* 1986; 25:143-57.

Fine J-D. Laboratory tests for epidermolysis bullosa. *Dermatol Clin.* 1994; 12:123-32.

Lin AN, Carter DM. Epidermolysis bullosa. *Ann Rev Med.* 1993; 44:189-99.

Sedano HO, Gorlin RJ. Epidermolysis bullosa. *Oral Surg Oral Med Oral Pathol.* 1989; 67:555-65.

Uitto J, Christiano AM. Inherited epidermolysis bullosa: clinical features, molecular genetics, and pathoetiologic mechanisms. *Dermatol Clin.* 1993; 11:549-63.

Wright JT, Fine J-D. Hereditary epidermolysis bullosa. *Semin Dermatol.* 1994; 13:102-7.

Wright JT, Fine J-D, Johnson LB. Hereditary epidermolysis bullosa: oral manifestations and dental management. *Pediatr Dent.* 1993; 15:242-8.

Wright JT, Fine J-D, Johnson LB. Oral soft tissues in hereditary epidermolysis bullosa. *Oral Surg Oral Med Oral Pathol.* 1991; 71:440-6.

ERYTHEMA MULTIFORME

Avakian R, Flowers FP, Araujo OE, Ramos-Caro FA. Toxic epidermal necrolysis: a review. *J Am Acad Dermatol.* 1991; 25:69-79.

Brice SL, Huff JC, Weston WL. Erythema multiforme minor in children. *Pediatrician.* 1991; 18:188-94.

Kaufman DW. Epidemiologic approaches to the study of toxic epidermal necrolysis. *J Invest Dermatol.* 1994; 102:31S-33S.

Lyell A. Drug-induced toxic epidermal necrolysis: I: an overview. *Clin Dermatol.* 1993; 11:491-2.

Parsons JM. Toxic epidermal necrolysis. *Int J Dermatol.* 1992; 31:749-68.

Roujeau JC. The spectrum of Stevens-Johnson syndrome and toxic epidermal necrolysis: a clinical classification. *J Invest Dermatol.* 1994; 102:28S-30S.

Roujeau JC. Drug-induced toxic epidermal necrolysis: II: current aspects. *Clin Dermatol.* 1993; 11:493-500.

Stampien TM, Schwartz RA. Erythema multiforme. *Am Fam Physician.* 1992; 46:1171-6.

Wilkins J, Morrison L, White CR. Oculocutaneous manifestations of the erythema multiforme/Stevens-Johnson syndrome/toxic epidermal necrolysis spectrum. *Dermatol Clin.* 1992; 10:571-82.

LUPUS ERYTHEMATOSUS

Blaszczyk M, Jablonska S, Chorzelski TP, Jarzabek-Chorzelska M. Clinical relevance of immunologic findings in cutaneous lupus erythematosus. *Clin Dermatol.* 1992; 10:399-406.

David-Bajar KM. Subacute cutaneous lupus erythematosus. *J Invest Dermatol.* 1993; 100:2S-8S.

Gately LE, Nesbitt LT. Update on immunofluorescent testing in bullous diseases and lupus erythematosus. *Dermatol Clin.* 1994; 12:133-42.

George PM, Tunnessen WW. Childhood discoid lupus erythematosus. *Arch Dermatol.* 1993; 129:613-7.

Laman SD, Provost TT. Cutaneous manifestations of lupus erythematosus. *Rheum Dis Clin North Am.* 1994; 20:195-212.

Jablonska S, Blaszczyk-Kostanecka M, Chorzelski T, Jarzabek-Chorzelska M. The red face: lupus erythematosus. *Clin Dermatol.* 1993; 11:253-60.

Norris DA. Pathomechanisms of photosensitive lupus erythematosus. *J Invest Dermatol.* 1993; 100:58S-68S.

Swaak AJ, Nossent JC, Smeenk RJ. Systemic lupus erythematosus. *Int J Clin Lab Res.* 1992; 22:190-5.

PROGRESSIVE SYSTEMIC SCLEROSIS

Eversole LR, Jacobsen PL, Stone CE. Oral and gingival changes in systemic sclerosis (scleroderma). *J Periodontol.* 1984; 55:175-178.

Haustein UF, Herrmann K, Bohme HJ. Pathogenesis of progressive systemic sclerosis. *Int J Dermatol.* 1986; 25:286-93.

Larrabee JH. Progressive systemic sclerosis: part 1: the disease and medical management. *ANNA J.* 1989; 16:489-93.

Reichlin M. Progressive systemic sclerosis. *Immunol Ser.* 1991; 54:275-87.

Sternberg EM. Pathogenetic approaches to management of progressive systemic sclerosis. *Concepts Immunopathol.* 1989; 7:196-209.

ANGIOEDEMA

Cooper KD. Urticaria and angioedema: diagnosis and evaluation. *J Am Acad Dermatol.* 1991; 25:166-74.

Davidson AE, Miller SD, Settipane G, Klein D. Urticaria and angioedema. *Cleve Clin J Med.* 1992; 59:529-34.

Greaves M, Lawlor F. Angioedema: manifestations and management. *J Am Acad Dermatol.* 1991; 25:155-61.

Huston DP, Bressler RB. Urticaria and angioedema. *Med Clin North Am.* 1992; 76:805-40.

Megerian CA, Arnold JE, Berger M. Angioedema: 5 years' experience with a review of the disorder's presentation and treatment. *Laryngoscope.* 1992; 102:256-60.

Oltvai ZN, Wong EC, Atkinson JP, Tung KS. C1 inhibitor deficiency: molecular and immunologic basis of hereditary and acquired angioedema. *Lab Invest.* 1991; 65:381-8.

Orfan NA, Kolski GB. Angioedema and C1 inhibitor deficiency. *Ann Allergy.* 1992; 69:167-72.

Robinson LC, Hart LL. Danazol in hereditary angioedema. *Ann Pharmacother.* 1992; 26:1251-2.

Soter NA. Acute and chronic urticaria and angioedema. *J Am Acad Dermatol.* 1991; 25:146-54.

CONTACT STOMATITIS

Corazza M, Virgili A, Martina S. Allergic contact stomatitis from methyl methacrylate in a dental prosthesis with a persistent patch test reaction. *Contact Dermatitis.* 1992; 26:210-1.

Torres V, Mano-Azul AC, Correia T, Soares AP. Allergic contact cheilitis and stomatitis from hydroquinone in an acrylic dental prosthesis. *Contact Dermatitis.* 1993; 29:102-3.

van Loon LA, Bos JD, Davidson CL. Clinical evaluation of fifty-six patients referred with symptoms tentatively related to allergic contact stomatitis. *Oral Surg Oral Med Oral Pathol.* 1992; 74:572-5.

Veien NK, Borchorst E, Hattel T, Laurberg G. Stomatitis or systemically-induced contact dermatitis from metal wire in orthodontic materials. *Contact Dermatitis.* 1994; 30:210-3.

CHEILITIS GLANDULARIS

Cohen DM, Green JG, Diekmann SL. Concurrent anomalies: cheilitis glandularis and double lip. *Oral Surg Oral Med Oral Pathol.* 1988; 66:397-9.

Rada DC, Koranda FC, Katz FS. Cheilitis glandularis: a disorder of ductal ectasia. *J Dermatol Surg Oncol.* 1985; 11:372-5.

Stuller CB, Schaberg SJ, Stokos J, Pierce GL. Cheilitis glandularis. *Oral Surg Oral Med Oral Pathol.* 1982; 53:602-5.

Swerlick RA, Cooper PH. Cheilitis glandularis: a re-evaluation. *J Am Acad Dermatol.* 1984; 10:466-72.

Yacobi R, Brown DA. Cheilitis glandularis: a pediatric case report. *J Am Dent Assoc.* 1989; 118:317-8.

Winchester L, Scully C, Prime SS, Eveson JW. Cheilitis glandularis: a case affecting the upper lip. *Oral Surg Oral Med Oral Pathol.* 1986; 62:654-6.

CHEILITIS GRANULOMATOSA

Allen CM, Camisa C, Hamzeh S, Stephens L. Cheilitis granulomatosa: report of six cases and review of the literature. *J Am Acad Dermatol.* 1990; 23:444-50.

Cranberg JA, Patterson R, Caro WA. Angioedema, elephantiasis nostras, and cheilitis granulomatosa. *Allergy Proc.* 1990; 1:79-82.

Kano Y, Shiohara T, Yagita A, Nagashima M. Treatment of recalcitrant cheilitis granulomatosa with metronidazole. *J Am Acad Dermatol.* 1992; 27:629-30.

Kuno Y, Sakakibara S, Mizuno N. Actinic cheilitis granulomatosa. *J Dermatol.* 1992; 19:556-62.

Lindelof B, Eklund A, Liden S. Kveim test reactivity in Melkersson-Rosenthal syndrome (cheilitis granulomatosa). *Acta Derm Venereol (Stockh).* 1985; 65:443-5.

Mesa M, Yan-xin Z, Worsaae N, Reibel J. Diagnostic problems between oral lesions of Crohn's disease and Melkersson-Rosenthal syndrome/cheilitis granulomatosa. *Clin Prev Dent.* 1985; 7:23-5.

Williams PM, Greenberg MS. Management of cheilitis granulomatosa. *Oral Surg Oral Med Oral Pathol.* 1991; 72:436-9.

Venable CE, Gaudio SA. Persistent swelling of the lower lip: cheilitis granulomatosa. *Arch Dermatol.* 1988; 124:1706, 1709.

Worsaae N, Christensen KC, Schiodt M, Reibel J. Melkersson-Rosenthal syndrome and cheilitis granulomatosa: a clinicopathological study of thirty-three patients with special reference to their oral lesions. *Oral Surg Oral Med Oral Pathol.* 1982; 54:404-13.

SARCOIDOSIS

DeRemee RA. Sarcoidosis and Wegener's granulomatosis: a comparative analysis. *Sarcoidosis.* 1994; 11:7-18.

Fidler HM. Mycobacteria and sarcoidosis: recent advances. *Sarcoidosis.* 1994; 11:66-8.

Fink SD, Kremer JM. Cutaneous and musculoskeletal features, diagnostic modalities, and immunopathology in sarcoidosis. *Curr Opin Rheumatol.* 1994; 6:78-81.

James DG. Epidemiology of sarcoidosis. *Sarcoidosis.* 1992; 9:79-87.

Mathur A, Kremer JM. Immunopathology, musculoskeletal features, and treatment of sarcoidosis. *Curr Opin Rheumatol.* 1993; 5:90-4.

Selroos O. Treatment of sarcoidosis. *Sarcoidosis.* 1994; 11:80-3.

Viskum K, Vestbo J. The prognosis of extrapulmonary sarcoidosis. *Sarcoidosis.* 1994; 11:73-5.

Weissler JC. Southwestern internal medicine conference: sarcoidosis: immunology and clinical management. *Am J Med Sci.* 1994; 307:233-45.

CONNECTIVE TISSUE LESIONS

FIBROUS TISSUE
Hyperplasias
Focal Fibrous Hyperplasia (Irritation Fibroma)
Peripheral Ossifying Fibroma
Peripheral Giant Cell Granuloma
Inflammatory Fibrous Hyperplasia
Inflammatory Papillary Hyperplasia
Hyperplastic Gingivitis
Hereditary Gingival Fibromatosis
Drug-Induced Gingival Hyperplasia
Indeterminate Proliferations
Fibromatosis/Desmoplastic Fibroma
Nodular Fasciitis
Benign Fibrous Histiocytoma

Malignancies
Fibrosarcoma/Malignant Fibrous Histiocytoma

NEURAL TISSUE
Hyperplasia
Traumatic Neuroma
Hamartomas
Multiple Endocrine Neoplasia Syndrome
Benign Neoplasms
Neurilemoma
Neurofibroma
Granular Cell Tumor

Congenital Gingival Granular Cell Tumor
Neuroectodermal Tumor of Infancy
Malignant Neoplasms
Neurogenic Sarcoma

MUSCLE TISSUE
Neoplasias
Leiomyoma
Rhabdomyosarcoma

ADIPOSE TISSUE
Neoplasia
Lipoma
Liposarcoma

VASCULAR TISSUE
Hyperplasia
Pyogenic Granuloma
Hamartomatous and Benign Neoplasms
Hemangioma
Lymphangioma
Angiosarcoma
Kaposi Sarcoma

OSSEOUS AND CARTILAGINOUS TISSUES
Developmental Lesions
Soft Tissue Osteoma
Osseous and Cartilaginous Choristoma
Reactive Lesions
Myositis Ossificans

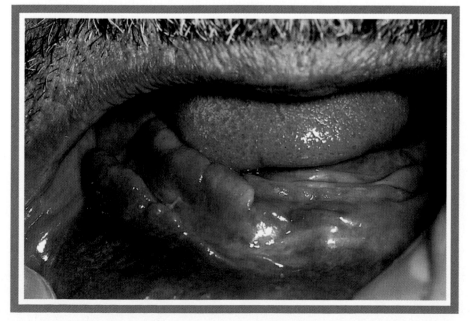

The term *tumor,* which literally means "a swelling," frequently causes confusion because it is used by some sources when referring to true neoplasms and by others to indicate the presence of any common overgrowth of tissue due to chronic injury. Within the oral cavity most of the so-called tumors are not true neoplasms but are hyperplastic reactions of connective tissue to chronic injury or irritation. The hyperplastic lesions are referred to as **reactive proliferations** because they represent self-limiting growths of fibroblastic tissue or a mixture of fibrous and vascular tissue resulting from chronic irritations such as cheek biting, ill-fitting dental appliances, or the negative pressure exerted by dentures. Within the oral cavity most local irritants are physical and stimulate the submucosal connective tissue, periodontal ligament, or the periosteum. The latter two locations become involved when the irritant is localized to the alveolus or gingival sulcus.

The true **benign neoplasms** of connective tissue found within the oral cavity arise from fibroblasts, endothelia, skeletal muscle, smooth muscle, lipocytes, nerve sheaths, and osteoprogenitor cells. Most are slow growing, but some are aggressive, causing extensive local destruction. Malignant connective tissue tumors, termed **sarcomas,** are rare. Their detection while still in the early stages of development is extremely important in providing the best opportunity for cure. As well as local aggressiveness, all sarcomas have the potential for metastasis. The degree of malignancy varies, and some are more life threatening than others. Unlike carcinomas that spread through the lymphatics, most sarcomas tend to spread via hematogenous routes, making dissemination more rapid and widespread. Box 9-1 lists benign and malignant connective tissue neoplasms found in the oral, head, and neck regions. Lesions of the oral connective tissue tend to be more common in some age groups and uncommon or even nonexistent in others (Box 9-2).

FIBROUS TISSUE

Fibrous proliferations occur as a result of reaction to injury, spontaneous benign neoplastic transformation, and malignant transformation of fibroblastic cells. The reactive hyperplasias are by far the most common growths encountered in the oral regions. True benign fibroblastic neoplasms or fibromas probably do not occur within the oral submucosa. The benign focal soft tissue growths found within the oral cavity are the result of reactive hyperplasias and are composed primarily of one or more of the following connective tissue components: mature collagen, focal bone formation, endothelial cells, and multinucleated giant cells.

■ BOX 9-1
Connective Tissue Neoplasms

Benign	Malignant
Desmoplastic fibroma	Fibrosarcoma
Benign fibrous histiocytoma	Malignant fibrous histiocytoma
Neurilemoma/neurofibroma	Neurogenic sarcoma
Granular cell tumor	Malignant granular cell tumor
Leiomyoma	Leiomyosarcoma
Rhabdomyoma	Rhabdomyosarcoma
Lipoma	Liposarcoma
Hemangioma	Angiosarcoma/Kaposi sarcoma
Lymphangioma	Lymphangiosarcoma

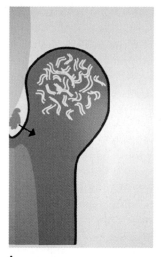 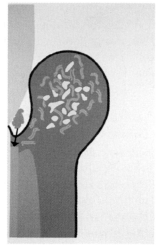 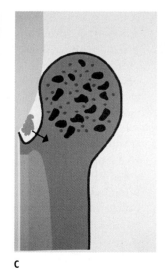 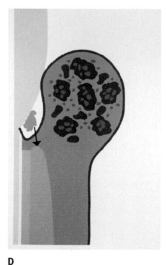

A   B   C   D

FIGURE 9-1

Diagram of distinguishing histologic features of a common reactive hyperplasia of gingival connective tissue clinically designated as an "epulis." Most lesions are thought to be reactive to a chronic irritant represented here as subgingival calculus. The *arrow* indicates the component of the gingival connective tissue that is stimulated. **A,** Peripheral fibroma: hyperplasia of superperiosteum resulting in overproduction of dense collagen *(white double lines)*. **B,** Peripheral ossifying fibroma: hyperplasia of periodontal membrane resulting in a cellular lesion consisting of fibroblasts and collagen *(green)* and "cemental" and bone deposits *(white)*. **C,** Pyogenic granuloma: hyperplasia of a vascular component of gingival connective tissue resulting in a cellular lesion composed of endothelial cells and small capillaries *(red)*. **D,** Peripheral giant cell granuloma: hyperplasia of the periosteum resulting in the overproduction of a vascular component *(red)* and mononuclear and multinucleated giant cells resembling osteoclasts *(blue)*.

When a reactive focal connective tissue proliferation is confined to the gingiva and its exact histologic nature is unknown, it is clinically designated as an **epulis.** The most common lesions referred to as epulides are peripheral fibroma, peripheral ossifying fibroma, pyogenic granuloma, and peripheral giant cell granuloma (Box 9-3); (Figure 9-1).

Even though the fibromatoses and fibrous histiocytomas are aggressive fibroblastic proliferations, they are considered by some sources to be reactive in nature instead of neoplastic. This is in spite of the fact that a history of injury to the area is seldom found. Therefore, because there is disagreement regarding their true nature, a group of connective tissue conditions, consisting of fibromatosis, nodular fasciitis, and benign fibrous histiocytoma, is considered to be **indeterminate,** that is, neither clearly reactive nor neoplastic. The malignant form of the fibroblast, fibrosarcoma, is an uncommon neoplasm encountered primarily in children and young adults. Most of the fibroblastic lesions arise within the soft tissue, but on occasion lesions are encountered within bone, mostly the mandible.

HYPERPLASIAS

Focal Fibrous Hyperplasia (Irritation Fibroma)

■ FOCAL FIBROUS HYPERPLASIA: hyperplasia of fibrous connective tissue that evolves in response to chronic irritation in which there is extensive elaboration of collagen resembling scar tissue.

■ **BOX 9-2**
Oral Connective Tissue Lesions by Age Groups

Infants
  Congenital gingival granular cell tumor
  Pigmented neuroectodermal tumor of infancy

Children
  Reactive hyperplasia
  Fibromatosis
  Neuroma
  Hemangioma
  Lymphangioma
  Sarcoma

Adults
  Reactive hyperplasia
  Neural tumors
  Granular cell tumor
  Lipoma
  Sarcoma

■ **BOX 9-3**
Common Reactive Hyperplasia of Gingival Connective Tissue (Epulis)

Peripheral fibroma
Peripheral ossifying fibroma
Pyogenic granuloma ("pregnancy tumor")
Peripheral giant cell granuloma

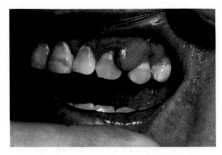

FIGURE 9-2

Focal fibrous hyperplasia. When located on the attached gingiva, lesions are referred to as peripheral fibroma.

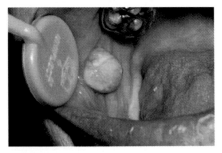

FIGURE 9-3

Focal fibrous hyperplasia. In other mucosal locations lesions are commonly referred to as irritation fibroma.

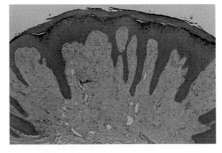

FIGURE 9-4

Focal fibrous hyperplasia. Microscopic appearance consisting of dense bundles of collagen. Because the lesion is usually chronically irritated, hyperorthokeratosis is commonly found on the surface of the epithelium.

A focal fibrous hyperplasia is not a true neoplasm of fibroblasts but an exuberant reaction to chronic injury in which the production of mature bundles of collagen predominates. Cheek and lip biting along with denture irritation are the most common contributing factors. The resulting lesion, commonly referred to as **irritation fibroma,** represents a pathologic overgrowth of both fibroblasts and their collagenous products. It is the most common *nodular* swelling found within the oral cavity.

CLINICAL

Focal fibrous hyperplasia is most often encountered in adults and is primarily located on the gingiva (Figure 9-2), lips, and buccal mucosa (Figure 9-3). Other common sites are the borders of the tongue. These nodular lesions usually occur on the soft tissue in the plane of the occlusal line. The clinical appearance of irritation fibroma is that of a domelike growth with a smooth mucosal surface of normal coloration. Ulceration is rare yet may occur if the patient continues to irritate the swelling. Surface hyperkeratosis is sometimes encountered and is probably due to a low-grade chronic irritation of the overlying epithelium. Lesions may remain the same size for many years. It is of importance that they cannot be positively diagnosed by clinical examination only because other mesenchymal tumors may show similar clinical features. When the irritant is removed, lesions often become slightly smaller as the inflammatory component diminishes yet they will not completely regress. For this reason it is usually recommended that they be excised and submitted for microscopic examination. When focal fibrous hyperplasia is on the attached gingiva in the area of the gingival sulcus or interdental papilla, it is sometimes termed **peripheral fibroma.** The term *peripheral* is used to distinguish this innocous lesion from the more aggressive fibrous lesion that may occur centrally within the jaws. It is surmised that the gingival reactive proliferations evolve from an irritant that becomes entrapped within the gingival sulcus. Toothpick fragments, food debris, and calculus are common causative factors. Unfortunately, often at the time of clinical examination there is no evidence of an exogenous irritant within the sulcus. By the time the lesion has evolved, the irritant has probably dissolved or has been extruded.

HISTOPATHOLOGY

The surface epithelium may be intact, exhibit hyperorthokeratosis, or show foci of ulceration. This epithelium overlies an underlying mass of dense, fibrous connective tissue composed of significant amounts of mature collagen in a scarlike pattern (Figure 9-4). The spindle-shaped fibroblasts, common in some of the indeterminate fibrous lesions, are sparse. The fibroblastic nuclei are monomorphic in character, and the overall appearance is one of hypocellularity.

A histologic variant of focal fibrous hyperplasia, referred to as **giant cell fibroma,** occurs in the oral mucosa and has a counterpart that is occasionally encountered on the skin and genitalia. The giant cell fibroma is also considered to be a reactive fibrous proliferation. The name given to this variant is based on the presence of binucleated and trinucleated fibroblasts that tend to occur in close proximity to the overlying epithelium. These binucleated and trinucleated cells have oval, monomorphic-appearing nuclei with copious eosinophilic cytoplasm. They often assume a stellate appearance, resembling a "manta ray." When ulceration occurs, some irritation fibromas become infiltrated by mononuclear inflammatory cells and other features of inflammation. The peripheral fibroma of the gingiva will usually show histologic features identical to the irritation fibroma located in other oral locations. A hypocellular fibrous reaction is encountered with mature collagen fibers.

TREATMENT

Local excision is the treatment of choice, and the lesions seldom recur. They will not involute spontaneously because the excess collagen found is permanent. The giant cell fibroma variant appears to be no different in behavior from the focal fibrous hyperplasia. The peripheral fibroma of the gingiva is also treated by local excision but must be accompanied by periodontal root planing to ensure that all sources of irritation are eliminated.

Peripheral Ossifying Fibroma

■ PERIPHERAL OSSIFYING FIBROMA: gingival nodule consisting of a reactive hyperplasia of connective tissue containing focal areas of bone.

The peripheral ossifying fibroma is a reactive fibrous proliferation, probably of periosteal or periodontal ligament origin. Because the periosteum and periodontal ligament contain cells that synthesize both bone and cementum, the proliferation includes cells with osteogenic potential. These lesions are related to other reactive gingival swellings because irritation is considered to play a significant role in the etiology.

CLINICAL

This reactive lesion is more common in women and tends to occur during the reproductive years, especially the third and fourth decades. It is usually not found in children and the elderly. Peripheral ossifying fibroma is an "epulis" that emanates from the interdental papillae, although occasionally it is seen to arise from the facial or lingual attached gingiva (Figure 9-5). Invariably, the mass originates from within the periodontal ligament, where an irritant is thought to be responsible for stimulating periodontal ligament fibroblasts that also possess osteogenic and cementogenic potential. The overlying mucosa may be smooth and of normal coloration, or there may be foci of surface ulceration. They are hard to palpate and are fixed to the underlying tissue. Dental radiographs will often disclose radiopacities within the soft tissue swelling.

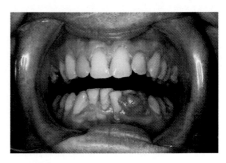

FIGURE 9-5

Peripheral ossifying fibroma. Lesions frequently become large and interfere with mastication.

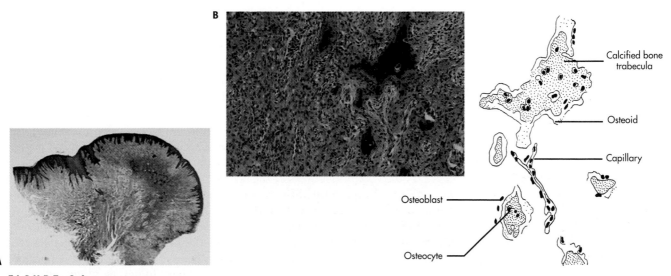

FIGURE 9-6

Peripheral ossifying fibroma. A, Low-power microscopy reveals a rounded mass with a zone of cellular connective tissue *(right side of lesion)*. **B,** High-power microscopy of cellular zone and accompanying tracing demonstrates the islands of calcified bone trabeculas, osteoid deposits, osteoblasts, and osteocytes that distinguish the lesion from a peripheral fibroma.

HISTOPATHOLOGY

Within the connective tissue are diffuse sheets of fibroblasts with plump monomorphic nuclei. The overall picture is one of hypercellularity, with the collagenous component somewhat hyalinized. There is no true capsule; the hypercellular zones slowly merge with mature fibrous and granulation tissues around the periphery (Figure 9-6, A). In focal areas osteoid deposits can be identified, and although some may contain lacunae with osteocyte nuclei, others are acellular (Figure 9-6, B). Rarely, thick mature trabeculas of bone are seen. The hypercellular component usually extends into the periodontal ligament.

TREATMENT

Peripheral ossifying fibroma must be excised to include the periodontal ligament. Thorough periodontal root planing is recommended to remove irritants trapped within the sulcus.

Peripheral Giant Cell Granuloma

> ◼ PERIPHERAL GIANT CELL GRANULOMA: an extraosseous nodule composed of a proliferation of mononuclear and multinucleated giant cells with an associated prominent vascularity found on the gingiva or alveolar ridge.

The peripheral giant cell granuloma is a hyperplastic reaction of the gingival connective tissue in which the histiocytic and endothelial cellular components predominate. These two cell types are intermingled and arranged in a lobular pattern separated by a fibrous connective tissue containing large sinusoidal blood vessels. The name of the lesion is derived from the tendency of the mononuclear histiocytes to form large multinucleated giant cells; the peripheral (extraosseous) location of the lesion in contrast to the larger, more aggressive central (intraosseous) giant cell lesions; and their clinical course of the gingival lesions, which is similar to a reactive granulomatous response. The factors that initiate the lesions are unknown. Lesions containing similar giant cell tissue are found in other parts of the body but are mainly within bone. These central boney lesions may be associated with hyperparathyroidism ("brown tumor"), other benign fibro-osseous lesions, a hereditary condition ("cherubism"), or exist as a neoplasm (giant cell tumor).

CLINICAL

Peripheral giant cell granuloma is found in all age groups, with a slight peak in incidence in adults around 30 years of age and in children during the mixed dentition stage. It is more common in females and is nearly equally distributed between the mandible and maxilla. Although it occurs in both anterior and posterior regions, most are found anterior to the molars. Occasionally, lesions are found on the edentulous areas of the alveolar ridges.

Lesions begin as a reddish or purplish dome-shaped swelling of the interdental papillae or alveolar ridge (Figure 9-7). In the dentulous patient they are often more reddish due to the ulceration that occurs when food is masticated and impinges on the thinned epithelium of the extruded mass. Larger lesions usually encircle one or more teeth, often involving the periodontal ligament including the apex of the teeth (Figure 9-8, A). These lesions produce loosening and movement of the teeth. In the edentulous areas the lesions are domed, purple, and usually with an intact surface. A periapical radiograph commonly reveals a superficial saucer-shaped loss of cortical bone, and the more central area of the bone remains uninvolved.

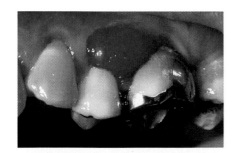

FIGURE 9-7

Peripheral giant cell granuloma. Lesions are commonly located in the interdental papilla.

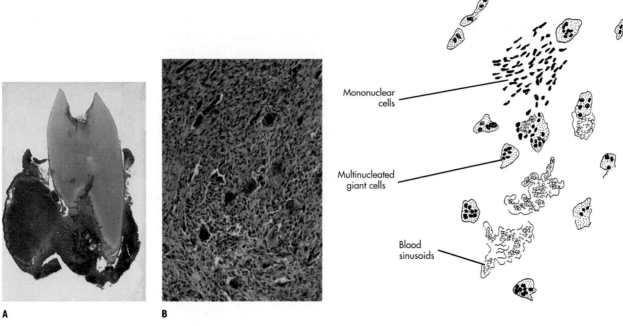

A   **B**

FIGURE 9-8

Peripheral giant cell granuloma. A, Low-power microscopy illustrating giant cell tissue within the periodontal membrane and surrounding the tooth. **B,** High-power microscopy and accompanying tracing of features of giant cell tissue illustrating the mononuclear and multinucleated giant cells and the irregularly shaped sinusoidal spaces.

HISTOPATHOLOGY

The microscopic appearance reveals a nodular arrangement of giant cell tissue separated by fibrous septa. The giant cell tissue consists of a mixture of mononuclear and multinucleated giant cells against a background of extravasated red blood cells (Figure 9-8, *B*). Some capillary vessels and sinusoidal spaces are usually present. The fibrous stroma may be loose or dense and contains large, thin-walled vascular structures. Heavy deposits of hemosiderin are common within the giant cell tissue and the surrounding fibrous component.

TREATMENT

Peripheral giant cell granuloma is treated by surgical excision. Removal must include all the giant cell tissue because recurrences are common. In the dentulous patient this usually requires removal of one or more teeth and curettage of the socket.

Inflammatory Fibrous Hyperplasia

■ **INFLAMMATORY FIBROUS HYPERPLASIA:** proliferation of fibrous connective tissue with an associated chronic inflammation in response to chronic injury.

Ill-fitting dentures with overextended flanges or older dentures that irritate vestibular tissue following alveolar ridge resorption may stimulate fibroblastic proliferation and collagen synthesis. These hyperplastic processes are most frequently found adjacent to denture flanges and tend to be multilobulated and diffuse. When they result from the impingement of an overextended flange, lesions usually contain an elongated trough with a linear ulcer (fissure) at its base. In the past it was commonly referred to as **"epulis fissuratum."**

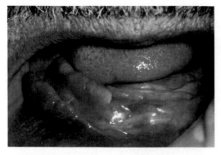

FIGURE 9-9

Inflammatory fibrous hyperplasia. With the denture removed the lesion reveals two linear folds of hyperplastic connective tissue with a central trough that is frequently ulcerated, thus contributing to the often accompanying intense inflammation. This lesion is commonly referred to as epulis fissuratum.

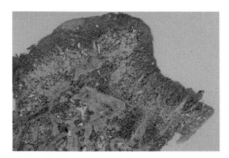

FIGURE 9-10

Inflammatory fibrous hyperplasia. Low-power microscopy exhibiting an abundance of dense fibrous connective tissue interspersed with focal accumulations of inflammatory cells and an increase in vascularity, all of which contribute to the excessive tissue.

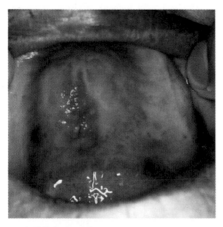

FIGURE 9-11

Inflammatory papillary hyperplasia. The lesion occurred under a denture that had been ill fitting for a prolonged period. The erythematous densely compacted nodules near the midline of the hard palate give the tissues a cobblestone appearance.

CLINICAL

Denture-induced fibrous hyperplasia is usually encountered in the maxillary or mandibular anterior vestibule where it is associated with an ill-fitting denture that has overextended denture flanges. The hyperplastic tissue is frequently lobulated or in folds and may be fissured where the denture flange impinges on the tissue at the base of the linear troughs (Figure 9-9). Most of these hyperplastic growths are erythematous due to the areas of ulceration. Occasionally, they may be normal in color. They are consistently flabby, soft, and movable and may occur anywhere along the margins of the prosthesis; the anterior locations are most common.

HISTOPATHOLOGY

The surface stratified squamous epithelium is frequently hyperplastic, demonstrating acanthosis with elongated rete ridges. Occasionally, zones of ulceration are encountered and the ulcerated areas are occupied by fibrin with entrapped leukocytes. The bulk of the tissue is composed of mature, fibrous connective tissue that is hypocellular. Spindle-shaped fibroblasts are interposed between dense collagen fibers in a scarlike pattern (Figure 9-10). When the fibrous hyperplasia extends into the lip and buccal mucosa, minor salivary gland lobules may be identified and will usually show acinar degeneration and ductal dilatation with inflammatory cell infiltration (chronic sclerosing sialadenitis).

TREATMENT

Diffuse inflammatory fibrous hyperplasia associated with an irritating dental prosthesis will not resolve completely on its own, even if the denture irritation is corrected or the denture is withdrawn. Lesions often become smaller when the denture is withdrawn, altered, or rebased due to the reduction in the inflammation. The permanently formed fibrous component will remain, resulting in an irregular, unstable area of soft tissue. For new prosthetic appliances to be satisfactory, the residual fibrous masses must be excised in their entirety before fabrication of a new dental prosthesis.

Inflammatory Papillary Hyperplasia

■ **INFLAMMATORY PAPILLARY HYPERPLASIA:** multiple small nodules that consist of a proliferation of fibrous connective tissue with an associated chronic inflammation found under ill-fitting dentures.

Some loose and ill-fitting maxillary dentures will initiate a hyperplastic response on the tissue of the palatal vault. This response is even more intense in dentures that have been made with a so-called palatal relief whereby negative pressure is placed against the palate. The palatal tissue responds by producing numerous small areas of erythematous focal fibrous hyperplasia that resemble the surface of a papilloma.

CLINICAL

Inflammatory papillary hyperplasia is confined to the palatal vault, seldom progressing onto the alveolar ridge. This is an important clinical observation because verrucous carcinoma, an aggressive epithelial proliferation, usually involves the alveolar ridge and vestibule and may extend to the palate, thereby resembling papillary hyperplasia. Inflammatory papillary hyperplasia is usually encountered under full dentures but occasionally occurs under the palatal coverage of partial dentures. The hyperplastic nodules are characteristically 3 to 4 mm in diameter with a generalized erythematous cobblestone pattern resembling a field of confluent reddish pink mushrooms (Figure 9-11). When probed with a dental instrument it can be seen that each polyp is independently attached.

HISTOPATHOLOGY

Tissue sections disclose an obvious polypoid appearance with multiple smooth, round nodules covered with stratified squamous epithelium. Where two papillary projections meet at their base, the epithelium is usually quite hyperplastic and displays acanthosis with elongated, anastomosing rete ridges (pseudoepitheliomatous hyperplasia). The individual epithelial cells fail to show any atypical cytologic features. The hyperplastic response is not confined to the connective tissue but also involves the overlying epithelium. Supporting each polypoid projection is a dense core of fibrous connective tissue that is traversed by capillaries. Scattered mononuclear inflammatory cells are usually dispersed throughout the connective tissue. This inflammatory component is quite variable and may be minimal in some cases.

TREATMENT

The hyperplastic tissue should be removed before fabrication of a new maxillary partial or complete denture. This may be achieved with a scalpel, a fluted burr on a rotary instrument, electrocautery, or laser surgery.

Hyperplastic Gingivitis

> ■ HYPERPLASTIC GINGIVITIS: focal or generalized fibrous hyperplasia of the marginal gingiva with an associated inflammatory response.

While the gingiva may be edematous and somewhat enlarged in chronic gingivitis and periodontal disease, it rarely becomes conspicuously enlarged. Such an occurrence is referred to as hyperplastic gingivitis and represents an exuberant inflammatory fibrous hyperplastic response usually to calculus and plaque that often is intensified by the patient's hormonal status.

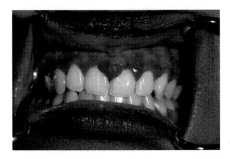

FIGURE 9-12

Focal hyperplastic gingivitis. The lesion is typically an erythematous enlargement of the interdental papilla of the gingiva. Milder degrees of gingivitis may be present in other areas.

CLINICAL

There is a predilection for this form of gingivitis in females because it is encountered with increased frequency during puberty and pregnancy **(puberty gingivitis** and **pregnancy gingivitis).** Conceptually it is postulated that hyperplastic gingivitis represents an excessive fibrous hyperplasia with an associated inflammatory cell infiltration that occurs in response to elevated estrogen and other hormone metabolites. The enlargements are centered in the interdental papillae where the tissue may be spongy and erythematous with a tendency to bleed with minimal provocation (Figure 9-12).

HISTOPATHOLOGY

The surface epithelium exhibits parakeratosis with marked acanthosis and epithelial hyperplasia characterized by elongated and anastomosing rete ridges. Transmigration by neutrophils into the epithelium is common. The submucosal connective tissue accounting for the zones of enlargement are represented by a unremarkable-appearing fibrous connective tissue with prominent vascularity. Disbursed throughout this tissue are mononuclear inflammatory cells—mainly plasma cells and lymphocytes. The clinical enlargement is due to both fibrous hyperplasia and mononuclear inflammatory cell infiltration.

TREATMENT

Dental prophylaxis with scaling and polishing may produce some resolution; however, the fibrotic gingiva usually fails to return completely to normal contour. Attempts to surgically remove the enlarged tissue will result in recurrence as long as the hormonal influences remain. In pregnancy gingivitis definitive treatment should not be performed until after delivery. Persistent enlargement that interferes with function can be managed by gingivoplasty.

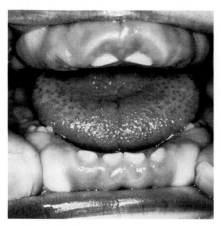

FIGURE 9-13

Hereditary gingival fibromatosis. The gingiva is firm, normal in color, and exhibits a generalized overgrowth that in some areas exceeds the height of the crowns of the teeth.

Hereditary Gingival Fibromatosis

■ HEREDITARY GINGIVAL FIBROMATOSIS: hereditary form of generalized gingival hyperplasia in which the autosomal dominant form may be associated with hypertrichosis, craniofacial deformities, epilepsy, and mental retardation.

Diffuse gingival hyperplasia may occur as a hereditary disorder. Although the precise mechanism of the disease is unknown, it appears to be restricted to the fibroblasts that populate the gingiva. The hyperplastic response does not involve the periodontal ligament and occurs peripheral to the alveolar bone within the attached gingiva. There appear to be at least two modes of inheritance, autosomal dominant and autosomal recessive.

CLINICAL

The gingiva becomes markedly enlarged and may cover the crowns of the teeth (Figure 9-13). The autosomal dominant form is most often associated with hypertrichosis and other defects including corneal dystrophy, cranial/facial deformities, nail defects, and deafness. In the forms occurring in children, epilepsy and mental retardation are sometimes present. In the autosomal recessive form facial anomalies with hypertelorism have been observed, but most forms are without defects other than the gingival enlargement. Consanguinity has been observed in the recessive forms of the disease.

In most patients the gingival enlargement begins at puberty and shows progressive proliferation that involves both the interdental papilla and the attached gingiva. Lingual and labial gingiva tissues may be involved. Clinically the gingiva is bulbous, firm, and hard yet usually retains its normal coloration. There is no sex predilection. The gingival enlargement is usually minimal but may be massively fibrotic, covering the crowns of the teeth. Eruption of teeth is normal.

HISTOPATHOLOGY

The surface epithelium exhibits elongated thin rete ridges. The fibrous connective tissue is densely collagenous with scattered mature spindle-shaped fibroblasts. There are significant numbers of mast cells associated with the fibroblastic proliferation. Inflammatory cells are essentially lacking. The tissue reaction is usually indistinguishable from other forms of gingival fibromatosis, including those associated with medications.

TREATMENT

Gingivectomy is the treatment of choice for patients in whom the gingiva becomes massively enlarged and covers the clinical crowns. Following surgery the tissue will recur but may take many months or even years to reach the massive size observed in patients who develop severe forms of the disease. Better oral hygiene practices do not appear to influence the degree of hyperplasia.

Drug-Induced Gingival Hyperplasia

■ DRUG-INDUCED GINGIVAL HYPERPLASIA: generalized increase in the fibrous component of the gingiva in patients who have been taking long-term doses of, cyclosporine and nifedipine.

The three pharmaceutical agents that most commonly have an effect on gingival fibroblast proliferation are phenytoin (Dilantin); cyclosporine; and nifedipine, a calcium channel blocker. Persistent dental plaque and gingival irritation appear to increase the severity of the hyperplasia.

CLINICAL

The gingival enlargement encountered due to Dilantin and nifedipine are clinically similar. They tend to begin in the interdental area involving the papilla and progressively enlarge until the crown is obscured (Figure 9-14). Clinically, the enlargement is diffuse and firm. Inflammatory changes are variable and the enlargement appears to be more severe among patients who do not maintain good oral hygiene. Cyclosporine is frequently administered as an immunosuppressive agent in transplant patients. The hyperplasia associated with this drug is usually less severe than that encountered with Dilantin and nifedipine. The gingiva may assume a multinodular or papillary appearance. In most instances drug-induced gingival hyperplasia becomes obvious within the first year of drug administration. As the gingival enlargement progresses, periodontal **pseudopockets** form around the crowns of the teeth. The disease is restricted to the gingiva when Dilantin and nifedipine are the associated agents. In addition to the gingiva, cyclosporine is known to induce fibrosis in other organ systems including the retroperitoneum and the kidneys.

HISTOPATHOLOGY

The microscopic features of drug-induced gingival hyperplasia are similar to those seen in hereditary gingival fibromatosis. The epithelium is thin and the rete ridges are markedly elongated and delicate, showing anastomosis. The connective tissue is composed of dense mature collagenous fibers with widely dispersed spindle-shaped fibroblasts (Figure 9-15). Inflammatory infiltration is variable, usually depending on the extent of the patient's oral hygiene.

TREATMENT

Most patients cannot withdraw their medication, and therefore local treatment must be provided. Gingivectomy and gingivoplasty are often required for functional and cosmetic reasons. The fibrotic changes will slowly recur. Since the recurrence rate is accelerated by the accumulation of plaque and calculi, regular dental prophylaxis and rigid home care are mandatory.

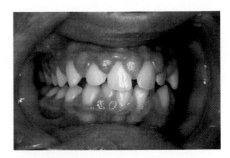

FIGURE 9-14
Drug-induced gingival hyperplasia. Patient with generalized gingival hyperplasia due to the administration of cyclosporine.

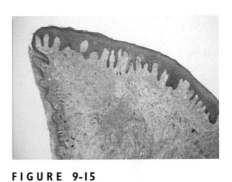

FIGURE 9-15
Drug-induced gingival hyperplasia. Microscopic features reveal elongated sulcular epithelium *(right side)* and hyperplasia due to excessive production of dense bundles of collagen in a scarlike pattern.

INDETERMINATE PROLIFERATIONS

Fibromatosis/desmoplastic fibroma, nodular fasciitis, and fibrous histiocytoma are considered **indeterminate proliferations.** Although these three forms histologically resemble the fibrous proliferations that arise in reaction to injury, they are slightly more aggressive, behaving more like benign neoplasms. Regardless of whether they are considered reactive proliferations or neoplasms, some proliferate rapidly, becoming large and displacing large portions of normal tissue. Although the lesions are aggressive and locally destructive, they do not metastasize. They are characterized by a cellular proliferation of fibroblasts and the elaboration of collagen fibers. It is the large increase in the number of fibroblasts that distinguishes this group of lesions from the more innocuous reactive fibrous hyperplasias that have been discussed previously.

Fibromatosis/Desmoplastic Fibroma

■ F I B R O M A T O S I S : benign diffuse infiltrative proliferation of fibroblasts and mature collagen occurring within the *soft tissues* of the head and neck in young patients.

■ D E S M O P L A S T I C   F I B R O M A : benign diffuse infiltrative proliferation of fibroblasts and mature collagen occurring primarily within the *mandible* in young patients.

The fibromatoses may occur anywhere in the body, yet certain sites such as the palms of the hands and the lateral neck are favored locations. A fibromatosis of the oral soft tissue is uncommon compared with the other reactive fibrous hyperplasias due to chronic irritation. The fibromatosis occuring within the bone of the mandible is a distinct, aggressive proliferation termed desmoplastic fibroma.

CLINICAL

Fibromatoses tend to occur in patients during the first and second decades of life; however, some are present at birth. There is no significant sex predilection. In the neck they appear as nodular masses within the deeper tissue, usually on either side of the sternomastoid muscle. They tend to grow slowly but sometimes show rapid enlargement. On palpation they are firm and may be movable. Some are markedly indurated and run the entire length of the lateral neck. When a neck lesion occurs bilaterally, it is referred to as **torticollis.** Individuals suffering from this form of fibromatosis appear to have a "webbed neck."

Similarly, oral submucosal fibromatosis is an aggressive lesion that can become large in a short period. Lesions in this area are firm, usually diffuse, and fixed to the surrounding tissue. They may involve the buccal mucosa, tongue, and submandibular regions. Most fibromatoses of the oral regions arise in the cheek or in the submandibular areas. When adherence to the mandibular periosteum occurs, it is common to have superficial erosion of the underlying bone (Figure 9-16).

Central (intraosseous) fibromatosis of the jaws is often referred to as **desmoplastic fibroma** of bone. Similar to soft tissue fibromatoses, the central fibrous proliferations arise in young patients and are aggressive. They cause bony expansion, displacement of the teeth, and resorption of the roots. Radiographically, a unilocular or multilocular radiolucency is observed, and the margins of the radiographic defect are usually relatively well demarcated. The mid-body of the mandible is the most common location for this tumor.

HISTOPATHOLOGY

Fibromatosis is characterized by a hypercellular proliferation of fibroblasts with accompanying mature collagen fibers. The individual fibroblasts are monomorphic, elongated, and typically spindle shaped (Figure 9-17). Cytologic atypia and mitotic activity are not encountered. The cellularity may predominate, and the elaboration of the collagenous product may be a relatively minor component. The elaborated collagen fibers are relatively thick and mature. In other lesions or even other fields of the same lesion, the collagenous component is more prominent and has a desmoplastic (scarlike) appearance. Fibromatoses may be relatively well demarcated; however, they are not encapsulated, and most tumors will infiltrate into neighboring muscle and other connective tissue, giving the impression of invasion. In torticollis of the neck, desmoplasia is a frequent feature.

TREATMENT

The behavior of these lesions varies depending on the site. Tumors arising in the lateral neck show continued proliferative capabilities, whereas in torticollis the proliferation appears to slow down and even arrest after puberty. A solitary fibromatosis is usually treated by a wide local excision to include normal adjacent tissue. Twenty-five percent of the tumors treated in this manner will recur. In the mandible the affected teeth must be extracted before the tumor is removed by curettage. Large expansile lesions require en bloc resection.

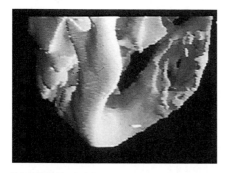

FIGURE 9-16

Oral submucosal fibromatosis. Computer generated 3-D CT radiograph of the mandible illustrating the erosion of the lingual cortical plate resulting from an adjacent fibromatosis in a young patient.

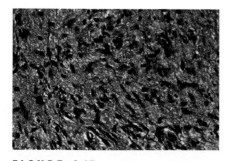

FIGURE 9-17

Oral submucosal fibromatosis. Microscopic features illustrating the uniform pattern of abundant spindle-shaped fibroblasts and mature collagen.

Nodular Fasciitis

■ NODULAR FASCIITIS: localized, benign lesion composed of fibroblasts and myofibroblasts that is often clinically mistaken for a malignancy.

Also termed "pseudosarcomatous fasciitis," nodular fasciitis represents a benign fibroblastic proliferation of the soft tissue. It exhibits unique microscopic features that allow differentiation from other fibroblastic proliferations. Nodular fasciitis is more commonly encountered in the extremities, with about 15% to 20% appearing in the head and neck regions.

CLINICAL

Within the oral cavity the lesion appears as a rapidly growing firm submucosal mass. Despite its rapid onset, its growth potential is limited. It may arise elsewhere within the upper respiratory system and the parotid gland. There is no sex predilection and the average age of a patient is 35 years. On palpation the tumor is firm and usually less than 5 cm in diameter and may even appear to be partially encapsulated.

HISTOPATHOLOGY

Confusion with fibrosarcoma is the most frequently encountered problem with nodular fasciitis because the cells exhibit some degree of pleomorphism and hypercellularity. The primary cell type is spindle or stellate in shape with the tissue demonstrating a tendency for a fascicular or swirled arrangement. Tissue spaces filled with extracellular mucin that have a myxoid appearance are prominent (Figure 9-18). Multiple mitotic figures may be encountered. In some instances multinucleated giants cells are present. Despite the high cellularity, individual nuclei are essentially monomorphic and uniform in appearance. Immunocytochemical marker research indicates that most of the fibroblastic cells are myofibroblasts because they stain positively for muscle-specific actin, smooth muscle actin, and vimentin.

TREATMENT

Local excision is the treatment of choice. Local recurrences have been recorded but are uncommon. Those that recur do so within a few months of the initial surgery and are usually the result of an incomplete excision.

Benign Fibrous Histiocytoma

■ BENIGN FIBROUS HISTIOCYTOMA: benign neoplasm of fibroblasts with a propensity to differentiate into histiocytes.

A benign fibrous histiocytoma is a fibrous proliferation that exhibits histiocytic differentiation. These lesions can be quite aggressive and are considered to represent true benign neoplasms of facultative fibroblasts. Facultative fibroblasts are mesenchymal cells that have the potential to differentiate into both fibroblastic and histiocytic cells. Some sources contend that benign fibrous histiocytomas are reactive proliferations, whereas others consider them benign neoplasms. A malignant variant is recognized.

CLINICAL

Benign fibrous histiocytoma may occur anywhere in the head and neck areas including the soft tissue of the oral regions. They are usually well demarcated and movable yet firm or even indurated on palpation (Figure 9-19).

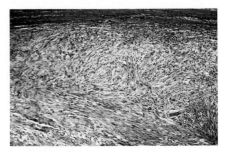

FIGURE 9-18

Nodular fasciitis. Low-power microscopy reveals a capsulelike outer boundary and a fibrous lesion containing abundant spindle and stellate cells against a slightly myxoid (loose) background with mucinous tissue spaces.

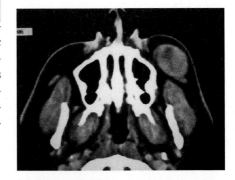

FIGURE 9-19

Benign fibrous histiocytoma. Radiograph of lesion overlying the zygomatic process.

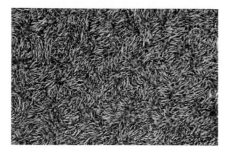

FIGURE 9-20

Benign fibrous histiocytoma. Tissue exhibiting the storiform pattern of the spindle-shaped fibroblasts and mature collagen.

HISTOPATHOLOGY

Fibrous histiocytoma is composed of elongated, spindle-shaped fibroblasts that elaborate mature collagen and large cells with oval nuclei and copious amounts of cytoplasm representing histiocytes. The borders are often infiltrative yet may be partially encapsulated or well delineated. The tumor cells are arranged in fascicles and whorls and are often tightly interwoven with hypercellularity. Those lesions located more superficially within the tissue will frequently show fibroblastic cellular arrays that resemble a "pinwheel." This is referred to as a *storiform pattern* and is characteristic of fibrohistiocytic lesions. In other tumors the fibroblastic element is more loosely arranged and forms alternating fascicles and whorls (Figure 9-20). Mitotic figures are uncommon. Interposed among the fibroblastic elements, often in isolated groupings, are histiocytic cells, which may show pleomorphic nuclei. Some of these cells have intensely stained cytoplasms and may be multinucleated; others will have foamy cytoplasms, which is accounted for by the presence of intracytoplasmic lipids. These latter cells are referred to as "xanthoma cells."

TREATMENT

Fibrous histiocytomas are aggressive proliferations that may become multinodular and reach large dimensions. Some appear to be self-limiting in their growth potential. Wide local excision is the treatment of choice; approximately 20% will recur within the first 2 years.

MALIGNANCIES

Fibrosarcoma/Malignant Fibrous Histiocytoma

■ **FIBROSARCOMA**: malignant neoplasm of fibroblastic cells.

■ **MALIGNANT FIBROUS HISTIOCYTOMA**: malignant neoplasm of fibroblasts with a propensity to differentiate into histiocytic and fibrohistiocytic cells.

When fibroblasts become malignant, the resulting lesion is aggressive and destructive and is referred to as a **fibrosarcoma**. In some cases the malignant fibroblasts differentiate along histiocytic lines, and the tumor is termed a **malignant fibrous histiocytoma**.

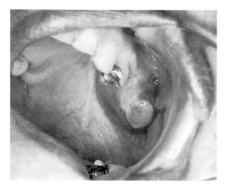

FIGURE 9-21

Fibrosarcoma. Extraosseous lesion of the posterior left maxillary gingiva.

CLINICAL

Although both fibrosarcoma and malignant fibrous histiocytoma occur most frequently in the neck, they also occur within the oral soft tissue, where they may involve the gingiva (Figures 9-21 and 9-22), tongue, buccal mucosa, or floor of the mouth. There is no sex predilection. The age distribution varies between these two tumors because fibrosarcomas tend to occur in children, whereas middle age adults are more often affected by malignant fibrous histiocytoma. Both tumors are rapidly proliferating and are firm and indurated on palpation. They lack encapsulation and become fixed to adjacent tissue. Larger lesions may be associated with ulceration of the surface epithelium.

Both of these malignancies of fibroblasts can arise within bone. Fibrosarcomas are more often encountered within the mandible where they appear as sharply defined radiolucencies. Root resorption, tooth displacement, and cortical expansion are frequent. Malignant fibrous histiocytoma is the most common sarcoma to involve the maxillary sinus. Lesions are thought to arise from fibro-

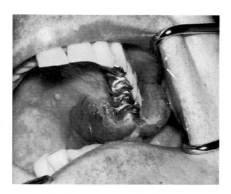

FIGURE 9-22

Malignant fibrous histiocytoma. Lesion of the posterior left alveolar ridge exhibiting ulceration.

histiocytic cells within the submucosal lining of the sinus. Malignant fibrous histiocytoma is rarely found within the mandible.

HISTOPATHOLOGY

Fibrosarcoma is a highly cellular tumor composed of anaplastic spindle-shaped nuclei with an eosinophilic cytoplasm that blends with delicate collagen fibers. Mitotic figures are numerous and many are atypical (Figure 9-23, *A*). The cells are arranged in fascicles, often with a "herringbone" pattern. The high mitotic rate and hypercellularity distinguish this lesion from other benign fibroblastic tumors.

Malignant fibrous histiocytoma is a highly pleomorphic fibroblastic tumor composed of spindle cells and a mixture of pleomorphic and multinucleated cells with copious eosinophilic cytoplasm. Foam cells may also be identified. The nuclei show marked pleomorphism, high mitotic activity, and bizarre or atypical mitotic figures (Figure 9-23, *B*). Fibrosarcoma and malignant fibrous histiocytoma lack a capsule and show borders that infiltrate adjacent tissue.

TREATMENT

Fibrosarcoma and malignant fibrous histiocytoma are aggressive, rapidly proliferating tumors that tend to metastasize to distant sites through vascular routes. Regardless of the therapeutic regimen, the prognosis is generally not good. Radical wide excision is the treatment of choice. In the jaws radical resection is recommended.

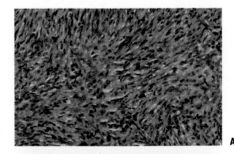

A

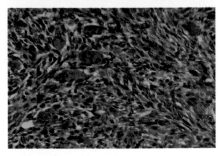

B

FIGURE 9-23

Medium-power microscopy features fibrosarcoma consisting of anaplastic spindle cells in a "herringbone" pattern **(A)** and malignant fibrous histiocytoma exhibiting pleomorphic and multinucleated spindle cells and abnormal mitotic figures **(B)**.

NEURAL TISSUE

The head and neck area contains the highest concentration of sensory nerve fibers of any location in the body. Reactive and neoplastic proliferations originating from the cells that ensheathe the neural axis cylinder are relatively common within the oral cavity and neck. When nerve fibers are injured, they undergo wallerian degeneration, whereby the distal axis cylinder segment degenerates and the proximal segment attempts to reroute itself through the existing Schwann cell sheath. This regeneration phenomenon is uncomplicated when the proximal segment is able to track itself into a juxtaposed distal nerve sheath. Alternatively, when the two ends are displaced, or lost completely as occurs with an amputation, a reactive hyperplasia of nerve and accompanying Schwann cells may develop during the futile attempt to rejoin with the distal nerve sheath. This hyperplastic response is termed **traumatic** or **amputation neuroma.**

The benign neoplasms derived from the cells that constitute the nerve sheath include **neurilemoma** and **neurofibroma.** Not only do these tumors arise from the nerve sheath, but they also differentiate in a manner that emulates the cells from which they were derived. The axis cylinder is enveloped by Schwann cells that form a continuous layer around the axis cylinder, much like insulation around an electric wire. These Schwann cells are capable of synthesizing myelin, which contributes to the insulating effect of the sheath. The neoplasm that is derived from the Schwann cell is the neurilemoma. The neuroectodermal tissue cells that synthesize collagen and create a binding network that envelops all of the individual axis cylinders with their associated Schwann cells are referred to as perineural fibroblasts. Within the nerve proper these cells resemble fibroblasts and constitute the endoneurium. These same cells, or their derivatives, also form an outer sheath around the entire nerve, referred to as the perineurium. These perineural fibroblasts are thought to give rise to the neurofibroma. The granular cell tumor, common in the tongue, may also arise from nerve sheath cells, although the sarcolemma of skeletal muscle may also be the cell of origin.

Most oral nerve sheath tumors are located in the tongue; however, because nerves are present throughout the oral cavity, any mucosal site may be affected. In the head and neck areas, nerve tumors are most commonly located along the course of the auditory nerve in the temporal bone or in the lateral neck. Whereas most of these tumors are solitary, neurofibromas can be multiple, constituting the syndrome referred to as **multiple neurofibromatosis** or **von Recklinghausen disease.**

HYPERPLASIA

Traumatic Neuroma

■ TRAUMATIC NEUROMA: painful nodular proliferation of nerve and fibrous tissue of the nerve sheath resulting from the futile attempt of nerve fibers to reunite with their severed distal portion.

Traumatic neuroma, also referred to as amputation neuroma, evolves when a nerve is severed and the proximal segment seeks to reunite with the distal nerve sheath in the process of regeneration. When the two nerve segments are displaced, the proximal segment undergoes axis cylinder elongation with the accompanying nerve sheath, which includes both Schwann cells and perineural fibroblasts. This vain attempt to reunify with the distal segment results in a tortuous proliferation of nerve tissue that clinically appears as a submucosal fibrous mass.

CLINICAL

Within the oral cavity the most common site for traumatic neuroma is along the distribution of the mental nerve, particularly in the area around the mental foramen (Figure 9-24). There is usually a history of laceration or trauma to the area. Traumatic neuromas in the neck may occur after trauma or surgery. The submucosal or subcutaneous neuroma is usually firm and painful on palpation. These hyperplastic nerve nodules are usually well encapsulated and movable within the underlying tissue.

HISTOPATHOLOGY

Because traumatic neuroma represents a hyperplasia of normal nerve and neural sheath elements, the microscopic features closely resemble that of normal nerve

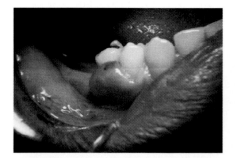

FIGURE 9-24

Traumatic neuroma. Lesion located over the mental foramen is usually firm and painful when palpated.

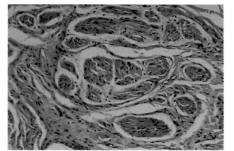

FIGURE 9-25

Traumatic neuroma. Medium-power microscopy reveals tortuous nerve bundles separated by dense fibrous connective tissue (scar tissue).

tissue and fibrous tissue, which are present in abundance. Multiple nerve bundles can be identified with axis cylinders, associated Schwann cells, and an enveloping perineurium. These nerve bundles are oval or elongated, tortuous, and separated from one another by mature fibrous connective tissue (Figure 9-25). Silver stains can be used to disclose the presence of axis cylinders.

TREATMENT

Because traumatic neuromas are often painful, surgical excision is recommended. A diagnosis cannot be based on clinical features alone but requires histopathologic examination. Simple surgical excision is the treatment of choice. Although recurrence is possible, most such lesions do not recur after complete excision.

HAMARTOMAS

Multiple Endocrine Neoplasia Syndrome

■ MULTIPLE ENDOCRINE NEOPLASIA SYNDROME: autosomal dominant condition involving the parathyroids, pancreas, thyroid, and adrenals with one variant (MEN-IIB) that has an oral manifestation consisting of multiple neuromas on the mucosal surfaces.

Syndromes consisting of multiple neoplasms involving different endocrine glands are inherited as an autosomal dominant trait. These syndrome complexes are collectively referred to as the *multiple endocrine neoplasia syndrome (MEN)*. Various endocrine tissues including the parathyroids, pancreas, thyroid, and adrenal tissues may be involved by either hyperplastic proliferations or malignant neoplasms. Only the variant of the MEN syndrome categorized as MEN-IIB exhibits oral manifestations. Patients with this variant of the syndrome develop malignant neoplasms, specifically a calcitonin-secreting medullary carcinoma of the thyroid gland and a catecholamine-secreting pheochromocytoma of the adrenal medulla. These endocrine tumors arise in association with the multiple mucosal neuromas that occur within the oral cavity and in the region of the eyelids.

CLINICAL

MEN-IIB is usually inherited as an autosomal dominant trait and has been associated with a mutation on chromosome 10. Occasional sporadic cases are also encountered. The oral neuromas appear as multiple submucosal nodules, revealing a smooth surface and measuring under 1 cm in diameter. These nodules are located in the submucosa of the upper and lower lips and on the anterior aspect of the tongue (Figure 9-26). Similar nodules may be encountered in the palpebral submucosa. These neuromas are hamartomatous nodules of neural tissue, and once they grow to a given size, they stop growing. Importantly, the oral neuromas are a harbinger for the development of endocrine neoplasia in the thyroid and adrenal glands. The neuromas usually occur during childhood, whereas the thyroid and adrenal tumors evolve during the second decade. The thyroid and adrenal tumors are malignant and have a potentially fatal outcome.

HISTOPATHOLOGY

The mucosal neuromas of MEN-IIB are remarkably similar in their microscopic appearance to traumatic neuroma. Intact nerve fibers represented by axis cylinders and accompanying Schwann cells are enveloped within a single perineurial capsule. Nerve cluster are separated from one another by mature fibrous connective tissue. The nerves of the neuromas of MEN-IIB are less tortuous than

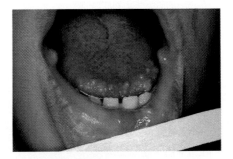

FIGURE 9-26

Multiple mucosal neuromas. Multiple small submucosal nodules of nerve tissue with smooth surfaces are present on the lips and tongue in patients with MEN-IIB syndrome.

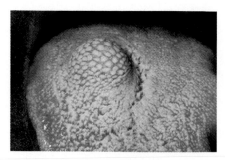

FIGURE 9-27

Neurilemoma. The dorsal surface of the tongue is a common intraoral location of this raised, firm, and movable lesion.

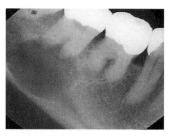

FIGURE 9-28

Intraosseous neurilemoma. Radiograph of lesion that is well demarcated and centered over the inferior alveolar nerve.

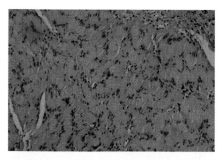

FIGURE 9-29

Neurilemoma. Medium-power microscopy features Antoni A tissue with its usual organoid pattern consisting of a central pink amorphous zone surrounded by palisaded spindle cells (Verocay bodies).

those of the traumatic or amputation neuroma; however, the two lesions may appear remarkably similar. Therefore the diagnosis is often based on the clinician's ability to detect multiple lesions within the oral cavity and on the eyelids.

TREATMENT

The mucosal neuromas are self-limiting hamartomatous lesions that usually require no treatment. Removal may be indicated for cosmetic reasons or when nodules interfere with mastication and speech. The recognition of the syndrome and the detection of the potentially fatal endocrine neoplasms of adrenal and thyroid glands is most important. These tumors are generally detectable utilizing imaging techniques. Surgical treatment is indicated.

BENIGN NEOPLASMS

Neurilemoma

■ NEURILEMOMA: well-demarcated, benign lesion consisting of a fibroblastic proliferation of the nerve sheath cell (Schwann cell) producing distinctive patterns referred to as Antoni A and Antoni B tissue.

CLINICAL

Neurilemomas typically occur as smooth, firm, raised, movable nodules within the oral soft tissue. They are common on the dorsal surface of the tongue (Figure 9-27). Lesions may also arise from the inferior alveolar nerve as a central lesion of the mandible. Central neurilemoma of the jaws presents as an expansile, well-demarcated radiolucency (Figure 9-28) centered around the inferior alveolar nerve. Large lesions may be multiloculated and cause tooth root divergence and bony expansion. Neurilemomas of the acoustic nerve, commonly referred to as *acoustic neuromas*, will often cause hearing loss. On the other hand, neurilemomas arising within the connective tissue of the neck may become large yet do not elicit pain, sensory deficit, or paralysis.

HISTOPATHOLOGY

Neurilemomas are composed of collagenous products. Myelin is not present because there are no axis cylinders to induce myelin formation by the neoplastic Schwann cells. Lesions are well defined with the presence of a true capsule or a pseudocapsule of fibrous connective tissue. The basic cell is spindle-shaped with an elongated nucleus. The cytoplasm cannot be readily delineated due to blending with the surrounding tissue. There are two distinct patterns that are pathognomonic for neurilemoma. The first pattern is referred to as the *Antoni A* tissue, which is represented by parallel rows of palisading nuclei. Frequently there are two palisaded configurations that are separated from one another by a cell-free zone, which is characterized by linear paralleling arrays of collagen fibers. These unique configurations are arranged in organoid swirls and are referred to as *Verocay bodies* (Figure 9-29). The second pattern is the *Antoni B* tissue, which is characterized by oval nuclei with surrounding collagen and distinctly vacuolated extracellular spaces. The *Antoni A* tissue forms multiple nodules that are interspersed by the *Antoni B* tissue (Figure 9-30).

A somewhat unique histologic variant, **palisaded and encapsulated neuroma,** occurs superficially and is well encapsulated and small. Lesions are solitary, firm, and sessile and found in middle-age adults. They are most common on the hard palate but have been found on other intraoral soft tissues. Nuclear palisading is quite prominent; however, the cell-free zones typical of *Antoni A* tissue are not conspicuous. Palisaded and encapsulated neuroma is thought to arise from tactile end organ fibers (Meissner corpuscles).

TREATMENT

Surgical excision is the treatment of choice for neurilemoma. Because tumors are well demarcated and encapsulated, they are easily dissected from the surrounding tissue. The recurrence for neurilemoma after excision or enucleation is less than 10%.

Neurofibroma

> ■ NEUROFIBROMA: demarcated or diffuse benign proliferation of perineural fibroblasts that are oriented in either a random pattern with a myxoid background or a nodular (plexiform) pattern.

> ■ MULTIPLE NEUROFIBROMATOSIS: autosomal dominant hereditary condition consisting of multiple neurofibromas of the skin and mucosa and associated café au lait pigmentations of the skin with the potential for producing disfigurement and malignant transformation.

The neurofibroma is derived from perineural fibroblasts and occurs with a variety of histologic subtypes. Some are diffuse and infiltrating, whereas others are multinodular and encapsulated. The majority of neurofibromas encountered within the oral cavity and neck are solitary. Occasionally, oral neurofibromas are a component of *multiple neurofibromatosis* (von Recklinghausen disease). This disease arises in patients who inherit a mutation in the NF gene, which encodes a tumor suppressor factor.

CLINICAL

Within the oral cavity neurofibroma is most frequently found in the tongue, followed by the buccal mucosa and the lips. Overall, solitary lesions of neurofibroma are most common on the skin (Figure 9-31). Most lesions are first noted in adults and show no sex predilection. They occur as relatively well-demarcated submucosal nodules. Depending on the degree of collagenization, they may be soft or firm on palpation. In the buccal mucosa they are either localized and freely movable or soft and diffuse.

In **multiple neurofibromatosis** neurofibromas may be encountered on both the skin and mucosal surfaces. Neurofibromatosis is inherited as an autosomal dominant trait with various subtypes. They are classified depending on the character and multiplicity of the tumors and the association with skin pigmentations. The neurofibromas in multiple neurofibromatosis may be nodular or diffuse. The nodular lesions vary in size from a few millimeters to many centimeters, are spherical, and produce a domelike elevation of the skin. The number of tumors per patient will vary from several to hundreds. Within the oral cavity they frequently are present as multiple diffuse soft tissue enlargements (Figure 9-32). The diffuse form can be quite grotesque with formation of pendulous tumor masses that may envelope an entire extremity. In the head and neck areas tumors of this nature may result in massive, flabby soft masses that emanate from the neck or involve the subcutaneous tissues of the face and scalp. This form of the disease has been publicized in the movie *Elephant Man*, which is about such a patient; the name is now attached to the disease by laypersons. Another classic feature of the disease is the presence of one or more large diffuse

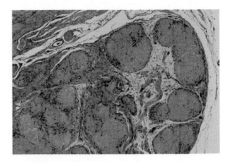

FIGURE 9-30

Neurilemoma. Low-power microscopy features Antoni A tissue *(nodules)* and Antoni B tissue *(background loose myxoid tissue)*.

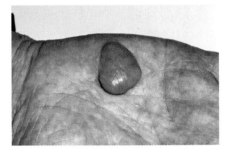

FIGURE 9-31

Solitary neurofibroma. Lesion of the palmar skin that is raised, firm, and smooth surfaced.

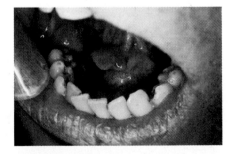

FIGURE 9-32

Multiple neurofibromatosis. Patient has multiple soft intraoral lesions of the floor of the mouth, lingual gingiva, and right retromolar area.

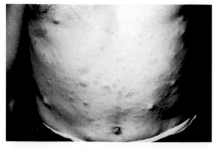

FIGURE 9-33

Multiple neurofibromatosis. Same patient as in Figure 9-32 with multiple neurofibromas and large pigmented macular lesions (café au lait spots).

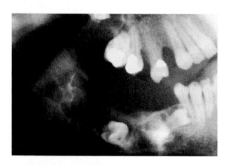

FIGURE 9-34

Intraosseous neurofibroma. Radiograph of a large, well-demarcated central (intraosseous) lesion of the posterior mandible that has displaced a molar.

macular brown pigmentations on the skin, referred to as the café au lait spots (Figure 9-33). The macular pigmentations represent a focal increase in the synthesis of melanin similar to skin freckles or melanotic macules. Rarely are café au lait spots seen on the oral mucosa. Repeated surgical excision of a neurofibroma may predispose the site to a malignant transformation into neurogenic sarcoma. Indeed, approximately 6% of patients with multiple neurofibromatosis will manifest malignant nerve sheath tumors.

The mandible is the most common site for intraosseous nerve sheath tumors, referred to as **central neurofibroma.** No other bone in the skeleton contains a neurovascular bundle as long as that which is present within the mandible. The presence of an intraosseous central neurofibroma is rarely associated with paresthesia or pain. These tumors are usually brought to the attention of the patient by a swelling of the mandible. Some tumors are found when the clinician investigates a radiolucency observed during routine procurement of dental radiographs. Radiographically, the central neurofibroma is relatively well demarcated, radiolucent, and may be unilocular or multilocular (Figure 9-34). As the tumor expands, it may cause root divergence.

HISTOPATHOLOGY

There are a variety of histologic patterns encountered in neurofibroma. The cells are spindle shaped and resemble fibroblasts. The clinically diffuse lesions are characterized by haphazardly arranged spindle-shaped cells that elaborate a delicate collagenous product. The cells fail to show any specific orientation (Figure 9-35, B). In some tumors a ground substance is a prominent finding, yielding a myxoid appearance. Tumors of this nature are frequently referred to as **myxoid neurofibromas** (Figure 9-35, B). Another variant is the **plexiform neurofibroma.** The plexiform variant is characterized by multiple nodules of fibroblastic tissue with a prominent myxoid appearance. Each nodule appears to have a pseudocapsule resembling the perineurium. When these encapsulated nodules are predominantly myxoid in appearance, the lesion is referred to as **nerve sheath myxoma.** The plexiform and diffuse myxoid variants are seen in multiple neurofibromatosis. Central neurofibromas are more often fibromyxomatous, lacking the multinodular encapsulated foci typical of the plexiform variant. The café au lait pigmentations are represented by basilar melanosis without the proliferation of melanocytes.

TREATMENT

The solitary neurofibroma is usually managed by excision. Because many of these tumors are diffuse, lacking discrete encapsulation, wide excision including

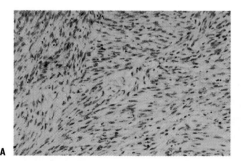
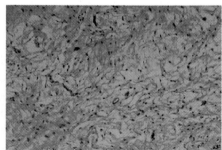

A   B

FIGURE 9-35

Neurofibroma. Medium-power microscopy features the two most common tissue patterns found in this lesion. **A,** Loose, delicate fibrous tissue containing haphazardly arranged spindle cells. **B,** Abundant mucinous ground substance with scattered spindle cells forming a myxoid connective tissue.

adjacent clinically normal tissue is the treatment of choice. Surgical removal of neurofibromas encountered in multiple neurofibromatosis may result in recurrence. Multiple recurrences have been associated with malignant transformation to neurogenic sarcoma. For this reason the neurofibromas in this condition are usually left untreated.

Granular Cell Tumor

■ GRANULAR CELL TUMOR: submucosal mass consisting of diffuse sheets of large cells of either nerve or muscle origin with a cytoplasm of densely packed eosinophilic granules (lysosomal bodies) and commonly found on the dorsal surface of the tongue.

Granular cell tumors are benign, submucosal neoplasms composed of large, oval cells containing prominent eosinophilic granules and small, round, monomorphic nuclei. Ultrastructural research has disclosed that the granules represent lysosomal or autophagic bodies. These cytoplasmic structures are ordinarily encountered in phagocytic cells and cells undergoing degeneration but in small amounts. The derivation of granular cells has been controversial with evidence supporting an origin from Schwann cells, whereas another line of evidence supports derivation from skeletal muscle. Because these cells show no specific features of differentiation other than the accumulation of autophagic vacuoles, it may be that they can arise from either Schwann cells or the sarcolemma of skeletal muscle. Regardless of their origin, granular cell tumors are benign. Even though they lack encapsulation, they rarely recur after excision.

CLINICAL

The granular cell tumor arises most frequently in the submucosa of the tongue, where it may be located in either the dorsal or lateral aspects (Figure 9-36). Uncommonly, it is also found on the ventral surface and in the soft palate. The lesion is extremely rare in other oral mucosal sites. It is of interest to note that of all areas in the body, the tongue is the most common site for this unique tumor. In the tongue and the soft palate a granular cell tumor presents as a firm, submucosal nodule or plaque, often with a yellow or orange tinge, that is nonmovable and lacks encapsulation. The surface mucosa is usually intact; however, on the dorsum of the tongue, the usual tongue papillae may be replaced by a smooth (atrophic) mucosal surface. Men are more commonly affected than women. Rarely, multiple granular cell tumors may be encountered in the oral mucosa and on the skin.

HISTOPATHOLOGY

Within the submucosa are diffuse sheets of large oval cells with distinct cytoplasmic membranes and discrete, punctate, eosinophilic granules. These sheets of cells are well delineated but lack encapsulation. In most granular tumors the granular cells extend upward to the epithelium and are present between the rete pegs. It is not uncommon for an epithelial proliferation to occur in response to these cells. The response is referred to as pseudoepitheliomatous hyperplasia and is characterized by elongated and branched rete pegs resembling the pattern of a neoplastic growth. (Figure 9-37). The epithelial cells lack cytologic atypia, a feature that differentiates this phenomenon from carcinoma. An erroneous diagnosis of squamous cell carcinoma has occasionally been rendered when insufficient submucosal connective tissue has been submitted for microscopic evaluation. Toward the inferior margin, continuity with the underlying skeletal muscle fibers is often apparent and frequently the granular cells appear to be emanating from individual skeletal muscle fibers. In other tumors the same granular cells

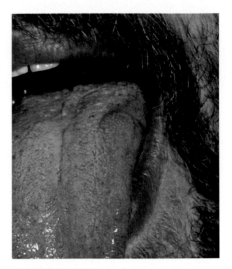

FIGURE 9-36

Granular cell tumor. Lesion located on the left lateral border of the tongue is raised, firm, and smooth surfaced.

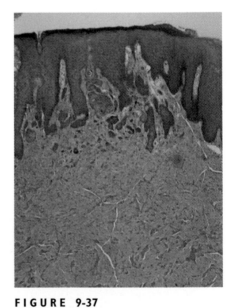

FIGURE 9-37

Granular cell tumor. Low-power microscopy of granular cells and overlying stratified squamous epithelium exhibiting pseudoepitheliomatosis hyperplasia.

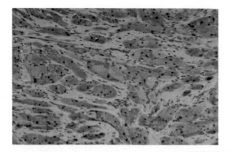

FIGURE 9-38

Granular cell tumor. High-power microscopy features granular cells intermingled with muscle cells and staining positive *(brownish color)* for S-100 protein.

are often found to emanate from nerve sheath cells. A small amount of fibrous stoma intervenes between the granular cells, although small vascular channels are present. When specific immunohistochemical markers are applied, the granular cells are strongly positive for the S-100 protein (Figure 9-38) yet often show positivity for skeletal muscle components including actin and myoglobin.

TREATMENT

The granular cell tumor may be treated by simple local excision. Recurrence is rare.

Congenital Gingival Granular Cell Tumor

■ CONGENITAL GINGIVAL GRANULAR CELL TUMOR: pedunculated growth on the anterior maxilla or mandible of newborns that is composed of granular cells.

The congenital gingival granular cell tumor is also referred to as *congenital epulis of the newborn* and *congenital granular cell epulis.* Although the cells appear to be similar to those of the granular cell tumor frequently found in the adult when viewed with light microscopy, there are some minor differences when studied ultrastructurally and immunohistochemically. As with the granular cell tumor, the tissue of origin is still controversial.

CLINICAL

Lesions are found only in the newborn, predominantly in the anterior maxilla (Figure 9-39), with occasional lesions in the anterior mandible. They occur far more frequently in females than males. The lesions are pedunculated, emanating from the crest of the alveolar ridge, have a smooth surface, and measure up to several centimeters in diameter.

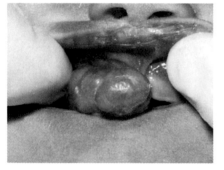

FIGURE 9-39

Congenital gingival granular cell tumor. A 7-day-old infant with a pedunculated, multilobular lesion of the anterior alveolar ridge.

HISTOPATHOLOGY

Contrary to the previously discussed granular cell tumor in adults, there is not only an absence of pseudoepitheliomatous hyperplasia of the overlying epithelium in the congenital gingival granular cell tumor but the epithelium is also usually atrophic (Figure 9-40, *A*). The lesion is composed of sheets of large cells with a granular cytoplasm and a vascular, noncollagenous stroma (Figure 9-40, *B*). The ultrastructural features of the congenital gingival granular cell tumor differ by not exhibiting angulate bodies in the cytoplasm; however, both lesions contain autophagic vacuoles. Lesions are negative for the S-100 protein.

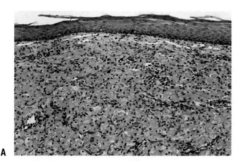 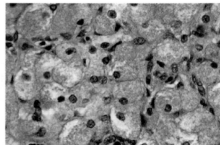

A   B

FIGURE 9-40

Congenital gingival granular cell tumor. A, Low-power microscopy of a lesion exhibiting a uniform pattern of granular cells with an outer surface of atrophic stratified squamous epithelium. **B,** High-power microscopy of large, rounded cells with granular cytoplasm and rounded nuclei.

TREATMENT

Lesions are treated by surgical excision that includes the base of the stalk. Recurrences are rare.

Neuroectodermal Tumor of Infancy

■ NEUROECTODERMAL TUMOR OF INFANCY: benign, usually pigmented neoplasm commonly of the anterior maxilla and composed of two cell types arranged in alveolar patterns and derived from embryonic neural crest tissue.

The neuroectodermal tumor of infancy is a benign congenital lesion derived from tissue of the primative neural crest. Its true origin was not revealed until recently when it was discovered that patients with lesions also had high urinary levels of vanilmandelic acid as is found in patients with neuroblastoma and pheochromocytoma conditions, with lesions that are known to be of neuroectodermal origin.

CLINICAL

Lesions occur as pigmented swellings, commonly of the anterior maxilla. They appear in infants usually before the age of 6 months, presenting as an elevation of the lip. The surface may have a brown or black pigmentation, reflecting the melanin produced by the large cell component of the lesion (Figure 9-41). Radiographs often exhibit an intraosseous radiolucency with displacement of tooth buds. Approximately one quarter of the lesions found within the oral cavity occur in the mandible. Other sporadic locations include the shoulder, scapula, anterior fontanel, cerebellum, and mediastinum.

HISTOPATHOLOGY

The tissue is composed of two cell types against a dense fibrous connective tissue background. One type is large with an open nucleus and a lightly staining cytoplasm that occasionally contains melanin granules. The other cell type is small with a dark, dense nucleus and scant cytoplasm, resembling lymphocytes. The cells are commonly clustered and arranged in alveolar patterns (Figure 9-42).

TREATMENT

The neuroectodermal tumor of infancy is treated surgically and can be effectively eradicated with thorough curettage or conservative surgical resection. Recurrences are uncommon.

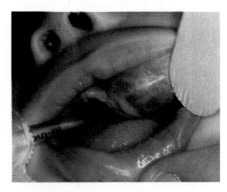

FIGURE 9-41

Neuroectodermal tumor of infancy. Lesion of a newborn producing a deformity of the anterior maxilla and lip. The mucosal surface exhibits a small amount of the pigmentation commonly found in these lesions. (Courtesy Dr. M. Rohrer, Dr. S. Young, and Dr. F. Rubin.)

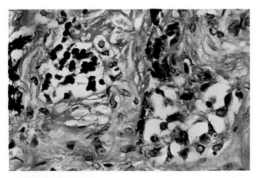
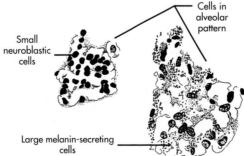

FIGURE 9-42

Neuroectodermal tumor of infancy. High-power microscopy exhibits two cell types arranged in alveolar patterns: small dark cells with a dense nucleus *(left)* and large clear cells with open nuclei and producing melanin granules *(right)*.

MALIGNANT NEOPLASMS

Neurogenic Sarcoma

■ NEUROGENIC SARCOMA: malignant neoplasm with a poor prognosis of perineural fibroblasts or Schwann cells with a propensity to rapidly extend along the associated nerve trunk.

Although malignant nerve sheath tumors are occasionally encountered in the deep connective tissue of the neck, they are extremely rare in the oral cavity and jaws.

CLINICAL

As mentioned previously, malignant transformation can occur in neurofibromas, particularly those that have been subjected to repeated surgical excision for recurrence in patients with multiple neurofibromatosis. Most malignant nerve sheath tumors of the head and neck regions are encountered in the deep soft tissue of the neck and arise de novo. Oral submucosal neurogenic sarcoma is extremely rare; but when such a tumor occurs, it grows rapidly and is indurated and nonmovable. Neurogenic sarcoma is more common within the mandible than in the soft tissue arising from the nerve sheath cells of the inferior alveolar nerve. Radiographically, it frequently manifests as a fusiform widening of the inferior alveolar canal, as evidenced by a radiolucent appearance. Root resorption is not prominent. Clinically, the patient may complain of paresthesia of the lower lip, and expansion of the mandible is usually observed.

HISTOPATHOLOGY

Neurogenic sarcoma is characterized by a highly cellular tumor composed of fascicles of spindle-shaped nuclei (Figure 9-43). These fascicles sometimes show a resemblance to Antoni A tissue, but most are indistinguishable from fibrosarcoma. Therefore the diagnosis must be based on identifying that the tumor is in direct continuity with a nerve trunk. The nuclei are pleomorphic, and numerous mitotic figures are seen. An important feature of this lesion is the extension of the malignant neoplasm along the course of the involved nerve. Central neurogenic sarcomas of the mandible frequently extend along the inferior alveolar nerve, out the lingula, and superior toward the cranial base and gasserian ganglion.

TREATMENT

Soft tissue neurogenic sarcoma must be treated by wide surgical excision. Local recurrence is a common complication, and hematogenous metastasis occurs in over 50% of the cases. Central neurogenic sarcoma of the mandible must be treated by mandibulectomy with wide excision and dissection along the nerve trunk up to the base of the skull. Despite aggressive surgery, local recurrence is common and distant metastases may ensue. The tumor is resistant to radiation therapy, and chemotherapeutic approaches have not proven effective.

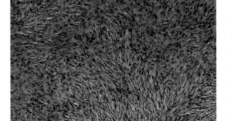

FIGURE 9-43

Neurogenic sarcoma. Medium-power microscopy reveals fascicles of malignant spindle cells resembling fibrosarcoma.

MUSCLE TISSUE

Both benign and malignant tumors of muscle origin can arise within the oral cavity and in the regions of the head and neck, but they are uncommon. Only the granular cell tumor occurs with any degree of frequency in the tongue, and its origin from muscle cells is somewhat controversial. True tumors of striated muscle occur most frequently in the heart and are termed **rhabdomyomas** (Figure 9-44); the tongue is the second most common site for these rare tumors. The other benign muscle tumor, the **leiomyoma,** is derived from smooth muscle. These lesions are very common in the uterine cervix, where they are referred to as *fibroids.* Elsewhere in the body most leiomyomas, including those within the oral cavity, arise from the smooth muscle surrounding arteries or arterioles. When origin from blood vessel walls is apparent, these lesions are referred to as **vascular leiomyomas.** Malignant neoplasms of either skeletal or smooth muscle are extremely rare within the oral cavity; however, when the malignancy of skeletal muscle, **rhabdomyosarcoma,** arises, it is usually in the periorbital tissue of children or the deep connective tissue of the neck in adults.

NEOPLASIAS

Leiomyoma

> ■ LEIOMYOMA: benign neoplasm of smooth muscle within the oral cavity, usually of the blood vessels, that appears as a firm, movable, submucosal nodule.

Leiomyomas are benign tumors of smooth muscle. Within the oral cavity they are usually derived from the smooth muscle component of the blood vessels.

CLINICAL

Although the most common site within the oral cavity is the tongue, lesions also occur on the palate (Figure 9-45) and the lips. Leiomyoma arises during the adult years and has no sex predilection. In addition to the usual source of smooth muscle cells from the wall of blood vessels, it is conceivable that pleuripotential mesenchymal cells within the connective tissue may give rise to this tumor. Leiomyoma is uncommon and usually appears as a smooth-surfaced submucosal nodule. The overlying epithelium lacks ulceration and may have a yellowish appearance. On palpation, the tumors are firm and usually well delineated. In the loose tissues of the lip and buccal mucosa, they are freely movable.

HISTOPATHOLOGY

Leiomyomas are composed of spindle-shaped smooth muscle cells with elongated nuclei that resemble fibroblasts. Because leiomyoma cells lack distinct cell margins, the cytoplasm of one cell appears to be fused to the adjacent cells. The elongated nuclei generally show blunt ends, resulting in a "cigar-shaped" appearance. These neoplastic cells are arranged in parallel fascicles, and lesions are either encapsulated or well delineated from the surrounding tissue. An intervening fibrous stroma is not evident, and only small capillaries are observed between the tumor cells. Differentiation from neurofibroma is often difficult. Because smooth muscle cells and fibroblastic cells are normally pink with routine hematoxylin and eosin (H&E) staining, differentiation between these two lesions is assisted by applying a trichrome stain. This latter stain differentiates the cytoplasmic elements of smooth muscle cells *(pink)* from the collagenous structures of fibroblasts *(blue or green).* Monoclonal antibodies to muscle-specific actin are also useful in confirming the diagnosis. Because most oral leiomyomas arise from perivascular cells, they show concentric laminations around endothelial-lined lumens (Figure 9-46). The vascular element is minimal and the laminated smooth muscle cells dominate the histologic fields.

TREATMENT

Local excision including adjacent normal-appearing tissue is the treatment of choice. These benign, smooth muscle tumors rarely recur when completely excised.

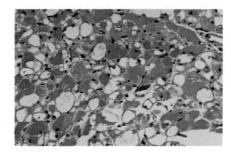

FIGURE 9-44

Rhabdomyoma. Medium-power microscopy of this rare benign neoplasm exhibits large round muscle cells rather than the elongated strap cells of normal muscle.

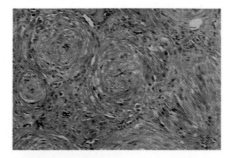

FIGURE 9-45

Vascular leiomyoma. The lesion is located on the palate as a firm submucosal swelling with a smooth intact surface.

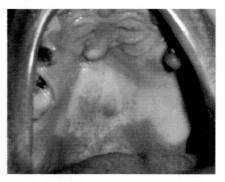

FIGURE 9-46

Vascular leiomyoma. Medium-power microscopy demonstrates the concentric laminations of smooth muscle cells around vascular channels that are nearly completely obliterated and a surrounding cellular fibrous connective tissue.

Rhabdomyosarcoma

> ■ RHABDOMYOSARCOMA: rare, rapidly growing malignant neoplasm of striated muscle that occurs in three histologic patterns (embryonal, alveolar, and pleomorphic); all have a poor prognosis.

Rhabdomyosarcoma is the malignant neoplasm of skeletal (striate) muscle. It is subcategorized into three microscopic variants, some of which arise in children and others in adults. The *embryonal rhabdomyosarcoma* tends to arise in children and may be identified within the head and neck area. *Alveolar rhabdomyosarcoma* is rarely seen in the oral region. *Pleomorphic rhabdomyosarcoma* is more often encountered in adults where the cells bear a close resemblance to skeletal muscle fibers. These neoplasms may arise from an existing skeletal muscle bundle or be derived from pleuripotential mesenchymal cells of connective tissue. In the latter case they are not necessarily localized within a muscle per se.

CLINICAL

In the head and neck areas the periorbital region is the most common site for rhabdomyosarcoma. These tumors occur during childhood and are usually of the embryonal type. Both sexes are equally affected. These tumors exhibit rapid growth with displacement of the eye. The tumors are indurated, fixed, and frequently ulcerated. Pleomorphic rhabdomyosarcoma is more often encountered in adults and may arise within the oral cavity.

HISTOPATHOLOGY

Rhabdomyosarcomas are composed of malignant rhabdomyoblasts. The **embryonal type** of rhabdomyosarcoma is characterized by small round cells with hyperchromatic, relatively monomorphic-appearing nuclei. Mitotic figures are common. Around the periphery of the tumor the anaplastic rhabdomyoblasts become condensed, whereas in the central regions the tissue is looser. The cytoplasm is usually wispy and indistinct. Small capillaries course throughout the tumor. The **alveolar rhabdomyosarcoma** is so named because the rhabdomyoblasts form conglomerate groups that assume a pattern similar to the lung alveoli or organoid structures. Individual cells resemble the round cells seen in embryonal rhabdomyosarcoma. **Pleomorphic rhabdomyosarcoma** is a more highly differentiated form, showing primitive muscle fiber formation. The nu-

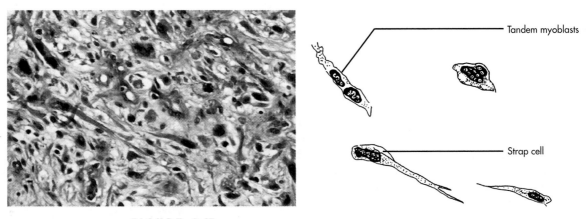

FIGURE 9-47

Rhabdomyosarcoma. Medium-power microscopy of the pleomorphic type of rhabdomyosarcoma exhibiting randomly distributed primitive and anaplastic muscle fibers, many of which are tadpole-shaped strap cells, whereas others are multinucleated with the cells in a linear pattern (tandem myoblasts).

clei are extremely pleomorphic and may contain prominent nucleoli. The tumor cells frequently assume a tadpole appearance, with a large pleomorphic nucleus and a brightly eosinophilic tail of cytoplasm (Figure 9-47). Many of these cells may show cross-striations that are demonstrated with a phosphotungstic acid–hematoxylin stain. Immunomarkers for skeletal muscle tumors, including desmin, muscle-specific actin, and myoglobin, stained positively in all three types of rhabdomyosarcoma.

TREATMENT

Rhabdomyosarcoma is a rapidly proliferating neoplasm with a marked tendency for hematogenous spreading and a poor prognosis. Embryonal rhabdomyosarcoma has a worse prognosis than the pleomorphic type. Surgery and radiation and combination drug chemotherapy are the modalities employed to treat these malignancies.

ADIPOSE TISSUE

Lipoma and liposarcoma are connective tissue tumors of adipose tissue origin. Lipoma is one of the most common benign neoplasms to arise in the neck and is frequently seen within the oral cavity. Lipoma is histologically identical to normal adipose tissue. Liposarcomas are rarely seen in the head and neck areas and are even rarer in the oral soft tissue.

NEOPLASIA

Lipoma

■ LIPOMA: benign neoplasm of normal fat cells that appears as a soft, movable swelling, often with a slight yellowish coloration.

The common lipoma is a benign neoplasm of adipose tissue composed of mature fat. Some variations exhibit more embryonic-appearing fat yet are still benign in nature. One such tumor occurs in multiple sites and is referred to as **multiple lipoblastomatosis.**

CLINICAL

Lipomas are usually relatively well defined, soft on palpation, and freely movable within the underlying connective tissue. There is no sex predilection. Most lesions occur in adults. In the neck they are usually encountered in the lateral regions along the sternomastoid muscle. Most oral lipomas arise within the superficial submucosal connective tissue (Figure 9-48). Some arise within the deeper tissue of the cheek and are detected only by palpation. The more superficial lipomas are often yellow and display a smooth overlying surface that may be telangiectatic. Fatty tissue within the buccal fat pad may herniate through the buccinator muscle. As the fatty tissue herniates through the damaged muscle fibers, it protrudes into the oral cavity as a buccal mucosal swelling. These **herniated buccal fat pads** reveal both clinical and histopathologic features that are indistinguishable from lipoma and are therefore diagnosed by obtaining a history of trauma.

HISTOPATHOLOGY

Lipomas are distinctive on gross examination because they are yellow and float in aqueous solutions such as the formalin fixative. Lipomas are usually well de-

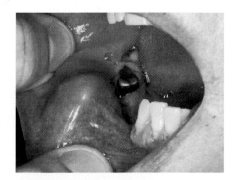

FIGURE 9-48

Lipoma. The lesion is a soft, movable submucosal mass of right buccal mucosa.

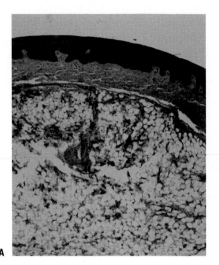
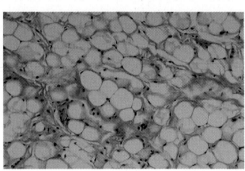

A

B

FIGURE 9-49

Lipoma. A, Low-power microscopy demonstrates the sharply demarcated nodular mass of normal-appearing adipose tissue. **B,** Medium-power microscopy reveals the clusters of normal fat cells with the nucleus barely visible.

fined, although they may not display a surrounding capsule. The adipocytes are identical to normal fat cells and exhibit a round, vacuolated clear cytoplasm with an eccentrically placed nucleus. Most lipomas have lobules of fat cells that are separated by fibrous septa (Figure 9-49). This same appearance is identifiable in herniated buccal fat pads. Occasionally, lipomas contain benign lipoblasts. These cells are characterized by a soap bubble appearance of vacuoles within the cytoplasm and multinucleated cells with nuclei arranged in a floret pattern. These are sometimes mistaken for malignant cells. This variant is referred to as **pleomorphic lipoma.** In some benign lipomas there may be significant amounts of myxomatous tissue in addition to the fat cells.

TREATMENT

Simple excision is the treatment of choice. Lipomas located deep within the tissue rarely recur after enucleation. Those arising in the submucosa of the oral cavity are usually treated by excision.

Liposarcoma

> ■ LIPOSARCOMA: rare, malignant neoplasm of the oral cavity composed of a wide spectrum of histologic patterns of the fat cells.

Liposarcomas are usually encountered in the extremities and are infrequently observed in the head and neck regions. They are derived from cells that differentiate along adipose tissue lines and show some evidence of fat synthesis.

CLINICAL

Malignant neoplasms with adipose tissue differentiation are usually multilobular and vary from firm to soft. There is usually a history of rapid growth. Liposarcomas usually arise de novo rather than through a malignant transformation of a preexisting lipoma. In the head and neck areas, they are more often encountered in the deep tissue of the neck. Within the oral cavity they may arise in the sublingual or buccal mucosa regions.

HISTOPATHOLOGY

There is a wide variation of morphologic patterns in liposarcoma, but common to all of them is the presence of lipoblasts. Some liposarcomas are composed of poorly differentiated round cells with only focal evidence of cytoplasmic vacuolization. Others display cells with a signet ring appearance in which the nucleus is prominently displaced to the side of a large vacuole. Some liposarcomas are highly anaplastic, whereas others show clear evidence of fatty differentiation (Figure 9-50).

TREATMENT

Like other sarcomas, liposarcomas tend to metastasize to distant sites such as the lungs, bone, and brain. The treatment of choice is surgical intervention with radical excision.

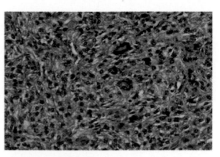

FIGURE 9-50

Liposarcoma. Medium-power microscopy exhibiting primitive lipoblasts with little evidence of fat production along with pleomorphic and multinucleated anaplastic cells.

VASCULAR TISSUE

Most vasoproliferative masses within the oral cavity are forms of reactive granulation tissue in response to injury. The neoplasms are derived from the lining of the endothelial cells of blood vessels and are referred to as **hemangiomas** and those derived from lymphatic vessels as **lymphangiomas.** Because hemangiomas are composed of numerous proliferating vascular channels containing erythrocytes, they usually appear clinically as red, purple, or blue lesions. Some hemangiomas are flat or macular, representing a superficial proliferation of vessels that fails to generate a tumefaction. Others are obvious swellings. Lymphangiomas contain lymphatic fluid, tend to be superficial, and appear as yellowish masses whereas the less common deeper lesions are usually of normal coloration. Some hemangiomas lie deep within the tissue, particularly those that are interposed between muscle fibers, so-called "intramuscular hemangioma." These lesions may have no discoloration of the surface mucosa or skin and are much more difficult to manage.

The mandible is the most common site in the body for vascular proliferations located within bone. These proliferations commonly evolve in patients early in life and represent arteriovenous anastomoses in which an intervening capillary bed is lacking. Lymphatic malformations of a similar nature do not occur within the mandible or maxilla.

HYPERPLASIA

Pyogenic Granuloma

> ■ PYOGENIC GRANULOMA: fast-growing reactive proliferation of endothelial cells commonly on the gingiva and usually in response to chronic irritation.

A focal reactive growth of fibrovascular or granulation tissue with extensive endothelial proliferation is termed a **pyogenic granuloma.** The term would imply that such lesions react to infection with pyogenic microorganisms. In fact, there is no relationship between bacteria and the emergence of these reactive proliferations. The tissue is infiltrated with many neutrophils, accounting for the erroneous interpretation of a bacterial etiology. Pyogenic granulomas can occur anywhere in the body and are common on the fingers and toes around the nail beds. Within the oral cavity pyogenic granulomas are frequently localized to the gingiva, where they are included as part of the differential diagnosis of an "epulis." An **epulis** is a collective clinical term for focal growths of the gingiva. Trauma or

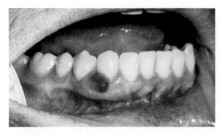

FIGURE 9-51

Pyogenic granuloma. This erythematous exophytic lesion is located in the interdental papilla where it receives continuous chronic irritation, resulting in an ulcerated surface.

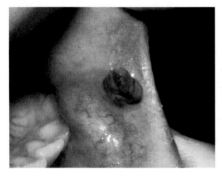

FIGURE 9-52

Pyogenic granuloma. A purplish pedunculated nodular lesion of the commissure area of the buccal mucosa.

introduction of foreign material into the gingival sulcus may provide the stimulus for this proliferative hyperplasia.

CLINICAL

Within the oral cavity pyogenic granuloma is most often encountered in the interdental papilla region (Figure 9-51). These lesions may extend from the buccal to the lingual or palatal gingiva; however, they are most often limited to either the buccal or the facial surface. Because they are extremely vascular, they are usually fiery red and will often show a grey pseudomembrane over the surface, secondary to ulceration of the overlying epithelium. There is a significant female predilection, and lesions tend to occur more often during the second and third trimesters of pregnancy. These lesions are often referred to as **pregnancy tumors.** Although they are benign hyperplastic reactions, they may grow at an alarming rate, reaching 1 to 2 cm in diameter within 4 to 7 days. Adjacent periodontal inflammation may be identified; however, pyogenic granuloma is unrelated to the regular forms of gingivitis and periodontitis. Pyogenic granulomas occur as exuberant granulation tissue responses after the removal of teeth, particularly the third molars. As such, the lesion emanates from the extraction sites, usually in response to an irritant that has fallen into the socket such as calculus, food, tooth fragments, or bone spicules. Pyogenic granulomas occur in other mucosal sites unrelated to the gingival sulcus, particularly on the tongue, lips, and buccal mucosa (Figure 9-52). In these locations it is assumed that biting of the tissue serves as the irritation that stimulates the hyperplastic response.

HISTOPATHOLOGY

Pyogenic granuloma is composed of granulation tissue, typified by a plethora of anastomosing endothelial-lined vascular channels engorged with erythrocytes and nodules of endothelial cells in medullary patterns (Figure 9-53). The endothelial cells are usually plump and vesicular, indicating active proliferation. Often the cells will have a pleomorphic character, and rarely, some of these actively proliferating hyperplasias closely resemble Kaposi sarcoma. Portions of the epithelium overlying the surface are usually ulcerated, leaving a fibrinous exudate with entrapped leukocytes. The loose connective tissue dispersed throughout the fibrovascular tissue and interposed between vascular channels is infiltrated predominantly by neutrophils and histiocytes.

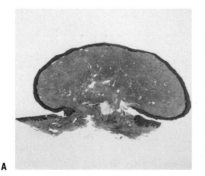
A

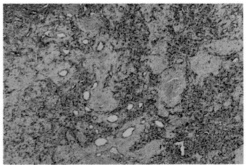
B

FIGURE 9-53

Pyogenic granuloma. A, Low-power microscopy demonstrating a raised lobular lesion with a thin stalk. **B,** Medium-power microscopy exhibiting a medullary pattern of endothelial cells intermingled with small vascular spaces and loose fibrous connective tissue. When ulcerated, lesions will also have acute and chronic inflammatory cells diffusely distributed throughout.

TREATMENT

Although these are reactive hyperplasias, they have a relatively high rate of recurrence after simple excision. If the patient is pregnant, recurrence is common. Whereas many pyogenic granulomas are quite large, gingival lesions usually have a single stalk. After surgical excision the underlying tissue should be thoroughly curetted and root planing should be undertaken. Recurrence after surgery of pyogenic granulomas in extragingival sites is uncommon.

HAMARTOMATOUS AND BENIGN NEOPLASMS

Hemangioma

> ■ HEMANGIOMA: a proliferation of large (cavernous) or small (capillary) vascular channels occurring commonly in children; individual lesions have variable clinical courses.

Hemangiomas are relatively common benign proliferations of vascular channels that may be present at birth or arise during early childhood (Figure 9-54). Some slowly evolve, stabilize in size, and then either remain for life (hamartomatous) or slowly resolve to normal. Others may have a gradual but continous growth pattern (benign).

Most are located within the skin, where they may be flat or raised. Flat (macular) hemangiomas can be relatively large, covering significant areas of the skin; these lesions are often referred to as "birthmarks." Approximately 90% of such hemangiomas spontaneously involute by the time the patient has finished puberty. The remainder do not and are considered hamartomas. Vascular lesions of the lips and oral mucosa may arise in adulthood (Figure 9-55) and represent focal venous dilatations that may become hyperplastic (Figure 9-56). This lesion is considered to be a reactive proliferation and is referred to as a **varix**.

CLINICAL

Hemangiomas of the oral mucosa are usually raised, often multinodular, and distinctly reddish, blue, or purple. They most often occur in children and have no sex predilection. Compression with a glass microscopic slide against the lesion will usually cause blanching because the erythrocytes are compressed out of the vascular channels. Hemangiomas may arise in any mucosal site but are most common in the tongue. Frequently, the multinodular character yields a racemose or polypoid appearance over the dorsal surface (Figure 9-57). These he-

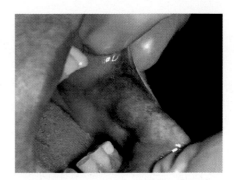

FIGURE 9-54

Hemangioma. Congenital hemangioma of the lower lip exhibiting the usual bluish coloration and nodularity.

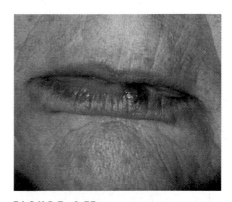

FIGURE 9-55

Varix. A lesion of the lower lip in an older adult is raised, soft, and bluish-purple.

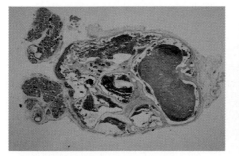

FIGURE 9-56

Varix. Low-power microscopy demonstrating a circumscribed collection of irregularly shaped dilatated venous structures with one vessel on the right side exhibiting thrombosis.

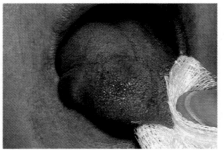

FIGURE 9-57

Cavernous hemangioma. Large multilobular lesion of the dorsal and lateral tongue.

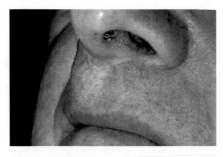

FIGURE 9-58

Intramuscular hemangioma. Lesion of the right upper lip exhibits swelling and some distortion; however, because the lesion is deep seated, the skin is normal in color.

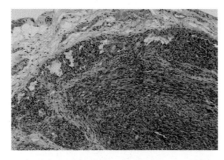

FIGURE 9-59

Port-wine stain capillary hemangioma. Congenital lesion following the distribution of the upper divisions of the trigeminal nerve on the right side of the face.

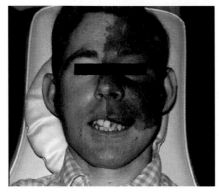

FIGURE 9-60

Capillary hemangioma. Low-power microscopy exhibiting a medullary pattern of a proliferation of endothelial cells forming numerous, small, densely packed capillaries with some larger vessels in the periphery.

mangiomas frequently extend deep into the intrinsic muscles of the tongue. Whereas many of these mucosal lesions will resolve once the patient has reached maturity, some remain constant, neither increasing in size nor undergoing involution.

Intramuscular hemangiomas may be encountered anywhere in the soft tissues of the head and neck. Within the oral cavity, they are usually seen on the tongue and lips. When they are deep seated, the surface tissue is often of normal coloration. Intramuscular hemangiomas cause a distortion of the area and have a spongy texture on palpation (Figure 9-58).

A unique type of hemangioma, referred to as the **port-wine stain,** is sometimes encountered on the face. These are usually unilateral and appear to follow one, two, or all three of the divisions of the trigeminal nerve (Figure 9-59). Although there may be occasional nodular elevations, most port-wine stains are purplish, diffuse macules with irregular borders that are sharply demarcated from the normal skin.

A specific syndrome is sometimes identified with unilateral port-wine stains on the face when the individuals also have intracranial hemangiomas and epilepsy. This is termed **encephalotrigeminal angiomatosis,** also referred to as *Sturge-Weber syndrome.* The intracranial hemangiomas will often develop calcifications within the walls of the meningeal vessels, leading to a unique radiographic appearance of parallel radiopaque lines that have been termed "tramline" calcifications.

Arteriovenous (AV) malformations occur in the head and neck and may involve both soft and hard tissues. Central mandibular arteriovenous malformations are more common in females and are usually first detected during childhood. These rare lesions slowly expand the mandible and are painless. Auscultation with a stethoscope will frequently reveal a bruit. The bruit is accounted for by the flow of blood through the anomalous vascular pathways. Teeth overlying these vascular malformations are often compressible with a spongy sensation, and there may be a spontaneous hemorrhage around the gingival crevice. Aspiration with a large-bore needle will yield bright red blood and frequently the syringe fills spontaneously without manipulation of the plunger. This feature is indicative of the considerable arterial pressure that exists within AV malformations. The classic radiographic appearance of central AV malformation is that of a multilocular radiolucency. Importantly, the radiolucencies are quite small, appearing as worm holes in wood. Anatomically, the radiolucencies represent the tortuous course of the vascular channels through the bone. True **hemangiomas of bone** are also encountered. These vascular proliferations are under capillary or venous pressure and represent benign vascular proliferations identical to the ordinary hemangioma of the soft tissue. Central hemangiomas may also expand bone with a multilocular radiographic appearance; however, a bruit is not detected.

HISTOPATHOLOGY

Hemangiomas are composed of multiple, small capillary channels or large tortuous dilated vascular spaces densely packed with erythrocytes. The former are referred to as **capillary hemangiomas,** whereas the lesions with large channels are termed **cavernous hemangiomas.** The capillary hemangioma is represented by numerous small endothelial-lined channels (Figure 9-60). The endothelial-lined cells are either spindle shaped or slightly elongated and plump. Whereas well-formed capillaries are present throughout, there may be foci of proliferating endothelial cells forming small aggregates that lack any attempt at lumen formation. A fibrous stroma is usually not prominent. Capillary hemangiomas closely resemble pyogenic granulomas histologically. Unless irritated, inflammatory cells are not a usual component of hemangiomas, whereas inflammation is a typical finding in pyogenic granuloma. The cavernous hemangioma consists of large, irregularly shaped, dilated endothelial-lined channels that contain large aggregates of erythrocytes (Figure 9-61). The vascular channels are of variable calibers, usually separated by a mature fibrous stroma. As a rule, cavernous hemangiomas lack a muscular coat, although occasionally some of these vessels will show a smooth muscle circumferential media. The macular hemangiomas, such as port-wine stain, are composed of small caliber channels similar to capillary hemangioma; however, the vessels are usually separated from one another by a mature fibrous tissue stroma.

Central hemangiomas of the bone are usually of the cavernous type. The AV malformation is rarely subjected to biopsy because surgical intervention can lead to profound hemorrhaging, which can result in death. These lesions are usually diagnosed with imaging studies such as Doppler angiography or contrast time-lapse angiography. Histologically, the arteriovenous malformation shows juxtaposed large vascular channels, most of which have either muscular or adventitial fibrous coats. These vascular channels replace the bone marrow, and the adjacent osseous trabeculas show evidence of osteoclastic resorption.

TREATMENT

Most hemangiomas in children are left untreated until puberty, anticipating spontaneous involution. Hemangiomas that persist into adult life usually become arrested in their growth potential and are often considered to represent **hamartomas** rather than true neoplasms. Lesions that appear to involve deeper structures are usually left untreated. In some cases for functional or cosmetic reasons, surgical excision may be attempted or the use of sclerosing agents may be employed. Many mucocutaneous hemangiomas, particularly the port-wine stains, are responsive to laser therapy.

Within bone a central multilocular radiolucency that yields blood upon aspiration may represent a central arteriovenous malformation, central hemangioma, or aneurysmal bone cyst. The arteriovenous malformation contains blood under high pressure, and time-lapse angiography will disclose the high flow that is encountered in these lesions. To prevent further destruction the treatment of choice is "induced embolization" administered through the feeder vessels. Frequently, the malformation receives a bilateral vascular supply and mandibular lesions may even have feeder vessels derived from the vertebral arteries, further complicating attempts at treatment. Treatment is often essential because spontaneous hemorrhage due to tooth loss could easily result in death.

Lymphangioma

■ LYMPHANGIOMA: benign proliferation of lymphatic vessels that occurs as a focal superficial lesion within the oral cavity and as a massive diffuse lesion of the neck (cystic hygroma).

Lymphangiomas are excessive vascular proliferations of the lymphatic system. Like hemangiomas, most lymphatic vessel proliferations arise during childhood. There is no sex predilection. There are two major types of lymphangiomas that occur in the head and neck. In the oral mucosa the tumors are usually self-limiting, whereas in the lateral neck, they may be quite massive and are referred to as **cystic hygroma.**

CLINICAL
Oral mucosal lymphangiomas are usually encountered in the tongues of children (Figure 9-62) where they may spontaneously involute at puberty or reach a given size and persist without further growth. Clinically, they are often racemose, es-

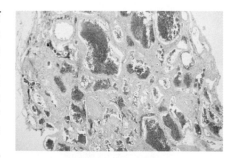

FIGURE 9-61
Cavernous hemangioma. Low-power microscopy demonstrating a circumscribed accumulation of large, irregularly shaped, thin-walled blood vessel engorged with red blood cells.

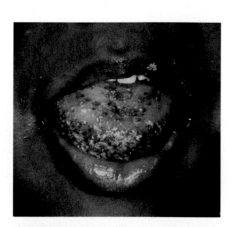

FIGURE 9-62
Lymphangioma. Lesion involves the entire tongue and exhibits multiple small surface nodules resulting in macroglossia.

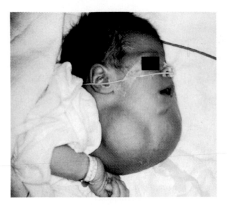

FIGURE 9-63

Cystic hygroma. The potentially life-threatening congenital, large, diffuse lymphangioma involves the deep structures of the neck of an infant.

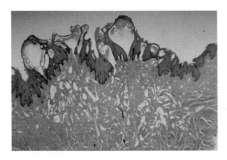

FIGURE 9-64

Lymphangioma. Low-power microscopy of a superficial mucosal lesion exhibiting the numerous clear spaces throughout the submucosa and extending between the rete pegs producing small delicate surface nodules.

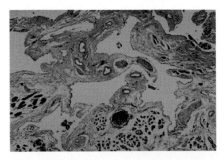

FIGURE 9-65

Lymphangioma. Low-power microscopy of large tortuous lymphatic spaces extending between the muscle bundles. Occasional vessels engorged with blood *(lower center)* are normally found in these lesions.

pecially when they occur on the dorsal tongue. The grapelike clusters may have a yellowish appearance and are soft on palpation. The lips are the second most common site for intraoral lymphangioma. **Cystic hygroma** presents as a massive swelling of the lateral neck (Figure 9-63). These tumors are usually covered by normal-appearing skin and may be quite pendulous, being several centimeters in diameter. They usually arise during the first or second years of the patient's life; and on palpation they have a decided cystic, fluctuant consistency. The proliferating lymphatic vessels frequently extend between muscle fibers and fascial planes, making their surgical removal problematic.

HISTOPATHOLOGY

The proliferating vessels of lymphangioma are thin walled and lined by plump endothelial cells. The lumens contain an eosinophilic proteinaceous coagulum with occasional erythrocytes and leukocytes. In lymphangioma of the tongue, the cavernous lymphatic channels usually extend between the rete ridges of the epithelium, producing papillomatous-like nodules on the surface. The lymphatic channels abut the epithelium without any intervening fibrous tissue (Figure 9-64). In cystic hygroma the histologic appearance is similar to lymphangioma of the oral submucosa. The channels are often quite large and of variable calibers, extend deep into the tissue, and traverse between muscle fibers and fibrous connective tissue (Figure 9-65). Although the lesion is infiltrative, it generally does not cause the destruction of neighboring structures.

TREATMENT

Lymphangiomas often spontaneously involute during puberty and are usually left untreated until the child reaches 18 years of age. Those that fail to involute usually demonstrate a cessation of growth and may be left untreated. Surgical excision is often deferred because many of the tumors will recur due to inability to completely excise all of the vascular channels. Cryosurgery and laser surgery have been used with some success.

Angiosarcoma

■ ANGIOSARCOMA: malignant, rare, rapidly growing lesion of endothelial cells that is more common in young patients and has a poor prognosis.

Malignant neoplasms of vascular endothelium are referred to as angiosarcomas. These tumors are extremely rare and may arise from the endothelial cells of either blood or lymphatic vessels. The **hemangioendothelioma** and **hemangiopericytoma** (Figure 9-66) are quasi-malignant neoplasms of vascular endothelium and vascular pericytes, respectively. These neoplasms are extremely cellular and represent proliferations of the individual cells rather than blood channels per se, as encountered in hemangiomas. They are quite aggressive, tend to occur in children and young adults, and have a tendency for recurrence, although distant metastases are rare. The most commonly encountered angiosarcoma within the oral cavity is **Kaposi sarcoma,** which is associated with the human immunodeficiency virus (HIV) epidemic. These tumors are usually multiple, and whereas some are self-limiting in their growth potential, others are capable of becoming large. Angiosarcomas other than Kaposi sarcoma are rapidly growing tumors with aggressive behaviors and high propensities for hematogenous metastases. These tumors are extremely rare in the head and neck regions and only a few cases of tumors within the oral cavity have been reported.

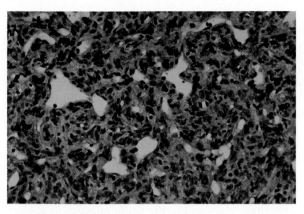

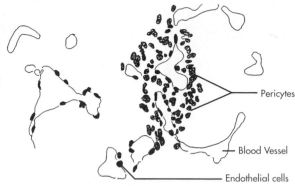

Pericytes

Blood Vessel

Endothelial cells

FIGURE 9-66

Hemangiopericytoma. Medium-power microscopy of cellular proliferation of the perivascular cells (periocyte) causing distortion of the endothelial-lined vascular spaces.

Kaposi Sarcoma

■ **KAPOSI SARCOMA**: a unique form of angiosarcoma that occurs in elderly and HIV-positive patients and has a predilection for the palate.

Kaposi sarcoma (KS) that occurs in the absence of HIV infection is extremely rare. These tumors typically arise in the palate and lower extremities among elderly males. HIV-associated Kaposi sarcoma is commonly seen on the skin and within the oral cavity. The tumor is associated with a gamma herpesvirus referred to as KS-associated herpesvirus or Herpes virus type 8. The homosexual risk group is most often involved, with very few cases occurring in intravenous drug users or female patients with HIV infection. When KS occurs in an HIV-infected patient, it usually carries the diagnosis of AIDS.

CLINICAL
On the skin KS lesions evolve through a flat, macular plaque phase of purple discoloration that progresses into a nodular tumor configuration that is red, blue, or purple. The palate is the most common site for KS within the oral cavity, and both hard and soft palatal mucosas may be affected. As on the skin the early lesions are macular, red or blue, and well demarcated (Figure 9-67). These macular angiomatous proliferations frequently progress to large nodular tumefactions (Figure 9-68) that can become quite pendulous. They maintain their vascular pigmentation and are often associated with brown discoloration due to the deposition of hemosiderin pigment within the tumor mass. The facial gingiva is the second most common location for intraoral KS. Lesions usually fail to blanche on compression because well-defined vascular channels are usually lacking.

HISTOPATHOLOGY
In the early plaque stage numerous slitlike vascular channels are encountered, and the endothelial cells often assume a beaded configuration along the vascular lumens. The nodular lesions are hypercellular and composed of two cellular elements: spindle cells with somewhat pleomorphic nuclei and endothelial cells ori-

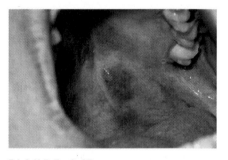

FIGURE 9-67

Kaposi sarcoma. Macular presentation of a lesion on the palate of an HIV-positive patient.

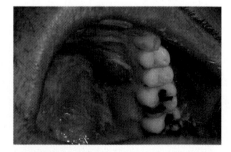

FIGURE 9-68

Kaposi sarcoma. Nodular form of a lesion on the palate of an HIV-positive patient.

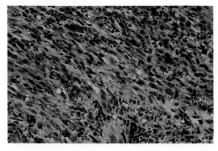

FIGURE 9-69

Kaposi sarcoma. Medium-power microscopy exhibiting the hyperchromatic and pleomorphic spindled endothelial cells found around partially formed vascular spaces against a background of extravasated red blood cells.

ented around sinusoidal slitlike vascular channels (Figure 9-69). Round capillary configurations may be admixed with the more sinusoidal-appearing cell population. Mitotic figures are not commonly seen, and cytologic atypia is usually evident yet relatively mild. Erythrocytes are encountered within the slitlike vascular channels, and many are extravasated. In addition, hemosiderin pigment granules are disbursed throughout the tumor.

TREATMENT

KS occurring in HIV-positive individuals is a multicentric disease. Patients often present with multiple sites of involvement, and these multiple tumors represent a multicentric distribution rather than metastases from a primary tumor. Experimental research discloses that these tumor cells proliferate in response to various growth factors that are secreted in an autocrine or paracrine manner. A variety of treatments have been investigated, including local treatment and systemically administered growth factor inhibitors. Mucosal lesions less than 2 centimeters commonly resolve after injection with sclerosing agents or chemotherapeutic agents. Low-dose radiation therapy has also been shown to cause shrinkage of these vascular proliferations.

OSSEOUS AND CARTILAGINOUS TISSUES

Bone- and cartilage-forming tumors of the jaws are discussed in Chapter 4. Occasionally, osseous or cartilaginous tissue may develop within subcutaneous or submucosal connective tissue. Formation of normal-appearing cartilage and bone in soft tissue located away from the osteoprogenitor cells in bone is referred to as a **choristoma.** Choristomas are similar to hamartomas because they tend to reach a given size and cease growing. Two reactive lesions are commonly derived from osteoprogenitor cellular elements of the gingiva. They are the peripheral ossifying fibroma and the peripheral giant cell granuloma and represent reactive hyperplasias with elaboration of bone and giant cells resembling osteoclasts respectively. Another bone-forming reactive process that occurs within the substance of muscle is myositis ossificans. A true osteoma of the soft tissue is probably nonexistent; nevertheless, compact bony nodules, referred to as osteomas may be encountered in the soft tissue around the jaws and in the sinuses in Gardner syndrome. Some osteogenic sarcoma may arise from the periosteum of the jaws, giving the clinical appearance of a soft tissue mass.

DEVELOPMENTAL LESIONS

Soft Tissue Osteoma

■ SOFT TISSUE OSTEOMA: focal growth of normal-appearing bone developing within the submucosal connective tissue; commonly found in patients with Gardner syndrome.

True osteomas of the soft tissue do not occur. As mentioned earlier, most of these represent choristomas. In **Gardner syndrome** ossified structures with the appearance of mature, compact bone may arise within the soft tissue or adhere to the periosteum of the jaws. The syndrome is characterized by supernumerary impacted teeth, facial bone osteomas, cutaneous nodules, and intestinal polyps that are premalignant. Other conditions in which calcified bodies occur within the soft tissue are calcinosis cutis and metastatic calcification, which may accompany hypercalcemia.

CLINICAL

The so-called osteomas of Gardner syndrome may arise in the mandibular area. These calcified masses usually adhere to the periosteum and appear as nodules along the angle or inferior border of the mandible. They can be identified on panoramic radiographs as well-delineated or lobular spherical calcifications that usually measure 1 to 2 cm. These calcified bodies are also frequently identified within the paranasal sinuses; the frontal and maxillary sinuses are the more common locations. Dental radiographs will disclose the presence of from one to four supernumerary teeth, which are usually impacted. Multiple subcutaneous nodules of a fibrous nature representing fibrous hamartomas can be identified on the skin, usually located on the extremities. The most significant aspect of the syndrome involves the intestinal mucosa. Multiple polyps occur within the colon, and predictably, adenocarcinoma arises from these polyps.

HISTOPATHOLOGY

The osteomas have a similar microscopic appearance to osseous choristomas. Compact lamellar bone containing osteocyte nuclei within the lacunas is observed, and a fibrous or adipose marrow component can usually be identified, although most of these osseous bodies are dense with formation of haversian systems.

TREATMENT

It may be necessary to extract the supernumerary impacted teeth because they may cause malocclusion of the remaining dentition. The osteomas can be excised if they are cosmetically or functionally problematic. Otherwise, they are self-limiting in their growth and do not usually continue to enlarge during adult years. Many oncologists recommend prophylactic resection of the colon in the areas involved with polyps.

Osseous and Cartilaginous Choristoma

> ■ OSSEOUS AND CARTILAGINOUS CHORISTOMA: raised, firm, movable soft tissue nodule containing a central nidus of bone and/or cartilage with self-limiting growth.

Osseous and cartilaginous choristomas are soft tissue masses in which normal-appearing bone and cartilage are found. They are benign and are self-limiting in their growth potential.

CLINICAL

Osseous and cartilaginous choristomas occur most frequently in the tongue, with a predilection for the ventral surface of the submucosa. They are also seen in the floor of the mouth yet are quite rare in other mucosal locations. There is no sex predilection, and most of these lesions are initially detected in adults. On palpation they are extremely hard and may be mistaken for a sialolith within a minor salivary gland. While indurated, they are usually easily movable.

HISTOPATHOLOGY

Osseous and cartilaginous choristomas are characterized by the formation of mature bone and/or cartilage. Mature osseous trabeculas contain lacunas with osteocytes. The trabeculas may resemble endostea or may be more compact with the appearance of cortical bone. In such cases haversian systems can be identified. The intervening connective tissue resembles normal bone marrow, being either fibrous or adipose. Hematogenous marrow is rarely identified in osseous choristomas. In cartilaginous choristoma, hyalin cartilage can be identified, showing its usual basophilic hyalinized appearance. Lacunas contain chondrocyte nuclei, which are small, pyknotic, and monomorphic. The periphery is usually round, smooth, and enveloped by mature fibrous connective tissue. Some of these choristomas demonstrate endochondral bone formation.

TREATMENT
Enucleation is the treatment of choice, and recurrence is rare.

REACTIVE LESIONS

Myositis Ossificans

> ■ MYOSITIS OSSIFICANS: rare reaction to injury of a muscle consisting of fibrosis and an associated deposition of bone resulting in pain, swelling, and limitation of motion.

In the maxillofacial complex myositis ossificans is most often encountered in the masseter or pterygoid muscles. A history of blunt trauma can sometimes be obtained. These reactive lesions tend to be self-limiting yet may cause dysfunction of the affected muscle.

CLINICAL
Myositis ossificans is a rare reactive lesion of muscle characterized by fibroblastic proliferation and elaboration of osseous trabeculas. The affected muscle has limitation of motion, is usually swollen, and may be tender on palpation. When palpated, the mass is considerably indurated. In the masseter and pterygoid muscles, limited jaw opening and/or closing may be observed. Radiographs will disclose multiple foci of ossification within the substance of the musculature. CT scans with a bone window are ideal for demonstrating these lesions. The ossification is usually dense and appears as a radiopacity on routine radiographs.

HISTOPATHOLOGY
Within the substance of skeletal muscle is a diffuse proliferation of fibroblastic spindle cells with an elaboration of either delicate or thin collagen fibers. The lesion is not well demarcated and may appear to infiltrate between contiguous skeletal muscle fibers. In the central area osteogenesis is identifiable with an elaboration of delicate osseous trabeculas undergoing various stages of calcification. Older lesions may show more compact bone. This osseous tissue is mature and benign.

TREATMENT
Once myositis ossificans has been diagnosed, surgical intervention is usually deferred. Removal of the involved muscle would not provide any improvement, and function could probably be worsened. Alternatively, if the mandible is completely restricted in motion, it may be advisable to debulk the involved area.

ADDITIONAL READING

FOCAL FIBROUS HYPERPLASIA

Bhaskar SN, Jacoway JR. Peripheral fibroma and peripheral fibroma with calcification: report of 376 cases. *J Am Dent Assoc.* 1966; 73:1312-20.

Bouquot JE, Gundlach KK. Oral exophytic lesions in 23,616 white Americans over 35 years of age. *Oral Surg Oral Med Oral Pathol.* 1986; 62:284-91.

Eversole LR, Rovin S. Reactive lesions of the gingiva. *J Oral Pathol Med.* 1972; 1:30.

Houston GD. The giant cell fibroma: a review of 464 cases. *Oral Surg Oral Med Oral Pathol.* 1982; 53:582-587.

PERIPHERAL OSSIFYING FIBROMA

Baumgartner JC, Stanley HR, Salomone JL. Peripheral ossifying fibroma. *J Endod.* 1991; 17:182-5.

Buchner A, Hansen LS. The histomorphologic spectrum of peripheral ossifying fibroma. *Oral Surg Oral Med Oral Pathol.* 1987; 63:452-61.

Hassan MA, Hamed S. Peripheral fibroma: clinical, histological and histochemical study. *Egypt Dent J.* 1985; 31:247-63.

Kenney JN, Kaugars GE, Abbey LM. Comparison between the peripheral ossifying fibroma and peripheral odontogenic fibroma. *J Oral Maxillofac Surg* 1989; 47:378-82.

Levin LS, North AF. Peripheral ossifying fibroma: a case report. *J Md State Dent Assoc.* 1985; 28:89-90.

McGinnis JP. Review of the clinical and histopathologic features of four exophytic gingival lesions—the pyogenic granuloma, irritation fibroma, peripheral giant cell granuloma, and peripheral ossifying fibroma. *J Okla Dent Assoc.* 1987; 77:25-30.

Zain RB, Fei YJ. Peripheral fibroma/fibrous epulis with and without calcifications: a clinical evaluation of 204 cases in Singapore. *Odontostomatol Trop.* 1990; 13:94-6.

Zain RB, Janakarajah N. Peripheral ossifying fibroma/ossifying fibrous epulis. *Dent J Malays.* 1988; 10:17-9.

PERIPHERAL GIANT CELL GRANULOMA

Giansanti JS, Waldron CA. Peripheral giant cell granuloma: review of 720 cases. *J Oral Maxillofac Surg.* 1969; 27:787.

Katsikeris N, Kakarantza-Angelopoulou E, Angelopoulos AP. Peripheral giant cell granuloma: clinicopathologic study of 224 new cases and review of 956 reported cases. *Int J Oral Maxillofac Surg.* 1988; 17:94-9.

Sapp JP. Ultrastructure and histogenesis of peripheral giant cell reparative granuloma of the jaws. *Cancer.* 1972; 30:119-129.

Smith BR, Fowler CB, Svane TJ. Primary hyperparathyroidism presenting as a peripheral giant cell granuloma. *Oral Maxillofac Surg.* 1988; 46:65-9.

INFLAMMATORY FIBROUS HYPERPLASIA

Cutwright DE. The histopathologic findings in 583 cases of epulis fissuratum. *Oral Surg Oral Med Oral Pathol.* 1974; 37:401-411.

Jha T, Mathur RM. Inflammatory fibrous hyperplasia. *J Pierre Fauchard Acad* 1990; 4:155.

Thomas GA. The immunohistochemical detection of involucrin in denture induced fibrous inflammatory hyperplasia of oral mucous membrane. *Aust Prosthodont J.* 1991; 5:29-34.

INFLAMMATORY PAPILLARY HYPERPLASIA

Wright SM, Scott BJ. Prosthetic assessment in the treatment of denture hyperplasia. *Br Dent J.* 1992; 172:313-5.

HYPERPLASTIC GINGIVITIS

Takagi M, Yamamoto H, Mega H, Hsieh KJ and others. Heterogeneity in the gingival fibromatoses. *Cancer.* 1991; 68:2202-12.

Van Dis ML, Allen CM, Neville BW. Erythematous gingival enlargement in diabetic patients: a report of four cases. *J Oral Maxillofac Surg.* 1988; 46:794-8.

HEREDITARY GINGIVAL FIBROMATOSIS

Bakaeen G, Scully C. Hereditary gingival fibromatosis in a family with the Zimmermann-Laband syndrome. *J Oral Pathol Med.* 1991; 20:456-9.

Chadwick B, Hunter B, Hunter L, Aldred M and others. Laband syndrome. *Oral Surg Oral Med Oral Pathol.* 1994; 78:57-63.

Clark D. Gingival fibromatosis and its related syndromes: a review. *J Can Dent Assoc.* 1987; 53:137-40.

DRUG-INDUCED GINGIVAL HYPERPLASIA

Daley T, Wysocki G, Day C. Clinical and pharmacologic correlations in cyclosporin-induced gingival hyperplasia. *Oral Surg Oral Med Oral Pathol.* 1986; 16:417-21.

Hassell TM, Hefti AF. Drug-induced gingival overgrowth: old problem, new problem. *Crit Rev Oral Biol Med.* 1991; 2:103-37.

Seymour RA, Jacobs DJ. Cyclosporin and the gingival tissues. *J Clin Periodontol.* 1992; 19:1-11.

Seymour RA. Calcium channel blockers and gingival overgrowth. *Br Dent J.* 1991; 170:376-9.

FIBROMATOSIS

Bridge JA, Rosenthal H, Sanger WG, Neff JR. Desmoplastic fibroma arising in fibrous dysplasia: chromosomal analysis and review of the literature. *Clin Orthop.* 1989; 272-8.

Farrel C, Haibach H, Gaines RW. Demoplastic fibroma of bone. *Mo Med.* 1986; 83:681-3.

Kwon PH, Horswell BB, Gatto DJ. Desmoplastic fibroma of the jaws: surgical management and review of the literature. *Head Neck.* 1989; 11:67-75.

Vally IM, Altini M. Fibromatoses of the oral and paraoral soft tissues and jaws: review of the literature and report of 12 new cases. *Oral Surg Oral Med Oral Pathol.* 1990; 69:191-8.

NODULAR FASCIITIS

Batsakis JG, Rice DH, Howard DR. The pathology of head and neck tumors: spindle cell lesions (sarcomatoid carcinomas, nodular fasciitis, and fibrosarcoma) of the aerodigestive tracts: part 14. *Head Neck Surg.* 1982; 4:499-513.

Davies HT, Bradley N, Bowerman JE. Oral nodular fasciitis. *Br J Oral Maxillofac Surg.* 1989; 27:147-51.

Shimizu S, Hashimoto H, Enjoji M. Nodular fasciitis: an analysis of 250 cases. *Pathology.* 1984; 16:161-66.

FIBROSARCOMA

Argyle JC, Tomlinson GE, Stewart D, Schneider NR. Ultrastructural, immunocytochemical, and cytogenetic characterization of a large congenital fibrosarcoma. *Arch Pathol Lab Med.* 1992; 116:972-5.

Batsakis JG, Rice DH, Howard DR. The pathology of head and neck tumors: spindle cell lesions (sarcomatoid carcinomas, nodular fasciitis, and fibrosarcoma) of the aerodigestive tracts: part 14. *Head Neck Surg.* 1982; 4:499-513.

Fletcher CD, McKee PH. Sarcomas—a clinicopathological guide with particular reference to cutaneous manifestation: III: angiosarcoma, malignant haemangiopericytoma, fibrosarcoma and synovial sarcoma. *Clin Exp Dermatol.* 1985; 10:332-49.

Oppenheimer RW, Friedman M. Fibrosarcoma of the maxillary sinus. *Ear Nose Throat J.* 1988; 67:193-8.

FIBROUS HISTIOCYTOMA

Chang P, Ferandez V. Malignant fibrous histiocytoma of the skin. *Int J Dermatol.* 1994; 33:50-1.

D'Costa GF, Nagle SB, Wagholikar UL. Angiomatoid malignant fibrous histiocytoma. *Indian J Pathol Microbiol.* 1990; 33:280-3.

Hayashi Y, Kikuchi-Tada A, Jitsukawa K, Sato S and others. Myofibroblasts in malignant fibrous histiocytoma—histochemical, immunohistochemical, ultrastructural and tissue culture studies. *Clin Exp Dermatol.* 1988; 13:402-5.

Perez-Bacete MJ, Llombart-Bosch A. FU-3 monoclonal antibody: a specific marker for malignant fibrous histiocytoma? An analysis of 32 malignant soft tissue and bone sarcomas. *Virchows Arch.* 1994; 424:243-7.

Regezi J, Zarbo R, Tomich C. Immunoprofile of benign and malignant fibrohistiocytic tumors. *J Oral Pathol.* 1987; 16:260-65.

Singh B, Shaha A, Har-El G. Malignant fibrous histiocytoma of the head and neck. *J Craniomaxillofac Surg.* 1993; 21:262-5.

Thompson S, Shear M. Fibrous histiocytomas of the oral and maxillofacial regions. *J Oral Pathol.* 1984; 13:282-94.

Weerapradist W, Punyasingh J. Fibrous histiocytoma: report of a case of the oral mucosa. *J Dent Assoc Thai.* 1984; 34:263-9.

TRAUMATIC NEUROMA

Alexander IJ, Johnson KA, Parr JW. Morton's neuroma: a review of recent concepts. *Orthopedics.* 1987; 10:103-6.

Chau MN, Jonsson E, Lee KM. Traumatic neuroma following sagittal mandibular osteotomy. *Int J Oral Maxillofac Surg.* 1989; 18:95-8.

Lipkin AF, Coker NJ, Jenkins HA, Alford BR. Intracranial and intratemporal facial neuroma. *Otolaryngol Head Neck Surg.* 1987; 96:71-9.

MULTIPLE ENDOCRINE NEOPLASIA SYNDROME

Calmettes C, Ponder BA, Fischer JA, Raue F. Early diagnosis of the multiple endocrine neoplasia type 2 syndrome: consensus statement. *Eur J Clin Invest.* 1992; 22:755-60.

Feingold KR, Elias PM. Endocrine-skin interactions: cutaneous manifestations of adrenal disease, pheochromocytomas, carcinoid syndrome, sex hormone excess and deficiency, polyglandular autoimmune syndromes and multiple endocrine neoplasia syndromes. *J Am Acad Dermatol.* 1988; 19:1-20.

Schenberg ME, Zajac JD, Lim-Tio S, Collier NA and others. Multiple endocrine neoplasia syndrome—type 2b: case report and review. *Int J Oral Maxillofac Surg.* 1992; 21:110-4.

Solcia E, Capella C, Fiocca R, Rindi G and others. Gastric argyrophil carcinoidosis in patients with Zollinger-Ellison syndrome due to type 1 multiple endocrine neoplasia. *Am J Surg Pathol.* 1990; 14:503-13.

NEURILEMOMA

Chauvin PJ, Wysocki GP, Daley TD, Pringle GA. Palisaded encapsulated neuroma of oral mucosa. *Oral Surg Oral Med Oral Path.* 1992; 73:71-74.

Cherrick HM, Eversole LR. Benign neural sheath neoplasms of the oral cavity: report of thirty-seven cases. *Oral Surg Oral Med Oral Pathol.* 1971; 32:900-09.

DiCerbo M, Sciubba JJ, Sordill WC, DeLuke DM. Malignant schwannoma of the palate: a case report and review of the literature. *J Oral Maxillofac Surg.* 1992; 50:1217-21.

Elias MM, Balm AJ, Peterse JL, Keus RB and others. Malignant schwannoma of the parapharyngeal space in von Recklinghausen's disease: a case report and review of the literature. *J Laryngol Otol.* 1993; 107:848-52.

NEUROFIBROMA

Polak M, Polak G, Brocheriou C, Vigneul J. Solitary neurofibroma of the mandible: case report and review of the literature. *J Oral Maxillofac Surg.* 1989; 47:65-8.

Skouteris CA. Incidence of solitary intraosseous neurofibroma of the maxilla. *J Oral Maxillofac Surg.* 1993; 51:688-90.

Skouteris CA, Sotereanos GC. Solitary neurofibroma of the maxilla: report of a case. *J Oral Maxillofac Surg.* 1988; 46:701-5.

GRANULAR CELL TUMOR

Baden E, Divaris M, Quillard J. A light microscopic and immunohistochemical study of a multiple granular cell tumor and review of the literature. *J Oral Maxillofac Surg.* 1990; 48:1093-9.

Naik R, Kamath AS. Granular cell tumor: a clinicopathological study. *Indian J Pathol Microbiol.* 1993; 36:227-32.

Okada H, Yamamoto H, Kawana T, Katoh T and others. Granular cell tumor of the tongue: an electron microscopical and immunohistochemical study. *J Nihon Univ Sch Dent.* 1990; 32:35-43.

Park SH, Kim TJ, Chi JG. Congenital granular cell tumor with systemic involvement: immunohistochemical and ultrastructural study. *Arch Pathol Lab Med.* 1991; 115:934-8.

Stewart CM, Watson RE, Eversole LR, Fischlschweiger W and others. Oral granular cell tumors: a clinicopathologic and immunocytochemical study. *Oral Surg Oral Med Oral Pathol.* 1988; 65:427-35.

CONGENITAL GINGIVAL GRANULAR CELL TUMOR

Fuhr AH, Krough JA. Congential epulis of the newborn: centennial review of the literature and a report of a case. *J Oral Maxillofac Surg.* 1972; 30:30.

Rohrer MD, Young SK. Congential epulis (gingival granular cell tumor): ultrastructural evidence of origin from pericytes. *Oral Surg Oral Med Oral Pathol.* 1982; 53:56-63.

Regezi J, Zarbo R, Courtney R, Crissman J. Immunoreactivity of granular cell lesions of skin, mucosa and jaw. *Cancer.* 1989; 64:1455-60.

NEUROECTODERMAL TUMOR OF INFANCY

Cutler LS, Chaudhry AP, Topazian R. Melanotic neuroectodermal tumor of infancy: an ultrastructural study, literature review, and reevaluation. *Cancer.* 1981; 48:257-70.

Dehner LP, Sibley RK, Sauk JJ, Vickers RA and others. Malignant melanotic neuroectodermal tumor of infancy: a clinical, pathologic, ultrastructural and tissue culture study. *Cancer.* 1979; 43:1389-410.

Handley GH, Peters GE. Melanotic neuroectodermal tumor of infancy. *South Med J.* 1988; 81:1170-2.

Mosby EL, Lowe MW, Cobb CM, Ennis RL. Melanotic neuroectodermal tumor of infancy: review of the literature and report of a case. *J Oral Maxillofac Surg.* 1992; 50:886-94.

Pierre-Kahn A, Cinalli G, Lellouch-Tubiana A, Villarejo FJ and others. Melanotic neuroectodermal tumor of the skull and meninges in infancy. *Pediatr Neurosurg.* 1992; 18:6-15.

Shah RV, Jambhekar NA, Rana DN, Raje NS and others. Melanotic neuroectodermal tumor of infancy: report of a case with ganglionic differentiation. *J Surg Oncol.* 1994; 55:65-8.

LEIOMYOMA

McMillian M, Ferguson J, Kardos T. Mandibular vascular leiomyoma. *Oral Surg Oral Med Oral Pathol.* 1985; 62:427-33.

Savage NW, Adkins KF, Young WG, Chapman PJ. Oral vascular leiomyoma: review of the literature and report of two cases. *Aust Dent J.* 1983; 28:346-51.

RHABDOMYOSARCOMA

Diller L. Rhabdomyosarcoma and other soft tissue sarcomas of childhood. *Curr Opin Oncol.* 1992; 4:689-95.

Hays DM. Rhabdomyosarcoma. *Clin Orthop.* 1993; 289:36-49.

Lazzaro B, Schwartz D, Lewis J, Weiss W. Rhabdomyosarcoma involving the oral cavity, mandible, and roots of the third molar: a clinical-pathologic correlation and review of literature. *J Oral Maxillofac Surg.* 1990; 48:72-7.

Maurer Hm, Ruymann FB, Pochedly C. *Rhabdomyosarcoma and Related Tumors in Children and Adolescents.* Boca Raton, Fla: CRC Press; 1991.

Peters E, Cohen M, Altini M, Murray J. Rhabdomyosarcoma of the oral and paraoral region. *Cancer.* 1989; 63:963-6.

Samaddar RR, Sen MK. Rhabdomyosarcoma of the head and neck in children—a review of literature. *Indian J Med Sci.* 1992; 46:250-4.

LIPOMA

Chen SY, Fantasia JE, Miller AS. Myxoid lipoma of oral soft tissue: a clinical and ultrastructural study. *Oral Surg Oral Med Oral Pathol.* 1984; 57:300-7.

Rapidis AD. Lipoma of the oral cavity. *Int J Oral Surg.* 1982; 11:30-5.

LIPOSARCOMA

Sadeghi EM, Sauk JJ. Liposarcoma of the oral cavity: clinical, tissue culture, and ultrastructure study of a case. *J Oral Pathol.* 1982; 11:263-75.

HEMANGIOMA

Rossiter JL, Hendrix RA, Tom LW, Potsic WP. Intramuscular hemangioma of the head and neck. *Otolaryngol Head Neck Surg.* 1993; 108:18-26.

Sadeghi E, Gingrass D. Histopathologic appraisal of an oral hemangioma treated with a sclerosing agent. *Compendium.* 1991; 12:288-90.

Toeg A, Kermish M, Grishkan A; Temkin D. Histiocytoid hemangioma of the oral cavity: a report of two cases. *J Oral Maxillofac Surg.* 1993; 51:812-4.

Wolf GT, Daniel F, Krause CJ, Kaufman RS. Intramuscular hemangioma of the head and neck. *Laryngoscope.* 1985; 95:210-3.

ENCEPHALOTRIGEMINAL ANGIOMATOSIS (STURGE-WEBER SYNDROME)

Marti-Bonmati L, Menor F, Mulas F. The Sturge-Weber syndrome: correlation between the clinical status and radiological CT and MRI findings. *Childs Nerv Syst.* 1993; 9:107-9.

Oakes WJ. The natural history of patients with the Sturge-Weber syndrome. *Pediatr Neurosurg.* 1992; 18:287-90.

Pascual-Castroviejo I, Diaz-Gonzalez C, Garcia-Melian RM, Gonzalez-Casado I and others. Sturge-Weber syndrome: study of 40 patients. *Pediatr Neurol.* 1993; 9:283-8.

LYMPHANGIOMA

Goldberg MH, Nemarich AN, Danielson P. Lymphangioma of the tongue: medical and surgical therapy. *J Oral Maxillofac Surg.* 1977; 35:841.

White B, Adkins WY. The use of the carbon dioxide laser in head and neck lymphangioma. *Lasers Surg Med.* 1986; 6: 293-5.

PYOGENIC GRANULOMA

Bucci FA, Wiener BD. The pyogenic granuloma. *Ariz Med.* 1984; 41:794-6.

Muench MG, Layton S, Wright JM. Pyogenic granuloma associated with a natal tooth: case report. *Pediatr Dent.* 1992; 14:265-7.

Vilmann A, Vilmann P, Vilmann H. Pyogenic granuloma: evaluation of oral conditions. *Br J Oral Maxillofac Surg.* 1986; 24:376-82.

ANGIOSARCOMA

Mark RJ, Tran LM, Sercarz J, Fu YS and others. Angiosarcoma of the head and neck: the UCLA experience 1955 through 1990. *Arch Otolaryngol Head Neck Surg.* 1993; 119:973-8.

Panje WR, Moran WJ, Bostwick DG, Kitt VV. Angiosarcoma of the head and neck: review of 11 cases. *Laryngoscope.* 1986; 96:1381-4.

KAPOSI SARCOMA

Searles GE, Markman S, Yazdi HM. Primary oral Kaposi's sarcoma of the hard palate. *J Am Acad Dermatol.* 1990; 23(pt 1):518-9.

Eversole LR, Leider AS, Jacobsen PL, Shaber EP. Oral Kaposi's sarcoma associated with acquired immunodeficiency syndrome among homosexual males. *J Am Dent Assoc.* 1983; 107:248-53.

Green TL, Beckstead JH, Lozada-Nur F, Silverman S and others. Histopathologic spectrum of oral Kaposi's sarcoma. *Oral Surg Oral Med Oral Pathol.* 1984; 58:306-14.

Kuntz AA, Gelderblom HR, Winkel T, Reichart PA. Ultrastructural findings in oral Kaposi's sarcoma (AIDS). *J Oral Pathol.* 1987; 16:372-9.

Lucatorto FM, Sapp JP. Treatment of oral Kaposi's sarcoma with a sclerosing agent in AIDS patients. *Oral Surg Oral Med Oral Pathol.* 1993; 75:192-8.

Lumerman H, Freedman PD, Kerpel SM, Phelan JA. Oral Kaposi's sarcoma: a clinicopathologic study of 23 homosexual and bisexual men from the New York metropolitan area. *Oral Surg Oral Med Oral Pathol.* 1988; 65:711-6.

Regezi JA, MacPhail LA, Daniels TE, DeSouza YG and others. Human immunodeficiency virus-associated oral Kaposi's sarcoma: a heterogeneous cell population dominated by spindle-shaped endothelial cells. *Am J Pathol.* 1993; 143:240-9.

Regezi JA, MacPhail LA, Daniels TE, Greenspan JS and others. Oral Kaposi's sarcoma: a 10-year retrospective histopathologic study. *J Oral Pathol Med.* 1993; 22:292-7.

OSSEOUS AND CARTILAGINOUS CHORISTOMA

Cabbabe EB, Sotelo-Avila C, Moloney ST, Makhlouf MV. Osseous choristoma of the tongue. *Ann Plast Surg.* 1986; 16:150-2.

Hodder SC, MacDonald DG. Osseous choristoma of buccal mucosa: report of a case. *Br J Oral Maxillofac Surg.* 1988; 26:78-80.

Ishikawa M, Mizukoshi T, Notani K, Iizuka T and others. Osseous choristoma of the tongue: report of two cases. *Oral Surg Oral Med Oral Pathol.* 1993; 76:561-3.

Long DE, Koutnik AW. Recurrent intraoral osseous choristoma: report of a case. *Oral Surg Oral Med Oral Pathol.* 1991; 72:337-9.

Shimono M, Tsuji T, Iguchi Y, Yamamura T and others. Lingual osseous choristoma: report of 2 cases. *Int J Oral Surg.* 1984; 13:355-9.

MYOSITIS OSSIFICANS

el-Labban NG, Hopper C, Barber P. Ultrastructural finding of vascular degeneration in myositis ossificans circumscripta (fibrodysplasia ossificans). *J Oral Pathol Med.* 1993; 22:428-31.

Clapton WK, James CL, Morris LL, Davey RB and others. Myositis ossificans in childhood. *Pathology.* 1992; 24:311-4.

Merchan EC, Sanchez-Herrera S, Valdazo DA, Gonzalez JM. Circumscribed myositis ossificans: report of nine cases without history of injury. *Acta Orthop Belg.* 1993; 59:273-7.

SALIVARY GLAND DISORDERS

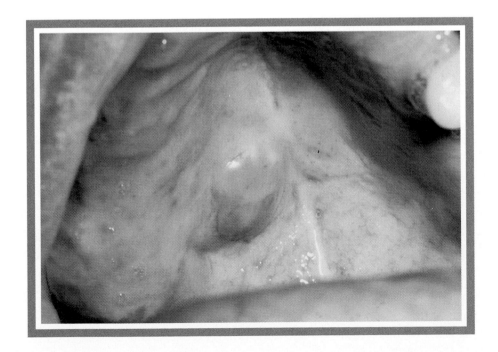

T

he diseases that occur in the major and minor salivary glands of the oro-facial structures are also encountered in the submucosal glands of all the upper air passages, including the mucus-secreting glands of the nose, paranasal sinuses, and larynx. The basic disease processes that affect the seromucous glands are *reactive* and *obstructive lesions, infections, immunopathologic disorders,* and *neoplasms.* A common feature of all of these processes is swelling of the gland. Pain is a common accompanying symptom in infectious and obstructive lesions, whereas immunologic and neoplastic disorders are usually characterized by painless enlargement.

Because most salivary gland diseases affect the ductal and secretory components and most neoplastic diseases arise from various cell types of the glandular tree, it is helpful in the understanding of these pathologic processes to be familiar with the normal histology of these glands (Figure 10-1).

Salivary glands, whether major or minor, arise embryologically from the primitive ectoderm of the stomatodeum. The gland primordia penetrate the submucosa as tubular invaginations that ultimately differentiate into end-bulbs with secretory capabilities. A mature gland may contain three types of acinar (secretory) cells: mucous, seromucous, and serous. In some glands mucous acini are capped by serous or seromucous demilunes. The acinar cells are enveloped by contractile myoepithelial cells that are surrounded by a basement membrane. The secretory fluids and proteins enter the small cuboidal-lined terminal or intercalated ducts and progress to the mitochondrial-rich striated ducts. These two ductal elements residing within the salivary gland proper are components of the intralobular ducts. Numerous acinar clusters secrete their products into these ducts that collectively drain into much larger ducts composed of basilar reserve cells, stratified epithelium, and luminally oriented cuboidal or columnar cells. These larger ducts exit the lobule as extralobular secretory ducts that eventually converge into the major salivary ducts. As these ducts reach the surface, they are lined by stratified squamous epithelium, although some still have luminally oriented cuboidal cells. Most tumors of the salivary glands are classified according to the histologic components they resemble.

Secreting into the oral cavity are three major glands—*parotid, submandibular,* and *sublingual*—and numerous *mucosal minor salivary glands.* The minor glands are distributed throughout the oral cavity, with the exception of the dorsal tongue and attached gingiva. It is estimated that on the average, there are 450 minor glands in the hard palate, 220 in the soft palate, and 8 in the uvula. It is important to realize that the posterior-lateral aspect of the hard palate is the most common location for salivary neoplasms within the oral cavity.

Deficient secretion occurs when the ductal drainage system is severed or blocked. Additionally, xerostomia may evolve as a consequence of acinar damage from infectious, immune, or sclerotic changes that occur secondary to obstructive disease. Salivary swellings are seen when the glands become infiltrated by leukocytes as occurs in obstruction or immunopathologic disease, edema associated with infection, fatty infiltration, or neoplastic processes.

Because the parotid gland overlies the facial (VII) nerve, tumors arising in this site may cause nerve paresis with attending facial weakness. This is an ominous sign because it may be the harbinger of a malignant parotid tumor that has invaded the nerve.

Clinical examination has been demonstrated to be valuable when attempting to reveal the basic nature of a salivary disease process. Palpation of swellings of the major glands or of the oral mucosa containing minor glands is diagnostically useful because soft or fluctuant swellings are the usual features of benign processes, whereas fixed and indurated swellings are more indicative of malignancy.

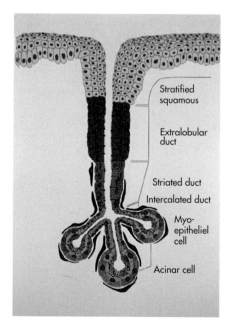

FIGURE 10-1

Components of the adult salivary gland secretory unit. Acinar secretions move from the intercalated ducts to the larger striated duct, both lined by cuboidal epithelium. The saliva is further transported, with aid from contractile myoepithelial cells, into the stratified, columnar, extralobular ducts, ultimately emerging from the mucosa through the excretory duct lined by stratified squamous epithelium.

REACTIVE LESIONS

Salivary glands react to injury or obstruction by undergoing atrophic degeneration and necrosis with replacement of the parenchyma by inflammatory cells and, ultimately, fibrous scarring. Certainly bacterial or viral infections of the gland or immunologic reactions to autoantigens may culminate in the same processes of degeneration, necrosis, and fibrosis. Those diseases that are considered to be reactive in nature are noninfectious; they represent responses to direct trauma or obstruction to the flow of saliva. A few are of unknown etiology.

Obstruction to flow may occur as a consequence of duct *blockage* by an object in the ductal lumen, *stricture* of a duct with narrowing of the lumen, or *severance* of a duct with pooling of mucin within the tissue. In all three instances, salivary obstruction evolves and as glandular secretions accumulate within the ductal lumina, back pressure changes evolve leading to acinar atrophic degeneration. As acinar cells progressively degenerate subsequent to obstruction, apoptosis and necrosis ensue. These degenerate changes are subtle, evolving over weeks or months, and are such that histologic evidence of frank necrosis is generally absent. Rather, the degenerating secretory units disappear, and as cells die a mild chronic inflammatory cell infiltrate composed of lymphocytes and plasma cells appears. Once acini are no longer evident, the parenchyma undergoes a progressive fibrosis (sclerosis), a process common to all reactive lesions. In the salivary glands it is referred to as **chronic sclerosing sialadenitis** (Box 10-1). It is notable that the ductal system is more resistant to the obstructive process than the acini. When tissue from chronic sclerosing sialadenitis is viewed microscopically, the ductal elements are often seen to remain whereas the acini are completely degenerated (Figure 10-2). The remaining ducts have little ability to generate secretion products resulting in a greatly reduced outward flow. This stasis predisposes the development of retrograde bacterial infections.

> ■ **BOX 10-1**
> **Common Causes of Chronic Sclerosing Sialadenitis**
>
> Excretory obstructions
> Infections
> Radiation
> Autoimmune diseases
> Systemic and metabolic conditions
> Medications and drugs

MUCOCELE

■ **MUCOCELE**: tissue swelling composed of pooled mucus that escaped into the connective tissue from a severed excretory duct.

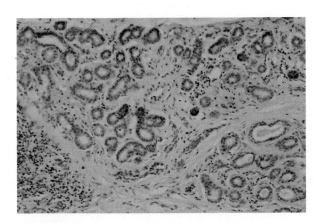 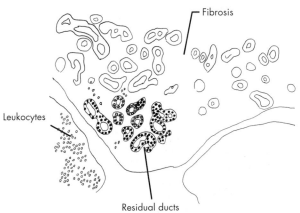

FIGURE 10-2

Chronic sclerosing sialadenitis. The intralobular ducts remain intact and dilatated. The acini have degenerated and are replaced by leukocyte infiltration and fibrosis of the salivary lobule.

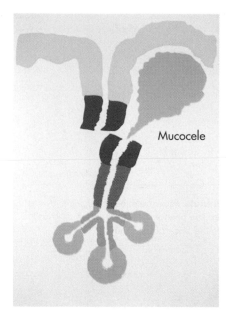

FIGURE 10-3

Mucocele. Mucus escapes from a severed duct and accumulates within the submucosal connective tissue.

When a salivary duct is severed, the acinar cells will continue to secrete saliva into the severed duct. At the site of severance the secretory products escape into the connective tissue forming a pool of mucus that distends the surrounding tissue (Figure 10-3). This mucus escape (extravasation) phenomenon is commonly termed a **mucocele.** The minor salivary glands of the lower lip are most prone to severance as a consequence of injury or biting of the mucosa, although other intraoral or even laryngeal minor mucous glands can be affected. Mucoceles of the major salivary glands are quite rare. Occasionally, such mucus extravasation reactions will occur in the floor of the mouth as a consequence of minor sublingual gland duct severance. These mucoceles have the finely vascularized, distended appearance of a frog's belly and are referred to as **ranulas.** When the major submandibular duct (Wharton duct) is punctured or severed, massive mucus extravasation may occur deeply within the submental, submandibular, or sublingual region. Mucus extravasation of this nature is termed **plunging mucocele** or **ranula.** Plunging mucoceles are of concern because they are capable of causing a severe compromise of the airway.

Whereas mucoceles do not cause direct obstruction to the flow of saliva, the amount of secretions that can be extravasated is limited by the distensibility of the surrounding tissue. Although mucoceles can become large, most are of limited size. As they enlarge, the gland that supplies mucin through the severed duct (the "feeder gland") becomes compressed and eventually obstructive changes develop.

On occasion, radiographs of the maxillary sinuses will reveal focal nodular hyperplastic enlargements of the maxillary sinus lining mucosa. They are sometimes referred to as "antral mucoceles," when in fact such lesions represent inflammatory polyps.

There are some neoplastic lesions that may clinically resemble mucoceles most notably mucoepidermoid carcinoma. This fact alone dictates that all suspected mucoceles should be submitted for microscopic examination. Others have an appearance similar to a cavernous hemangioma. When mucoceles are superficial, they may clinically and histologically resemble blisters seen in some bullous/desquamative diseases; however, the latter are usually multifocal.

CLINICAL

Mucoceles are most often encountered in children and young adults, although they may occur at any age. Almost two thirds of all mucoceles occur during the first three decades of life. Both males and females are equally affected. The mucosal surface of the lower lip is the favored site (Figure 10-4), followed by the buccal mucosa, the floor of the mouth, ventral tongue, and palate. Although the upper lip is traumatized as frequently as the lower lip, mucoceles in this location are uncommon. It should be recalled that minor salivary glands are ubiquitous within the oral cavity with the exception of the anterior dorsal tongue and facial attached gingiva. Therefore mucoceles can arise in any oral location that harbors minor salivary tissue.

The clinical appearance of a mucocele is dependent on its location within the submucosa. More superficial zones of mucous extravasation present a fluctuant mass with a bluish translucent appearance. In some mucoceles the trauma that initiated the ductal severance or the continued trauma by the dentition may result in hemorrhage. When the extravasated mucin is admixed with erythrocytes, an ecchymotic mucocele develops and may appear deep blue or reddish purple, resembling a cavernous hemangioma. More deep-seated accumulations may simply present as a soft or fluctuant submucosal nodule of normal mucosal coloration. There is usually a history of injury to the area, followed by progressive swelling over a 2- to 4-day period. Commonly, patients will describe a fluctuation in size; however, after the initial traumatic episode pain is seldom a com-

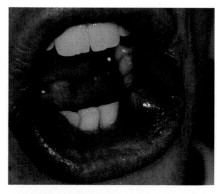

FIGURE 10-4

Mucocele of the lower lip. Lesion is soft and fluctuant on palpation.

plaint. The amount of the fluctuation may be barely noticeable or significant to the point that the lesion disappears only to recur to its original size within a few days. Under these circumstances the patient will probably reinjure the area, allowing the mucin to escape through the thinned mucosal epithelium. After the small puncture heals, the secretions reaccumulate, resulting in the recurrence. Initially, mucoceles are well circumscribed. With repeated trauma they may become nodular, more diffuse, and more firm on palpation. In the floor of the mouth ranulas are generally located laterally and tend to be quite translucent with surface vascular markings readily apparent (Figure 10-5).

The plunging ranula is deep seated and results from extravasation of saliva through the mylohyoid musculature into the submandibular or submental space. These lesions are soft on palpation, fluctuant, and often clinically evident as submental or submandibular swellings. Extension deep into the neck to involve the juxtahyoid region can compromise the airway.

HISTOPATHOLOGY

The surface epithelium is distended by an underlying pool of mucin. This mucin is generally walled by a rim of either granulation tissue or, in long-standing lesions, by condensed collagen that gives an encapsulated appearance. An epithelial lining is lacking (Figure 10-6). The mucinous material is basophilic or amphophilic and contains neutrophils and large, round to oval, foam cell histiocytes. These same cells infiltrate the granulation tissue wall. Occasionally, the base of the mucocele on a fortuitous tissue section will reveal the presence of the feeder duct. The underlying salivary lobules that supply secretions through the feeder duct show varying degrees of chronic sclerosing sialadenitis depending on the duration of the process. Long-standing mucoceles will show extensive acinar degeneration with fibrosis and minimal inflammation, whereas more recently traumatized lesions will show mononuclear infiltration with very little fibrosis.

Mucoceles that have been present for many weeks or those that are repeatedly traumatized to allow mucus escape often show histologic evidence of organization, an attempt at healing. The zone of mucus extravasation will be infiltrated by budding vascular channels and granulation tissue, lacking the unilocular encapsulated appearance of the uncomplicated mucocele. Likewise, plunging

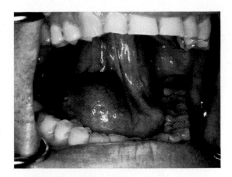

FIGURE 10-5

Ranula. Patient exhibits a fluctuant mucus escape phenomenon located off the midline in the floor of the mouth.

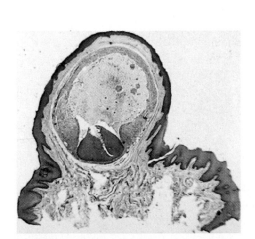
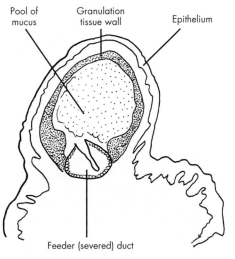

Pool of mucus

Granulation tissue wall

Epithelium

Feeder (severed) duct

FIGURE 10-6

Mucocele. Microscopic appearance showing pooled mucin, a granulation tissue wall, distended overlying epithelium, and remnants of the severed feeder duct.

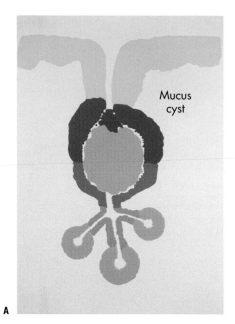

Mucus
cyst

A

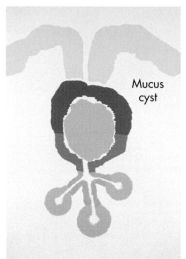

Mucus
cyst

B

FIGURE 10-7

Mucus retention cyst. A, Some are hypothesized to arise as ductal dilatations from obstruction by mucus plugs. **B,** Other salivary mucus cysts are thought to occur as isolated blind cysts.

mucoceles are characterized by diffuse foci of mucin admixed with granulation tissue, neutrophils, and foamy histiocytes. This mucus extravasation often extends between salivary lobules and along fascial and muscle planes.

TREATMENT

The typical minor gland mucocele will not resolve of its own accord and must be surgically excised. To minimize the chance for recurrence, the underlying feeder glands should be removed in continuity with the mucocele or extirpated from the base of the surgical bed after the removal of the lesion. Oral floor ranulas can also be excised; however, deroofing or "marsupialization" has been advocated as an alternative procedure. The rationale for marsupialization is predicated on the presence of an epithelial-lined cavity of mucus retention. Because true mucus cysts are rarely encountered in this location and most ranulas are mucoceles that lack an epithelial lining, marsupialization is to be discouraged. Plunging ranulas should be attended to quickly because airway obstruction may ensue. The mucinous material should be removed by aspiration and/or surgery to relieve airway compression, followed by cannulation and repair of the major duct when possible.

MUCUS RETENTION CYST

> ■ MUCUS RETENTION CYST: swelling caused by an obstruction of a salivary gland excretory duct resulting in an epithelial-lined cavity containing mucus.

True mucus retention cysts, sometimes referred to as true mucoceles or sialocysts, are aneurysm-like dilatations of salivary ducts containing mucus. Alternatively, some of these lesions may represent true blind cysts that are not in continuity with the ductal system (Figure 10-7). Unlike a mucocele that is surrounded by granulation tissue, the mucus retention cyst is lined by epithelium. These cysts rarely involve the major salivary glands; when they do, they are often mul-

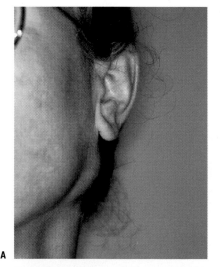

A

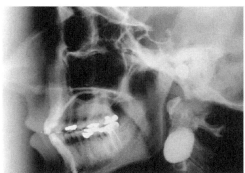

B

FIGURE 10-8

Dysgenic polycystic disease. A, Clinical appearance of a fluctuant parotid mass located beneath the earlobe and distal to the angle of the mandible. **B,** Injected opaque dye defines the cyst as a rounded radiopacity *(lower right)*.

tiple (dysgenic or polycystic disease of the parotid gland) (Figure 10-8). More often, mucus retention cysts arise in the oral minor salivary glands where they are solitary but may be either unilocular or multilocular lesions. Clinically, a mucus retention cyst is indistinguishable from a mucocele and may resemble low-grade mucoepidermoid carcinoma.

CLINICAL

True mucus retention cysts are more often encountered among adults throughout the third to eighth decades, although they may occur at any age. Those cysts located in the major salivary glands show a marked predilection for the parotid gland, which accounts for almost 90% of cysts of the major glands. When cysts occur in this location, the mean age of patients is 45 years. Parotid cysts are usually located in the superficial lobe and present as fluctuant, well-defined masses anterior to the ear or overlying the angle of the mandible. A history of slow progressive enlargement is usually noted. Within the oral cavity the floor of the mouth is the most common site, followed by the buccal mucosa and the lower lip. The lesions are painless, cystic, fluctuant, and generally superficial. In these instances they have a translucent, bluish appearance. Deep-seated cysts may be detectable only during bimanual palpation. A specific histologic type of cyst that involves the minor salivary glands is the **oncocytoid cyst,** which is most frequently seen in the buccal mucosa and lips in older patients (mean age is 60 years). The oncocytoid cysts are usually identified as painless, sessile, dome-shaped masses of normal coloration that are located just below the surface in the buccal mucosa, vestibule, and lips. This type of cyst often has a history of fluctuation in size.

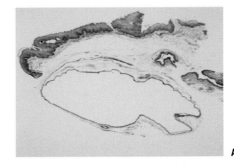

HISTOPATHOLOGY

The surface stratified squamous mucosal epithelium of the oral cavity is distended by a cystic cavity that is lined by cuboidal or, occasionally, columnar ductlike epithelium (Figure 10-9, *A*). The cytoplasm of these ductal lining cells is either eosinophilic or clear, and some may show evidence of mucous differentiation. Whereas 70% of these cells are unilocular, 30% show multilocular patterns, sometimes with small papillary projections into the cystic lumens (Figure 10-9, *B*). The surrounding fibrous tissue may be compressed yet is rarely inflamed. The underlying gland lobules sometimes show evidence of chronic sclerosing sialadenitis. Those cysts arising in the parotid gland usually have a well-defined fibrous capsule that separates the cyst from the parotid parenchyma. Whether the mucus retention cyst is a true cyst of salivary duct origin or a focal dilatation due to obstruction is not always clear; indeed, the two processes are not mutually exclusive. Nevertheless, although the cyst cavity may contain congealed mucin, there may not be evidence of a stone or another readily identifiable source of obstruction that might result in a focal, aneurysmal, ductal dilatation. The oncocytoid cyst, which favors older individuals, shows a distinctive, histologic appearance. The lining cells are columnar and often pseudostratified and their cytoplasm is strikingly eosinophilic, typical of oncocytes. The lumen is filled with eosinophilic, proteinaceous material thought to represent inspissated mucin. The adjacent gland lobules show evidence of obstructive chronic sclerosing sialadenitis. Oncocytic changes are often seen in the ducts of the adjacent glands. Rare varieties of mucus retention cysts occur that are multilobular with papillary projections and may be confused with cystic adenomas.

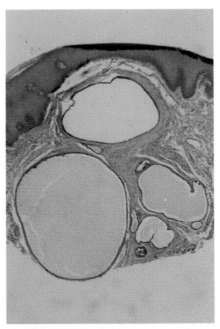

TREATMENT

Simple excision is the treatment of choice. Care must be taken to avoid rupturing the delicate cystic sac at the time of surgery. Recurrence is rare; however, damage to adjacent glands may result in the formation of a mucocele.

FIGURE 10-9

Mucus retention cyst. Lesions are located in the submucosa. **A,** Unilocular. **B,** Multilocular.

SIALOLITHIASIS

■ SIALOLITHIASIS: presence of one or more oval or round calcified structures (salivary stones) in a duct of a major or minor salivary gland.

Salivary stones can form within the lumens of major and minor salivary glands. In the major salivary glands the submandibular gland is most commonly involved; the consequences of duct blockage in the major salivary glands are more significant than when stones form in oral mucosal minor salivary gland ducts. In the major salivary glands prolonged blockage can lead to complete degeneration of parenchyma with secretory shutdown. During the process of obstruction, salivary retention with ductal dilatation results in pain and swelling. Glands that are no longer functional become subject to retrograde bacterial infections that can cause severe pain.

Stones that develop in other ductal systems of the body, such as uroliths (kidney stones) and choleliths (gall stones), have individual mineral contents and are associated with specific underlying predisposing conditions. Cholelithiasis is associated with bile secretion changes, infection, and stasis in the biliary tree. Gall stones are composed of either cholesterol or bilirubin. Kidney stones are usually calcium containing and develop as a consequence of hypercalciuria with or without hypercalcemia. Conversely, salivary stones are not associated with hypercalcemia; no specific secretory predisposing condition has been identified in sialolithiasis. For unknown reasons it is assumed that congealed mucin, protein, and desquamated ductal epithelial cells form a small nidus on which calcium salts precipitate (Figure 10-10). The small nidus then allows concentric lamellar crystalizations to occur; the sialolith increases in diameter as layer after layer of salts becomes deposited, much like growth rings in a tree. Microliths would probably be expelled easily in the saliva. Those that are not expelled usually continue to enlarge until a duct branch or even the major duct becomes occluded.

CLINICAL

About 80% of all sialoliths affect the major salivary glands; 75% of these have a predilection for the more viscous-secreting submandibular gland. The parotid gland is involved in 20% of the cases with only 5% involvement of the sublingual gland (Table 10-1). Rare bilateral cases have been observed. Whereas the main duct is usually the site of the stone, multiple sialoliths can develop within ductal branches throughout the gland and long-standing lesions may result in complete calcification of the entire gland. Stones are rare in children. The average age of patients with sialolith formation is 45, and there is no sex preference. Although some stones are asymptomatic and are detected on dental radiographs taken for other purposes, most will cause symptoms. The chief complaints are pain and swelling. Swelling is the consequence of ductal dilatation caused by retention of mucin in the blocked ducts. The swelling is most often observed at

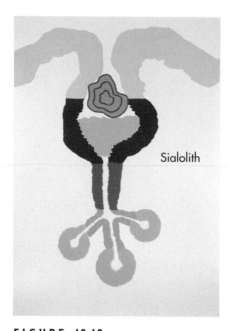

FIGURE 10-10

Sialolithiasis. Sialoliths obstruct the flow of mucin as they slowly enlarge.

TABLE 10-1			
Incidence of Sialolithiasis in Major and Minor Salivary Glands			
Major Glands	**Incidence**	**Minor Glands**	**Incidence**
Submandibular gland	73%	Lips	37%
Parotid gland	23%	Buccal mucosa	34%
Sublingual gland	4%	Floor of the mouth	9%
		All other sites	20%

mealtimes or on direct stimulation of saliva production with a lemon drop candy. A persistent swelling eventually evolves in patients with chronic obstruction as the enlargement becomes a chronic sialadenitis containing inflammatory cells and interstitial edema. The pain is described as a pulling, drawing, or stinging sensation that can be quite uncomfortable if the entire duct is blocked. Partial obstruction occurs when pressure increases but saliva can escape around the stone or when only a duct branch rather than the main duct is blocked. In these situations the symptoms are mild or transient.

When a submandibular gland becomes symptomatic, unilateral glandular enlargement can be seen medial to the inferior border of the mandible. On palpation the swelling is firm yet tender (Figure 10-11, *A*). An occlusal radiograph will typically disclose the presence of a calcification in the floor of the mouth along the course of the major duct (Figure 10-11, *B*). If only branches of the duct at the level of the submandibular gland are affected, a posterior occlusal film, submental vertex, or lateral jaw film may be required to disclose the stone. Panoramic radiographs are also used to demonstrate submandibular duct stones; however, they are often projected over the image of the mandible, masquerading as intrabony opacities. Parotid stones, which usually cause firm swellings over the ramus of the mandible, are also more prevalent during meals and can usually be visualized on a panoramic film. When radiographs fail to disclose the presence of calcified bodies in the parotid gland, sialography may be indicated. Not all sialoliths are sufficiently calcified to become radiographically demonstrable.

The recoverability and regenerative capacity of an obstructed gland depends on the degree of acinar necrosis and lobular fibrosis. When the secretory capacity is destroyed and normal secretions cannot flush the ducts, a retrograde infection ensues. In these instances pyogenic infections can result in persistent swelling with acute persistent pain, fever, and malaise. Often, the affected gland and distended ducts become filled with purulent exudate.

Minor salivary gland sialolithiasis is most often seen in the upper lip and buccal mucosa. Because minor salivary glands are small, a transient enlargement is not seen during meals. Rather, the stone itself is often clinically obvious or is readily palpable as a hard, movable nodule within the submucosa.

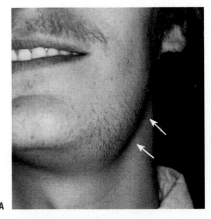
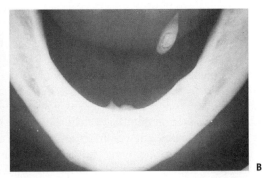

A   B

FIGURE 10-11

Submandibular sialolithiasis. A, Swelling below the mandible *(arrows)*, indicative of mucus retention and sialadenitis of the submandibular gland. **B,** Occlusal radiograph disclosing an oval stone in Warthin duct.

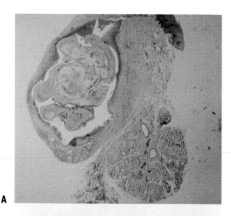

A

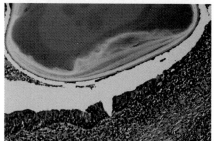

B

FIGURE 10-12

Sialolithiasis. A, Low-power photomicrograph of a large sialolith completely blocking a distended excretory duct of a minor salivary gland. **B,** Medium-power photomicrograph of a portion of a sialolith that exhibits lamination. The ductal wall is infiltrated by leukocytes.

HISTOPATHOLOGY

On gross examination most sialoliths are yellowish-white, round to oval, and heavily calcified. Some are multinodular, whereas others are found in aggregates. After decalcification the stones exhibit lamination with concentric rings of basophilic bands. The material is otherwise acellular and amorphous. The outer margin may contain aggregates of microbial colonies. When the glandular elements are submitted for microscopic examination, the ductal lining that surrounds the sialolith shows a variety of reactive changes including squamous and mucus cell metaplasia whereby the duct lining thickens into a stratified squamous type of epithelium that contains numerous mucus goblet cells in the more luminally oriented superficial layers. Occasionally, the columnar cells show true cilia. The periductal connective tissue is often densely infiltrated by lymphocytes and plasma cells (Figure 10-12). The rest of the gland will usually show varying progressive consequences of obstruction. In early disease the acini show degenerative changes with the dilatation of intralobular ducts. At this stage, lymphocytic and plasmacytic infiltration is spotty and some acinar degeneration may be present within lobules. As more pressure changes evolve, the ductal ectasia becomes more pronounced and acinar atrophy progresses with few secretory units remaining. Rather, the lobules become intensely infiltrated with mononuclear cells and the ducts remain intact yet dilated. Eventually, the infiltrate wanes and the lobules become progressively collagenized. Obstructed glands that become complicated by retrograde acute bacterial sialadenitis show tissue infiltration by neutrophils with purulent material in the ductal lumens.

TREATMENT

Many major salivary gland sialoliths can be removed by manual manipulation of the stone through the major duct orifice. When manual maneuvers fail, a surgical "cut-down" into the main duct is needed. Intraglandular stones, multiple stones within the gland proper, diffuse glandular calcifications, and longstanding obstructions will usually require removal of the stone along with sialoadenectomy. Minor salivary gland stones are well localized and are best treated by simple surgical excision of the stone and the surrounding ductal and minor salivary gland lobular tissues.

When signs and symptoms of an acute pyogenic infection exist, incision and drainage with antibiotic therapy should precede or accompany sialoadenectomy.

CHRONIC SCLEROSING SIALADENITIS

> ■ SIALADENITIS: inflammatory response of salivary gland tissue to a wide spectrum of etiologic factors.

> ■ CHRONIC SCLEROSING SIALADENITIS: chronic inflammation of salivary gland tissue resulting in replacement of acini by lymphocytes, plasma cells, and fibrous tissue but sparing much of the ductal architecture.

An inflammation of either a major or minor salivary gland is termed sialadenitis. Most are chronic and result in the formation of a substantial amount of fibrous replacement of parenchyma and occur as a consequence of mucus extravasation or duct blockage from salivary stones. Also, direct trauma or compression of the glands and/or ducts can cause sialadenitis. In addition to injuries, hyperplasias and neoplasms can lead to a secondary glandular inflammation. Regardless of the source or cause, when degeneration with fibrous replacement and chronic inflammation occurs, the process is referred to as **chronic sclerosing sialadenitis.**

CLINICAL

Chronic sclerosing sialadenitis is most often the consequence of direct compression or ductal obstruction. The clinical features of obstructive salivary disease that are reactive to sialoliths and mucus extravasation have been discussed. The obstructed major salivary gland becomes enlarged due to the accumulation of secretions within the duct system and later as a consequence of inflammatory cell infiltration (Figure 10-13). The enlarged gland is generally firm yet freely movable. The firmness may increase with time as more and more fibrotic replacement of acini occurs. In the minor salivary glands, various surface epithelial proliferations such as papilloma or squamous cell carcinoma and submucosal fibrous enlargements such as fibrous hyperplasia may obstruct the minor duct lumen or compress the extralobular ducts that exit from the gland proper. The flanges of dental prostheses, if overextended, can compress minor salivary glands in the vestibule, resulting in a sialadenitis. In addition, salivary gland neoplasms can compress adjacent normal glands, resulting in obstruction. As a consequence, minor gland chronic sclerosing sialadenitis will evolve, although it may not be clinically obvious.

One of the major causes of sialadenitis is radiation therapy used to treat head and neck cancer. The radiation ports often include the major salivary glands within the treatment field, particularly when the cancer is located in the oral cavity or oropharynx. Destruction of acini occurs early in the course of radiotherapy. When dose levels reach 50 centagrey, most secretory function will be lost. In these early phases acinar cell destruction begins and is accompanied by an increase in serum amylase. After a full course of radiation, exposed glands ultimately lose much of their acini and become fibrosed. This usually results in a permanent loss of secretory activity (xerostomia) and leads to cervical caries, oral mucositis, and candidiasis.

HISTOPATHOLOGY

The microscopic changes that are typically found in the affected glands of patients with sialolithiasis are also present in chronic sclerosing sialadenitis caused by other etiologic factors (see Figure 10-2). The acinar units degenerate as mononuclear leukocytes, chiefly plasma cells and lymphocytes, infiltrate the lobules. In radiation sialadenitis the earliest changes include loss of secretory granules, cloudy swelling with edema, and neutrophilic infiltration, which is soon followed by mononuclear infiltrates. With time all acini are lost and the gland is no longer functional. The ductal elements remain intact, showing ectasia and sialodochitis, whereas the parenchyma becomes progressively fibrotic. These glands, particularly the major salivary glands, may then be subject to retrograde bacterial acute sialadenitis.

TREATMENT

The primary cause of the sialadenitis must be identified before treatment can be initiated. Sources of irritation and obstruction must be removed. If it is ascertained that a major salivary gland is no longer functional, it can be surmised that parenchymal destruction is complete and the gland is fibrosed. Because these glands are prone to acute infections within the persistent duct tree, sialoadenectomy will be necessary. Complete loss of salivary function as a result of the chronic sclerosing sialadenitis that occurs following radiation therapy has many attending complications. The chief dental complication of xerostomia is root caries. Daily fluoride gels should be prescribed, and meticulous oral hygiene must be instilled. Saliva substitutes offer some benefit for the dryness; and if some degree of salivation persists, electrostimulatory devices may increase salivary flow. Pilocarpine may also stimulate salivary flow when not all acinar units are destroyed.

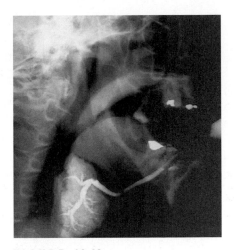

FIGURE 10-13

Sialadenitis. This sialogram shows an enlarged submandibular gland with prominent ductal ectasia.

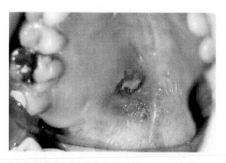

FIGURE 10-14

Necrotizing sialometaplasia. Lesion in typical location appearing as a deep ulcer of the palate.

NECROTIZING SIALOMETAPLASIA

■ **NECROTIZING SIALOMETAPLASIA**: spontaneous condition of unknown etiology, usually of the palate, in which a large area of surface epithelium, underlying connective tissue, and associated minor salivary glands become necrotic while ducts undergo squamous metaplasia.

Necrosis due to obstructive disease of the salivary glands generally occurs slowly. In necrotizing sialometaplasia, acute necrosis of entire lobules of minor salivary tissue occurs in a short period. It is believed that this process is due to infarction. Although the cause of infarction is unknown and is unrelated to systemic microvascular occlusion or thromboembolic disease, the preservation of cellular outlines, characteristic of the coagulative necrosis seen in infarction, is evident in this disease. Importantly, this benign spontaneously healing lesion may be mistaken for a malignant salivary gland neoplasm, clinically and microscopically.

CLINICAL

Usually located at the hard-soft palate junction, necrotizing sialometaplasia is characterized by a deep-seated ulceration that generally lacks a raised or rolled border (Figure 10-14). Rather, the ulcer is punched out and within its deep crater are gray, granular lobules that represent necrotic minor salivary glands. The ulcer often measures 2 to 3 cm in diameter. Whereas some patients complain of numbness or burning pain, others are completely asymptomatic. The palate is the most common site of involvement, and in most cases the ulcer evolves spontaneously without antecedent trauma; however, a few reports have mentioned occurrence after a local palatal anesthetic injection. The lesion rarely occurs in other sites but has been reported in the tongue, retromolar pad, nasal cavity, antrum, and major salivary glands. In these nonpalatal sites the disease is often traced to an etiologic factor such as surgery, trauma, or radiation. The fact that ischemic necrosis accounts for the pathologic features is supported by the experimental replication of the process in laboratory animals. Ligation of vessels reducing blood supply to the salivary glands recapitulates the same microscopic changes that occur in human tissue.

Most cases of necrotizing sialometaplasia occur in adults who have a broad age range and a mean age of about 47, although women seem to be affected at a somewhat younger age. Males are afflicted slightly more often than females.

HISTOPATHOLOGY

The microscopic features are distinctive and specific. In the palate the surface epithelium is lacking in the zone of ulceration and is replaced by fibrin and granulation tissue. Lobules of minor salivary acini that exhibit features of coagulation necrosis underlie this thin granulation tissue covering. The cytoplasmic borders of the cells of the acinar bulbs are intact. These acinar cells lack nuclei, are distended, and appear pale and basophilic. Entire lobules are similarly affected with the result that the lobular architecture of the minor salivary glands is still maintained although the cells are nonvital.

Scattered neutrophils and foamy histiocytes are often found in the zones of necrosis where mucin has accumulated or leaked from the necrotic acinar cells. Dispersed around the periphery of the necrotic lobules are ductal elements, many of which show squamous metaplasia (Figure 10-15). These metaplastic foci are typically represented by round or oval epithelial islands composed of benign squamous cells. Lumens are no longer evident in most of these islands. This represents a reactive process akin to pseudoepitheliomatous hyperplasia. Whereas some of the squamous islands are surrounded by necrotic "ghosts" of acinar elements, others show an enveloping fibrous stroma. The histologic features are similar to those encountered in mucoepidermoid carcinoma. In the lat-

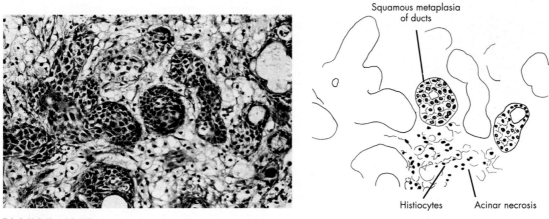

Squamous metaplasia
of ducts

Histiocytes   Acinar necrosis

FIGURE 10-15

Necrotizing sialometaplasia. Ductal structures undergo transformation from cuboidal to squamous cells (squamous metaplasia) yielding nodules of epithelium, whereas acini cells undergo necrosis.

ter case the epithelial component is not oriented into multiple round or oval islands; rather, more diffuse anastomosing sheets of squamous cells are encountered and surround the luminal spaces. Mucus, clear, and intermediate cells are also present. Furthermore, mucoepidermoid carcinoma is not associated with lobular necrosis.

TREATMENT

No treatment is necessary once the diagnosis is microscopically confirmed. The ulcerated area heals slowly, usually within 1 to 3 months.

INFECTIONS

ACUTE PAROTITIS

Acute infections of the salivary glands may be of either viral or bacterial origin. Endemic parotitis or mumps is the most commonly encountered form of infectious sialadenitis. Pyogenic bacterial infections are uncommon and may be seen after major abdominal surgery or in glands that have been obstructed. Chronic infections such as tuberculous sialadenitis and cat-scratch fever are rarely encountered.

VIRAL (ENDEMIC) PAROTITIS

Viral or endemic parotitis is an acute sialadenitis caused by an RNA virus of the paramyxoviridae family referred to as the mumps virus. Other viruses may infect the salivary glands including the cytomegalovirus (salivary inclusion disease), coxsackie viruses, ECHO virus, and influenza and parainfluenza virus; however, the mumps virus is the main cause of acute parotitis.

MUMPS

CLINICAL

The mumps virus is transmitted by airborne droplets. It primarily affects the parotid glands but may also infect the submandibular gland. Children between

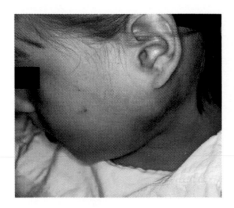

FIGURE 10-16

Endemic parotitis. Child with painful parotid swelling.

the ages of 5 and 18 are most often infected with this disease, which tends to become epidemic. Once exposed, patients will manifest the disease in 2 to 3 weeks. Onset is characterized by rapid bilateral swelling of the parotid gland with acute pain, particularly during salivation (Figure 10-16). The earlobe is often elevated from the underlying glandular enlargement. A purulent exudate can sometimes be expressed from the main parotid duct orifice but is usually clear and unremarkable. As acini become infected, salivary amylase leaks into the interstitium and is absorbed into the blood stream thereby raising serum levels of the enzyme. Complement-fixing antibodies to the mumps "S" and "V" antigens can be assayed to confirm the diagnosis. The disease usually persists for 7 to 10 days; whereas most cases are uncomplicated, some individuals experience dissemination to the testis or develop encephalitis with attending deafness. Severe forms of mumps orchitis can result in sterility. Because most children in industrialized countries are vaccinated against mumps, the disease is only rarely encountered.

HISTOPATHOLOGY

In mumps the acini develop cloudy swellings and the interstitial connective tissue becomes edematous and infiltrated with plasma cells and lymphocytes. Ductal ectasia is a feature, and the lumens often contain desquamated cell debris and leukocytes. In acute bacterial sialadenitis the interstitial regions are infiltrated by neutrophils and the ductal lumina also contain necrotic material and neutrophilic leukocytes. Acinar cell degeneration and necrosis can also be seen.

TREATMENT

There are no effective antiviral agents for the treatment of mumps. Patients are given analgesics and antipyretics to control pain and fever. A liquid diet with vitamin supplementation should be considered along with bed rest. Acute bacterial sialadenitis should be managed with antibiotics selected on the basis of sensitivity testing. Under local anesthetic, probing and dilatation of the main duct exiting the gland may facilitate drainage of purulent exudate.

BACTERIAL SIALADENITIS

Bacterial sialadenitis may occur after major surgery, usually abdominal surgery (Figure 10-17). Although the predisposition is unknown, it may be related to a temporary lack of ductal outflow that can develop with the administration of atropine sulfate while delivering general anesthetics, allowing an ascending infection. Similarly, obstructed glands can become infected by pyogenic bacteria, usually staphylococci and streptococci. The gland enlarges and is painful on palpation. In classic cases, purulent exudate can be expressed from the duct orifice. This material should be subjected to culture and sensitivity so that the appropriate antibiotic can be selected.

IMMUNE-MEDIATED DISEASE

Autoimmune diseases may have multiorgan involvement or affect only a single organ. When an autoimmune disease affects the major salivary glands (autoimmune sialadenitis), it is usually associated with a similar lacrimal gland disease and rheumatoid polyarthritis. The immunologic process that occurs within the salivary tissue is chronic and progressive with the eventual destruction of acini by inflammatory cells. The glands become enlarged bilaterally and are functionally deficient, leading to xerostomia. Xerophthalmia also occurs because the lacrimal glands are similarly affected. The histopathologic pattern is one of infil-

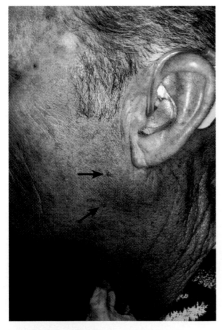

FIGURE 10-17

Bacterial parotitis. Infection causing painful parotid enlargement anterior and inferior to earlobe *(arrows)*.

tration with T lymphocytes that mediate the acinar cell destruction and a reactive proliferation of the ductal epithelium. The tissue changes are a classic process in salivary glands and are referred to as a *benign lymphoepithelial lesion (BLL)*. It is the hallmark of the multisystem disease referred to as *Sjögren syndrome (SS)*.

BENIGN LYMPHOEPITHELIAL LESION

■ BENIGN LYMPHOEPITHELIAL LESION: progressive autoimmune chronic inflammatory process primarily of the parotid glands in which dense infiltrates of T lymphocytes replace the acini and the residual ductal elements are stimulated to undergo hyperplasia, forming irregularly shaped islands of squamous epithelium (epimyoepithelial islands).

Whether gland enlargement is present or not, the tissue changes of BLL are usually indicative of eventual development of SS. The benign lymphoepithelial lesion has also been associated with multiple salivary cysts in patients with HIV infection. In addition, lymphocytic infiltration of the salivary glands with clinical evidence of parotid gland enlargement may occur in mucosa-associated lymphoid tissue lymphoma (**MALToma**) and as an independent organ-restricted autoimmune form of sialadenitis referred to as **Mikulicz disease.** When **sarcoidosis** involves the parotid glands (Heerfordt syndrome) a painless bilateral enlargement also occurs, mimicking the benign lymphoepithelial lesion clinically. Histologically, sarcoidosis differs greatly from the benign lymphoepithelial lesion in that the salivary parenchyma is replaced by noncaseating granulomatous inflammation consisting of macrophages and multinucleated giant cells.

SJÖGREN SYNDROME

■ SJÖGREN SYNDROME: group of autoimmune conditions with a marked predilection for women that has an intense T lymphocyte-mediated autoimmune process in the salivary and lacrimal glands as one of its most prominent components.

In Sjögren syndrome (SS) there is progressive T lymphocyte infiltration and replacement of the glandular parenchyma that leads to **xerostomia** and **xerophthalmia.** The characteristic histologic appearance is that of BLL. The hypersensitivity reaction in the parotid and lacrimal parenchymal glands is considered to be a cell-mediated immunologic reaction to native antigens on specific glandular epithelial cells (for example, autoimmune sialadenitis). This reaction accounts for the dryness that eventually develops in the eyes and oral cavity, the so-called "sicca (dry) complex." **Rheumatoid arthritis** is the third and a variable component of the syndrome.

Clinical
SS occurs in 0.5% to 1.0% of the population; whereas the disease is not hereditary, associations with certain HLA genotypes have been noted (HLA-B8 and HLA-DR3). Over 80% of patients with SS are women. If the disease affects only salivary and lacrimal glands without other coexisting systemic autoimmune diseases, it is termed *primary Sjögren syndrome*. Patients will show keratoconjunctivitis sicca, characterized by corneal keratotic lesions that stain pink when rose bengal dye is used. There is a reduction in tear meniscus and breakup time. The Schirmer test is used to assess lacrimal flow and is positive when the flow is reduced to less than 5 mm during a 5-minute sample period. This test utilizes a

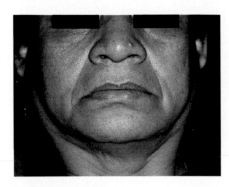

FIGURE 10-18

Sjögren syndrome. Patient exhibits bilateral parotid enlargements.

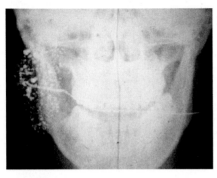

FIGURE 10-19

Sjögren syndrome. Sialogram of parotid enlargement of patient exhibiting characteristic pattern of pooling of dye in areas of damage to the ductal architecture.

strip of filter paper that is placed between the eye and the eyelid to determine the degree of tearing, which is measured in millimeters. *Secondary Sjögren syndrome* occurs when other signs or symptoms of autoimmune disease are present, the most common being rheumatoid arthritis. Other collagen-vascular diseases may occur in secondary SS, including lupus erythematosus, systemic sclerosis, dermatomyositis, and mixed connective tissue disease. Other extrasalivary/lacrimal diseases that have been identified in either primary or secondary forms of SS include Raynaud disease, interstitial nephritis, interstitial pneumonitis, purpura, and polymyopathy. There is also an increased risk for the development of extrasalivary malignant lymphoma. Specific laboratory findings are most often encountered in secondary SS and include an elevated erythrocyte sedimentation rate, hypergammaglobulinemia, and positive serologic tests for rheumatoid factors and antinuclear antibodies (ANA)—anti-Ro (anti–SS-A) and anti-La (anti–SS-B).

The basic etiology of SS is unknown. The signs and symptoms of dryness and swelling are the result of the immunologic reaction that occurs in the parenchymal tissue with consequential acinar loss and lymphocytic infiltration. The antigens that stimulate this immune mechanism are not well defined. A viral origin has been suggested whereby immunologic responses to viral proteins crossreact with host cell proteins in salivary epithelia. Some evidence has been forwarded to suggest that a retrovirus may be involved.

Parotid gland enlargement is observed in approximately 45% of SS patients, and the glands feel firm yet doughy (Figure 10-18). When enlargement is seen, it is usually bilateral and because the parotids are the primary major salivary glands to be involved, some patients also have submandibular gland involvement. Imaging with contrast sialography, pertechnetate scintigraphy, computed tomography, or magnetic resonance will often assist with the diagnosis because these techniques will usually demonstrate inflammatory rather than neoplastic imaging features. None of these imaging techniques are specifically diagnostic for SS because any sialadenitis may reveal the same features. Despite the progressive loss of acini and secretory activity, it is rare for the salivary glands of SS patients to develop an acute bacterial sialadenitis. Sialogram reveals a characteristic appearance of pooling of the opaque dye that resembles "shotgun pellets" throughout the gland (Figure 10-19).

The manifestations of SS that are of most significance to the patient are dry mouth (xerostomia) and dry eyes (xerophthalmia). The dry sensation is very annoying because the mucosa in both the mouth and the eyes become thinned, inflamed, and painful with a burning sensation. The dry mucosa is also very susceptible to candidiasis. One of the major consequences of xerostomia is the predilection for root caries, usually at the cementoenamel junction (CEJ) on the facial aspects of the teeth.

Biopsy of the labial mucosa minor salivary glands has proven to be a reliable adjunct in the diagnosis of SS. This simple procedure requires a sample of six to eight minor salivary gland lobules harvested from the lower lip. Lymphocyte aggregates within the minor glands are enumerated to generate a focus score. The diagnosis of SS is supported when the focus score exceeds that of normal glandular tissue.

HISTOPATHOLOGY

The microscopic features of SS are those of the benign lymphoepithelial lesion because it is the pathologic hallmark of SS in the parotid gland. Although immunomarker studies have identified the presence of both B and T lymphocytes, the latter are the most abundant. With increasing numbers of infiltrating lymphocytes there is progressive destruction and loss of acinar units. Once entire lobules have been infiltrated, it is not uncommon for germinal centers to form

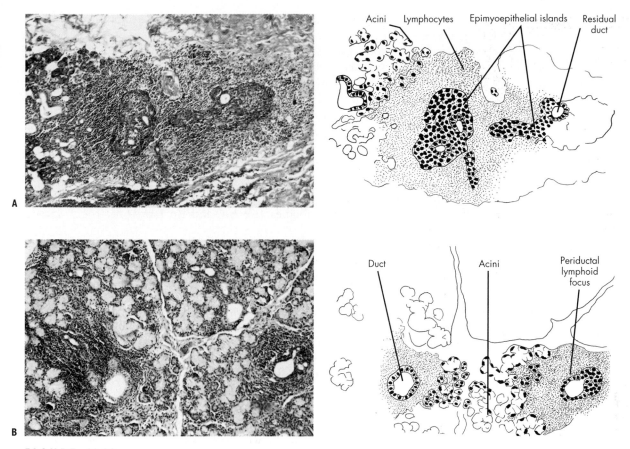

FIGURE 10-20

Benign lymphoepithelial lesion in Sjögren syndrome. A, Lymphocyte replacement of acini with formation of epimyoepithelial islands. **B,** Periductal lymphoid aggregates in a lower lip minor gland.

with a surrounding mantle of small lymphocytes resembling lymphoid hyperplasia in a node. The ductal elements are not eliminated by these infiltrating cells. Indeed, the ductal and periductal myoepithelial cells undergo hyperplasia, resulting in islands of epithelial cells that no longer contain well-defined ductal lumens. These epithelial foci are termed *epimyoepithelial islands* (Figure 10-20, *A*). The combination of acinar loss, lymphocytic infiltration, and epimyoepithelial islands constitute BLL. Although MALToma may show similar features, the infiltrating lymphocytes of BLL are histiocytoid or plasmacytoid and immunohistochemical markers are positive for B lymphocytes.

The histopathologic changes seen in the minor salivary glands in SS consist of aggregates of lymphocytes oriented around intralobular ducts (Figure 10-20, *B*). Normal salivary glands show very few lymphoid foci, and those that are present are composed of only a few cells. Foci with more than 50 lymphocytes are significant; however, when one or more of these aggregates is identified in a 4 mm² area of glandular parenchyma, a diagnosis of SS is supported. These lymphoid foci are primarily composed of T lymphocytes.

TREATMENT

There is no effective therapy for SS. Unfortunately, the dryness becomes progressively worse although some patients retain some degree of secretory function. The complications of xerostomia are difficult to treat satisfactorily, but the patient can be helped to cope with the discomfort. The development and progression of root caries can be minimized by daily application of topical fluoride gels and meticulous dental hygiene. Candidiasis can be managed with the use of antifungal medications. Salivary substitutes or lemon flavored glycerin/water can be carried and constantly sipped to offer some relief for the sensation of dryness. Pilocarpine and transmucosal neurostimulatory devices may stimulate secretions in those patients who retain some degree of secretory function. Secondary SS with accompanying collagen diseases will often require additional forms of therapy, including immunosuppressive agents.

BENIGN SALIVARY GLAND TUMORS

The tumors that arise from salivary glands may be derived from salivary epithelium (parenchymal) or the supportive stroma (mesenchymal). The stromal, or mesenchymal, tumors are generally seen in children and most are benign neoplasms of vascular or fibrohistiocytic origin. The parenchymal tumors may occasionally be encountered among children but more often arise during adulthood. Salivary gland tumors affect 1 to 3 individuals per 100,000 population, except for northern native peoples who experience a fivefold to tenfold increase in risk. The major glands account for over 70% of all salivary gland tumors; less than 30% arise in the minor glands (Table 10-2).

As a group the benign parenchymal tumors are **adenomas,** whereas malignant salivary gland tumors are classified as **adenocarcinomas.** These tumors may arise in patients at any age; the majority are encountered in the fifth to seventh decades. Females are afflicted more often than males. In the parotid gland almost 70% of salivary parenchymal tumors are benign adenomas; whereas tumors arising in the submandibular gland and minor glands of the oral, nasal, and paranasal sinus cavities show an equal predilection for benign and malignant tumors. Intraoral minor salivary tumors are most often encountered in the palate, followed by the upper lip and buccal mucosa. Whereas palatal and buccal mucosa glands harbor as many malignant as benign tumors, the lip neoplasms are more often benign adenomas. Salivary tumors arising from glands located in the tongue, lower lip, and retromolar areas are more often adenocarcinomas.

TABLE 10-2
Anatomic Distribution of Benign and Malignant Salivary Gland Tumors

	Benign	Malignant
MAJOR GLANDS		
Parotid	70%	30%
Submandibular	60%	40%
Sublingual	30%	70%
MINOR GLANDS		
Palate	50%	50%
Buccal mucosa	50%	50%
Upper lip	75%	25%
Oropharynx	60%	40%
Lower lip	40%	60%
Tongue	15%	85%
Retromolar	10%	90%
Floor of the mouth	10%	90%

Salivary tumors may arise from any of the cellular components of the glandular tree including basal or reserve ductal cells, striated ducts, intercalated ducts, acini, and myoepithelial cells. The various neoplasms are named according to the differentiation of the tumor cells. Some tumors elaborate a wide variety of secretory, ductal, and myoepithelial cells; whereas others are more monomorphic and composed of ductal or acinar cells only. The histopathologic patterns assumed by these salivary tumors are a reflection of their route of differentiation and should not be misconstrued as being indicative of the cells of origin. All salivary tumors arise from salivary epithelia yet they differ according to the line of differentiation that the cell population follows.

Unlike carcinomas in other locations (for example, squamous cell carcinoma), salivary adenocarcinomas usually fail to exhibit significant cytologic anaplasia or atypism. Importantly, most benign adenomas are well demarcated, not infiltrative, and encapsulated; whereas being nonencapsulated, the adenocarcinomas collectively show evidence of invasion into adjacent connective tissue (Figure 10-21). The diagnosis is made based on growth pattern characteristics and differentiation features. As a group, salivary adenocarcinomas are capa-

B

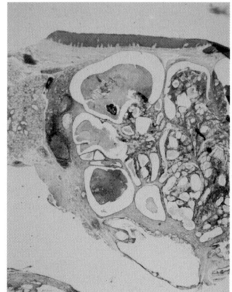

A

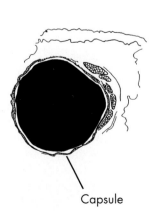

C

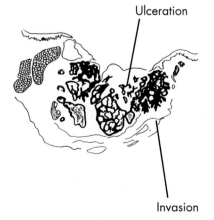

ENCAPSULATED   **DEMARCATED**   **NONENCAPSULATED**

Solid component   Ulceration

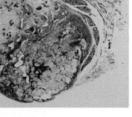   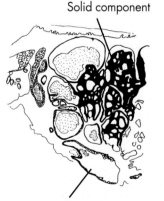

Capsule   Cystic component   Invasion

TABLE 10-3
Distinguishing Features of Benign and Malignant Salivary Gland Tumors

	Benign	Malignant
CLINICAL FEATURES	Smooth, uniform surface	Nodular surface
	Normal surface coloration	Surface telangiectasia
	Round, dome shaped	Irregularly shaped
	Intact overlying mucosa/skin	Ulcerated
	Movable	Fixed and indurated
	Asymptomatic	Occasional nerve deficits
MICROSCOPIC FEATURES	Distinct and intact capsule	Lacks encapsulation
	Uniformity of cells	Cells irregular in size and shape
	Tissue structures resemble normal	Altered tissue patterns
	Neoplastic cells displace nerves	Neoplastic cells invade nerves
	Normal stroma	Lacks sufficient stroma
	No necrotic areas	Occasional areas of necrosis

ble of locally aggressive behavior with a tendency for recurrence after treatment and may metastasize via lymphatic and/or hematogenous routes (Table 10-3).

Among benign tumors, **pleomorphic adenoma** is the most common. **Monomorphic adenoma, oncocytoma,** and **papillary cystadenoma lymphomatosum** are also relatively common. Rare types of adenomas include sebaceous adenoma, intraductal papilloma, sialadenoma papilliferum, and cystadenoma. The most commonly encountered malignant tumors are **mucoepidermoid carcinoma, adenoid cystic carcinoma, polymorphous low-grade adenocarcinoma,** and **acinic cell carcinoma.** Rare malignancies arising in salivary glands include clear cell carcinoma, epithelial-myoepithelial carcinoma of intercalated ducts, papillary cystadenocarcinoma, basal cell adenocarcinoma, undifferentiated carcinoma, mucinous carcinoma, malignant mixed tumor (pleomorphic adenoma with cytologic features of malignancy), carcinoma ex mixed tumor (an adenocarcinoma arising from a preexisting benign pleomorphic adenoma), squamous cell carcinoma of salivary origin, adenosquamous carcinoma, and salivary duct carcinoma. Melanoma and lymphoma also occur within the major salivary glands.

PLEOMORPHIC ADENOMA

■ PLEOMORPHIC ADENOMA: most common of the benign salivary gland tumors composed basically of a proliferation of myoepithelial cells and a wide spectrum of epithelial and mesenchymal tissue components and surrounded by a distinctive fibrous capsule.

The most common benign salivary gland tumor is the pleomorphic adenoma (PA), or **mixed tumor.** The term *pleomorphic* refers to the wide variation in parenchymal and stromal differentiation shown by the tumor cells and should not be confused with the nuclear pleomorphism exhibited by many malignant neoplasms. On the contrary, the individual cells of pleomorphic adenoma show bland, normal, and uniform nuclei regardless of their degree of differentiation.

The often-used term, *mixed tumor,* implies that a wide mixture of different tissue types are observed within individual tumors. The term was originally applied because it was thought that the neoplastic growth arose from multiple germ layers that gave rise to the epithelial and mesenchymal components of salivary tissue. It is now documented that this is not the case because the origin of the varied cellular elements is from the epithelial and/or myoepithelial cell. The myoepithelial cell is present in periductal locations and has a potential to differentiate into epithelial or connective tissue structures.

Pleomorphic adenoma accounts for 60% of all parotid gland tumors, 50% of submandibular gland tumors, and only 25% of sublingual gland neoplasms. Fifty percent of all oral minor gland tumors are mixed tumors of which 55% arise in the palate, 25% in the lip (mostly upper lip), 10% in the buccal mucosa, and 10% from all other oral and oropharyngeal sites.

CLINICAL

Like other benign tumors the pleomorphic adenoma has a slow growth rate and is well delineated. It is soft or only slightly firm on palpation and in the larger major salivary glands is freely movable. In the parotid gland the tumor is generally spherical and more often arises in the superficial lobe as an obvious mass anterior to the ear or overlying the angle of the mandible (Figure 10-22). Deep lobe tumors are not always detected as a facial mass because they may protrude into the lateral wall of the oropharynx. Occasionally, tumors that have been present for many years will become lobulated or multinodular, a feature shared with tumors that recur after incomplete surgical excision. In the oral minor glands the most common presentation is a soft to slightly firm swelling of the hard or soft palate without ulceration or telangiectasia of the overlying mucosa (Figure 10-23). Although rare, some palatal pleomorphic adenomas will become ulcerated. In the buccal mucosa and lip, pleomorphic adenomas are encapsulated, well defined, and movable on palpation. The overlying mucosa is usually intact.

Pleomorphic adenoma is encountered in patients of all ages; however, 60% of the cases occur in the third to fifth decades (mean age is 40 years). Less than 10% occur in children. The female/male ratio exceeds 2:1.

Magnetic resonance imaging (MRI) is a reliable diagnostic approach to determining the extent of the disease, particularly in the major salivary glands. The signal is intense, probably owing to the amount of myxoid stroma in these tumors. The images of mixed tumors appear as well-defined spherical or multinodular masses (see Figure 10-22, *B*).

HISTOPATHOLOGY

The histologic variations both within an individual lesion and between different pleomorphic adenomas can be extensive. The most constant finding in pleomorphic adenoma is the presence of a pronounced *fibrous capsule* (see Figure 10-21, *A*). This is an extremely important histologic feature when distinguishing benign from malignant salivary tumors. Some lesions of long duration may be multinodular or multifocal; however, each nodule or foci is enveloped by a distinct fibrous capsule. Although the tumor cells may show a wide variation, there are usually two dominant patterns of differentiation: *ductal* and *myoepithelial* (Figure 10-24). Many pleomorphic adenomas will contain diffuse sheets (medullary pattern) of monomorphic epithelial cells; others appear as interlacing cords (trabecular pattern). Almost all have ductal-tubular elements composed of cuboidal cells oriented around a lumen and associated spindle-shaped myoepithelial cells that appear to spin off of the ductal elements. In some tumors the *myoepithelial spindle cells* are included in a stromal myxomatous pattern, which may constitute its major component. Rarely, squamous differentiation with keratin production and mucus-secreting cells may be seen; these cell types are never predominant. Sheets of myoepithelial cells in many tumors lose their typical spindle-shaped appearance, becoming polygonal. The polygonal myoepithelial cells often show eccentric nuclei with hyalinized cytoplasms and are referred to

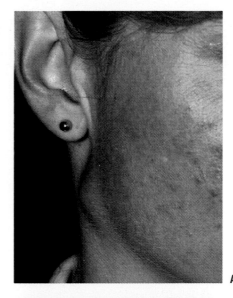

A

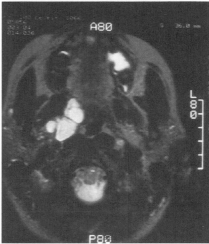

B

FIGURE 10-22

Pleomorphic adenoma of the parotid gland. A, Clinical appearance. **B,** Magnetic resonance imaging (MRI) shows a nodular mass of a recurrent pleomorphic adenoma in the deep lobe of the left parotid gland (*right side of image*).

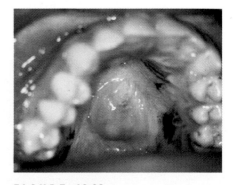

FIGURE 10-23

Pleomorphic adenoma of the palate.

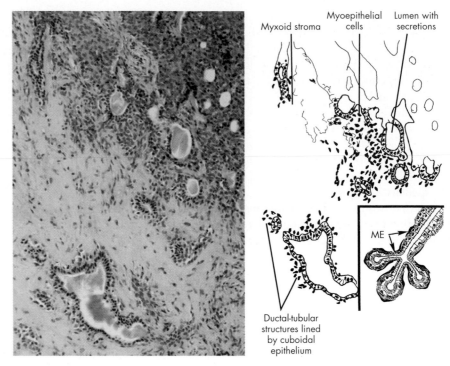

Myxoid stroma Myoepithelial cells Lumen with secretions

ME

Ductal-tubular structures lined by cuboidal epithelium

FIGURE 10-24

Pleomorphic adenoma. Ductal structures are lined by cuboidal cells. Myoepithelial cells *(ME)* are elongated and become loosely dispersed in the connective tissue stroma.

as *plasmacytoid myoepithelial cells.* The fibrous stroma usually blends with the spindle-shaped myoepithelial component. In some tumors the stroma becomes densely hyalinized; whereas in others, chondroid, adipose and even osseous stromal elements are encountered. The wide variation in the stromal elements are thought to evolve from inductive biochemical signals from the salivary epithelial and myoepithelial tumor cells.

Importantly, although pleomorphic adenomas are well encapsulated, it is not uncommon for neoplastic nests of cells to perforate the capsule, creating a new tumor focus. This event leads to the multinodularity sometimes observed in these tumors. If the tumors are simply enucleated, extracapsular foci may be incompletely removed, thereby leading to a recurrence. In less than 1% of cases malignant transformation occurs in a pleomorphic adenoma, especially those that have undergone multiple recurrences. These tumors are termed *carcinoma ex pleomorphic adenoma.*

TREATMENT

Pleomorphic adenomas arising in the major glands are treated by lobectomy or sialoadenectomy. Because recurrences are common due to the presence of extracapsular foci of the disease, simple enucleation is contraindicated. Within the oral cavity the palatal lesions, overlying mucosa, and underlying periosteum should also be excised. Pleomorphic adenomas of the lip and buccal mucosa rarely recur after simple enucleation; however, the incidence of recurrence is minimized or eliminated in all locations by excising the tumor with a margin of normal tissue.

MONOMORPHIC ADENOMA

■ MONOMORPHIC ADENOMA: group of benign salivary gland tumors composed of a proliferation of a single epithelial cell type that has a distinctive architectural pattern and is surrounded by a well-defined fibrous capsule. The two most common types are basal cell adenoma and canalicular adenoma.

The other salivary gland adenomas lack the wide cellular diversity encountered in pleomorphic adenomas. They are composed of a single cell type and are classified as *monomorphic adenomas*. Although these salivary gland adenomas are slow growing and encapsulated, similar to pleomorphic adenoma, they differ by having a lower propensity for recurrence. There are two distinct entities in this group that exhibit different clinicopathologic features: the **basal cell adenoma**, usually found in the parotid gland, and the **canalicular adenoma**, typically located in the submucosa of the upper lip.

CLINICAL

The *basal cell adenoma* is localized to the parotid gland in 75% of the cases. Less than 20% of these tumors are found within the oral cavity; those that arise from intraoral minor glands are usually found within the upper lip and buccal mucosa. The tumor is seen in adults and has a peak predilection for the seventh decade; females are affected more often than males. In the parotid gland these neoplasms are clinically indistinguishable from pleomorphic adenomas because they also tend to arise in the superficial lobe, are well encapsuled, and movable. On palpation basal cell adenomas are firmer than mixed tumors. Most are small tumors less than 3 cm in diameter.

Canalicular adenoma occurs in older patients, commonly in the seventh decade, with females affected more often than males. It rarely occurs in children. Approximately 75% of canalicular adenomas occur in the upper lip. The remaining tumors are found in the buccal mucosa; occurrence in the major glands or other oral minor glands is extremely rare. Most canalicular adenomas are single tumors less than 2 cm in diameter. They are freely movable and encapsulated. The overlying mucosa is smooth, intact, and usually normal in color but can show a slight bluish tinge.

HISTOPATHOLOGY

The **basal cell adenoma** is surrounded by a fibrous capsule. Within the tumor, cells cluster in oval nests that are separated by mature fibrous stroma. The outermost layer of cells that surround each cell nest are usually cuboidal, whereas the more centrally located cells within the cell nests are uniform and resemble basal cells in stratified squamous epithelium (Figure 10-25). In some tumors the individual tumor nests are small and well defined, resembling those seen in basal cell carcinoma of skin. In others the diffuse sheets of basaloid cells may be encountered with some exhibiting keratin pearl formation. A *trabecular* pattern may predominate in which elongated anastomosing cords of basal cells are surrounded by mature connective tissue stroma. *Tubular* patterns may prevail and are characterized by basaloid nests that surround cuboidal-lined ductal spaces filled with an eosinophilic secretion product. Occasionally, basal cell adenomas show islands of tumor cells that are enveloped by a prominent hyalinized basal lamina, the so-called *membranous* or *dermal analogue* adenoma. This type of adenoma resembles the dermal eccrine cylindroma, hence the term *dermal analogue tumor*. Both salivary and cutaneous tumors may occur in a given patient.

The **canalicular adenoma** has a histologic pattern that is usually unique and distinct. It is featured by the presence of a capsule that surrounds the prolif-

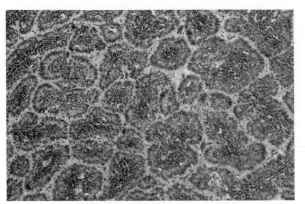
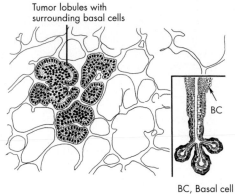

Tumor lobules with
surrounding basal cells

BC

BC, Basal cell

FIGURE 10-25

Basal cell adenoma. This variant of monomorphic adenoma is composed of solid nests of cells rimmed by basal cells *(BC)*.

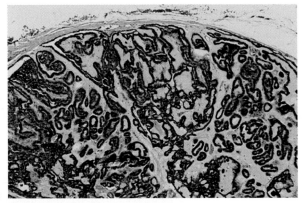

A

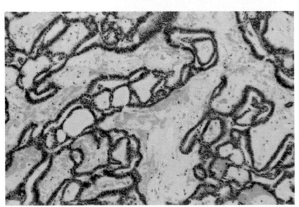
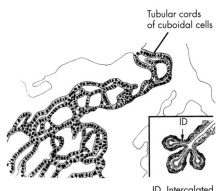

Tubular cords
of cuboidal cells

ID

B

ID, Intercalated
duct cells

FIGURE 10-26

Canalicular adenoma. A, Low-power photomicrograph exhibiting a capsule and cord arrangement of the epithelial component. **B,** High-power photomicrograph reveals the anastomosing cords of cuboidal cells accompanied by a delicate immature stroma typical of this variant.

erating monomorphic single-layered cuboidal and/or columnar ductal cells that are arranged in elongated anastomosing chords (Figure 10-26). The nuclei are oval or elongated and monomorphic. Ductal lumina are often prominent with the nuclei polarized toward the basement membrane. The stroma is classically myxomatous and composed of an eosinophilic-staining hypocellular mucoid matrix that is traversed by prominently dilated capillaries. The extensive ductal and anastomosing network of cuboidal and columnar cells gives the impression of multiple interconnecting canals, hence the term *canalicular*. Some tumors show cystic areas into which papillary fronds of the canalicular pattern of cells project. Multicentric tumors are occasionally seen, and even with single lesions adjacent salivary lobules may show minute multiple foci of tumor cells surrounded by normal acini.

TREATMENT

Simple excision is the treatment of choice for both basal cell and canalicular types of monomorphic adenoma. It is recommended that the excision include some surrounding normal tissue. Recurrence is uncommon.

PAPILLARY CYSTADENOMA LYMPHOMATOSUM

> ■ PAPILLARY CYSTADENOMA LYMPHOMATOSUM: benign salivary gland lesion with limited growth potential primarily occurring in the tail lobe of the parotid gland that is composed of cystic spaces with intraluminal projections lined by a double cell layer of eosinophilic columnar cells and contains abundant lymphoid tissue in the underlying connective tissue.

Of all the tumors that occur in the salivary glands, papillary cystadenoma lymphomatosum, also referred to as the *Warthin tumor*, is the most benign with self-limited growth potential. Because of their limited growth, these tumors are considered by most pathologists and clinicians to be hamartomas rather than true neoplasms. The unique aspect of this tumor is the mixture of cystic salivary ductal elements and normal lymphoid tissue. It is proposed by some that the lesion arises from ductal cells that have permeated and proliferated within parotid gland lymph nodes or lymphoid aggregates. Others suggest that the presence of the cystic adenomatous proliferation initiates a secondary lymphoid reactive response in the stroma.

CLINICAL

The papillary cystadenoma lymphomatosum primarily occurs in the parotid gland, accounting for about 5% of all parotid salivary tumors. It is extremely rare in other major or minor glands. Unlike other salivary tumors it has a slight predilection for males. Most cases are discovered in patients who are in the sixth and seventh decades of life. Approximately 10% of the cases are bilateral. Multiple lesions within one of the parotid glands are also encountered. The tumor is consistently found overlying the angle of the mandible in the superficial lobe and is well encapsuled and movable. It has a characteristic feel on palpation. When compressed with the fingers, the tumor usually feels "doughy." Technetium^{99m} pertechnetate radioisotope scanning is often helpful because the tumor readily takes up the isotope and appears as a *"hot nodule."*

HISTOPATHOLOGY

Before microscopy the gross examination of a sectioned tumor reveals a characteristic appearance. The tumor has a dense fibrous capsule with the internal structures exhibiting multiple confluent cystic compartments containing clear,

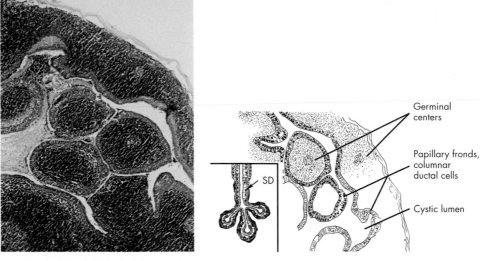

FIGURE 10-27

Papillary cystadenoma lymphomatosum. Present are intraluminal projections *(papillary fronds)* with an outer two cell layer covering of eosinophilic ductal cells resembling striated duct cells *(SD)* and central lymphoid follicles, some with *germinal centers.*

yellow, or brown viscous material. The microscopic appearance demonstrates cystic spaces lined by pseudostratified columnar cells with a very distinct eosinophilic cytoplasm (columnar oncocytes) (Figure 10-27). These cells resemble those normally found in striated ducts of salivary glands and are in a double row with the nuclei oriented in the basilar area of the bottom row and in the superior aspect of the upper row. These cells cover papillary fronds that extend into the cystic spaces. The papillary fronds are supported by large amounts of lymphoid tissue with widely scattered germinal centers. Rarely, mucous goblet cells are interposed among the oncocytic columnar epithelial cells. Rare cases of malignant transformation into adenocarcinoma have been reported.

TREATMENT

Simple enucleation is probably adequate for most papillary cystadenoma lymphomatosum tumors; however, due to the potential for multicentricity, most surgeons recommend superficial lobectomy to prevent recurrence or emergence of a new tumor at a later time. A true assessment of recurrence rate is difficult to ascertain because a perceived recurrence may simply represent a second new tumor. The rate of recurrence is less than 10%.

ONCOCYTOMA

■ ONCOCYTOMA: benign salivary gland tumor occurring primarily in the parotid gland that is composed of clusters of eosinophilic granular cells (oncocytes) containing abundant mitochondria arranged in an organoid pattern and surrounded by an intact fibrous capsule.

An oncocyte is an abnormal cell with a prominent eosinophilic and granular cytoplasm. Occasional oncocytes are found in many other glands; however, when they constitute the primary cell population of a neoplastic process, they are termed *oncocytoma*. The oncocytes are commonly seen in the normal salivary ducts of older patients where they resemble enlarged striated duct cells. The prominent cytoplasmic eosinophilic granules are mitochondria. An oncocyte is essentially an epithelial cell with excessive proliferations of mitochondria. The majority of oncocytomas arise in the parotid gland; only 10% are found in other major salivary glands.

CLINICAL

Oncocytoma shows a female predilection and tends to occur in older patients; most tumors arise in the eighth decade. It accounts for only 1% of all of the salivary gland tumors. The lesion is usually located anterior to the ear or over the mandibular ramus. It may be multinodular but is usually singular. On palpation it appears as a freely movable nodular mass. Occasionally, the tumor arises in the deep lobe of the parotid gland where it may lie adjacent to branches of the facial nerve. As with papillary cystadenoma lymphomatosum, technetium[99m] pertechnetate concentrates in oncocytomas, causing a "hot" appearance during radioisotope scanning.

HISTOPATHOLOGY

Oncocytoma contains a distinct capsule and may have a unilobular or multilobular pattern. The individual cells are polygonal or cuboidal and are usually arranged in an organoid or acinar pattern. Although discrete ductal lumina are not prominent, some oncocytomas have organoid cell clusters that form cords or "doughnut-shaped" circular configurations (Figure 10-28). The cell clusters are characteristic because they stain intensely eosinophilic. Each cell exhibits a copious amount of granular cytoplasm with centrally placed nuclei, usually small and pyknotic but occasionally vesicular. A characteristic feature is the lack of a fibrous stroma. The tumor cells are clustered, and each cluster is surrounded by fine vascular septae.

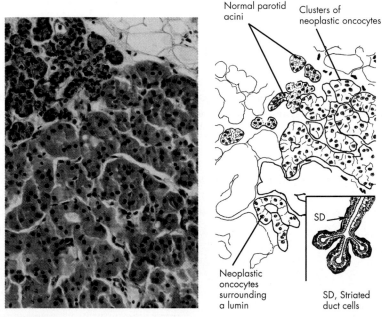

FIGURE 10-28

Oncocytoma. Tumor cells are prominently eosinophilic, granular, and uniform with centrally placed nuclei resembling striated duct cells *(SD)*.

A clear cell variant occurs in which the typical granular eosinophilic cytoplasm is not present. The cells in **clear cell oncocytoma** are vacuolated with only whispy remnants of cytosol. The rest of the tumor architecture is identical to the common form of oncocytoma.

TREATMENT

Surgical excision by lobectomy with preservation of the facial nerve is the treatment of choice. Simple enucleation without removal of the entire lobe will result in incomplete removal with recurrence in 10% of the cases.

MALIGNANT SALIVARY GLAND TUMORS

MUCOEPIDERMOID CARCINOMA

> ■ MUCOEPIDERMOID CARCINOMA: malignant salivary gland tumor of varying degrees of aggressiveness, composed of mucus-secreting and stratified squamous (epidermoid) epithelial cells and lacking a capsule.

All malignant salivary gland tumors are a form of adenocarcinoma. Adenocarcinomas of the salivary glands differ from some of the other groups of adenocarcinomas in the body. There is a wide variation in the behavioral patterns between each type of adenocarcinoma; some are almost benign, and others have a very poor prognosis. Mucoepidermoid carcinoma differs in its general behavior from other adenocarcinomas of salivary gland origin and also by exhibiting distinctive behavioral differences within its own histopathologic spectrum. Consequently, mucoepidermoid carcinoma is subcategorized based on its histopathologic features into *high-grade, intermediate-grade* and *low-grade* varieties; the high-grade type of mucoepidermoid carcinoma is the most aggressively malignant. The neoplastic cells of mucoepidermoid carcinoma differentiate along both mucous cell and squamous cell lines, thereby showing cell types that mimic mucous acinar cells and extralobular ductal cell elements. This malignancy arises in both major and minor salivary glands. On rare occasions it has been found within the mandible where it is thought to arise from odontogenic epithelium.

CLINICAL

Mucoepidermoid carcinomas can occur in patients throughout their adult life, with approximately equal numbers occurring from the third to the seventh decades. Although they are occasionally encountered in teenagers, they rarely occur during the first decade of life. There is a significant female predilection, particularly for tumors arising in the tongue and retromolar minor glands. Nearly half of mucoepidermoid carcinomas are found in the parotid gland, and the palate accounts for almost 20%. Of the lesions arising from the minor glands within the oral cavity, almost half of the cases are located in the palate (Figure 10-29). The buccal mucosa, lips, tongue, mandible, and retromolar areas are other favored sites.

In the parotid gland the tumors usually arise in the superficial lobe where they appear as relatively well-defined focal nodules. They may be movable, which is an uncommon feature for a malignant lesion. The low-grade lesions are often fluctuant, whereas high-grade tumors are usually indurated and fixed to adjacent tissue. These tumors usually range from 1 to 4 cm in diameter when first diagnosed. Facial nerve involvement, manifested as facial weakness or paralysis, is uncommon but when present is usually a harbinger of a high-grade le-

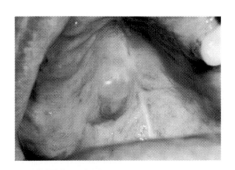

FIGURE 10-29

Mucoepidermoid carcinoma. Lesion of the palate revealing a smooth, nonulcerated appearance similar to a mucocele.

sion. Within the oral cavity most low-grade tumors are submucosal masses that have an intact, nonulcerated surface. Low-grade lesions, which are often composed of multiple cystic structures containing mucin, may yield a bluish tinge to the overlying mucosa and are easily mistaken for mucoceles. High-grade intraoral tumors may show surface ulceration. MRI is useful in demonstrating the extent of disease. Low-grade tumors with high mucin content will exhibit a high signal intensity on T2 weighted images.

Central (intraosseous) mucoepidermoid carcinoma of the jaws is most often located in the mandible; however, some maxillary cases have been observed. Approximately 4% of all mucoepidermoid carcinomas arise in the central region in bone. Whereas some of these tumors are detected due to osseous expansion and clinically evident bony enlargement, others are observed on routine dental radiographs. The central lesions may be unilocular or multilocular radiolucencies, occurring most frequently in the mandibular third molar region. An impacted tooth is often associated with the neoplasm, suggesting a relationship to odontogenic tissue. Unlike other intraosseous jaw malignancies, paresthesia is rarely a complaint.

HISTOPATHOLOGY

Mucoepidermoid carcinomas have three dominant cell types: mucous, epidermoid, and intermediate. These cellular elements are arranged in nests and diffuse sheets that may surround cystic spaces. A true capsule is generally lacking, although in some regions the leading edge of the tumor is often well demarcated (see Figure 10-21, *B*). It is common for focal areas to exhibit infiltration into the normal salivary tissue, connective tissue, or muscle. The individual cells show neither significant cytologic features of malignancy nor evidence of increased mitotic activity. Tumors with a preponderance of mucus cells and multiple cystic spaces are classified as low-grade; whereas those with more solid islands, fewer mucus-secreting cells, and a high proportion of stratified squamous epithelial (epidermoid) cells are classified as high-grade tumors. Intermediate-grade tumors fall between these two extremes.

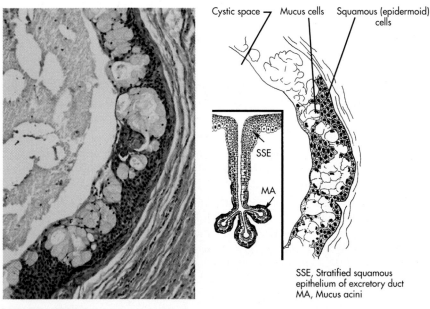

Cystic space ⌐ Mucus cells   Squamous (epidermoid) cells

SSE

MA

SSE, Stratified squamous epithelium of excretory duct
MA, Mucus acini

FIGURE 10-30

Low-grade mucoepidermoid carcinoma. A cystic space is lined by squamous (epidermoid) cells and clusters of mucus-secreting cells.

Low-grade mucoepidermoid carcinoma has limited metastatic potential. The multiple cystic spaces are lined by goblet mucus-secreting cells and columnar ductal cells (Figure 10-30). Papillary fronds surfaced by both mucous and columnar cells are commonly encountered with only focal nests of squamous cells that generally lack keratin pearl formation. The tumor islands and cystic structures are separated from one another by a mature fibrous stroma. Commonly, the marginal tissue is infiltrated by lymphocytes with occasional germinal center formation. These lymphoid foci seem to be a reaction to the tumor and should not be confused with metastatic disease to a lymph node. Intermediate-grade tumors also show cystic spaces; however, they are neither numerous nor large. The so-called *intermediate cells*, which are polygonal but lack true squamous differentiation, are often arranged in diffuse sheets that intervene between the ductal, mucous, and squamous cells. In high-grade tumors the proliferating squamous cells predominate, few cystic spaces are encountered, and only occasional nests of mucus-secreting cells are noted. The high-grade tumors resemble squamous cell carcinoma to some extent but usually do not show the keratin pearl formation and the severe cytologic atypia of that lesion. Nevertheless, some degree of pleomorphism and hyperchromatism are usually seen in high-grade tumors. A **clear cell variant** exists and is characterized by sheets of vacuolated cells that fail to stain for mucin. These clear cells merge with the squamous cells. The usual distinguishing features of mucoepidermoid carcinoma are generally found in neighboring fields. The clear cell variant is classified as intermediate to high grade.

Central mucoepidermoid carcinoma of the jaws is usually of the low-grade variety. These tumors are believed to arise from odontogenic epithelium because dentigerous cysts sometimes show areas of mucous metaplasia within their stratified squamous epithelial lining. Approximately half of all central mucoepidermoid carcinomas show a coexistent odontogenic epithelial lining from which tumor transformation is demonstrable. An odontogenic cyst with extensive mucus cell metaplasia and the glandular or sialo-odontogenic cyst share many histologic features with low-grade central mucoepidermoid carcinoma, often making the diagnosis difficult.

TREATMENT

The management of mucoepidermoid carcinoma must be tailored to the type of tumor, its location, and grade of malignancy. It is noteworthy that low-grade mucoepidermoid carcinoma of the *major* salivary glands has a greater propensity to metastasize to the regional lymph nodes than similarly low-grade tumors of the *minor* salivary glands. Distant hematogenous metastasis of low-grade tumors is extremely rare. Conversely, high-grade tumors, regardless of the site of origin, are aggressive with recurrences approaching 75% with local metastasis to regional nodes and distant hematogous metastasis to the lungs, brain, and skeleton. The initial 5-year survival rate for high-grade tumors is over 70%; however, it drops to below 50% at 10 years and to 33% at 15 years. Death attributed to low-grade tumors is unusual.

In the parotid gland treatment of mucoepidermoid tumors is lobectomy with cervical node dissection when regional nodes are palpable. For high-grade tumors, regional node dissection in the absence of detectable disease has been advocated (elective neck dissection). Postoperative radiotherapy is often advocated for high-grade tumors, and it may control tumors that cannot be adequately removed surgically. In the palate low-grade tumors can be treated by wide local excision to include palatal bone, whereas high-grade carcinomas require more radical procedures such as palatectomy or partial maxillectomy. Of all intraoral sites the tongue carries the worst prognosis for mucoepidermoid carcinoma. Hemiglossectomy is indicated along with neck node dissection. Central tumors of the jaws, which are usually low grade, should be treated by en bloc resection, ensuring tumor-free margins of bone.

ADENOID CYSTIC CARCINOMA

■ ADENOID CYSTIC CARCINOMA: malignant salivary gland tumor composed of cuboidal cells in a solid, cribriform ("Swiss cheese" appearance) or tubular pattern with a predilection for invading perineural lymphatic spaces.

Adenoid cystic carcinoma is a malignant salivary tumor that may arise in either major or minor salivary glands. Because of its frequent microscopic appearance resembling cross sections of tubular structures (cylinders), it was previously referred to as "cylindroma." The individual tumor cells resemble the intercalated ducts of normal glands. This tumor is prone to recur after surgery. Although the 5-year survival rate is quite good, long-term follow-up discloses a low cure rate with recurrences appearing 10 to 15 years after initial treatment.

CLINICAL

Although adenoid cystic carcinoma may occur in persons of any age, the peak incidence is in the sixth decade of life with a slight female predilection. It is rare in children. Clinically, adenoid cystic carcinoma is most common in the parotid gland and is typically detectable as a subcutaneous mass anterior to or below the ear. Almost as many cases arise in the submandibular gland as in the parotid gland. Adenoid cystic carcinoma of the submandibular gland may become quite large before the patient notices its presence. Despite its malignant nature, its growth rate is slow. Over time the mass becomes indurated and fixed. Because it has a marked propensity to surround nerve trunks, when in the parotid gland the involvement of the facial nerve is quite common. Involvement of the facial nerve is clinically apparent as weakness of facial muscles or paralysis. Although minor salivary gland tumors occur nearly as often as parotid and submandibular gland tumors, the most common intraoral site is the palate (Figure 10-31). The minor salivary glands of the tongue, buccal mucosa, lips, and floor of the mouth may also give rise to this tumor. In the palate adenoid cystic carcinoma appears as an eccentric nodule that is usually ulcerated. There may be some palatal paresthesia due to involvement of the greater palatine branch of the trigeminal nerve.

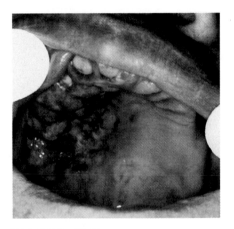

FIGURE 10-31

Adenoid cystic carcinoma. Diffuse large ulcerated lesion of the right palate.

HISTOPATHOLOGY

Most adenoid cystic carcinomas show classic microscopic patterns that allow for a straightforward diagnosis. However, the polymorphous low-grade adenocarcinoma shares many features with adenoid cystic carcinoma; occasionally a distinction between the two is problematic. The typical adenoid cystic carcinoma is composed of oval nests of cuboidal or polygonal epithelial cells with hyperchromatic nuclei. Mitotic figures are rare. There are three patterns of growth, all of which may be encountered in a single tumor, although one pattern usually predominates. The **cribriform pattern** is classic (Figure 10-32). The tumor islands are punctuated with multiple prominent microcytic spaces that divide the lobules into numerous *cylinders* yielding a *Swiss cheese* or *honeycomb* appearance. These cylindric spaces contain either eosinophilic or basophilic secretion products that react positively with mucin stains. The cells oriented around the microcysts are not well polarized into true ductal cells. The stoma is mature and often hyalinized. A **tubular pattern** may dominate the tumor, showing only a few foci of cribriform elements. Small ductal elements prevail and are usually lined by 1 to 3 layers of basaloid cells. These tubuloductal formations are identified in both cross and longitudinal arrays with an intervening hyalinized stroma. The

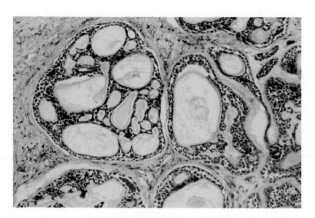
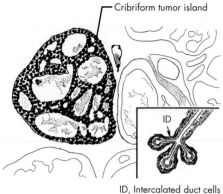

Cribriform tumor island

ID

ID, Intercalated duct cells

FIGURE 10-32

Adenoid cystic carcinoma. Cribriform pattern with a "Swiss cheese" appearance.

basaloid pattern consists of solid nests of basal cells that resemble those seen in basal cell carcinoma or basal cell adenoma. The nuclei, however, show evidence of atypia including hyperchromatism and pleomorphism and increased mitotic activity. Most basaloid cylindromas will contain foci of cribriform or tubular configurations. Immunomarkers disclose the presence of cytokeratins and muscle-specific actin, indicating both ductal and myoepithelial differentiation. Common to all forms of adenoid cystic carcinoma is the tendency for perineural invasion. Tubular concentric laminations of tumor cells wrap themselves around the perineurium of nerve cells (Figure 10-33) where they have actually invaded the perineural lymphatic vessels. This neurotropism is characteristic yet not pathognomonic. It accounts for the high local recurrence seen after surgery because tumor cells may spread along nerve trunks for a considerable distance from the main tumor mass.

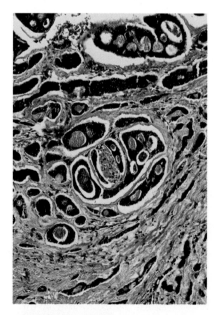
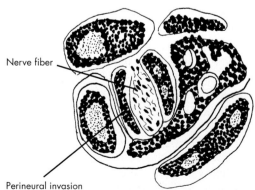

Nerve fiber

Perineural invasion

FIGURE 10-33

Adenoid cystic carcinoma. Affinity for perineural invasion by tumor cells (neurotropism) is evident.

TREATMENT

Adenoid cystic carcinoma is a slow-growing adenocarcinoma with a tendency for neural involvement, a phenomenon that contributes greatly to its ability to recur many years after the initial surgery. Commonly, the 5-year survival rate is good; however, recurrences are common after 10 to 15 years. There is a tendency for both regional and hematogenous tumor spread, and nearly 40% of the patients develop metastasis. Distant spread to the lungs and bone is more common than nodal disease. Even so, the most troublesome consequence of adenoid cystic carcinoma is its persistence and tendency to recur locally (Figure 10-34). In the major glands, total sialoadenectomy is the treatment of choice and frozen section samples of the surrounding neural bundles should be evaluated at the time of surgery for the presence of perineural invasion. Involved nerves must be evaluated until tumor cells are no longer identifiable. Palatal adenoid cystic carcinomas may extend into the pterygomaxillary space via the greater palatine nerve. Partial maxillectomy is the treatment of choice. Lymph node metastasis at the time of initial diagnosis is usually not common; when detectable clinically or with special imaging techniques, node dissection may be indicated. Postoperative radiation therapy is usually advocated because the tumor is radiosensitive and any remaining undetected tumor foci may be eliminated in this manner.

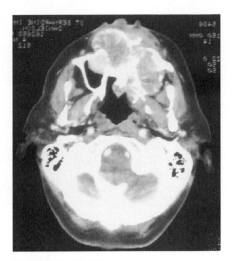

FIGURE 10-34

Recurrent adenoid cystic carcinoma. Computed tomography axial image shows extensive involvement of the anterior maxilla and antrum *(top right area)*.

ACINIC CELL CARCINOMA

■ **ACINIC CELL CARCINOMA**: malignant salivary gland tumor primarily of the parotid gland and composed of pale-staining acini cells usually in a solid or follicular pattern with little visible stroma.

Acinic cell carcinoma is usually found in the parotid gland and is uncommon in the other major and minor salivary glands. After mucoepidermoid carcinoma, it is the second most common malignant salivary gland tumor of the parotid gland. The tumor cells consist of either serous or mucous acinar cells with few ductal or myoepithelial cell elements. The tumor is a low-grade malignancy with slow growth potential; however, like adenoid cystic carcinoma, there is a tendency for local recurrence long after initial therapy.

CLINICAL

The parotid gland is the site of origin in over 80% of acinic cell carcinomas, and intraoral localization is encountered in 15% (Figure 10-35). Unlike most oral salivary tumors that tend to occur in the palate, the few tumors that arise from oral minor glands are most often located in the buccal mucosa and lips. Women are affected more frequently then men, and there is no age predilection. The tumor occurs with equal frequency in patients throughout the second to seventh decades; rare cases are seen in young children. Most acinic cell carcinomas are well demarcated and movable. In the parotid gland some may feel fluctuant because cystic spaces can occasionally be present. The overlying skin or mucosa is intact. At the time of initial examination most tumors are smaller than 3 cm in diameter and rarely exhibit facial nerve compression and paralysis. In the lip and buccal mucosa a firm and well-defined submucosal mass is detected, either visually or by palpation.

HISTOPATHOLOGY

The cells of acinic cell carcinoma resemble the secretory units of salivary tissue and may be mucous, serous, or seromucous. Microscopy shows that the individual cells usually are rich in cytoplasm and the contents stain lightly basophilic or amphophilic. In the common forms of acinic cell carcinoma, zymogen granules

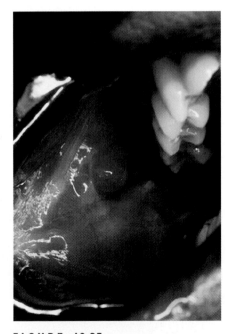

FIGURE 10-35

Acinic cell carcinoma. Smooth, nonulcerated lesion of minor salivary gland located on the buccal mucosa.

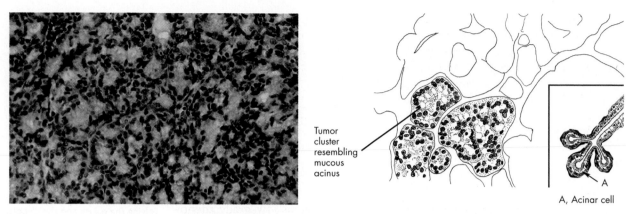

Tumor cluster resembling mucous acinus

A, Acinar cell

FIGURE 10-36

Acinic cell carcinoma. Sheets and clusters of neoplastic acinar cells with little supportive connective tissue stroma.

are rare. In the unusual zymogen-secreting tumors, the acinar cell components are stippled with richly basophilic granules. Most acinic cell neoplasms elaborate a more seromucous material, which is not granular. The mucosubstances stain with periodic acid-Schiff (PAS) and are diastase resistant, indicating that they do not contain large amounts of glycogen. These acinar cells are arranged in a variety of growth patterns, which can be described as *solid, microcystic, papillary cystic,* and *follicular* (Figure 10-36). These patterns have no prognostic significance. In the solid type fine capillary septa divide sheets of acinar cells into indistinct lobules. This same pattern is encountered in the microcystic variant except that varying sizes of microcysts are scattered throughout. In the papillary cystic form, large cystic spaces are seen and large papillary fronds of solid and microcystic acinar configurations protrude into the cystic spaces. A characteristic finding in microcystic and papillary cystic foci are acinar cells that appear to be beaded or yield a *hobnail* pattern when they line a cystic space. The stroma of acinic cell carcinoma is very scant. The outer margin of the tumor is lobulated, relatively well demarcated, and sometimes may actually be partially encapsulated. Lymphoid tissue with germinal centers is commonly encountered around the periphery and may represent residual parotid lymphoid tissue or a lymphoid reaction to the tumor itself.

TREATMENT

In the short term, acinic cell carcinoma masquerades as a benign tumor because very few problems are encountered in the first few years after surgical excision. Long-term follow-up, however, discloses that 30% may recur and 15% will metastasize. The 5-year survival rate after surgery is over 80% but drops to less than 65% at 10 years. Tumors located in the superficial lobes of the parotid gland may be treated by lobectomy, whereas total parotidectomy is advocated for deep lobe neoplasms. Neck dissection is indicated only when there is evidence of regional metastasis. The tumor is radioresistant.

POLYMORPHOUS LOW-GRADE ADENOCARCINOMA

■ **POLYMORPHOUS LOW-GRADE ADENOCARCINOMA:** malignant salivary gland tumor with a predilection for the minor glands that is composed of a wide variety of lobular and cribriform patterns in the central areas and laminated single-file tubular patterns in the periphery and that has a low potential for metastasis.

Polymorphous low-grade adenocarcinoma generally occurs in the minor salivary glands of the oral cavity and only rarely arises within the major salivary glands. Some adenocarcinomas arising in preexisting pleomorphic adenoma (carcinoma ex pleomorphic adenoma) will show growth patterns strikingly similar or identical to polymorphous low-grade adenocarcinoma. The population of tumor cells is quite varied with many growth patterns encountered, hence the term *polymorphous*. Most of the cells resemble the intercalated or terminal salivary ducts. Confusion with adenoid cystic carcinoma may occur in some cases because both tumors have some common cellular configurations, which can be seen microscopically.

CLINICAL

There is a significant female predilection for polymorphous low-grade adenocarcinoma. Most tumors are found in patients who are in the sixth to eighth decades. At present, none has been found in patients in the first two decades of life. The tumor occurs in the palate 60% of the time, 35% are found in the lips and buccal mucosa, and only a few tumors are found in other oral mucosal sites (Figure 10-37). They are painless masses, firm on palpation, and fixed when in the palate. Surface ulceration is rarely seen. There is a history of slow growth, and most tumors are smaller than 3 cm in diameter.

HISTOPATHOLOGY

Confusion with adenoid cystic carcinoma on the basis of microscopically viewed features can be problematic; however, most polymorphous low-grade adenocarcinomas have distinctly different growth patterns. The tumor is usually well de-

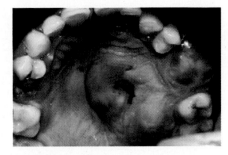

FIGURE 10-37

Polymorphous low-grade adenocarcinoma. Large, nodular ulcerated lesion involving the palate and the alveolar bone.

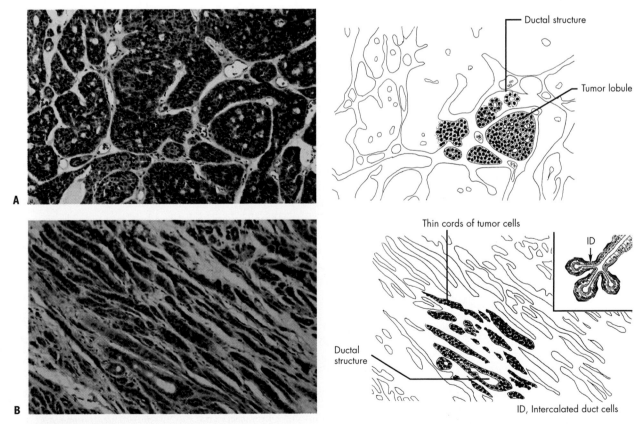

FIGURE 10-38

Polymorphous low-grade adenocarcinoma. A, Lobular pattern of basaloid tumor cells with lumen formation. **B,** Parallel tubular structures (thin cords) found at periphery of the lesion.

marcated but is not encapsulated. Invasive tumor nests are generally seen around the periphery with extension into adjacent minor salivary gland lobules or muscle fibers, depending on the location. Two basic growth patterns are encountered (Figure 10-38, *A*). The **lobular** pattern is composed of ovoid or round nests of basaloid cells with monomorphic nuclei. The connective tissue stroma is scant and mature. The **cribriform pattern** is similar to that of adenoid cystic carcinoma and has a Swiss cheese appearance because the tumor lobules are riddled with multiple microcysts. Perhaps the most distinguishing feature of polymorphous low-grade adenocarcinoma is found around the periphery of the lesion. In this region the tumor cells are arranged in parallel arrays of elongated, single-file tubular formations (Figure 10-38, *B*). These single-file tubular structures appear to be stacked upon one another, producing an onionskin or laminated appearance. Perineural invasion may also be seen and is therefore not a reliable feature in differentiating this tumor from adenoid cystic carcinoma.

TREATMENT

Polymorphous low-grade adenocarcinoma, as the name indicates, is a low-grade, indolent malignancy. At present, only a single death has been reported from a local recurrence. Recurrences are commonly due to incomplete excision. Distant hematogenous metastases do not occur. Only 5% have been reported to spread locally. Surgical excision including wide margins is the treatment of choice. Any identifiable nerve fibers passing into the tumor should be surgically tracked, and frozen section samples should be evaluated. In the palate a partial maxillectomy is recommended.

ADDITIONAL READING

GENERAL

Batsakis JG. *Tumors of the Head and Neck: Clinical and Pathological Considerations.* 2nd ed. Baltimore: Williams & Wilkins; 1979.

Ellis GL, Auclair PL, Gnepp DR. *Surgical Pathology of the Salivary Glands: Vol 25: Major Problems in Pathology.* Livolsi VA, Series ed. Philidelphia: WB Saunders Co; 1991.

Seifert G, Donath K. Classification of the pathohistology of diseases of the salivary glands: review of 2,600 cases in the salivary gland register. *Beitr Path Bd.* 1976; 159:1-32.

MUCOCELE/MUCUS RETENTION CYST

Blitzer A. Inflammatory and obstructive disorders of salivary glands. *J Dent Res.* 1987; 66:675-679.

Bodner L, Tal H. Salivary gland cysts of the oral cavity: clinical observation and surgical management. *Compendium.* 1991; 12:150, 152, 154-6.

Eversole RL. Oral sialocysts. *Arch Otolaryngol Head and Neck Surg.* 1987; 113:51-56.

SIALOLITHIASIS

Bodner L. Salivary gland calculi: diagnostic imaging and surgical management. *Compendium.* 1993; 14:572.

Daley TD, Lovas JG. Diseases of the salivary glands: a review. *J Can Dent Assoc.* 1991; 57:411-4.

Jensen JL, Howell FV, Rick GM, Correll RW. Minor salivary gland calculi: a clinicopathologic study of forty-seven new cases. *Oral Surg Oral Med Oral Pathol.* 1979; 47:44-50.

Mandel L, Fatehi J. Minor salivary gland sialolithiasis: review and case report. *N Y State Dent J.* 1992; 58:31-3.

White AK. Salivary gland disease in infancy and childhood: non-malignant lesions. *J Otolaryngol.* 1992; 21:422-8.

CHRONIC SCLEROSING SIALADENITIS

Matthews TW, Dardick I. Morphological alterations of salivary gland parenchyma in chronic sialadenitis. *J Otolaryngol.* 1988; 17:385-393.

Narang R, Dixon RA. Surgical management of submandibular sialadenitis and sialolithiasis. *Oral Surg Oral Med Oral Pathol.* 1977; 43:201-210.

St. Clair EW. New developments in Sjögren's syndrome. *Curr Opin Rheumatol.* 1993; 5:604-1.

NECROTIZING SIALOMETAPLASIA

Abrams AM, Melrose RJ, Howell FV. Necrotizing sialometaplasia: a disease simulating malignancy. *Cancer.* 1973; 32: 130-135.

Brannon RB, Fowler CB, Hartman KS. Necrotizing sialometaplasia: a clinicopathologic study of sixty-nine cases and review of the literature. *Oral Surg Oral Med Oral Pathol.* 1991; 72:317-25.

Sneige N, Batsakis JG. Necrotizing sialometaplasia. *Ann Otol Rhinol Laryngol.* 1992; 101:282-4.

INFECTIONS

ACUTE PAROTITIS

Loughran DH, Smith LG. Infectious disorders of the parotid gland. *N J Med*. 1988; 85:311-4.

Myer C, Cotton RT. Salivary gland disease in children: a review. Part 1: acquired non-neoplastic disease. *Clin Pediatr (Phila)*. 1986; 25:314-22.

Fox PC. Bacterial infections of salivary glands. *Curr Opin Dent*. 1991; 1:411-4.

IMMUNE-MEDIATED DISEASE

SJÖGREN SYNDROME

Atkinson JC, Fox PC. Sjögren's syndrome: oral and dental considerations. *J Am Dent Assoc*. 1993; 124:74-6, 78-82, 84-6.

Aziz KE, Montanaro A, McCluskey PJ, Wakefield D. Sjögren's syndrome: review with recent insights into immunopathogenesis. *Aust N Z J Med*. 1992; 22:671-8.

Chisholm DM, Waterhouse JP, Mason DK. Lymphocytic sialadenitis in the major and minor glands: a correlation in postmortem subjects. *J Clin Pathol*. 1970; 23:690-694.

Daniels TE, Fox PC. Salivary and oral components of Sjögren's syndrome. *Rheum Dis Clin North Am*. 1992; 18:571-89.

Fox RI, Kang HI. Pathogenesis of Sjögren's syndrome. *Rheum Dis Clin North Am*. 1992; 18:517-38.

Greenspan JS, Daniels TE, Talal N, Sylvester RA. The histopathology of Sjögren's syndrome in labial salivary gland biopsies. *Oral Surg Oral Med Oral Pathol*. 1974; 37:217-229.

St. Clair EW. New developments in Sjögren's syndrome. *Curr Opin Rheumatol*. 1993; 5:604-12.

BENIGN SALIVARY GLAND TUMORS

Attie JN, Sciubba JJ. Tumors of major and minor salivary glands: clinical and pathologic features. *Curr Probl Surg*. 1981; 18:65-155.

Batsakis JG, Kraemer B, Sciubba JJ. The pathology of head and neck tumors: the myoepithelial cell and its participation in salivary gland neoplasia: part 17. *Head Neck Surg*. 1983; 5:222-33.

Dardick I. A role for electron microscopy in salivary gland neoplasms. *Ultrastruct Pathol*. 1985; 9:151-61.

Goldblatt LI, Ellis GL. Salivary gland tumors of the tongue: analysis of 55 new cases and review of the literature. *Cancer*. 1987; 60:74-81.

Luna MA, Batsakis JG, el-Naggar AK. Salivary gland tumors in children. *Ann Otol Rhinol Laryngol*. 1991; 100:869-71.

Seifert G, Sobin LH. The World Health Organization's Histological Classification of Salivary Gland Tumors: a commentary on the second edition. *Cancer*. 1992; 70:379-85.

Shikhani AH, Johns ME. Tumors of the major salivary glands in children. *Head Neck Surg*. 1988; 10:257-63.

Waldron CA, el-Mofty SK, Gnepp DR. Tumors of the intraoral minor salivary glands: a demographic and histologic study of 426 cases. *Oral Surg Oral Med Oral Pathol*. 1988; 66:323-33.

PLEOMORPHIC ADENOMA

Dardick I, van Nostrand AWP. Myoepithelial cells in salivary gland tumors: revisited. *Head Neck Surg*. 1985; 7:395-408.

Gnepp DR. Malignant mixed tumors of the salivary glands: a review. *Pathol Annu*. 1993; 28(pt 1):279-328.

MONOMORPHIC ADENOMA

Batsakis JG, Brannon RB, Scuibba JJ. Monomorphic adenomas of major salivary glands: a histologic study of 96 tumours. *Clin Otolaryngol*. 1981; 6:129-143.

Cho KJ, Kim YI. Monomorphic adenomas of the salivary glands: a clinico-pathologic study of 12 cases with immuno-histochemical observation. *Path Res Pract*. 1989; 184:614-20.

Dardick I, Lytwyn A, Bourne AJ, Byard RW. Trabecular and solid-cribriform types of basal cell adenoma: a morphological study of two of an unusal variant of monomorphic adenoma. *Oral Surg Oral Med Oral Pathol*. 1992; 73:75-83.

Feinmesser M, Feinmesser R, Okon E, Freeman JL and others. A monomorphic adenoma of the minor salivary glands presenting at the base of the tongue: a case report and review of the literature. *J Otolaryngol*. 1993; 22:110-2.

PAPILLARY CYSTADENOMA LYMPHOMATOSUM

Dardick I, Claude A, Parks WR, Hoppe D and others. Warthin's tumor: an ultrastructural and immunohistochemical study of basilar epithelium. *Ultrastruct Pathol*. 1988; 12:419-32.

Eveson JW, Cawson RA. Warthin's tumor (cystadenolymphoma) of salivary glands: a clinicopathological investigation of 278 cases. *Oral Surg*. 1986; 61:256-262.

Hartwick R, Batsakis JG. Non-Warthin's tumor oncocytic lesions. *Ann Otol Rhinol Laryngol*. 1990; 99:674-7.

ONCOCYTOMA

Chang A, Harawi SJ. Oncocytes, oncocytosis and oncocytic tumors. *Pathol Annu*. 1992; 27(pt 1):263-304.

Damm DD, White DK, Geissler RH, Drummond JF and others. Benign solid oncocytoma of intraoral minor salivary glands. *Oral Surg Oral Med Oral Pathol*. 1989; 67:84-6.

MALIGNANT SALIVARY GLAND TUMORS

Batsakis JG, Luna MA. Undifferentiated carcinomas of salivary glands. *Ann Otol Rhinol Laryngol*. 1991; 100:82-4.

Gates GA. Current concepts in otolaryngology: malignant neoplasms of the minor salivary glands. *N Engl J Med*. 1982; 25:306, 718-22.

Hunter RM, Davis BW, Gray GF, Rosenfeld L. Primary malignant tumors of salivary gland origin: a 52-year review. *Am Surg*. 1983; 49:82-9.

Luna MA, Batsakis JG, Ordonez NG, Mackay B and others. Salivary gland adenocarcinomas: a clinicopathologic analysis of three distinctive types. *Semin Diagn Pathol*. 1987; 4:117-35.

Seifert G. Histopathology of malignant salivary gland tumours. *Eur J Cancer B Oral Oncol*. 1992; 28B:49-56.

Spiro RH, Armstrong J, Harrison L, Geller NL and others. Carcinoma of major salivary glands: major trends. *Arch Otolaryngol Head and Neck Surg*. 1989; 115:316-321.

ADENOID CYSTIC CARCINOMA

Batsakis JG, Luna MA, el-Naggar A. Histopathologic grading of salivary gland neoplasms: III: adenoid cystic carcinomas. *Ann Otol Rhinol Laryngol.* 1990; 99:1007-9.

Brookstone MS, Huvos AG, Spiro RH. Central adenoid cystic carcinoma of the mandible. *J Oral Maxillofac Surg.* 1990; 48:1329-33.

Nascimento AG, Amaral ALP, Prado LAF, Kligerman J and others. Adenoid cystic carcinoma of salivary glands: a study of 61 cases with clincopathologic correlation. *Cancer.* 1986; 57:312-319.

Perzin KH, Gullane P, Clairmont AC. Adenoid cystic carcinoma arising in salivary glands: a correlation of histologic features and clinical courses. *Cancer.* 1978; 42:265-282.

MUCOEPIDERMOID CARCINOMA

Batsakis JG, Luna MA. Histopathological grading of salivary gland tumors: I: mucoepidermoid carcinoma. *Ann Otol Rhinol Laryngol.* 1990; 99:835-838.

Chaudhry AP, Cutler LS, Leifer C, Labay G and others. Ultrastructural study of the histogenesis of salivary gland mucoepidermoid carcinoma. *J Oral Pathol Med.* 1989; 18:400-9.

Dardick I, Daya D, Hardie J, van Nostrand AWP. Mucoepidermoid carcinoma: ultrastructural and histogenic aspects. *J Oral Pathol.* 1984; 13:342-358.

ACINIC CELL CARCINOMA

Zbaeren P, Lehmann W, Widgren S. Acinic cell carcinoma of minor salivary gland origin. *J Laryngol Otol.* 1991;105:782-5.

Lewis JE, Olsen KD, Welland LH. Acinic cell carcinoma: clinicopathologic review. *Cancer.* 1991; 67:172-179.

POLYMORPHOUS LOW-GRADE ADENOCARCINOMA

Dardick I, van Nostrand AWP. Polymorphous low-grade adenocarcinoma: a case report with ultrastructural findings. *Oral Surg Oral Med Oral Pathol.* 1988; 66:459-465.

Norberg L, Dardick I. The need for clinical awareness of polymorphous low-grade adenocarcinoma: a review. *J Otolaryngol.* 1992; 21:149-52.

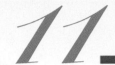

CHAPTER

11

PHYSICAL AND CHEMICAL INJURIES

PHYSICAL INJURIES
Teeth
  Attrition
  Abrasion
  Erosion
  Fracture
  Avulsion
  Internal Resorption
  External Resorption
  Ankylosis

Gingiva
  Toothbrush Trauma
  Toothpick Injury
Tongue
  Traumatic Atrophic Glossitis
  Benign Migratory Glossitis
  Chronic Ulcers
Mucosal Tissue
  Factitious Injuries
  Denture Injuries

Electrical Burns
Thermal Burns
Radiation Injuries
  Radiation Mucositis
  Xerostomia
  Radiation Caries
  Osteoradionecrosis
  Soft Tissue Injuries

CHEMICAL INJURIES
Teeth
  Tetracycline
  Congenital Porphyria
  Biliary Atresia
  Erythroblastosis Fetalis
Gingiva
  Phenytoin
  Cyclosporine
  Nifedipine
Mucosal Tissue
  Amalgam
  Graphite
Chemical Burns
  Acetylsalicylic Acid
  Other Medications

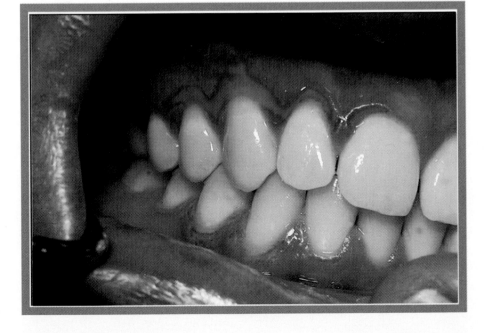

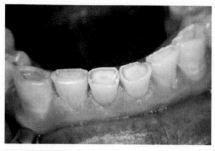

FIGURE 11-1

Attrition. Anterior lower teeth exhibit extensive wear on the incisal edges exposing the underlying sclerotic dentin.

PHYSICAL INJURIES

TEETH

Physical injuries are among the most common causes of tooth defects. Most of the injuries are self-induced or **factitious.** Although some of these are purposeful due to a neurosis, psychosis, or hereditary condition, most are inadvertent. Injuries due to overzealous daily habits are the most common, with abuse of oral hygiene practices being most notable. On occasion, environmental elements such as toxic levels of chemicals in the air contribute to the loss of tooth structure in light of normal hygiene practices. The physical injuries of teeth have been divided into three major categories: *attrition, abrasion,* and *erosion.*

Attrition

■ ATTRITION: loss of tooth structure due to the mechanical action of mastication.

Some degree of attrition is normal because it occurs naturally as an accumulative process over many years. It is normally present on the cuspal and incisal edges of the anterior teeth (Figure 11-1) and on the tips of the cusps of molars that are in occlusion. These changes become more pronounced with advanced age. Attrition is excessive and premature on the teeth of patients who habitually clench and grind their teeth **(bruxism).** The pattern of attrition will vary among these patients depending on the interocclusal contacts and the relationship of the arches. In patients with class II relationships the excessive wear tends to be on the molars, with the occlusal surfaces becoming nearly flat. A class III relationship will exhibit most of the wear on the incisal edges of the anterior teeth.

In some societies there is generally greater attrition due to dietary habits. This was particularly evident in past and primitive societies whose diets were more fibrous; abrasive particles became intermingled in the food during preparation. Excessive wear is still found in some cultures today where day-long chewing of certain substances such as betel nuts is a common custom.

Because attrition is generally a slowly progressive process, the dentin and pulp tissue have time to react to the loss of tooth tissue. The exposed dentin undergoes sclerosis of the dentinal tubules while the pulp deposits layers of calcified tissue, referred to as **tertiary** or **reparative dentin.** This process protects the pulp from irritants that might otherwise permeate the dentin, thus it remains viable even in situations where more that half the crown has been lost due to attrition.

Abrasion

■ ABRASION: abnormal loss of tooth structure due to nonmasticatory physical friction.

The most common cause of abrasion is overuse and misuse of the toothbrush (Figure 11-2, *A*) or the use of coarse abrasives while cleaning the teeth. In some cultures teeth are cleaned with implements that are more abrasive than the bristle brush and fine abrasives common in Western societies. In these societies the teeth commonly exhibit a characteristic pattern in which the buccal and labial surfaces exhibit excessive tooth loss, particularly of the cervical areas (Figure 11-2, *B*). Severe abrasion predominantly involves the anterior and premolar teeth of the arches, with the maxillary teeth more severely affected than the mandibular. In Western and other cultures the overuse of **toothpicks** to clean teeth or massage the gingiva often produces a distinctive pattern of interproxi-

A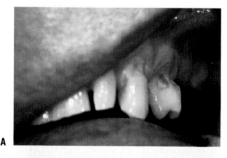

B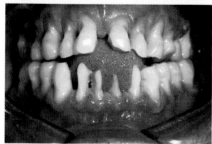

FIGURE 11-2

Abrasion. A, Excessive and improper use of a toothbrush, producing "notching" on the buccal surfaces at the cervicoenamel junction of the cuspid and premolars. **B,** Extensive loss of tooth structure in a compulsive patient in whom the teeth were overzealously cleaned with a wooden instrument and a coarse abrasive.

mal wear. Linear patterns of tooth loss on the exposed cementum of older patients occurs when **dental floss** is improperly used.

Other forms of nonhygienic habits will produce characteristic patterns of
abrasion. Notching of the incisal edges of the anterior teeth is common when
hairpins are constantly opened using the anterior teeth. A similar pattern of
tooth loss involving several anterior teeth of the left or right anterior arches occurs in habitual pipe smokers.

Erosion

EROSION: loss of tooth structure due to nonbacterial chemical causes.

The most common chemicals to contribute to erosive tooth loss are those with a
pH in the acidic range. The continuous contact of the enamel with these chemicals leads to leaching of the calcifying salts and a reduction in its hardness.
Tooth structure that has been weakened by this process is easily lost, even when
normal hygiene techniques are employed.

Most causes of erosions are known and can be attributed to an excessive diet
of foods with an acid pH such as **citrus fruits** and **carbonated beverages** (soft
drinks). These foods produce a unique pattern of smooth saucer-shaped cavita-
tions of the *labial* surfaces of the anterior teeth (Figure 11-3). Patients who suffer from regurgitation of acidic stomach contents develop erosions on the *lingual*
surfaces of the teeth, particularly the anterior teeth. This occurs frequently during **pregnancy** and in patients suffering from **bulimia** (Figure 11-4). Other
common causes of dental erosion are occupational. These are due to the presence of certain **atmospheric gases** that become mixed with the saliva, producing acid solutions. These erosions are also located on the labial surfaces of the
anterior teeth.

Fracture

Fractures of teeth occur under a wide variety of conditions. The most common
are those associated with acute trauma, particularly in young patients. These are
often caused by a fall or a sudden blow to the midface. Fractures may also occur
during normal use of the teeth because of one or more of the following predisposing factors: (1) the pulp has been rendered more brittle after it has become
devitalized, (2) the presence of internal resorption, (3) the presence of large in-
tracoronal restorations—particularly MOD (mesial-occlusal-distal) fillings in
premolars, and (4) teeth affected by dentinogenesis imperfecta or other congenital or acquired conditions that affect the integrity of the tooth structure.

The most commonly encountered tooth fractures are **crown fractures** of
anterior teeth. These fractures have been classified as involving (1) enamel only;
(2) enamel and dentin; and (3) enamel, dentin, and pulp. The most prevalent of
these are the fractures involving both enamel and dentin; most are oblique, involving one of the incisal corners. When dentin is exposed, bacterial invasion of
the tubules and penetration into the pulp ensues unless the patient obtains
prompt attention. Pain is usually associated with dentin exposure; however,
when the pulp has been severed, pain may be absent. This severe pulpal trauma
may not be reversible and usually requires immediate pulpal extirpation.

Root fractures represent a small percentage of the total number of tooth
fractures. Most are of traumatic origin, occurring in patients between the ages of
10 and 20 years. The majority are horizontal fractures in the middle third of the
root. The second most common root fracture occurs in the apical third of the
root (Figure 11-5). Most teeth become nonvital immediately when root fracture
occurs. Some root fractures may take other courses. They may heal by forming
an inner layer of reparative dentin on the pulpal wall, or they may replace the

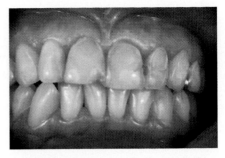

FIGURE 11-3

Erosion. The labial surfaces of the anterior
teeth exhibit thinning of the enamel and
rounding of the crowns with white opaque
areas of demineralization common in patients whose intake of highly acidic foods and
beverages is excessive.

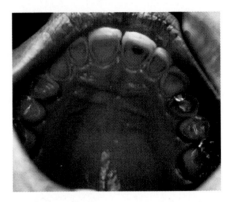

FIGURE 11-4

Bulimia. The lingual surfaces of the maxillary teeth show loss of enamel due to constant contact with regurgitated acidic stomach contents.

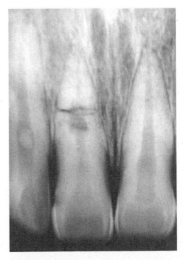

FIGURE 11-5

Root fracture. Fracture located at the
junction of the middle and apical third of the
root with a small area of resorption occurring adjacent to the fracture line in the coronal portion of the tooth fragment.

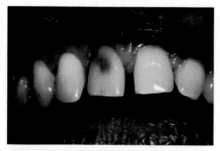

FIGURE 11-6

Internal resorption. Clinical appearance of a tooth with a large area of internal resorption as revealed by a "pink spot" in the cervical third of the crown.

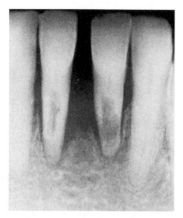

FIGURE 11-7

Internal resorption. Radiographic appearance of resorption that appears to be originating within the pulpal tissue of the root.

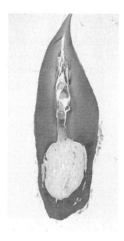

FIGURE 11-8

Internal resorption. Low-power microscopic appearance of an incisor containing characteristic vascular loose connective tissue within the area of root resorption.

hard tissue along the fracture line with granulation tissue that progresses to mature connective tissue. Others remain vital and proceed to round off the sharp fracture edges, separating the two fragments by connective tissue and bone. In some cases they may become nonvital with the fragments becoming surrounded by granulation tissue, which usually results in extensive resorption with eventual tooth loss. The chances of tooth resorption and loss are reduced if the tooth is immobilized for a time.

A traumatic event is not always of sufficient force to fracture the tooth but is still capable of producing a **cemental tear.** Cemental tears are small fractures of the cementum, usually the result of sudden torsional (rotational) forces. These usually are not of clinical significance because they seldom produce symptoms. They are occasionally observed as incidental findings during a histologic examination of periodontal tissue removed for other purposes.

Avulsion

> ■ AVULSION: the forceful displacement of a tooth in its socket.

Avulsion of teeth may be **partial**—the tooth is moved but has not become devitalized—or **total**—the tooth has become nonvital due to extensive movement of the apex or the tooth has been extruded from the socket, both of which result in severance of the apical blood supply. Avulsed teeth should be immediately repositioned, and a determination should be made regarding their vitality.

Internal Resorption

> ■ INTERNAL RESORPTION: form of tooth loss that begins within the pulpal chambers of intact teeth destroying dentin as it extends outward in a uniform pattern toward the tooth surfaces.

Most occurrences of internal resorption are within the crown of anterior incisors and are idiopathic. The affected tooth is usually asymptomatic with the lesion first detected by the appearance of a "pink spot" beneath the enamel surface (Figure 11-6). At this point there is usually extensive loss of tooth structure that greatly weakens the tooth, predisposing it to fracture.

The radiographic appearance of internal resorption is distinctive. It usually consists of a fusiform enlargement of the pulpal chamber of one or more teeth that appears in either the crown or root pulpal chambers (Figure 11-7).

In intact teeth histologic examination of the pulpal tissue in the area of the resorption reveals a loose connective tissue with increased vascularity and few inflammatory cells (Figure 11-8). When internal resorption is associated with caries exposure, pulpal treatments, or hairline fractures, the pulpal tissues will contain a granulation tissue that is densely infiltrated with acute and chronic inflammatory cells. If internal resorption has not progressed to the point of making the tooth structurally unsound, endodontic treatment can often halt the process.

External Resorption

> ■ EXTERNAL RESORPTION: loss of tooth structure that begins on the outer surface and extends inward toward the pulp.

There are several forms of external resorption. On an erupted tooth lesions commonly begin in the **cervical** areas where they are usually considered idiopathic (Figure 11-9, *A*); when they occur in the **midroot** area ((Figure 11-9, *B*),

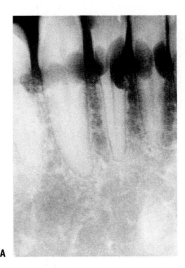
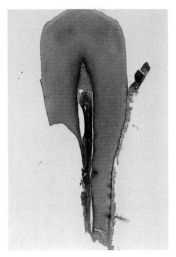

FIGURE 11-9

External resorption. A, Radiographic appearance of idiopathic external resorption involving the cervical area of multiple mandibular anterior teeth. **B,** Microscopic appearance of a decalcified tooth with an intact crown and external resorption of the middle and apical third of the root.

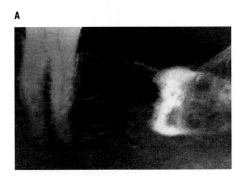
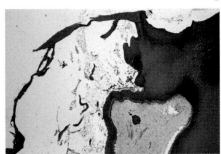

FIGURE 11-10

External resorption. A, Radiograph of an impacted tooth of long duration revealing mottling of crown and adjacent root. **B,** Microscopic appearance of a decalcified impacted molar with a large portion of the crown destroyed by external resorption. The pulpal tissue is unaffected by the process.

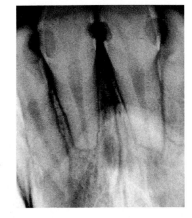

FIGURE 11-11

External resorption. Radiograph of anterior maxillary incisors with blunted apical areas indicative of previous period of active resorption. This form of resorption is commonly associated with prior orthodontic treatment, tumors, or cysts in the area.

they are commonly the result of a traumatic incident; and at the **apex** they commonly are the result of an encroaching inflammatory or neoplastic lesion. **Impacted teeth** of long duration can also undergo resorption. The resorption usually begins on the enamel of the crown (Figure 11-10), appearing as a mottled area with indistinct borders and progressing to the dentin. As with internal resorption the process is without pain or other symptoms.

Evidence of external resorption of the root apices may be found in either a regional (Figure 11-11) or a generalized pattern throughout the mouth. These patterns are commonly the result of overly aggressive **orthodontic movement** of the teeth at an earlier time. In some patients apical resorption of multiple teeth is in an active state. This is commonly due to a chronic form of excessive **traumatic occlusion.**

Transplanted and **reimplanted teeth** have a high incidence of developing external resorption. In the case of reimplantation it has been shown that the time between removal and subsequent reimplantation is of utmost importance in determining if the tooth will eventually be lost due to postimplant external resorption.

Ankylosis

> ■ ANKYLOSIS: fusion of the cementum or dentin to the surrounding alveolar bone after loss of the intervening periodontal membrane.

Within the dental arch ankylosis most commonly involves the primary second molar, although any tooth may undergo this process after a traumatic incident. The exact pathogenesis of tooth ankylosis is unknown. It appears that whenever the connective tissue of the periodontal membrane is lost allowing cementum and/or dentin to come in direct contact with alveolar bone, fusion of these two opposing calcified structures occurs (Figure 11-12). Ankylosis is also found when the normal physiologic resorption of the roots of deciduous teeth is interrupted or curtailed. When this occurs the granulation tissue surrounding the resorbing roots reverts to a fibrous tissue that goes on to become bone and fuses with the surrounding alveolar bone. Another cause of ankylosis is chronic or acute trauma, either of which can cause inflammation and destruction of the periodontal membrane. Autoimplanted or reimplanted avulsed teeth in which the periodontal membrane has been destroyed usually undergo some degree of ankylosis if they are not lost by external resorption. In general, nearly any factor that can cause external root resorption has the potential to result in ankylosis. This includes rapid orthodontic movement, periapical infections, and occlusal

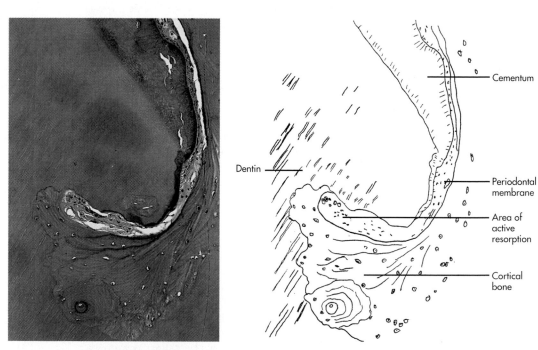

FIGURE 11-12

Ankylosis. Photomicrogarph of partially ankylosed tooth illustrating an area in which there is an absence of ankylosis with root dentin *(left)* containing cementum and a periodontal membrane in the coronal portion of the root and an area of ankylosis in the apical portion in which the root dentin is fused to mature alveolar bone *(right)* in the absence of a cementum layer and periodontal membrane. At the junction of the two *(center)*, a zone of active external resorption is present.

traumatism. On rare occasions long-standing impacted teeth will become anky-losed. Often the impacted tooth is not completely ankylosed but fused only in one or two areas.

The most common example of ankylosis is the **submerged (retained) de-ciduous molar,** usually located in the second mandibular premolar location (Figure 11-13). The submerged appearance occurs because the occlusal table of the retained smaller deciduous molar is located below the rest of the teeth in the arch. In many cases it is merely a deciduous tooth that has not yet undergone normal root resorption, allowing it to be shed in a timely manner. Eventually the surrounding earlier erupting permanent teeth lock the submerged deciduous molar in its original position, and the primary molar that may have had some physiologic resorption often eventually becomes ankylosed to the surrounding bone. In such situations if an underlying premolar is present, it will either re-main impacted or will eventually erupt buccally or lingually in the arch, result-ing in local malocclusion. Often, the deciduous molar becomes locked in posi-tion because there is a congenital absence of an underlying permanent premolar and thus a lack of stimulation for timely root resorption.

Making an accurate assessment that a tooth may be ankylosed is of utmost importantance when extraction by luxation is contemplated. Failure to do so usually results in root breakage and the possibility of fracture of the surrounding alveolar bone. The most effective aid to diagnosis is the availability of periapical radiographs that demonstrate the presence or absence of a uniform periodontal space.

GINGIVA

Toothbrush Trauma

Lesions of the marginal and attached gingiva created by the chronic physical ir-ritation of toothbrush bristles are usually confused with a number of other dis-ease processes. They may appear as white, red, or ulcerative lesions. Although any area of a quadrant can be involved, the lesions are most commonly present on the maxillary gingiva over the premolars and cuspids because these are the lo-cations that maximal pressure can be exerted during brushing (Figure 11-14). Lesions will be more severe on the left if the patient is right handed and vice versa.

The injury commonly appears as linear superficial erosions against a red background. These lesions are easily confused with several of the vesicular-ulcerative and infectious diseases; misdiagnosis and unsuccessful treatment are common problems.

When more severe forms of toothbrush injury occur, the lesions appear as deep clefts of the gingival margin with generalized severe gingival recession and deep horizontal notching of the dentin of the exposed root surfaces. In severe cases the underlying alveolar bone will be lost and does not return when the de-structive traumatic activity is reversed even though much of the gingival damage to the soft tissue improves (Figure 11-15).

Diagnosis often requires a tissue biopsy to rule out other disease processes. The histologic features of toothbrush injury are similar to those of a superficial ulcer due to excess pressure or other nonspecific causes. They consist of a focal loss of the overlying epithelium, a superficial zone of granulation tissue over fi-brous tissue, and a diffuse infiltrate of lymphocytes and plasma cells. Adjacent to the ulcers the epithelium exhibits mild hyperorthokeratosis and acanthosis.

Treatment consists of identifying the cause as a mechanical loss of the gin-giva and tooth structure and helping the patient recognize the factitious nature of the injuries and how maintenance of oral hygiene can be attained without in-jury to the soft tissues.

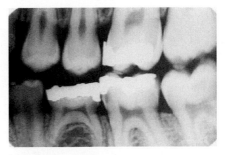

FIGURE 11-13
Submerged tooth. Radiograph of a re-tained deciduous second molar with its oc-clusal surface beneath the occlusal plane of the surrounding teeth.

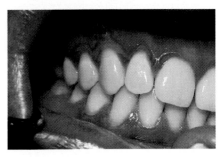

FIGURE 11-14
Toothbrush trauma. Areas of erosion and acute inflammation are present, typically lo-cated on the marginal gingiva in the cuspid and premolar areas.

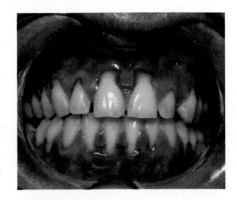

FIGURE 11-15
Toothbrush trauma. Chronic toothbrush abuse illustrating permanent loss of soft tis-sue, underlying bone, and tooth structure.

Toothpick Injury

Toothpick injury of the gingiva is closely related to the previously discussed toothbrush injury. It is also the result of habitual, overzealous use of a common utensil for oral hygiene. The clinical appearance of toothpick injury is different because there are usually only one or two lesions present. Lesions involve loss of soft and hard tissues. The interdental papilla in these areas is usually lost and replaced by a depression that includes both the buccal and lingual aspects of the gingiva. The injury to the tooth itself consists of loss of cementum, dentin, and cervical enamel on the mesial and distal portions of adjacent teeth.

TONGUE

Traumatic Atrophic Glossitis

■ TRAUMATIC ATROPHIC GLOSSITIS: focal sensitive erythematous areas of the tongue due to a habit in which the filiform papillae are lost, the fungiform papillae are enlarged and reddened, and the epithelium is thinned.

The most common location for traumatic atrophic glossitis is the anterior tip of the tongue (Figure 11-16). Less commonly, lesions are located on the lateral margins, extending onto the dorsal surfaces. They are frequently found in patients who have had recent restorations or other changes in their oral environment. Patients with atrophic glossitis usually overuse their tongues in a compulsive manner to explore recently placed restorations or other intraoral changes such as broken fillings, chipped cusps, or sharp incisal edges. The lesions located on the lateral tongue occur secondary to the extensive movement of the anterior tongue over the crowns of the cuspids and premolars.

Other causes of this condition are a loose upper denture that is constantly being reseated with the tongue, extensive calculus on the lingual surfaces of the mandibular teeth, and malaligned or crowded anterior teeth.

HISTOPATHOLOGY

The microscopic features of the lesions are those of a nonspecific inflammation of the mucosa (mucositis), which consists of thinned epithelium devoid of filiform papillae and connective tissue containing a diffuse infiltrate of lymphocytes and plasma cells and dilatated capillaries and venules.

Treatment consists of identifying the factors that become the focus of the patient's attention and correcting them and any other rough or uncomfortable areas such as exposed margins, protrusions, sharp edges, calculus deposits, or loose appliances. To ensure continued oral comfort, the patient must be made aware of the necessity to curtail compulsive movements of the tongue.

Benign Migratory Glossitis

■ BENIGN MIGRATORY GLOSSITIS: multiple sensitive irregularly shaped erythematous patches of the tongue with arcuate white rims that enlarge and change shape daily.

Benign migratory glossitis is also commonly referred to as *geographic tongue* because the clinical appearance of the tongue often resembles a map of the world. The cause of this lesion is still unknown; although many feel that chronic irritation, similar to that described as the cause of chronic atrophic glossitis, is a significant contributing factor. Many patients will have crowding of the lower arch with one or more mandibular premolars and/or anterior incisors in linguoversion that produces some degree of irritation of the tongue, even during normal

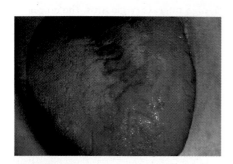

FIGURE 11-16

Traumatic atrophic glossitis. The tongue exhibits patchy loss of filiform papillae and erythema due to chronic excessive movement of the tongue. The tip of the tongue contains enlarged and reddened fungiform papillae.

movement. Periods of excessive tongue movement produce exacerbations of the condition.

CLINICAL

A distinctive clinical feature of benign migratory glossitis is the daily change in the size and shape of the lesions. Patients of all age groups have been found to exhibit these tongue lesions. New lesions commonly begin on the lateral borders and anterior tip of the tongue and gradually enlarge in a circumferential pattern. Individual lesions have a characteristic appearance consisting of a central atrophic area exhibiting loss of the filiform papillae. The atrophic areas are rimmed by an erythematous zone with a slightly raised distinct whitish line at the junction with the normal tissue (Figure 11-17). In ensuing days as the lesion ages, the epithelium regenerates and the central area of the lesion gradually develops a normal appearance. As the lesion enlarges, its borders gradually become less distinct.

Similar-appearing lesions consisting of circular or arcuate lesions of other oral mucosal surfaces such as the ventral tongue (Figure 11-18), floor of the mouth, and buccal vestibule are occasionally present and are referred to as **stomatitis areata migrans.**

The clinical behavior of both of these lesions is similar to that of benign migratory glossitis, although no associated traumatic factors are usually apparent.

HISTOPATHOLOGY

The microscopic appearances of benign migratory glossitis and stomatitis areata migrans are distinctive, consisting of an outer zone of subcorneal abscesses separating the normal from the atrophic epithelium. The underlying connective tissue contains an infiltrate of chronic inflammatory cells and an increase in the size and number of vascular structures (Figure 11-19).

TREATMENT

Treatment is empirical and consists of removing local sources of irritation and informing the patient of the factors and circumstances that may contribute to the exacerbation of the disease. Brushing of the tongue should be avoided because it tends to intensify and prolong the condition.

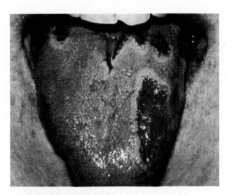

FIGURE 11-17

Benign migratory glossitis. The tongue demonstrates the typical erythematous patches with a distinctive white rim on the dorsal surface. The tip exhibits features of atrophic glossitis.

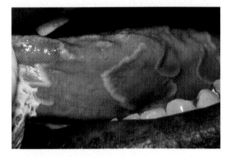

FIGURE 11-18

Stomatitis areata migrans. The ventral surface of the tongue exhibits arcuate raised lines against an erythematous background.

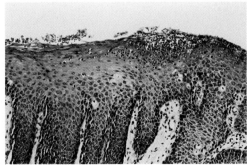

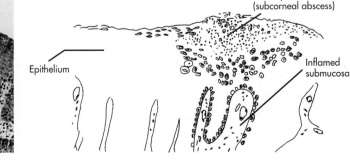

Neutrophil accumulation (subcorneal abscess)

Epithelium

Inflamed submucosa

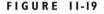

FIGURE 11-19

Benign migratory glossitis/stomatitis areata migrans. Microscopic features of both conditions are identical consisting of a localized zone in the parakeratin layer consisting of an accumulation of neutrophils (subcorneal abscess) that corresponds to the location of the distinctive arcuate white lines observed clinically.

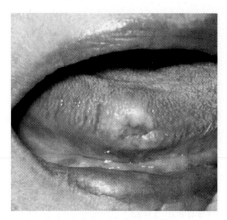

FIGURE 11-20

Chronic ulcer of the tongue. Deep ulcer located in the middle third of the lateral border of the tongue exhibits a raised indurated border resembling a malignant lesion.

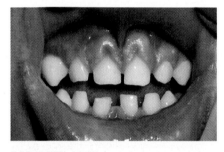

FIGURE 11-21

Factitious injury. Child exhibiting vertical clefting and reactive hyperplasia of fibrous tissue of the labial gingiva of the two maxillary anterior teeth due to habitual irritation with fingernail.

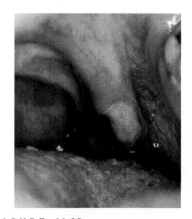

FIGURE 11-22

Factitious injury. Adult with a chronic non-healing ulcer of the anterior tonsillar pillar due to habitual scratching to relieve itchiness.

Chronic Ulcers

Chronic tongue ulcers differ from ulcers in other parts of the mouth because they may remain relatively unchanged for long periods. They are commonly found on the middle and posterior third of the lateral borders of the tongue where each appears as a shallow ulceration surrounded by a raised rolled border of fibrous tissue and an outer wide zone of induration (Figure 11-20). These nonhealing indurated lesions are easily mistaken for squamous cell carcinomas, which commonly occur in the same area and can have a similar appearance.

Management of chronic tongue ulcers can be demanding because identification of the irritating factors can be difficult. If a broken cusp, fractured restoration, or interfering denture clasp can be identified and corrected, healing may take place. In many cases injury is the result of lack of tongue coordination during mastication due to a prescribed medication or systemic conditions such as Parkinson disease or a stroke involving the cranial nerves. In other cases the tongue may be enlarged due to amyloidosis, acromegaly, hypothyroidism, hemangioma or lymphangioma, or allergic reactions. In some denture wearers, malpositioned posterior teeth on the denture base may be the contributing factor.

It is not uncommon for an ulcer to remain unhealed even after correction of the predisposing factors. This is thought to occur because of the presence of the large and continually active tongue muscles that are close to the epithelial surface. The normal constant motion of the tongue prevents re-epithelialization over the defect. In these cases surgical removal of the ulcer and its immediate surrounding fibrous tissue and the immobilization of the overlying epithelium by the use of ample numbers of sutures allow the defect to heal. The removed tissue also provides a specimen for microscopic evaluation to ensure the ulcer is not the result of a malignancy.

MUCOSAL TISSUE

Factitious Injuries

Factitious injuries are inflicted by the patient. They may be consciously undertaken, habitual, or inadvertent. The most common are injuries incidental to toothbrushing, flossing, and the use of toothpicks, which were previously discussed.

Fingernail injuries to the oral tissue are among the most common of the factitious injuries. Patients often indicate that their habit was initiated and perpetuated due to "itchiness" in the area. On the gingiva lesions are characteristic-appearing vertical clefts produced by forcing the free gingival margin apically. This habit results in root exposure on one or more teeth (Figure 11-21). In other accessible areas of the mucosa the habit produces a chronic nonhealing ulcer (Figure 11-22).

Cheek and lip biting are also forms of habitual factitious injuries. The lesions have a characteristic "shaggy" appearance and are only present in areas where the mucosal soft tissue can be grasped between the patient's teeth. The usual pattern is along the occlusal line of the buccal mucosa and the labial surfaces of the lips (Figure 11-23).

In some **emotionally disturbed patients** the secretive and purposeful production of oral lesions is performed to obtain continuous attention and compassion from family and healthcare workers. The lesions are usually in the mandibular sulcus or on the lips. They may be produced with fingernails or instruments. Attempts to heal the areas are often fruitless because the patients usually interfere with the process to ensure failure.

Patients with **Gilles de la Tourette syndrome** are prone to spontaneous erratic behavior and incoherent facial expressions and verbalizations. Part of the syndrome is the tendency for self-mutilation, which is often directed to the oral tissue either through the use of the teeth or fingernails (Figure 11-24).

Denture Injuries

Denture injuries may be either acute or chronic. Acute injuries most commonly occur when a prosthetic appliance is new and not completely adjusted for fit and even distribution of occlusal forces. These appliances produce excessive pressure on one or more focal areas of the soft tissue, causing stasis or ischemia of the blood supply and/or severe frictional activity over the tissue, resulting in ulceration and pain.

The chronic injuries are the result of gradual alteration in the supporting tissue while the denture base remains unchanged. In these situations the appliance becomes unstable and unevenly seated, leading to continuous mild frictional movements over the supporting tissue. The usual result is a large zone of reactive tissue changes, the most notable occurring on the palate as an **inflammatory papillary hyperplasia.** It has also been referred to as "denture papillomatosis." These lesions have a "raspberry" appearance consisting of multiple small erythematous nodules (Figure 11-25). The area may become secondarily infected with *Candida albicans* and become symptomatic; patients experience a burning sensation of the palate. It is more common in patients who wear their dentures continuously. Treatment consists of removing the appliances for prolonged periods, particularly at night, and using a tissue conditioner on the base of the denture. This is helpful in removing the inflammation and symptoms, particularly when used in combination with an antifungal agent. Unfortunately, the condition seldom resolves completely because the nodules are composed of dense fibrous tissue that do not return to normal. Some surgical intervention is often required before placement of the new prosthesis.

Over time as ridge support becomes diminished due to alveolar resorption, the denture flanges tend to gradually extend deeper in the sulcus, abnormally impinging on the soft tissue. In these areas a lesion is produced that is a combination of a chronic ulcer and a hyperplasia of the adjacent chronically inflamed connective tissue (Figure 11-26, *A*). This lesion is referred to as **inflammatory fibrous hyperplasia** or commonly as **epulis fissuratum.** After correction of the denture the lesion will have some reduction in size and may even return to normal color, but usually a residual nodule or mass of fibrous tissue (Figure 11-26, *B*) remains that requires surgical removal.

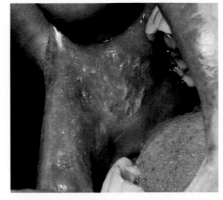

FIGURE 11-23

Factitious injury. Shaggy appearance of surface mucosa along the occlusal line and commissure area of the anterior buccal mucosa typical of chronic cheek biting.

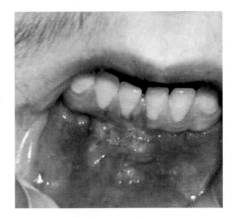

FIGURE 11-24

Factitious injury. Chronic self-mutilation of the anterior buccal vestibule with the fingernails in a patient with Gilles de la Tourette syndrome.

A

B

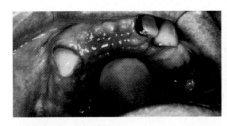 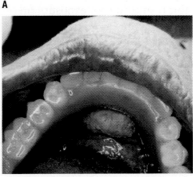

FIGURE 11-25

Denture injury. Focal erythema and diffuse nodular hyperplasia under an ill-fitting partial denture.

FIGURE 11-26

Denture injury. A, Single large area of fibrous hyperplasia (epulis fissuratum) in the location of a long-term impingement of a denture flange on the anterior floor of the mouth. **B,** Low-power photomicrograph of denture-induced fibrous hyperplasia exhibiting a centrally located sulcus that corresponds to denture flange impingement.

Electrical Burns

Electrical burns most commonly occur in young children between the ages of 2 and 4 years. Most burns are due to biting on the plugged cord of an appliance. The burns are produced by an arc that results from the electric current passing through the electrolyte-rich saliva. The arc reaches temperatures as high as 3000° C and is capable of quickly producing deep thermal burns and local tissue destruction. Less commonly, the damage occurs by sucking on the receptacle (female) end of an electrical extension cord. The severity of the injury depends on the voltage, amperage, and duration of the contact.

CLINICAL

Clinically, electrical burns differ from thermal burns by having one or more deep craters with a light yellow base, each measuring 1 to 3 cm in diameter. Lesions are commonly painless and bloodless. Often large areas will feel "cold" because normal-appearing tissue surrounding the crater is usually rendered ischemic. For 3 to 4 weeks the base of the crater and some of the surrounding tissue sloughs, leaving a large defect with ragged edges. The lower lip and angles of the mouth are most frequently involved. If untreated, patients may develop deformities that include microstomia, mucosal-alveolar adhesions, and morphologic alterations in the shape of the lips. If the alveolar ridges receive substantial current, development of the tooth buds in the area may be curtailed. Damage to the growth centers of bone results in failure of arch growth and shape, leading to malocclusion. Development of microstomia is of particular concern because the patient is unable to maintain adequate oral hygiene and have routine restorative procedures performed.

HISTOPATHOLOGY

The histologic features of electrical arc burns consist of a large area of necrosis, protein coagulation, and fat liquefaction surrounded by a zone of granulation tissue and abundant inflammatory cells. If bone is involved, areas of necrotic bone containing empty lacunae and the production of sequestra are common.

TREATMENT

Treatment of the area is often temporarily delayed to allow time to determine the extent of the injury because additional adjacent areas may not immediately appear to be severely damaged. Cosmetic reconstruction is often required in later years.

Thermal Burns

Most intraoral thermal burns are mild and result from contact with hot foods and beverages. The anterior tongue and palate are most frequently involved because they are the first anatomic structures to be contacted. With mild burns the areas may exhibit slight erythema for a short period and resolve. In more severe burns, as sometimes occurs when hot cheese contacts the palate, the area exhibits sloughing of the superficial layers of epithelium, revealing an erythematous base that becomes sensitive for a much longer period (Figure 11-27). It is rare that permanent damage results from burns caused by hot foods of any type.

More serious thermal burns can occur during dental procedures when hot instruments accidentally contact tissue. These burns are frequently located on the lips and in the commissure areas where they can cause a great deal of pain and heal with scar formation. Burns due to overheated hydrocolloid impression material occur primarily on the gingiva and can be diffuse and painful. Healing is often slow with some permanent defects possible.

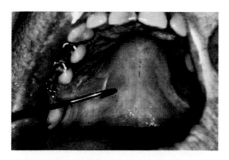

FIGURE 11-27

Thermal burn. Palate reveals erythema and superficial sloughing due to the ingestion of a hot beverage.

RADIATION INJURIES

Radiation injuries are due to the ionizing effects of electromagnetic waves or energized particles on cells. Radiation therapy is commonly used in the management of head and neck malignancies. In the process of eliminating the diseased tissue, normal oral tissue in or near the same field is also damaged but usually to a lesser extent, allowing for the selective elimination of the neoplasm.

Therapeutic electromagnetic waves may be low energy, less than 1000 KeV (orthovoltage), or high energy, 4 million to 25 million KeV (supervoltage). The low-energy waves are effectively used for superficial skin or mucosal lesions because energy absorption is at the point of initial contact with tissue. When high energy is used, the maximal energy absorption is located substantially beneath the surface, resulting in a beneficial "skin-sparing" effect. This is a useful tool for the treatment of deep tumors or metastatic lesions in lymph nodes. Particulate radiation consists mostly of electrons, protons, neutrons, or heavily charged ions. The particulate energy is generated with a linear accelerator and is commonly in the 6 million to 21 million eV range.

The amount of cell damage depends on the amount of energy the tissue absorbs. This is measured as the radiation absorbed dose *(rad)* or as a gray *(Gy)*. In these systems 1 rad is equivalent to the absorption of 100 ergs/g and 1 Gy equals 100 rads. Cell necrosis can occur as a result of *direct* damage to the larger cell molecules or *indirectly* by means of the toxic compounds produced by the ionizing radiation when energy is absorbed. The indirect process occurs through the production of free radicals that combine to form toxic substances such as hydrogen peroxide. This mechanism can be manipulated therapeutically by superoxygenating tissue to increase the production of hydrogen peroxide and the cancericidal activity, allowing the use of lower doses. With particulate radiation, cell necrosis is primarily the result of direct damage rather than the production of free radicals.

Other factors determine the effectiveness of radiation. The stage of the cell cycle is important because cells in G1/S and late G2 stages are very sensitive to radiation, whereas those in the other stages are relatively resistant. Because of this a single dose of radiation is effective only on a small number of cells; multiple exposures must be made as other cells go into their sensitive stages. Lesions that have a high index of mitotic activity, as occurs in the higher grades of malignancy, have more cells in the sensitive stages at any one time than the lower grades of malignancy and are usually more responsive to radiotherapy. Some lesions and tissues have little or no mitotic activity and are somewhat resistant to radiation. These are such tissues as nerve, muscle, bone, and mature cartilage. Other normal tissue contains cells that are as sensitive to radiation as the neoplastic cells that are being targeted, making it difficult to eliminate the lesion while sparing the surrounding tissue. These cells are lymphoblasts, bone marrow cells, germ cells of the ovaries and testes, and the epithelial cells of the mucosal lining of the stomach and intestines. Additionally, some cells have a greater capacity to repair themselves, and others are able to quickly repopulate the void produced. Many of the negative factors are diminished when the total cancericidal dose is properly fractionated.

Radiation Mucositis

Because the basal cell layer of the mucosal epithelium normally has a somewhat high mitotic activity, it is especially sensitive to radiation that passes through it en route to a neoplastic lesion. During the second week of fractionated treatments, the exposed mucosa will initially become atrophic and erythematous. This phase quickly progresses to a layer of necrotic cells. The affected areas of the mucosa clinically appear pale yellow and when mechanically removed reveal

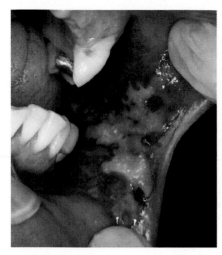

FIGURE 11-28

Radiation mucositis. The buccal mucosa exhibits an area of superficial white slough composed of necrotic epithelium against a background of erythematous atrophic mucosa.

an erythematous painful erosive area (Figure 11-28). In ensuing weeks many patients will develop superimposed bacterial and yeast (candidiasis) infections within the necrotic tissue, further increasing the degree of discomfort. By the end of the sixth week of treatment, particularly when large fields for treatment are used, the mucositis enlarges to include most of the oral cavity, nasopharynx, and esophagus. The mucositis persists at the same level of intensity for 2 additional weeks after the last treatment, and complete regeneration of normal epithelium occurs at the end of an additional month.

During all stages eating becomes progressively more painful and difficult as patients experience alteration or loss of taste and the saliva becomes thickened and stagnant. Symptoms are managed with frequent oral, warm saline and baking soda rinses. Often topical anesthetic is applied to allow the intake of food. Otherwise, the patient is restricted to a liquid diet.

Xerostomia

When there is greatly reduced saliva production in the mouth, the condition is referred to as xerostomia. It is a slowly evolving complication of radiation to the orofacial area, resulting from the damage to the parenchyma of the major and minor salivary glands in the path of the beam. Most radiation treatments intentionally include the lymph nodes because they may contain metastatic lesions; the submandibular glands and lower lobes of the parotids are included in that field. Glands receiving less than the usual cancericidal dose of 6000 rads will receive less permanent damage. The parenchymal cells will have altered pH and electrolytes and reduced secretion of immunoglobins. These alterations in the oral environment, particularly the loss of tissue immunoglobins, alters the commensal relationships of the oral flora, allowing the normally present *C. albicans* to proliferate and become infective. The candidal infection contributes to the intensification of the pain and discomfort already present during the acute stages of radiation mucositis and leads to a chronic sore mouth that may last for months or years. Treatment with slowly dissolving lozenges containing antifungal agents such as clotrimazole are often effective in controlling the yeast infection. When medication is withdrawn, there is often a recurrence until the saliva returns to normal.

Radiation Caries

There are no known deleterious effects on the teeth directly due to radiation. The dramatic increase in the caries activity during radiation treatments is a result of a major shift of the pH of saliva into the acidic range and an accompanying reduction in its buffering capacity due to changes in the electrolytes. All teeth in the mouth are affected by the increased caries incidence, regardless of whether they are within the treatment field. Caries secondary to radiation have a distinctive pattern prevalent at the cementoenamel junction of the buccolabial surfaces, locations normally resistant to caries (Figure 11-29). This pattern of caries often leads to amputation of the crowns if appropriate preventive measures are not implemented during the early stages of radiotherapy. The buccal and lingual smooth surfaces frequently develop white chalky or opaque areas due to the demineralization of the enamel. These areas occur as a result of severe demineralization that occurs when the saliva becomes acidic and loses the mineral content that normally replenishes ions lost from the enamel surface. After several months of negative ion exchange the surface softens, loses its translucency, and often crumbles, leaving shallow erosions and exposed softened dentin.

Management of the rampant caries and demineralization associated with radiotherapy require close monitoring by dental personnel. Oral hygiene must be meticulously maintained, and daily use of a fluoride gel is necessary.

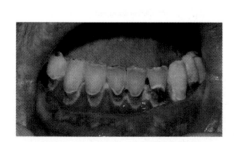

FIGURE 11-29

Radiation caries. Typical pattern of caries involvement after radiotherapy consisting of rampant caries circling the teeth at the cervical area and on the incisal edges. The teeth also exhibit a loss of translucency and appear whitish yellow and opaque. An acute candidiasis is evident on the soft tissue.

Osteoradionecrosis

■ OSTEORADIONECROSIS: an acute form of osteomyelitis with sequestrum formation due to severe radiation damage to intraosseous blood vessels predisposing to areas of refractory infection and necrosis that is most commonly found in the mandible.

The effect of radiation on bone is usually secondary to the changes induced in the walls of the blood vessels that nourish it. Some direct damage by ionizing radiation on the osteocytes does occur when the dose is high enough and usually when the malignancy is in close proximity to bone. Because bone normally has minimal vascularity, particularly the bones of the mandible, it is subject to severe infections that are slow to resolve. Further compromise of the vascular flow due to radiation-induced endarteritis often results in an acute osteomyelitis that results in the sequestration of large pieces of nonvital bone (Figure 11-30). Bacterial organisms initially enter the damaged bone through portals created by extractions, periapical abscesses, periodontal disease, traumatic breaks in the tissue during general anesthetic or surgical procedures, and the wearing of prosthetic appliances. Reducing these predisposing factors is of utmost importance in managing the oral cavity of patients receiving head and neck radiotherapy.

The management of osteoradionecrosis is difficult and often unsuccessful. Because the blood vessels are permanently damaged, it is difficult for nutrients and antibiotics to reach the bone and infectious microorganisms. Curettage of the necrotic tissues and attempts to obtain primary closure are often helpful. Otherwise, the use of frequent lavage of the defect to promote epithelialization is the only hope to halt the process. Prevention of further opportunities for penetration of the microorganism into the bone is necessary to increase chances of success. When possible, teeth should be restored or extracted and periodontal disease should be controlled before the initiation of radiotherapy. The use of fluoride gels and meticulous oral hygiene are necessary during and immediately after treatment to prevent the development of caries and periodontal disease.

Soft Tissue Injuries

The other oral soft tissues within the irradiated field will also incur some degree of damage. First to appear is a gradual loss in taste sensation that increases as

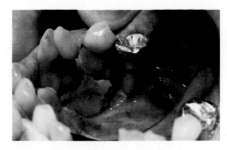

FIGURE 11-30

Osteoradionecrosis. Fragment of necrotic bone (sequestrum) exteriorized in an area of advanced periodontal disease in a patient who received radiotherapy to the region.

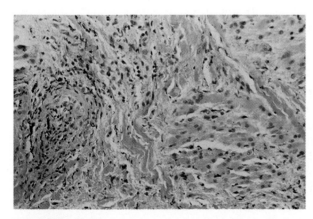 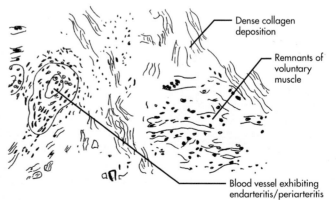

Dense collagen deposition

Remnants of voluntary muscle

Blood vessel exhibiting endarteritis/periarteritis

FIGURE 11-31

Soft tissue radiation injury. Photomicrograph of submucosal tissue within an irradiated field containing a blood vessel exhibiting severe endarteritis and periarteritis *(right)* and myositis with replacement of damaged tissues with scar tissue (fibrosis).

treatments continue. This complication is particularly distressing to patients because the intake of food is already a painful and difficult activity due to the acute mucositis. The return of taste acuity is very slow, only beginning several months after therapy ceases. Full recovery may take more than a year.

Muscle damage and eventual replacement with fibrous tissue occasionally develops (Figure 11-31). This, combined with fibrosis within the temporomandibular joint, can result in a reduced oral opening and trismus. Both conditions are difficult to correct and are best controlled by careful planning of the fields and fractionation of the dose of radiation and physiotherapy to the muscles during the recovery phase.

Of greater concern are the complications of posttreatment necrosis and gangrene of the soft tissue. Because blood vessels are particularly sensitive to ionizing radiation, endarteritis and periarteritis are common occurrences during treatment. These conditions result in permanently damaged vessels that have either significantly reduced blood flow or become completely blocked. Additionally, the capacity for new vessel formation in the affected tissue is reduced. On occasion, the mucosa becomes atrophic with the frequent development of ulcers that are slow to heal or may undergo ischemic necrosis followed by large areas of sloughing. The wearing of dentures or other appliances should be delayed for at least 1 year. Surgical procedures in areas previously irradiated should be avoided or conservatively undertaken due to the reduced vascularity and ability to heal.

CHEMICAL INJURIES

TEETH

Tetracycline

The ingestion of tetracycline during the mineralization of the organic matrix of developing deciduous and permanent teeth, bone, or cartilage results in permanent incorporation of the antibiotic into the mineral component of these tissues. Although this is not a serious problem in bone or cartilage since they are not visible, the teeth usually become cosmetically disturbing to the patient. The affected teeth exhibit yellowish to brownish-gray diffuse bands of discoloration that are located within the tooth structure and not on the surface. The intensity and distribution of color vary depending on the specific form of tetracycline taken and the duration of the administration. Chlortetracycline tends to cause a brownish-gray color (Figure 11-32, *A*), whereas oxytetracycline and tetracycline give a yellowish color (Figure 11-32, *B*), which is the least noticeable. In young teeth the color is most intense and unattractive but tends to fade slightly with time to a light brown. With the loss of intensity of the coloration, the ability to diagnose tetracycline staining when using ultraviolet light to demonstrate its fluorescent property also diminishes.

To prevent discoloration of the teeth, alternative types of antibiotics for treatment of infections is recommended for women who are in the second and third trimesters of pregnancy and should continue until the child is 7 years of age. External bleaching is of little value because the tetracycline is complexed with the calcium ions that are deposited during the mineralization of the enamel and the dentin and thus is not accessible like surface stains. The ability of tetracyclines to become incorporated into bones and teeth within hours of ingestion has been a useful experimental tool for labeling microscopic events according to time. When teeth are sectioned and examined microscopically with ultraviolet light, narrow bands or rings are seen coinciding with the part of the tooth developing at the time of administration (Figure 11-33).

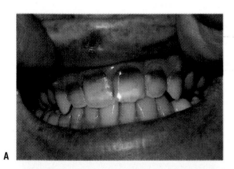

A

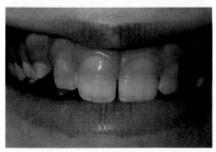

B

FIGURE 11-32

Tetracycline discoloration. Gray-brown **(A)** and yellowish-gray **(B)** discolorations of the cervical third of the maxillary anterior teeth in patients with chronic conditions requiring prolonged treatment with tetracycline during early childhood.

Congenital Porphyria

Although there are multiple types of porphyrias, only the congenital type produces the distinct discoloration of the teeth. Discoloration occurs because excess porphyrins are present in the blood during the mineralization of the teeth. Congenital porphyria is inherited as an autosomal recessive trait that is responsible for the development of a defective pathway for the metabolism of hematoporphyrins, resulting in the accumulation of excessive porphyrins in the blood and urine. The porphyrins become deposited in the skin and the developing teeth and bones. Affected teeth are pinkish brown and when viewed with ultraviolet light fluoresce bright scarlet. Sectioned teeth exhibit similar findings with normal and ultraviolet light and show the fluorescence in bands conforming to the incremental growth lines. The skin is also severely affected, becoming light brown and extremely sensitive to sunlight. The photosensitivity is expressed as large bullous lesions that often heal with scarring. It is not uncommon for patients with porphyria to have extensively scarred limbs and faces by the time they reach adulthood.

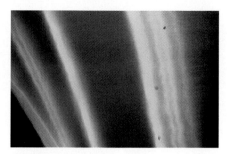

FIGURE 11-33

Tetracycline discoloration. Section of a nondecalcified tooth of a patient periodically treated with tetracycline during childhood viewed with ultraviolet light microscopy exhibiting dentin containing yellowish fluorescent bands of tetracycline deposited during the period of tooth development.

Biliary Atresia

Biliary atresia is an uncommon congenital condition in which there is narrowing of the ductal elements of the biliary system of the liver, resulting in elevated bilirubin levels in the blood. Complete or nearly complete congenital blockage is fatal and those most severely affected die within months of birth. Patients with lesser degrees of atresia appear jaundiced and will exhibit discolored teeth, particularly in the primary dentition. In these patients the teeth will have a dark greenish color with the roots more intensely stained than the crowns. The degree and distribution of tooth discoloration depends on the ability to manage the medical condition during tooth development in both the deciduous and permanent dentition.

Erythroblastosis Fetalis

Erythroblastosis fetalis is a hemolytic anemia that begins in utero. It results from incompatible factors in the blood of the mother and the fetus. An Rh-negative mother will develop antibodies against the erythrocytes of an Rh-positive fetus. The antibodies transgress the placental barrier, attacking and destroying the fetal erythrocytes. The result of the extensive hemolysis is the greatly elevated levels of the biliverdin and bilirubin blood pigments. These pigments become deposited in both the skin and the developing teeth of the fetus. Not all Rh incompatibilities result in tooth changes because the blood levels of pigment must be very high and present in the fetus between 4 and 7 months intrauterine. Only primary teeth are affected, with colors varying from green and bluish-green to yellowish-gray. The dentin is primarily affected. When dentin is severely involved, some enamel hypoplasia may also be present. The color fades in time but is still noticeable. With immediate blood transfusion at birth, discoloration is minimal. The permanent teeth are usually not affected.

GINGIVA

Chemical effects on gingiva may be in the form of (1) pigmentations that result from the ingestion of medications containing heavy metals such as bismuth, silver, mercury, gold, copper, and zinc or (2) hyperplasia of the collagenous component. Except for bismuth, the pigmentation effects of chemicals are rarely seen today because these compounds have been replaced as antimicrobials by antibiotics. Bismuth is still widely used as an antidiarrhea agent, but unless it is taken in excess, the only resulting pigmentation is in the form of a transitory brown staining of the dorsal tongue. If for some reason there is extensive intake of the heavy metals such as during occupational exposure, it usually is present in the marginal gingiva where it appears as a thin dark brown or gray line.

In recent years the medications that most commonly affect the gingiva are those that have the overproduction of collagen as a side effect. They are capable of inducing such extensive gingival hyperplasia that if left untreated will rapidly lead to advanced periodontitis with eventual premature loss of the dentition. These medications consist of phenytoin, cyclosporine, and calcium channel blocking medications such as nifedipine, each administered for different purposes in the management of systemic conditions.

Phenytoin

Phenytoin (Dilantin) is used to depress selected brain pathways without affecting the body's sensory functions. It is effective as an anticonvulsant and thus is widely used in patients with epilepsy, brain tumors, and other central nervous system (CNS) conditions that are prone to produce seizures.

The mechanism of the oral side effect of gingival enlargement is not completely known. Some research shows a direct effect by phenytoin on the fibroblasts responsible for collagen production. Other research indicates that phenytoin acts to destabilize the cell wall of the gingival mast cells, inducing excessive degranulation and release of histamine, heparin, and other ingredients that stimulate the fibroblasts to produce excessive collagen.

The incidence of gingival hyperplasia is in the range of 40% to 50%. In those patients subject to the side effect the hyperplastic condition becomes obvious 2 to 3 months after the administration of phenytoin, with the enlargement reaching its maximal severity in 12 to 18 months. There does not seem to be a close relationship between the dose of phenytoin and the severity of the enlargement. It has been generally thought that patients lacking adequate oral hygiene will develop a more rapid and severe form of the condition. Some patients develop extensive enlargements in the absence of gingivitis, developing lesions in edentulous areas. Hereditary factors are considered responsible for the degree to which some patients are affected and whether they become affected at all.

Enlargement begins in the interdental papillae as a bulbous or lobular growth, extending both buccally and lingually. The anterior part of the mouth usually becomes more involved than the posterior. The growths can enlarge to cover part or all of the crowns of the teeth, interfering with mastication. When not inflamed, the enlarged gingiva appears pink in color with a normally stippled surface. The enlargement is firm with little resiliency and does not bleed when probed. In contrast, inflamed gingiva not due to phenytoin enlargement is dark red, edematous, friable, and bleeds easily. Treatment consists of surgical removal of excessive tissue as necessary to allow function and maintenance of oral hygiene.

Cyclosporine

Cyclosporine, a compound derived from soil fungi, has a selective immunosuppressive effect on the T lymphocyte helper cells but without bone marrow suppression. It is used primarily to reduce the chance of rejection in organ transplant patients. It is occasionally used in the treatment of some autoimmune diseases. Because it has nephrotoxic and hepatotoxic effects, blood levels of patients who are taking the medication are carefully monitored.

Within the oral cavity it has the frequent side effect of inducing generalized gingival hyperplasia (Figure 11-34) and perioral hyperesthesia. In some clinical studies generalized gingival enlargement was found in 50% of all patients, with incidences approaching 100% of patients under 20 years of age. Some gingival enlargement is apparent within 1 to 3 months of the initiation of cyclosporine therapy, becoming maximized at about 1 year.

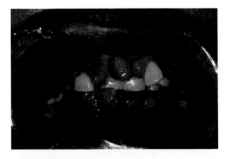

FIGURE 11-34

Cyclosporine-induced gingival hyperplasia. Renal transplant patient with generalized nodular gingival overgrowth.

The mechanism of cyclosporine-induced gingival hyperplasia is not well understood. Because not all patients exhibit gingival enlargement, selective stimulation of fibroblasts is suspected. In some cases an increase in the noncollagenous extracellular matrix has been found. This latter finding is consistent with the clinical observation that with cessation of the medication, gingival enlargement often subsides substantially.

The clinical appearance of cyclosporine-induced gingival hyperplasia is similar to that induced by phenytoin. It is more pronounced in the anterior aspect of the mouth and can enlarge to cover the crowns of the teeth. The extent of inflammation depends on the degree of local irritants. Because cyclosporine is an immunosuppressant, it is thought by some sources that the incidence of progressive periodontitis is enhanced due to the compromised defense system within the gingiva. At present, there is no experimental evidence that supports this.

The ideal treatment for cyclosporine-induced gingival hyperplasia is withdrawal of the medication; however, this is seldom possible. The enlargements can be minimized with meticulous oral hygiene. Periodically, enlargements that interfere with mastication will require surgical excision.

Nifedipine

Nifedipine is a commonly used calcium channel-blocking agent in the treatment of cardiovascular disorders such as angina pectoris and hypertension. It acts by inhibiting calcium ion influx in the smooth muscle of cardiac tissue and blood vessel walls without changing the serum calcium concentration. It is thus useful to selectively reduce contraction of some smooth muscles and is effective as a vasodilator. It enables the relaxation of blood vessels, thereby reducing vascular hypertension and the tendency for spasms in coronary arteries. This allows for better blood flow, thereby increasing oxygen levels to cardiac muscle. Because it acts on all smooth muscle, it has the generalized side effects of hypotension, weakness, dizziness, and syncope in some patients. The notable side effect within the oral cavity is a tendency for gingival enlargement.

The manner in which nifedipine and the other calcium channel blockers induce excessive gingival hyperplasia is thought to be through altered calcium influx into fibroblasts interfering with the production of collagenase. Thus collagen is not degraded and accumulates.

Between 25% and 50% of patients taking the medication will develop gingival enlargement. The enlargement begins 1 to 3 months after treatment begins and does not appear to be correlated with the dose. The gingival hyperplasia of nifedipine is clinically similar to that of phenytoin and cyclosporine. It is nodular and firm, originating in the interdental papillae of the anterior teeth (Figure 11-35). The enlargements are more severe when local irritants such as plaque, calculus, and defective fillings and crowns are present.

The best treatment for calcium channel blocker–induced gingival hyperplasia is the substitution of another vasodilator. If this is not possible, gingivectomy and meticulous oral hygiene can be used to control the severity of the condition.

MUCOSAL TISSUE

Amalgam

The accidental implantation of silver-containing compounds into the mucosal connective tissue usually results in a permanent grayish-black pigmentation, commonly referred to as *amalgam tattoo*. These pigmentations are notable because they are similar in appearance to melanin-containing pigmentations, which are of concern to the clinician and patient. The most common source of embedded silver compounds is amalgam, hence the name amalgam tattoo.

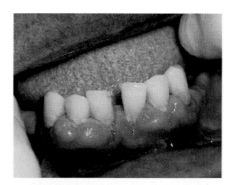

FIGURE 11-35

Nifedipine-induced gingival hyperplasia. Interdental gingiva exhibits nodular fibrous hyperplasia in the region of the mandible containing teeth.

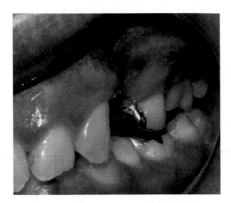

FIGURE 11-36

Amalgam tattoo. Focal gray-black pigmentation resembling a melanin-producing lesion on the buccal gingiva in the area of a previous extraction and large restoration.

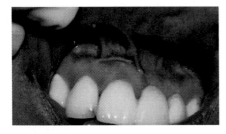

FIGURE 11-37

Amalgam tattoo. Diffuse area of blue-gray pigmentation of submucosal tissue over the apex of a nonvital central incisor previously treated by apicoectomy and an amalgam retrofil of the tooth apex.

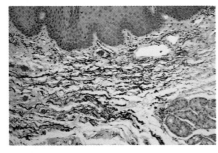

FIGURE 11-38

Amalgam tattoo. Microscopic appearance of submucosal tissue exhibiting linear staining of elastic and reticular fibers with a dark brown silver precipitate.

Amalgam is presently the most commonly used material for dental restorations and is composed of a mixture of silver, mercury, and tin. It enters the tissue accidentally, either through a laceration in the mucosa during a dental procedure, by falling into a socket during the extraction of a tooth, or by inadvertent compaction into the gingival sulcus while a restoration is placed (Figure 11-36). Amalgam is also used to seal the apex of a nonvital tooth after apicoectomy. Because this requires an intraosseous surgical procedure during which amalgam is intentionally placed within the bone and adjacent soft tissue, the pigmentation is often apparent on the surface (Figure 11-37). Larger fragments of amalgam may sometimes be discernible on radiographs. Absence of radiographic evidence of amalgam does not rule out the possibility of an amalgam tattoo because the particles are often too fine or widely dispersed to be visible. Clinical pigmented lesions that are not visible on radiographs should be biopsied to ensure that they do not represent an early melanoma.

The microscopic features of amalgam tattoos vary depending on the size of the particles and the quantity present. When larger fragments are present, a granuloma consisting of multinucleated giant cells, lymphocytes, and increased fibrosis surrounds the foreign material. When only smaller dustlike particles are present, they are usually engulfed by individual macrophages without the formation of distinctive granulomas. The fine particles are also found within the cytoplasm of a large number of cells and tissues including muscle, nerve, blood vessel walls, and collagen. Some tissues, particularly elastic fibers and the basement membrane, chemically interact with amalgam incorporating the liberated silver as a fine linear deposit of brown precipitate (Figure 11-38).

Once the diagnosis has been made, additional treatment is necessary only if the pigmentation is cosmetically unacceptable. In some instances if the amalgam particles are large, they should be removed to prevent a further foreign body response or a source of irritation, especially if a prosthetic appliance is to be placed over the area.

Graphite

Graphite pigmentations are similar to amalgam pigmentations in size and color but tend to occur in different locations. They are caused by accidental tissue punctures of the mucosa with a pencil. At the time of puncture, fine particles of carbon are permanently deposited in the submucosal tissue.

Most pigmentations of this origin are located in the anterior part of the mouth and on the soft palate where they may be associated with a perforation. The pigmentations are small, usually of several millimeters in diameter, grayish-black, and circular.

The microscopic appearance differs from that of an amalgam tattoo because there are no large fragments inducing a foreign body response. Inflammation, granuloma formation, and multinucleated giant cells often associated with amalgam are absent. Because graphite is an inert material, there is no chemical interaction with the elastic fibers or basement membrane as occurs with the silver contained within amalgam. The fine carbon particles are nearly all found within the cytoplasm of macrophages and other tissue cells capable of phagocytosis.

After biopsy no treatment is necessary unless the patient wishes the area removed for cosmetic reasons.

CHEMICAL BURNS

Acetylsalicylic Acid

The placement of acetylsalicylic acid (ASA) on the alveolar processes directly over the roots of a tooth that is the source of severe pain is a commonly held misconception. It is based on the belief that the analgesic is able to penetrate the

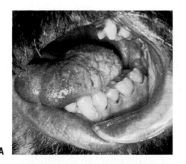

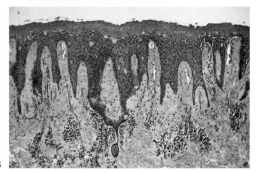

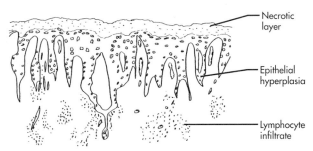

FIGURE 11-39

Aspirin burn. A, The lateral surface of the tongue and buccal mucosa with a white, wrinkled surface and an erythematous background resulting from prolonged contact with acetylsalicylic acid placed adjacent to a painful tooth. **B,** Microscopic appearance of chemically injured tissue demonstrating a superficial layer of necrotic epithelial cells and connective tissue diffusely infiltrated with plasma cells and lymphocytes.

Necrotic layer

Epithelial hyperplasia

Lymphocyte infiltrate

mucosa and cortical plate of bone and act directly on the nerve bundle of the offending tooth. Sometimes the ASA is placed within the cavitation of a carious tooth. In either location the tablet is slowly dissolved, liberating a concentrated acidic solution in the immediate area that becomes diluted and buffered in the saliva farther away from the painful area. Most of the relief that patients receive is believed to be due to the fact that the solution is swallowed and absorbed systemically.

Because in many cases the ASA is in direct contact with the tongue and buccal mucosa, the soft tissue will appear white and friable, superimposed against an erythematous background with associated symptoms of burning ("aspirin burn") (Figure 11-39, *A*). If the lesion is severe, removal of the superficial white layer may reveal a bleeding erosive base. The concentrated solution produces necrosis of the surface layers of the epithelium and an inflammatory response of the deeper connective tissue (Figure 11-39, *B*). Upon cessation of the practice, healing occurs in 1 to 2 weeks.

Other Medications

Many other medications used in dentistry can also produce chemical burns of the perioral facial skin and mucosal tissue if inadvertently dropped on these surfaces during use. Some medications such as phenol (carbolic acid), which is used as a disinfectant, or silver nitrate, which is often deployed as a cauterizing agent, are capable of superficial necrosis when dropped on the tissue in concentrated form. Other chemical agents are used as astringents (trichloroacetic acid) for gingival retraction and when overused result in tissue necrosis of the marginal gingiva. Some patients have misused denture cleansing agents that contain concentrated detergent and oxidating agents by placing the appliances in their mouths without properly rinsing off the excess cleaner (Figure 11-40). In some patients overuse of some types of mouthwash and toothpaste can cause a superficial necrosis of the superficial mucosa ("slough") (Figure 11-41). This can be easily wiped off temporarily by passing the finger over the mucosa. In all of these situations the severity of the condition depends on the concentration of the medication, the duration of the application, and the biologic differences in individuals.

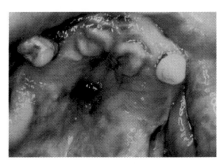

FIGURE 11-40

Severe chemical burn. Large area of superficial necrotic soft tissue developed after patient placed a partial denture in the mouth without removing denture cleansing agent.

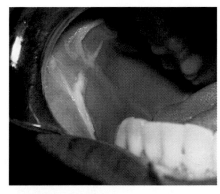

FIGURE 11-41

Mild chemical burn. Superficial thin, white membrane of necrotic epithelial cells on the buccal mucosa due to overuse of mouthwash. The mucosal slough can be easily removed by wiping with a finger or gauze.

ADDITIONAL READING

INJURIES TO TEETH

Addy M, Pearce N. Aetiological, predisposing and environmental factors in dentine hypersensitivity. *Arch Oral Biol.* 1994; 39(suppl):33S-38S.

Attanasio R. Nocturnal bruxism and its clinical management. *Dent Clin North Am.* 1991; 35:245-52.

Bevenius J, Evans S, L'Estrange P. Conservative management of erosion-abrasion: a system for the general practitioner. *Aust Dent J.* 1994; 39:4-10.

Bishop K, Briggs P, Kelleher M. The aetiology and management of localized anterior tooth wear in the young adult. *Dent Update.* 1994; 21:153-60.

Burke FJ, Whitehead SA, McCaughey AD. Contemporary concepts in the pathogenesis of the Class V non-carious lesion. *Dent Update.* 1995; 22:28-32.

Camp JH. Diagnosis and management of sports-related injuries to the teeth. *Dent Clin North Am.* 1991; 35:733-56.

Johansson A, Omar R. Identification and management of tooth wear. *Int J Prosthodont.* 1994; 7:506-16.

Johnson GK, Sivers JE. Attrition, abrasion and erosion: diagnosis and therapy. *Clin Prev Dent.* 1987; 9:12-6.

Johnson R. Traumatic dental injuries in children: part 1: evaluation of traumatic dental injuries and treatment of injuries to primary teeth. *Update Pediatr Dent.* 1989; 2:1-4, 6-7.

Johnson R. Traumatic dental injuries in children: part 2: treatment of injuries to permanent teeth. *Update Pediatr Dent.* 1989; 2:1-4, 6-8.

Levitch LC, Bader JD, Shugars DA, Heymann HO. Non-carious cervical lesions. *J Dent.* 1994; 22:195-207.

Milosevic A. Tooth wear: an aetiological and diagnostic problem. *Eur J Prosthodont Restor Dent.* 1993; 1:173-8.

Russell MD. The distinction between physiological and pathological attrition. *J Ir Dent Assoc.* 1987; 33:23-31.

Seligman DA, Pullinger AG, Solberg WK. The prevalence of dental attrition and its association with factors of age, gender, occlusion, and TMJ symptomatology. *J Dent Res.* 1988; 67:1323-33.

Spieler EL. Toothbrush abrasion: prevention and the Alert toothbrush. *Compendium.* 1994; 15:306, 308, 310-2.

Tyas MJ. The class V lesion—aetiology and restoration. *Aust Dent J.* 1995; 40:167-70.

Watkins KV. Self-inflected oral injuries and suicidal ideation secondary to loss of teeth. *N Y State Dent J.* 1991; 57:21-3.

AVULSION, TRANSPLANTATION, AND ANKYLOSIS

Burch J, Ngan P, Hackman A. Diagnosis and treatment planning for unerupted premolars. *Pediatr Dent.* 1994; 16:89-95.

Douglass J, Tinanoff N. The etiology, prevalence, and sequelae of infraclusion of primary molars. *ASDC J Dent Child.* 1991; 58:481-3.

Hammarstrom L, Pierce A, Blomlof L, Feiglin B and others. Tooth avulsion and replantation—a review. *Endod Dent Traumatol.* 1986; 2:1-8.

Jacobs SG. Ankylosis of permanent teeth: a case report and literature review. *Aust Orthod J.* 1989; 11:38-44.

Kehoe JC. Splinting and replantation after traumatic avulsion. *J Am Dent Assoc.* 1986; 112:224-30.

Tsukiboshi M. Autogenous tooth transplantation: a reevaluation. *Int J Periodontics Restorative Dent.* 1993; 13:120-49.

Vanarsdall RL. Complications of orthodontic treatment. *Curr Opin Dent.* 1991; 1:622-33.

RESORPTION

Carter LC. Resorption of tooth substance: diagnosis and management. *Compendium.* 1992; 13:1012-1016.

Goldman HM. An atlas of acquired dental defects. *Compend Contin Educ Dent.* 1982; 3:275-90.

O'Riordan MW, Ralstrom CS, Doerr SE. Treatment of avulsed permanent teeth: an update. *J Am Dent Assoc.* 1982; 105:1028-30.

Pierce AM. Experimental basis for the management of dental resorption. *Endod Dent Traumatol.* 1989; 5:255-65.

Torabinejad M, Bakland LK. Prostaglandins: their possible role in the pathogenesis of pulpal and periapical diseases, part 2. *J Endod.* 1980; 6:769-76.

Yaacob HB. Idiopathic external resorption of teeth. *J Can Dent Assoc.* 1980; 46:578-82.

TONGUE INJURIES

Beitman RG, Frost SS, Roth JL. Oral manifestations of gastrointestinal disease. *Dig Dis Sci.* 1981; 26:741-7.

Grinspan D, Fernandez Blanco G, Aguero S, Bianchi O and others. Ectopic geographic tongue and AIDS. *Int J Dermatol.* 1990; 29:113-6.

Nally F. Diseases of the tongue. *Practitioner.* 1991; 235:65-71.

Smith RG, Burtner AP. Oral side-effects of the most frequently prescribed drugs. *Spec Care Dentist.* 1994; 14:96-102.

DENTURE INJURIES

Arendorf TM, Walker DM. Denture stomatitis: a review. *J Oral Rehabil.* 1987; 14:217-27.

Budtz-Jorgensen E. Oral mucosal lesions associated with the wearing of removable dentures. *J Oral Pathol.* 1981; 10:65-80.

Devlin H, Watts DC. Acrylic "allergy"? *Br Dent J.* 1984; 157:272-5.

Jeganathan S, Lin CC. Denture stomatitis—a review of the aetiology, diagnosis and management. *Aust Dent J.* 1992; 37:107-14.

Lombardi T, Budtz-Jorgensen E. Treatment of denture-induced stomatitis: a review. *Eur J Prosthodont Restor Dent.* 1993; 2:17-22.

MacEntee MI. The prevalence of edentulism and diseases related to dentures: a literature review. *J Oral Rehabil.* 1985; 12:195-207.

Reeve CM, Van Roekel NB. Denture sore mouth. *Dermatol Clin.* 1987; 5:681-6.

ELECTRICAL BURNS

Bailey B, Gaudreault P, Thivierge RL, Turgeon JP. Cardiac monitoring of children with household electrical injuries. *Ann Emerg Med.* 1995; 25:612-7.

Patel A, Lo R. Electric injury with cerebral venous thrombosis: case report and review of the literature. *Stroke.* 1993; 24:903-5.

Thompson JC, Ashwal S. Electrical injuries in children. *Am J Dis Child.* 1983; 137:231-5.

THERMAL BURNS

Conine TA, Carlow DL, Stevenson-Moore P. The Vancouver microstomia orthosis. *J Prosthet Dent.* 1989; 61:476-83.

Edlich RF, Nichter LS, Morgan RF, Persing JA and others. Burns of the head and neck. *Otolaryngol Clin North Am.* 1984; 17:361-88.

RADIATION INJURIES

Berthrong M, Fajardo LF. Radiation injury in surgical pathology: part II: alimentary tract. *Am J Surg Pathol.* 1981; 5: 153-78.

Jacob RF. Management of xerostomia in the irradiated patient. *Clin Plast Surg.* 1993; 20:507-16.

Wright JM, Barton FE, Byrd DL, Dahl EW and others. Complications of the treatment of oral cancer. In: *Oral Cancer: Clinical and Pathological Considerations.* Boca Raton, Fla: CRC Press; 1988: chap 7.

OSTEORADIONECROSIS

Balogh JM, Sutherland SE. Osteoradionecrosis of the mandible: a review. *J Otolaryngol.* 1989; 18:245-50.

Bernier S, Clermont S, Maranda G, Turcotte JY. Osteomyelitis of the jaws. *J Can Dent Assoc.* 1995; 61:441-2, 445-8.

Carlson ER. The radiobiology, treatment, and prevention of osteoradionecrosis of the mandible. *Recent Results Cancer Res.* 1994; 134:191-9.

Dreizen S. Oral complications of cancer therapies: description and incidence of oral complications. *NCI Monogr.* 1990; (9):11-5.

Friedman RB. Osteoradionecrosis: causes and prevention. *NCI Monogr.* 1990; (9):145-9.

Maxymiw WG, Wood RE. The role of dentistry in head and neck radiation therapy. *J Can Dent Assoc.* 1989; 55:193-8.

Mealey BL, Semba SE, Hallmon WW. The head and neck radiotherapy patient: part 2: management of oral complications. *Compendium.* 1994; 15:446-52.

Nguyen AM. Dental management of patients who receive chemo- and radiation therapy. *Gen Dent.* 1992; 40:305-11.

Precious D, Dalton M, Hoffman D. Infection of facial bones. *J Otolaryngol.* 1990; 19:214-21.

Sanger JR, Matloub HS, Yousif NJ, Larson DL. Management of osteoradionecrosis of the mandible. *Clin Plast Surg.* 1993; 20:517-30.

Semba SE, Mealey BL, Hallmon WW. The head and neck radiotherapy patient: part 1: oral manifestations of radiation therapy. *Compendium.* 1994; 15:252-60.

Stevenson-Moore P, Epstein JB. The management of teeth in irradiated sites. *Eur J Cancer B Oral Oncol.* 1993; 29B:39-43.

TOOTH STAINING

Jensen JD, Resnick SD. Porphyria in childhood. *Semin Dermatol.* 1995; 14:33-9.

May BK, Dogra SC, Sadlon TJ, Bhasker CR and others. Molecular regulation of heme biosynthesis in higher vertebrates. *Prog Nucleic Acid Res Mol Biol.* 1995; 51:1-51.

Mello HS. The mechanism of tetracycline staining in primary and permanent teeth. *J Dent Child.* 1967; 34:478-87.

Paterson JR. Tetracycline stained vital teeth—review of literature. *J Indiana Dent Assoc.* 1979; 58:18-22.

With TK. Porphyrias in animals. *Clin Haematol.* 1980; 9:345-70.

CHEMICAL-INDUCED GINGIVAL HYPERPLASIA

Ellis JS, Seymour RA, Monkman SC, Idle JR. Gingival sequestration of nifedipine in nifedipine-induced gingival overgrowth. *Lancet.* 1992; 339:1382-3.

Fujii A, Matsumoto H, Nakao S, Teshigawara H and others. Effect of calcium-channel blockers on cell proliferation, DNA synthesis and collagen synthesis of cultured gingival fibroblasts derived from human nifedipine responders and nonresponders. *Arch Oral Biol.* 1994; 39:99-104.

Lucas RM, Howell LP, Wall BA. Nifedipine-induced gingival hyperplasia: a histochemical and ultrastructural study. *J Periodontol.* 1985; 56:211-5.

McCulloch CA, Knowles GC. Deficiencies in collagen phagocytosis by human fibroblasts in vitro: a mechanism for fibrosis? *J Cell Physiol.* 1993; 155:461-71.

Niimi A, Tohnai I, Kaneda T, Takeuchi M and others. Immunohistochemical analysis of effects of cyclosporin A on gingival epithelium. *J Oral Pathol Med.* 1990; 19:397-403.

Penarrocha-Diago M, Bagan-Sebastian JV, Vera-Sempere F. Diphenylhydantoin-induced gingival overgrowth in man: a clinico-pathological study. *J Periodontol.* 1990; 61:571-4.

Pernu HE, Knuuttila ML, Huttunen KR, Tiilikainen AS. Drug-induced gingival overgrowth and class II major histocompatibility antigens. *Transplantation.* 1994; 57:1811-3.

Pernu HE, Pernu LM, Knuuttila ML, Huttunen KR. Gingival overgrowth among renal transplant recipients and uraemic patients. *Nephrol Dial Transplant.* 1993; 8:1254-8.

Salo T, Oikarinen KS, Oikarinen AI. Effect of phenytoin and nifedipine on collagen gene expression in human gingival fibroblasts. *J Oral Pathol Med.* 1990; 19:404-7.

Seymour RA. Drug-induced gingival overgrowth. *Adverse Drug React Toxicol Rev.* 1993; 12:215-32.

Seymour RA, Jacobs DJ. Cyclosporin and the gingival tissues. *J Clin Periodontol.* 1992; 19:1-11.

Smith QT, Hinrichs JE. Phenytoin and 5-(p-hydroxyphenyl)-5-

phenylhydantoin do not alter the effects of bacterial and amplified plaque extracts on cultures of fibroblasts from normal and overgrown gingivae. *J Dent Res.* 1987; 66:1393-8.

Suresh R, Puvanakrishnan R, Dhar SC. Alterations in human gingival glycosaminoglycan pattern in inflammation and in phenytoin-induced overgrowth. *Mol Cell Biochem.* 1992; 115:149-54.

Walker CR, Tomich CE, Hutton CE. Treatment of phenytoin-induced gingival hyperplasia by electrosurgery. *J Oral Surg.* 1980; 38:306-11.

Willershausen-Zonnchen B, Lemmen C, Schumacher U. Influence of cyclosporine A on growth and extracellular matrix synthesis of human fibroblasts. *J Cell Physiol.* 1992; 152: 397-402.

Willershausen-Zonnchen B, Lemmen C, Zonnchen B, Hamm G and others. Influence of nifedipine on the metabolism of gingival fibroblasts. *Biol Chem Hoppe Seyler.* 1994; 375: 299-303.

Williamson MS, Miller EK, Plemons J, Rees T and others. Cyclosporine A upregulates interleukin-6 gene expression in human gingiva: possible mechanism for gingival overgrowth. *J Periodontol.* 1994; 65:895-903.

AMALGAM TATTOO

Hartman LC, Natiella JR, Meenaghan MA. The use of elemental microanalysis in verification of the composition of presumptive amalgam tattoo. *J Oral Maxillofac Surg.* 1986; 44:628-33.

McGinnis JP, Greer JL, Daniels DS. Amalgam tattoo: report of an unusual clinical presentation and the use of energy dispersive x-ray analysis as an aid to diagnosis. *J Am Dent Assoc.* 1985; 110:52-4.

Shiloah J, Covington JS, Schuman NJ. Reconstructive mucogingival surgery: the management of amalgam tattoo. *Quintessence Int.* 1988; 19:489-92.

Slabbert H, Ackermann GL, Altini M. Amalgam tattoo as a means for person identification. *J Forensic Odontostomatol.* 1991; 9:17-23.

Weaver T, Auclair PL, Taybos GM. An amalgam tattoo causing local and systemic disease? *Oral Surg Oral Med Oral Pathol.* 1987; 63:137-40.

CHEMICAL BURNS

Abrams RG, Josell SD. Common oral and dental emergencies and problems. *Pediatr Clin North Am.* 1982; 29:681-715.

Mills SW, Okoye MI. Sulfuric acid poisoning. *Am J Forensic Med Pathol.* 1987; 8:252-5.

Scott JC, Jones B, Eisele DW, Ravich WJ. Caustic ingestion injuries of the upper aerodigestive tract. *Laryngoscope.* 1992; 102:1-8.

Seals RR, Cain JR. Prosthetic treatment for chemical burns of the oral cavity. *J Prosthet Dent.* 1985; 53:688-91.

DISEASES OF BLOOD

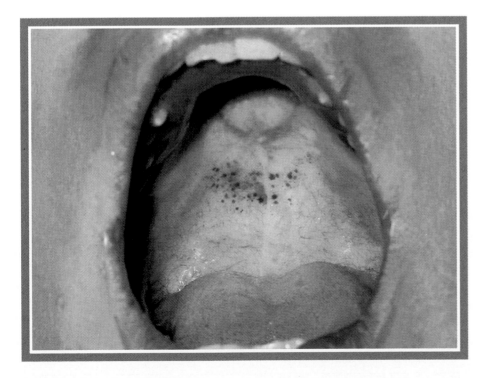

RED BLOOD CELLS

The average male has approximately 6 million red blood cells per cubic millimeter of whole blood, whereas the average female has somewhat less, about 5 million cells. Erythrocytes, by virtue of their hemoglobin content, transport oxygen to the tissue and are involved in the transport of CO_2 away from the tissue to be exhaled through the lungs. Deficiencies in the capacity to transport oxygen are referred to as **anemias** and may be due to a reduction in the number of red cells, the size of the individual cells, or the hemoglobin content. Most of the disorders affecting red blood cells are anemias. A neoplastic process of hematopoiesis in which erythrocytes are synthesized by the bone marrow in increased numbers is called **polycythemia.** Most of these red blood cell disorders cause generalized systemic changes; however, many may be associated with oral or osseous lesions, the latter of which may be observed on dental radiographs.

ANEMIA

Anemia occurs when the oxygen-carrying capacity of the erythrocyte is hampered. This can occur as a consequence of a decreased number of red cells, a decrease in their size, or a decrease in their hemoglobin content. The specific alterations may be induced by a variety of disease factors: (1) excessive blood loss due to trauma or internal hemorrhaging or to spontaneous hemolysis, which can be a consequence of autoimmune mechanisms in which antibodies attach to erythrocytes, fix complement, and lyse them; (2) genetic diseases in which the hemoglobin is defective, leading to a pathologic cell shape that predisposes them to lysis; and (3) nutritional deficiencies in which erythrocyte precursor substances are lacking in the diet or fail to be absorbed in the intestines.

In the laboratory anemia is assessed by (1) performing a red blood cell count, (2) measuring the total packed cell volume (the hematocrit), and (3) quantifying the amount of hemoglobin (Figure 12-1). These three parameters are formulated to yield the *red cell indices.* These indices represent calculations that aid in determining the size and hemoglobin content of an individual's red blood cell. Although the total red count may be within normal limits, the patient may still suffer from decreased oxygen transport capacity if the individual cells are too small. In this case the hematocrit would be decreased. Even though present in adequate numbers, because the test is measuring the total volume of smaller cells, it would show a lower volume or mass within the total blood sample. Anemia characterized by small cells is termed **microcytic anemia.** Alternatively, if the individual cells are of normal size but contain insufficient amounts of hemoglobin, the patient will still be anemic. Anemia due to decreased hemoglobin content within normal-sized cells is referred to as **hypochromic anemia.** When the total number of red blood cells is decreased and the bone marrow attempts to compensate by synthesizing larger cells with an increased concentration of hemoglobin, the anemia is said to be a **macrocytic and hyperchromic anemia.**

Genetic abnormalities of hemoglobin are assessed by more sophisticated laboratory procedures such as hemoglobin electrophoresis. When subjected to an electric current (electrophoresis), abnormal hemoglobins migrate at different rates and can be detected in this manner. The definitive diagnosis for a specific type of anemia is therefore based on an assessment of a variety of clinical and laboratory tests.

Iron Deficiency Anemia

■ IRON DEFICIENCY ANEMIA: lack of red blood cells and hemoglobin due to inadequate dietary intake of iron.

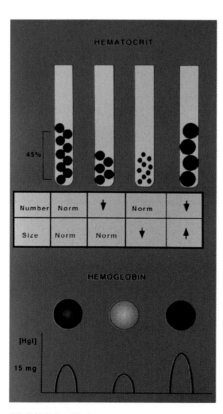

FIGURE 12-1

Anemia. *(Top)* The hematocrit represents the packed cell volume of red cells and is expressed as a percentage of whole blood. The hematocrit is decreased when the red cell count is decreased or when erythrocytes are small. *(Bottom)* The hemoglobin is a measure of the oxygen-carrying capacity of the erythrocyte and in any given cell may be *(left to right)* normal (normochromic), decreased (hypochromic), or elevated (hyperchromic).

The most common form of anemia is secondary to iron deficiency. This is most frequently encountered in women, particularly when the menstrual cycle is heavy and hematopoiesis takes place in the absence of adequate dietary iron intake. The erythrocytes of patients with the iron deficiency will be both hypochromic and microcytic. In addition, the total number of erythrocytes may be decreased. Therefore the red cell count, hematocrit, and hemoglobin will be at levels below normal.

CLINICAL

Patients suffering from iron deficiency anemia will manifest symptoms of tiredness, weakness, and malaise. Increased respiratory rate may also be a finding. The primary physical change will be tissue pallor, which may be more obvious on the mucous membranes than on the skin. Oral manifestations of iron deficiency anemia include bald tongue, atrophic mucositis, angular cheilitis (probably secondary to candidiasis), and aphthous ulcerations; signs are similar to those found more prominently in patients with pernicious anemia. In some patients with iron deficiency anemia, particularly those of Scandinavian descent, there is the occurrence of atrophic mucositis of the upper aerodigestive tract, including the oropharynx, which predisposes the patients to squamous cell carcinoma. The coexistence of iron deficiency anemia, mucosal atrophy, and carcinoma is quite rare and is referred to as the **Plummer-Vinson syndrome.**

LABORATORY

The blood exhibits a decrease in total red cell count, hematocrit, and hemoglobin. A stained microscopic slide of a blood smear may show evidence of microcytic erythrocytes. Iron levels are decreased in the blood. Serum iron binding capacity and transferrin saturation should be assessed, particularly when overt hypochromic microcytic anemia is not obvious. Serum iron decreases as the iron binding capacity increases with a concomitant drop in transferrin saturation. The dorsal surface of the tongue may exhibit histopathologic features of atrophy with loss of the usual tongue papillae. The spinous layer and submucosa in atrophic tongues show a mixed leukocytic infiltrate in the connective tissue.

TREATMENT

Once the diagnosis has been made, dietary iron supplementation is the usual treatment. Iron supplementation will generally reverse the anemia within a few weeks of therapy. Development of carcinoma in the Plummer-Vinson syndrome requires surgical and radiotherapeutic interventions.

Pernicious Anemia

■ PERNICIOUS ANEMIA: impaired red blood cell maturation secondary to insufficient vitamin B_{12} due to a defective intrinsic factor required for its absorption through the intestinal wall.

Erythrocyte maturation within the bone marrow depends on the availability of adequate amounts of folic acid and vitamin B_{12}. These cofactors are essential for the maturation of the erythrocyte. Whereas folic acid deficiency may be ameliorated by nutritional therapy, vitamin B_{12} deficiency is rarely the consequence of inadequate intake of the vitamin. Rather, in pernicious anemia the patient is affected by a defective absorption factor referred to as the *intrinsic factor*. This intestinal transport protein is required for absorption of vitamin B_{12}. The gastric mucosa is atrophic and fails to secrete appropriate amounts of hydrochloric acid, a condition referred to as **achlorhydria.** Both folate deficiency and B_{12} malabsorption are **megaloblastic anemias.**

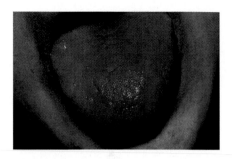

FIGURE 12-2

Pernicious anemia. Atrophy of the filiform papillae of the dorsal surface of the tongue ("bald tongue").

CLINICAL

Pernicious anemia can be a severe disease causing extreme malaise and tiredness. The patient will exhibit pallor and may also suffer sensory neurologic disorders manifested as paresthesia. Motor function may also be impaired. The neurologic symptoms are also related to the lack of vitamin B_{12}. A characteristic finding in pernicious anemia within the oral cavity, occurring in 50% of cases, is depapillation of the tongue, a condition known as **Hunter glossitis.** The filiform papillae undergo atrophy, and the tongue appears bald and smooth with an erythematous cast (Figure 12-2). The oral mucosa in general may be atrophic and exhibit pallor. Angular cheilitis is also seen and is usually associated with a chronic atrophic form of candidiasis. Other oral changes that are encountered in megaloblastic anemias are oral aphthouslike ulcerations, focal red macules, and mucosal pigmentations.

LABORATORY

The total red count is significantly decreased with a disproportionate change in the hematocrit and hemoglobin content. To compensate for the decrease in vitamin B_{12} the individual erythrocytes that are synthesized are large and incorporate greater than normal amounts of hemoglobin. Therefore pernicious anemia is classically a hyperchromic macrocytic anemia, a feature shared with folic acid deficiency. On blood smears the cells will be larger than normal and will stain darker, owing to their increased hemoglobin content. Bone marrow aspirates disclose the presence of megaloblasts, which are large erythrocyte precursor cells typical of folate and vitamin B_{12} deficiency anemias. Gastric analysis will reveal achlorhydria. Because folate and vitamin B_{12} deficiencies are characterized by macrocytic hyperchromic anemia, serum folate and B_{12} levels must be obtained to distinguish between the two types of anemia. Microscopically, the tongue exhibits a loss of fungiform and filiform papillae, epithelial atrophy, and submucosal inflammation.

TREATMENT

Pernicious anemia patients lack *intrinsic factor* necessary for absorption, and therefore increased dietary supplementation will not reverse the signs and symptoms. For this reason intramuscular injections of vitamin B_{12} must be initiated. Monthly injections are usually adequate to allow for normal hematopoiesis.

Sickle Cell Anemia

■ SICKLE CELL ANEMIA: inherited defect in the structure of the hemoglobin molecule causing the erythrocyte to assume a crescent shape ("sickle") and to undergo lysis.

Inherited as an autosomal recessive disease, sickle cell anemia is characterized by a point mutation in the hemoglobin gene, creating an abnormal hemoglobin molecule (Hg S). The point mutation causes a substitution of the amino acid valine for glutamine in the gene. The resultant hemoglobin is defective; the usual discoid shape is lost, leading the cells to assume a crescent or sickle shape. These cells are prone to agglutinate and clog the small caliber vascular channels. When such an event occurs, usually in the context of low oxygen pressure, a **sickle cell crisis** may evolve and can be fatal. More commonly, the sickle cells tend to hemolyze, causing jaundice.

Sickle cell anemia is encountered primarily among blacks; when it occurs as a heterozygous genotype (Hg A, Hg S), the affected individual shows only minor signs of the disease and is said to harbor the **sickle cell trait.** Individuals who inherit both recessive genes in the homozygous genotype manifest the full-blown hemolytic disease, sickle cell anemia (Hg S, Hg S). Other rare forms of sickling disease have been identified.

CLINICAL

Patients affected with the trait only rarely show any significant signs or symptoms but may have a slightly lowered red blood cell count. Those with the homozygous form of sickle cell anemia share signs and symptoms in common with other anemias, including malaise and weakness. The sclera may be yellowed, owing to the accumulation of unconjugated bilirubin within the blood as a consequence of hemolysis. As more cells hemolyze and the oxygen tension in the blood decreases, the tendency for sickling is greater. A sickle cell crisis is characterized by muscle rigidity and unconsciousness. Widespread ischemia may develop, leading to death.

There are no specific oral mucosa findings in sickle cell anemia; however, bone changes are frequently identified on dental and skull radiographs. A compensatory increase in hematopoiesis may occur, leading to osseous changes. In the skull numerous small icicle-like spicules may be identified across the calvarium, yielding a so-called *hair-on-end* effect. On dental radiographs, although not pathognomonic, *step-ladder trabeculas* are often seen between contiguous posterior teeth (Figure 12-3).

LABORATORY

The total red blood cell count, hemoglobin, and hematocrit are decreased; on differential smears, sickle cells may be identified. Characteristic concomitant findings include elevated unconjugated bilirubin and urine urobilinogen. Hemoglobin electrophoresis will disclose the presence of normal hemoglobin and hemoglobin S in those with the sickle cell trait, whereas the individuals with homozygous sickle cell disease will show a single hemoglobin S band on electrophoresis (Figure 12-4).

TREATMENT

There is no specific treatment for this genetic disease, although gene therapy may prove to be an important intervention in the future. At present, individuals with the disease must be closely monitored for the development of sickle cell crisis. In these instances hospitalization is required with administration of oxygen and blood transfusions.

Thalassemia

■ THALASSEMIA: inherited defect in either the α or β chain of the hemoglobin molecule resulting in hemolysis.

Also referred to as Mediterranean or Cooley anemia, thalassemia is a heritable disease in which the gene for the hemoglobin molecule is mutated with generation of defective forms of the α or β chain of hemoglobin A (Hg A). Individuals of Mediterranean region descent are the most prone to develop this form of anemia. Like sickle cell anemia, thalassemia is an autosomal recessive disease; therefore heterozygous individuals only carry the trait and are said to suffer from **thalassemia minor. Thalassemia major** occurs when both genes are affected, as in the homozygous genotype. Thalassemia major is lethal, whereas those with the minor form show no ill effects.

CLINICAL

Heterozygous individuals with thalassemia minor show lesser signs and symptoms of anemia. Those with homozygous disease are lethargic, manifesting weakness and malaise. Because the defective cells are prone to hemolysis, the pa-

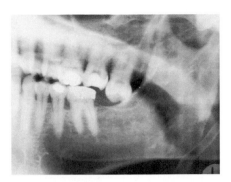

FIGURE 12-3

Sickle cell anemia. Radiographic appearance exhibiting abnormal trabecular pattern.

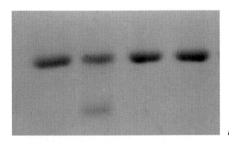

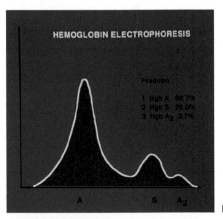

FIGURE 12-4

Sickle cell anemia. A, Hemoglobin electrophoresis. Lanes 1, 3, and 4 *(left to right)* have one band of normal hemoglobin A; lane 2 shows two bands—one for hemoglobin A and a second one for hemoglobin S, indicating the presence of a heterozygous sickle cell trait. **B,** Graph of findings of **A** showing two major peaks for hemoglobin A and hemoglobin S, respectively.

FIGURE 12-5

Thalassemia. Radiograph of characteristic honeycomb radiolucencies bilaterally in the mandible and in the left maxilla.

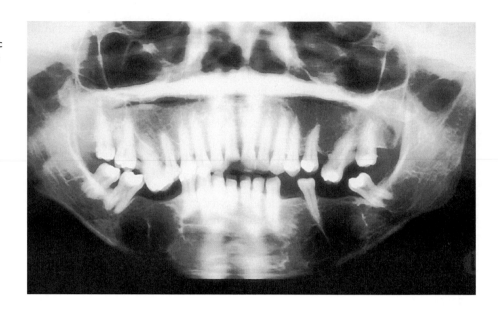

tients may show evidence of jaundice; death often occurs in adolescence.

Other than a tendency toward pallor, other soft tissue changes are not observed. Osseous changes are radiographically demonstrable in the jaws and on skull films. These changes are only seen in thalassemia major. The calvarium shows altered trabeculation with osteophyte formation, yielding a "hair-on-end" effect. On dental films the trabeculation may be markedly altered with an unusual honeycomb radiolucent appearance (Figure 12-5). Bones containing this multilocular configuration show no evidence of enlargement or expansion, unlike various tumors that cause similar radiologic changes. In some cases enlargement of the zygomatic bones can be seen, yielding a mongoloid facies.

LABORATORY

The hemoglobin, hematocrit, and red blood cell count will be decreased and the unconjugated bilirubin will be elevated. Hemoglobin electrophoresis will disclose the characteristic pattern for the various forms of thalassemia major.

TREATMENT

As with sickle cell anemia, there is currently no definitive treatment for thalassemia. Genetic intervention may hold promise for the future.

Fetal Erythroblastosis

■ FETAL ERYTHROBLASTOSIS: form of hemolytic anemia that occurs in utero when maternal antibodies develop against antigens on fetal red blood cells not present in the mother and intermingle with fetal blood.

Another form of hemolytic anemia is fetal erythroblastosis. As opposed to sickle cell and thalassemia anemias, erythroblastosis is not due to a genetic defect; rather, it represents an immunologic response with antibody- and complement-mediated hemolysis. Whereas the disease is often referred to as Rh-factor disease, the ABO blood group antigens may also initiate the adverse reaction. In the classic form of the disease the pregnant mother lacks the Rh factor, whereas the fetus inherits the Rh factor from his or her father. A minor tear in the placenta will allow fetal blood to be introduced into the maternal circulation, and the mother then makes antibodies to the Rh-positive erythrocytes. The first birth is usually of no consequence; however, when a second pregnancy occurs in a mother who now has circulating anti-Rh antibodies, mingling of blood may result in the passage of anti-Rh factor antibodies into the fetal circulation. These antibodies will attach to the fetal erythrocytes, fix complement, and cause hemolysis. As mentioned previously, a similar phenomenon may occur with ABO incompatibility between the fetus and mother. As erythrocytes continue to hemolyze, the bilirubin levels increase and kernicterus may develop, leading to neural damage and retardation. For this reason affected newborns are transfused immediately.

CLINICAL

Fetal erythroblastosis is diagnosed on delivery of the newborn. The affected infant will be cyanotic and jaundiced. Cyanosis is usually readily seen on the skin and mucous membranes; the oral and conjunctival areas will also show a bluish cast. Depending on the duration of hemolysis, bilirubin pigments may become deposited in the developing deciduous teeth. As these teeth erupt, they show a yellowish-green discoloration of the dentin, which is most obvious on the root surfaces.

LABORATORY

The hemoglobin, hematocrit, and red blood cell count are markedly decreased, and there is a significant increase in unconjugated bilirubin. The disease can be detected in utero by assessing a Coombs test of the mother's blood. This is an assay that detects maternal antibodies to the infant's erythrocytes.

TREATMENT

On delivery, the cyanotic neonate is subjected to rapid diagnostic tests; when fetal erythroblastosis is confirmed, blood transfusions are initiated. Once the maternal antibodies have been cleared from the infant's serum, the hemolysis will cease. Failure to act quickly may result in mental retardation or even death.

WHITE BLOOD CELLS

Leukocytes are formed within the bone marrow and are derived from partially differentiated stem cells. The neutrophil and monocyte are derived from a common precursor of the myelogenous series. The mononuclear cells derived from lymphoblasts differentiate into T and B subsets. Lymphoid stem cells reside in the marrow, lymph nodes, and the spleen. Factors that impact the bone marrow may have a deleterious effect on leukocyte histogenesis. A variety of chemicals and cytotoxic agents will inhibit mitosis of the formative leukocytes. When the leukocyte blast cells are crowded out by other pathologic processes (myelophthisic response), the total circulating white blood cells will decrease. In addition, other processes in which the etiology is unknown can cause defective leukocyte maturation. Conversely, there are a number of leukocyte proliferative responses that will increase the number of circulating white blood cells. Both inflammatory and neoplastic disorders of white blood cells fall into this group.

The most commonly employed indicator of leukocyte disease is the peripheral white blood cell count. The normal count in adults is 6000 to 9000 white blood cells per cubic millimeter of blood. The most prevalent circulating white cell is the neutrophil, followed by the lymphocyte; other circulating cells including eosinophils, basophils, and monocytes are usually present in low numbers. An increase in the total circulating white blood cell count is referred to as **leukocytosis** and a decrease is **leukopenia.** Although a leukocytosis may be due

FIGURE 12-6

Leukocytosis. The total white blood cell (WBC) count is elevated in infection (bacterial and viral) and leukemia. Pyogenic bacteria cause a neutrophilic leukocytosis, whereas viral and some chronic bacterial and fungal granulomatous infections induce a lymphocytic leukocytosis. In leukemia the differential white blood cell count will show primitive malignant blast cells.

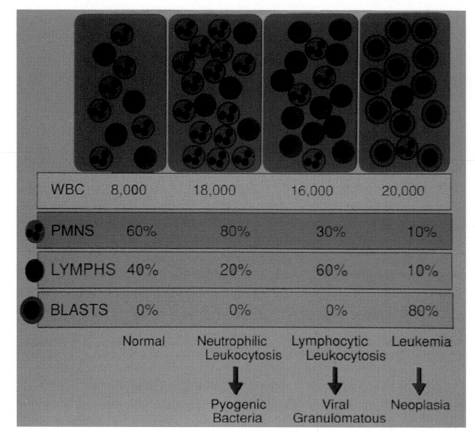

WBC	8,000	18,000	16,000	20,000
PMNS	60%	80%	30%	10%
LYMPHS	40%	20%	60%	10%
BLASTS	0%	0%	0%	80%
	Normal	Neutrophilic Leukocytosis	Lymphocytic Leukocytosis	Leukemia
		Pyogenic Bacteria	Viral Granulomatous	Neoplasia

to an increase in all types of leukocytes, more commonly, however, an absolute increase or decrease in a specific subpopulation of leukocytes accounts for the elevated white blood cell count. Therefore it becomes important to know the *absolute numbers* of each type of leukocyte or to compare the relative proportions of each on a *differential white cell count*. A leukocytosis may be seen in both leukemia and infection (Figure 12-6). In inflammatory responses due to infections the white cells retain their differentiated morphologic appearance and relative numbers, and there is simply an increase in the total number. In leukemia the immature malignant cells leave the bone marrow before being fully differentiated, and therefore blast cells are encountered in unusually high numbers within the peripheral blood.

LEUKOPENIA

Although leukopenias may be associated with an overall reduction in leukocytes, they are most commonly associated with a decreased ability to generate neutrophils. Therefore the most common form of leukopenia is agranulocytosis or neutropenia. Lymphopenia may be encountered but is rare. A decrease in circulating leukocytes implies that there has been an arrest of the maturation of the cells of the bone marrow, the hematopoietic elements have been replaced, or pharmaceutical agents have inhibited cell cycling.

Agranulocytosis

■ A G R A N U L O C Y T O S I S : marked decrease in circulating granulocytes, particularly neutrophils, attributable to a variety of causes.

Agranulocytosis implies a total or absolute deficiency in the number of granulocytes. In practice the term actually refers to a decrease in polymorphonuclear leukocytes or neutrophils (neutropenia) (Figure 12-7). The most common cause of agranulocytosis is cancer chemotherapeutic agents that arrest the cell cycle or interfere with the assembly of the mitotic spindle. In these instances other hematopoietic cells may be decreased, including erythrocytes and thrombocytes. An additional common cause of agranulocytosis is leukemia. As the bone marrow becomes overpopulated with malignant leukocytes, normal hematopoiesis can no longer proceed due to the encroachment. In this ironic situation there is a leukocytosis, represented by circulating malignant blast cells but a leukopenia of the normal blood elements. Because all of these cells are affected, agranulocytosis is usually coexistent with anemia and thrombocytopenia. There is also an idiopathic form of agranulocytosis in which neutrophils fail to mature at the physiologic rate. The **myelodysplastic syndrome** is one such condition; in many cases it represents an early form of myelogenous leukemia whereby the patient remains leukopenic for many years before a leukemic episode evolves.

CLINICAL

Because neutrophils are the main cellular line of defense against bacterial infections, agranulocytosis, if severe, can result in death due to secondary bacterial infection. These infections can involve any organ, and bacterial pneumonia is a frequently encountered complication.

Oral ulceration becomes a prominent finding when cancer chemotherapeutic drugs reach a toxic threshold and the white cell count precipitously drops (Figure 12-8). The ulcers may resemble the common aphthous ulcer and can be located anywhere within the oral mucous membrane. In other cases the ulcers are much larger and irregularly shaped. Within a few days the ulcerations continue to enlarge and extend down to the bone with resultant osteomyelitis and sequestration. When deep ulcers are encountered in agranulocytosis, the prognosis is extremely grave and a life-threatening infection is imminent.

LABORATORY

In agranulocytosis the total white blood cell count becomes greatly decreased and may be as low as 1000 cells per cubic millimeter. The differential count will reveal an absolute decrease in circulating neutrophils. The normal levels of 60% to 65% neutrophils may drop to 10% to 15%. When associated with myelodysplastic syndrome or an early phase of full-blown leukemia, the atypical blast cells should be evident on a peripheral blood smear. Bone marrow aspiration will determine which cells are neoplastic within the marrow.

Biopsy of an oral ulcer shows pathognomonic findings. The surface epithelium is ulcerated and replaced by a fibrin clot. Unlike most ulcerations that show leukocytic infiltration into the zone of ulceration, the agranulocytic ulcer is devoid of neutrophils.

TREATMENT

In acute agranulocytosis secondary to chemotherapy, the drug regimen should be immediately adjusted to avoid secondary and severe infection. Antibiotic therapy may be indicated, and transfusion with leukocytes should be considered. Recombinant leukocyte growth factors such as the granulocyte-monocyte colony-stimulating factor may be employed in immunosuppressed patients with agranulocytosis. Before treatment can commence, the cause for the agranulocytosis must be identified. Agranulocytosis secondary to leukemia must be managed by chemotherapeutic approaches that inhibit or eliminate the neoplastic leukocytes. Paradoxically, these same medications may also inhibit neutrophil production.

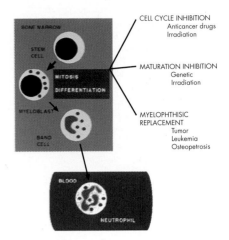

FIGURE 12-7

Agranulocytosis. Mature neutrophils circulating in the blood stream arise from stem cells of the marrow that undergo prior mitosis and differentiate into myeloblasts and band cells. A decrease in circulating neutrophils can be the consequence of mitotic inhibition, failure of cells to mature, and replacement of normal stem cells by cancer cells or increased osteogenesis in the marrow compartment.

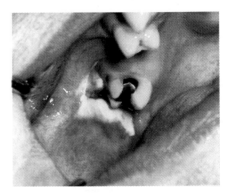

FIGURE 12-8

Agranulocytosis. Agranulocytic ulceration of the gingiva and buccal mucosa.

Cyclic Neutropenia

■ CYCLIC NEUTROPENIA: idiopathic disease in which episodic defects in neutrophil maturation in the bone marrow result in periodic decreases in circulating neutrophils.

Cyclic neutropenia is a rare condition that is characterized by an episodic fluctuation in the number of circulating neutrophils and is due to a bone marrow maturation arrest that occurs on a periodic basis. In most patients the cycle occurs every 30 days with a neutropenic phase that persists for 4 to 5 days. Otherwise, the number of circulating neutrophils in the interim is within normal levels.

CLINICAL

Children with cyclic neutropenia suffer from frequent recurrent respiratory tract infections, which are usually bacterial in origin. On a regular basis they may develop short-term fevers that spontaneously resolve once the neutrophil count returns to normal. Within a few days of the neutropenic phase aphthous-like oral ulcerations may appear, persisting for 2 to 3 days. These ulcerations may arise on either fixed or movable mucosa. In addition, premature periodontal disease is often encountered, and children and teenagers may experience alveolar bone loss and periodontal pockets. Periodontal abscesses are rarely encountered, probably because the neutrophil count returns to normal levels in a short period.

LABORATORY

The total white blood cell count may decrease to 3000 cells per cubic millimeter each month for a 5-day period. In the interim the white cell count approaches normal levels yet is usually slightly depressed. Therefore the diagnosis is made by obtaining weekly leukocyte counts over a 6-week period. The ulcers will show a decrease or absence of infiltrating neutrophils. The periodontal findings are histologically no different than those encountered in ordinary chronic inflammatory periodontal disease.

TREATMENT

There is no specific treatment for the disorder because the specific maturation defect has not been identified. Patients with a tendency for more severe infections may be placed on recombinant granulocyte-monocyte colony-stimulating factor.

NEUTROPHIL FUNCTION DISORDERS

Neutrophils exert their defensive role against infectious agents by functioning as phagocytes and by exercising various intracellular mechanisms of microbial killing that include the elaboration of myeloperoxidase, lysosomal enzymes, and other cytoplasmic and microsomal antimicrobial peptides. Inherited defects in neutrophil function are rare but when present predispose patients to unchecked infection by certain microorganisms. Although the disease entity **chronic granulomatous disease of childhood** is the most common of these functional defects, other rare functional deficiencies, including **glucose-6-phosphate dehydrogenase deficiency, myeloperoxidase deficiency,** and the **lazy leukocyte syndrome,** show similar clinical features. Oral mucosal infections can be seen in all of these diseases. Specific microbicidal motility and phagocytic function tests can be performed on blood samples taken from patients with suspected neutrophil function defects. Acquired functional defects can occur with drug administration, particularly corticosteroids.

Chronic Granulomatous Disease of Childhood

■ CHRONIC GRANULOMATOUS DISEASE OF CHILDHOOD: inherited disorder of neutrophil and monocyte function that predisposes patients to opportunistic infections.

Inherited as an X-linked disorder, chronic granulomatous disease of childhood represents a disease in which neutrophil microbicidal activity is defective. There are various forms of the disease, all of which involve a suboptimal respiratory burst in the neutrophils and monocytes; the consequences are a lack of free radical formation and decreased peroxide and superoxide release. The various forms of the disease all involve defects in the electron transport enzyme/coenzyme pathways.

CLINICAL

The disease evolves early in life with symptoms usually observed in children by age 2. It is characterized by susceptibility to a variety of opportunistic bacterial and fungal infections including *Staphylococcus*, *Streptococcus*, the coliform microorganisms, and *Candida*. Clinically, draining lymphadenitis, hepatosplenomegaly, abscesses, pneumonia, and osteomyelitis are evident. Males are affected in the X-linked variant, and females act as carriers. The oral mucosa is often infected with *Candida* in which white pseudomembranous and erythematous lesions may be encountered anywhere in the mouth; the tongue, soft palate, and buccal mucosa are the most frequently affected sites. An eczematous cheilitis is often present along with facial skin lesions. Cervical lymphadenitis is invariably detectable, and drainage may be seen. Generalized ulcerative stomatitis, acute gingivitis, and advanced periodontitis are also common manifestations of the disease.

LABORATORY

A variety of function tests can be performed. The most widely available test is the quantitative nitroblue tetrazolium test. This test employs a redox dye that is sensitive to neutrophil respiratory activity. The test is negative in affected patients yet is normal or slightly reduced in female carriers. Tests that show defects in leukocyte microbicidal activity are also used in the diagnosis. There is usually a neutrophilic leukocytosis, and hypergammaglobulinemia is detected. Biopsy of the oral mucosa in patients who develop candidiasis will disclose the presence of hyphae and yeast forms colonizing the superficial layers of the epithelium.

TREATMENT

Because the defects are inherited, a cure is not available. The therapeutic aim is to prevent or contain life-threatening infection. Combination antibiotic therapy is usually required, and abscesses should be cultured to assess antibiotic sensitivity. Antifungal therapy should be prescribed when oral candidiasis is present. Delta interferon, which increases the leukocyte respiratory burst, and continuous sulfisoxazole therapy have also been employed.

LEUKOCYTOSIS

In this section leukocytosis refers to disorders that evolve as a consequence of infectious diseases (Figure 12-9). An increase in circulating white blood cells occurring as a consequence of leukemia is discussed later. Because the blood leukocytes are critical cellular elements in the defense against infectious disease, they increase their numbers when an active infection exists. The total circulating white blood cells increase above 10,000 during active infection. **Neutrophilic**

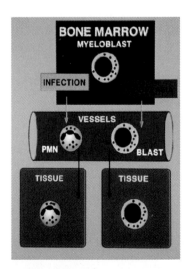

FIGURE 12-9

Leukocytosis versus leukemia. The myeloblast is stimulated to generate increased numbers of mature neutrophils (PMNs) into the circulation in defense against pyogenic organisms *(left)*. In myelogenous leukemia, increased numbers of immature (blastic) neutrophils enter the circulating blood due to neoplastic change in the myeloblast *(right)*.

leukocytosis evolves in response to pyogenic bacterial organisms such as *Streptococcus*, *Staphylococcus*, *Neisseria*, *Actinomyces*, and *Bacteroides*. **Mononuclear leukocytosis** may involve either lymphocytes, monocytes, or both. Because lymphocytes and monocytes are active defense elements against viral infections, mononuclear leukocytoses are usually indicative of a viral infection.

Bacteria-Associated Leukocytosis

■ **BACTERIA-ASSOCIATED LEUKOCYTOSIS:** marked elevation in levels of circulating neutrophils occurring as a result of an infection by pyogenic bacteria.

Pyogenic bacteria will initiate a neutrophilic leukocytosis and the white blood cell count will be elevated. There is a marked increase in mature neutrophils, approaching 85%, on the differential count. As the marrow releases neutrophils into the circulating blood, some immature forms will be found to exit the marrow prematurely. Specifically, nonlobulated nuclei are encountered, and these immature neutrophils are termed **band cells.** The appearance of immature neutrophil forms may include earlier precursors such as metamyelocytes. A neutrophilic leukocytosis with immature neutrophils is referred to as a **shift to the left.** This term refers to the traditional diagrams of cellular maturation whereby the immature forms are illustrated on the left with arrows showing differentiation and maturation proceeding to the right. Therefore a shift to the left indicates a retrogressive phenomenon with appearance of immature, less differentiated cells.

CLINICAL

Whereas an infection of any organ by pyogenic bacteria may induce a neutrophilic leukocytosis, it is important to realize that odontogenic and periodontal infections are bacterial and will cause the same type of reaction. The neutrophilic leukocytosis will usually be accompanied by constitutional signs and symptoms of infectious diseases, including malaise and fever (see Chapter 3).

LABORATORY

Mononuclear leukocytosis is occasionally noted in specific bacterial and fungal infections that induce chronic granulomatous inflammation. In tuberculosis and deep fungal infections, oral ulcerations may be encountered and are usually deep seated with rolled margins. Granulomatous oral ulcers simply represent dissemination from a systemic infection that is usually of pulmonary origin.

TREATMENT

Leukocytosis of a reactive nature resolves once the infection has cleared. The white blood cell count will usually return to normal levels within 1 to 2 days. Once the site of infection has been uncovered, culture and sensitivity are required to select the appropriate antibiotic. In the facial area if the leukocytosis is associated with a soft tissue abscess, resolution may be accelerated by incision and drainage (I & D). Alternatively, cellulitis, a more diffuse process, is not amenable to I & D.

Virus-Associated Leukocytosis

■ **VIRUS-ASSOCIATED LEUKOCYTOSIS:** marked elevation in circulating lymphocytes and monocytes in response to a viral infection.

Viruses, being intracellular parasites, elicit a defense response in which the inflammatory cells are predominantly lymphocytes and monocytes; neutrophils play a very small role in the elimination of viral agents. For this reason the leukocytoses that accompany viral infections are typically mononuclear in nature and include small lymphocytes, large lymphocytes, and monocytes. Although the prototype viral infection with a mononuclear leukocytosis is infectious mononucleosis, most other viral infections will be associated with an increase in the lymphocyte count as well (see Chapter 7). Those caused by the herpes simplex virus, varicella-zoster virus, and coxsackievirus manifest oral and facial vesicles that ultimately ulcerate, contributing to the intensity of the inflammatory response.

Infectious Mononucleosis

■ INFECTIOUS MONONUCLEOSIS: infectious disease of B lymphocytes caused by the Epstein-Barr virus that produces a marked mononuclear leukocytosis.

The Epstein-Barr virus possesses envelope molecules that bind to a B lymphocyte receptor. Infected B lymphocytes rapidly proliferate in response to the infection by the Epstein-Barr virus, thereby causing a mononuclear leukocytosis.

CLINICAL
Infectious mononucleosis is acquired through droplets and aerosol or direct contact, accounting for the term *kissing disease*. After exposure and an incubation period of 7 to 10 days, the patient begins to experience fever and weakness. This malaise might be quite severe, restricting the patient to bed. As the symptoms progress, lymphadenopathy becomes a prominent finding with the most severely affected nodes being the cervical, axillary, and inguinal. Enlarged tender swellings may be identified at the angle of the mandible and down the cervical chain. The infection primarily affects young adults and children. An oral manifestation, which is not invariably present, is the appearance of petechiae in the soft palate. Although minor abnormalities in platelet function have been reported, the petechiae are probably induced by suction when the patient clicks a sore or itchy soft palate against the tongue. The disease usually persists for approximately 2 weeks and then spontaneously resolves. The virus has also been linked to the chronic fatigue syndrome that affects adults, primarily females. The association between chronic fatigue syndrome and a chronic latent Epstein-Barr virus infection is tenuous.

LABORATORY
The white blood cell count may range from 15,000 to 20,000 cells per cubic millimeter with a marked increase in lymphocytes and monocytes. On the differential smear many of the lymphocytes appear to have undergone blastogenesis and appear atypical. These characteristically large lymphocytes are referred to as Downey cells, or simply atypical lymphocytes. A rapid serologic assay is the monospot test, which detects antibodies to the Epstein-Barr virus. A more specific quantitative assay is the heterophile antibody, or Paul-Bunnel test. Other specific antibodies to various components of the Epstein-Barr virus coat can be detected in the serum, including the Epstein-Barr virus early antigen (EA) and viral capsid antigen (VCA). Lymph node biopsy shows follicular hyperplasia with the appearance of many large reactive follicular center cell lymphocytes.

TREATMENT
There is no specific treatment for infectious mononucleosis, although the virus, which is a herpes group virus, will respond to systemically administered acyclovir. Treatment, however, does not usually speed resolution. General palliative

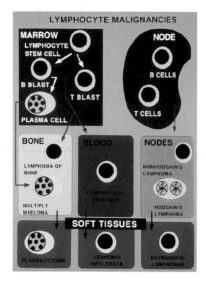

FIGURE 12-10

Lymphocyte malignancies. Lymphoid cells are generated in the bone marrow and in the lymph nodes. Bone marrow malignancies may take the form of leukemia or, within bone, lymphoma and plasma cell tumors (myeloma). Malignancies of lymph nodes may be either Hodgkin or non-Hodgkin lymphomas. All of these malignancies may infiltrate the soft tissue and with the exception of leukemia may arise in the soft tissue.

care is recommended, including bed rest, adequate nutrition, and administration of analgesics.

NEOPLASMS

Neoplastic processes of leukocytes result in an elevation of the white blood cell count. These leukocytoses are referred to as the **leukemias.** Because leukocyte progenitors lie within the bone marrow and lymph nodes, other nonleukemic forms of malignant leukocyte neoplasia may cause widespread osteolytic disease or lymph node swelling, respectively. The most common bone marrow malignancy is **multiple myeloma,** a neoplastic proliferation of B lymphocytes. Neoplastic lymphoid tumors associated with node enlargements are collectively referred to as the **lymphomas.** Although T-cells may undergo neoplastic transformation, most lymphomas are of B-cell origin (Figure 12-10).

Leukemia

■ LEUKEMIA: circulating malignant leukocytes of bone marrow or lymph node origin.

The leukemias are classified according to the specific leukocytic stem cell of origin. In this regard they are usually categorized in the granulocytic series, **myelogenous** or **granulocytic leukemia,** and in the lymphoid series, **lymphocytic leukemia.** Most leukemias among animals are caused by retroviruses. Whereas one form of leukemia, endemic to Japan, is associated with human T-cell lymphotropic virus type I, most leukemias in humans have not been definitively associated with a viral agent. Oncogene mutations and overexpression are implicated in the pathogenesis of leukemias. In 80% of patients with chronic myelogenous (granulocytic) leukemia, a chromosomal translocation is observed between chromosomes 9 and 22 and is commonly referred to as the **Philadelphia chromosome** (t[9:22]). This translocation causes a juxtaposition of the **c-abl proto-oncogene** from chromosome 9 to a breakpoint cluster region on chromosome 22 **(bcr).** The resultant translocated and hybrid oncogene is implicated in the mechanism of carcinogenesis. Many other chromosomal abnormalities and oncogenes have recently been identified and associated with the various forms of human leukemia.

Another classification is commonly used based on the severity of the leukemia, regardless of the cell type. **Acute leukemias** are rapidly progressing, usually fatal, and tend to occur in children. The **chronic leukemias** are more often encountered among adults, and although they are potentially fatal, many will undergo prolonged periods of remission with appropriate multidrug chemotherapy.

CLINICAL

One of the earliest signs of leukemia is chronic fatigue and malaise. Due to a myelophthisic response in the bone marrow, as malignant leukocytes crowd out the other hematopoietic precursors, a tendency for petechial hemorrhages secondary to thrombocytopenia evolves. Anemia is also frequently encountered in leukemia. In addition to generalized malaise, the patient may develop fevers of unknown origin or other identifiable infections of the upper respiratory or genitourinary tracts. Within the oral cavity petechial hemorrhages may also be identifiable. In both acute and chronic leukemias, gingival enlargement is encountered in 10% of untreated patients (Figure 12-11). Because the leukemic leukocytes are nonfunctional, all patients with leukemia are considered to be immunocompromised and are therefore susceptible to a variety of infectious dis-

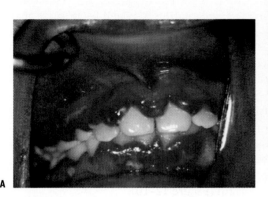
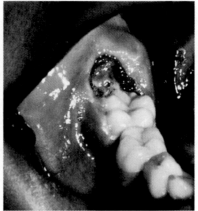

A   B

FIGURE 12-11

Leukemia. A, Generalized gingival swelling and erythema as an early clinical manifestation of acute myelogenous leukemia in a child. **B,** Ulcerated mass representing a localized leukemic infiltrate of myelogenous cells (granulocytic sarcoma) in a young adult.   (**A** Courtesy Dr. Donald Duperon.)

eases. Of major importance in dental practice is the propensity for a hemorrhagic diathesis due to the inability of platelets to be produced in the neoplastic bone marrow (myelophthisic thrombocytopenia).

LABORATORY

In leukemia the white count may fluctuate widely, varying from no increase in white cells or even a leukopenia to that of a marked leukocytosis. The differential smear, however, will usually disclose the presence of blast cells even in the leukopenic phase of leukemia, the so-called **aleukemic leukemia** phase. Invariably, a pronounced leukocytosis soon occurs as the malignant cells emanating from the marrow begin entering the circulating blood at a rapid pace. The leukocytosis of leukemia is easily differentiated from that of infection due to the appearance of large numbers of blast cells in the peripheral smear. Bone marrow aspiration is usually performed to specifically identify the cell type or lineage of the blast cells. Immunocytochemical markers and flow cytometry are often employed to refine the diagnosis. The diagnostic precision of immunomarkers and cytometry is of clinical importance because specific precursor cells respond differently to the various array of available chemotherapeutic agents.

HISTOPATHOLOGY

Biopsy of the enlarged gingiva will disclose the presence of a leukemic infiltrate. Separation from an inflammatory gingival hyperplasia is made by the presence of mononuclear blast cells that show cytologic atypia. Specific immunocytochemical markers may be necessary to ascertain whether the cells are of myelogenous or lymphocytic duration (Figure 12-12). Some forms of myelogenous leukemia are notorious for producing soft tissue infiltrates that can become quite large. Specifically, **granulocytic sarcoma** is a tumor mass that occurs when leukemic cells infiltrate the soft tissue in myelogenous leukemia. Utilizing immunohistochemistry, these cells can be identified as they are chloraceptate esterase positive.

TREATMENT

The treatment for leukemia is tailored according to the specific diagnosis, which is based on the cell of origin, degree of differentiation, and severity of disease. In general, most forms of leukemia are managed by multidrug regimens, which are

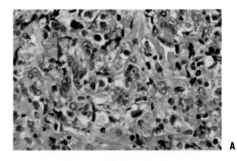

A

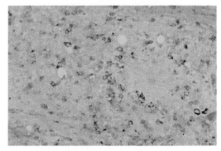

B

FIGURE 12-12

Leukemia. A, Atypical leukocyte blast cells infiltrating the connective tissue. **B,** Specific immunomarker for myeloid cells in the infiltrate indicates the patient has a myelogenous leukemia (granulocytic sarcoma).

employed until a remission evolves. Sometimes remissions last many months or even years before repeated chemotherapy is required. In intractable refractory leukemias the option for bone marrow transplantation is available. In these instances high potency cytotoxic drugs are combined with total body irradiation to eradicate all malignant cells. Donor marrow is then grafted into the recipient. **Graft-versus-host disease** is a predictable complication that must be controlled by the administration of such immunosuppressive drugs as steroids and cyclosporine. Because gingival enlargement is the consequence of leukemia cell infiltration, it will resolve as the patient responds to chemotherapy. If cyclosporine is used as the therapeutic agent, a gingival enlargement may again ensue due to medication-induced fibrosis rather than malignant cell infiltration. A platelet count should be assessed in all patients with leukemia before performing oral surgery.

Hodgkin Lymphoma

■ HODGKIN LYMPHOMA: malignant tumor of lymphocytes characterized by the appearance of Reed-Sternberg cells.

Hodgkin lymphoma is a malignancy of a specific type of lymphoid precursor cell that has not been completely identified. The cell is referred to as the **Reed-Sternberg** cell and exhibits a specific morphology that is identifiable on lymph node biopsies of patient's with Hodgkin lymphoma. There are four subtypes that are classified according to the variations in the lymphocyte cell population when observed microscopically (Table 12-1). Each of these subtypes conveys a unique prognosis. In addition to the histologic subtyping, all lymphomas are subjected to clinical staging (Table 12-2). *Stage 1* disease is characterized by involvement of a single group of lymph nodes in a given anatomic area, whereas *stage 2* disease represents nodal involvement in more than one region. *Stage 3* disease includes lymphoid evolvement above and below the diaphragm, whereas *stage 4* is reached when the malignant cells are disseminated and are no longer

TABLE 12-1
Classification of Hodgkin Lymphoma

Histologic type	Prognosis	5-year survival rate
Lymphocyte predominance	Very good	90%
Nodular sclerosis	Good	70%
Mixed cellularity	Fair	60%
Lymphocyte depletion	Poor	20%

TABLE 12-2
Clinical Staging of Lymphomas

Stage	Extent of disease
1	Single node region or single extranodal site
2	Two or more nodes localized on one side of diaphragm
2_E	Same as above (2) with contiguous extranodal extension
3	Nodes on both sides of diaphragm involved
3_S	Same as 3, including spleen
3_E	Same as 3, with contiguous extranodal extension
4	Disseminated disease with extranodal, noncontiguous tumor

confined to lymphoid tissue. Stage 1 lymphoma, regardless of the histopathologic type, has a relatively good prognosis when appropriate therapy is selected; whereas, stage 4 disease has a dire prognosis, and most patients will succumb to the disease regardless of treatment. The same clinical staging system applies to non-Hodgkin lymphomas.

CLINICAL

Hodgkin lymphoma is more common among males than females and has a predilection for the third decade of life. Hodgkin lymphoma begins in a single lymph node that becomes progressively enlarged and may be firm or rubbery on palpation. The cervical chain of lymph nodes is a common site for Hodgkin lymphoma; axillary and inguinal node groups may also be the initial sites. Patients often experience low-grade episodic fever and night sweats. With advancing stages of the disease additional node groups may be palpable and splenomegaly may be detected. The nodes of advanced disease are often multiple and confluent with a matted character. Because most lymph node enlargements are inflammatory in nature, it is important to realize that the early phases of Hodgkin disease may simulate an inflammatory process. When no infectious source can be identified and the affected node persists for over 1 month, fine needle aspiration biopsy should be undertaken.

Hodgkin disease rarely occurs as an extranodal process and is therefore not identified within the soft tissue of the oral cavity. Only in widely disseminated stage 4 disease might a tumor deposit be identified in the oral soft tissue or within the jaws.

HISTOPATHOLOGY

As mentioned previously, the diagnosis of Hodgkin disease is based on identification of the Reed-Sternberg cell. This cell has a characteristic morphologic appearance; it is binucleated, sometimes multinucleated, with the nuclei round to oval and quite large (Figure 12-13). The nuclear membrane is prominently stained, and the nucleoplasm is quite pale with a prominent, centrally placed nucleolus. This binucleated cell resides within a vacant lacunar space separated from the remaining sheets of lymphoid cells. There are four histopathologic classifications that are based on the ratio of Reed-Sternberg cells to the associated lymphocytic population. Common to all lymphomas is effacement of the

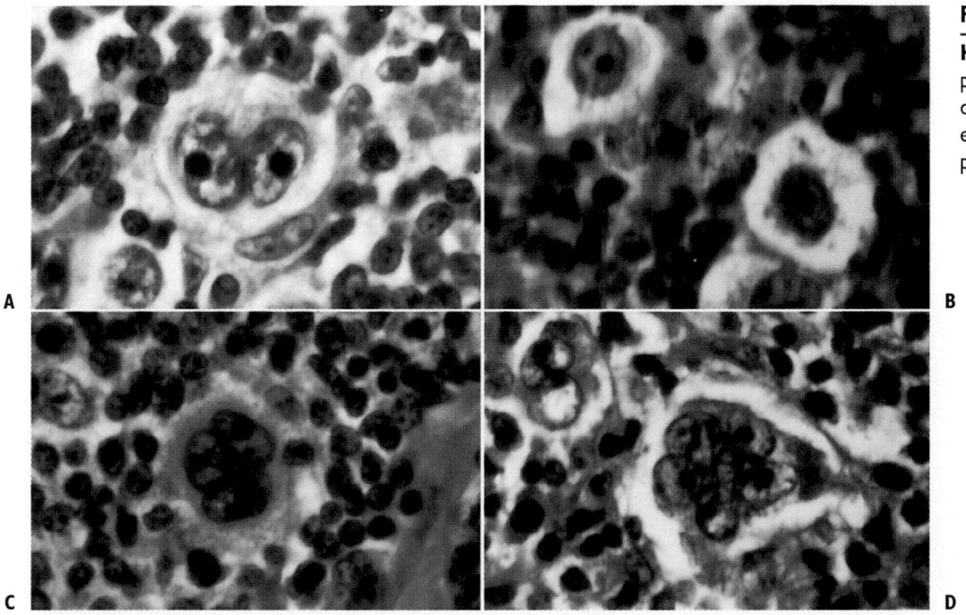

FIGURE 12-13

Hodgkin lymphoma. Four different appearances of the Reed-Sternberg cell that is diagnostic of this neoplasm. The classic "owl eyes" appearance is present in the upper left photomicrograph.

normal lymph node architecture with replacement of the germinal centers by diffuse sheets of lymphoid cells. The most favorable prognosis is associated with the **lymphocyte predominance type.** Reed-Sternberg cells are widely dispersed and few in number. The neoplasm is dominated by diffuse sheets of relatively monomorphic-appearing lymphocytes, although some may have enlarged nuclei (Figure 12-14, *A*). The **mixed cellularity type** is represented by scattered Reed-Sternberg cells within their lacunae and a polymorphous leukocytic population. Included in the mixed cell type are monocytoid cells, lymphocytes, and numerous eosinophils (Figure 12-14, *B*). **Nodular sclerosis** is represented by large confluent multinodular aggregates of lymphocytes and intervening collagen deposits. Reed-Sternberg cells are present in greater numbers (Figure 12-14, *C*). The worst prognosis is associated with the **lymphocyte depletion** variant of Hodgkin lymphoma. Reed-Sternberg cells dominate the microscopic fields with only scattered lymphocytes (Figure 12-14, *D*). In addition, large mononuclear lymphoblasts are identified that resemble the Reed-Sternberg cell by having a vesicular nucleoplasm with a prominent nucleolus. Mitotic figures are also commonly encountered.

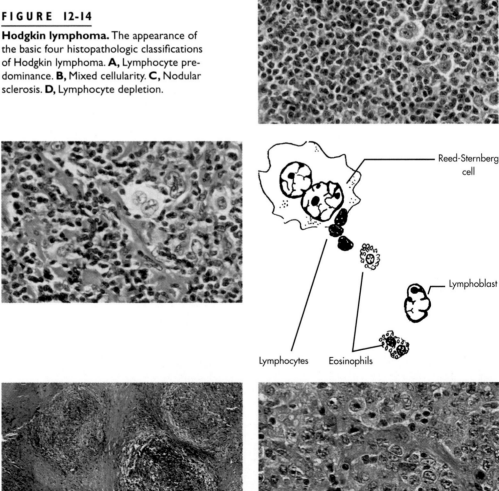

FIGURE 12-14

Hodgkin lymphoma. The appearance of the basic four histopathologic classifications of Hodgkin lymphoma. **A,** Lymphocyte predominance. **B,** Mixed cellularity. **C,** Nodular sclerosis. **D,** Lymphocyte depletion.

Reed-Sternberg cell

Lymphoblast

Lymphocytes   Eosinophils

TREATMENT

The treatment is based on the stage of disease and histomorphologic subtype. A stage 1 lymphocyte predominant Hodgkin lymphoma has an excellent prognosis, and most patients will survive the disease after radiotherapy and chemotherapy. Conversely, a stage 4 lymphocyte depletion type would carry the worst prognosis, and most individuals would not survive 12 months. Oncologists have selected and specified combination chemotherapeutic drugs for each type of Hodgkin lymphoma; radiation therapy plays a major role in the control of the disease.

Non-Hodgkin Lymphoma

■ **NON-HODGKIN LYMPHOMA:** malignant neoplasm of lymphocytes lacking Reed-Sternberg cells.

Lymphomas characterized by diffuse or nodular sheets of lymphocytes or lymphoblasts without the presence of Reed-Sternberg cells are classified as non-Hodgkin lymphoma. These lymphomas are clinically staged in similar fashion to Hodgkin lymphoma. As a group they carry a worse prognosis. As with Hodgkin lymphomas the non-Hodgkin lymphomas are diagnosed according to the cell population that predominates. Denoting the subtypes is important because all have different prognoses. The histopathologic classification schemes are numerous and quite complex (Box 12-1). Currently there are two major classifications that are more often used. Whereas most non-Hodgkin lymphomas are derived from B lymphocytes, a cutaneous form that originates from T-cells is encountered. This cutaneous T-cell lymphoma is extranodal and is referred to as **mycosis fungoides.** Rarely, cutaneous and lymphoid tissue are involved simultaneously, and the disease is referred to as the **Sézary syndrome.**

■ **BOX 12-1**
Classification Schemes for Non-Hodgkin Lymphomas

KIEL Classification (Europe)
LOW GRADE
ML—Lymphocytic (with *CLL)
ML—Lymphoplasmacytoid (immunocytic)
ML—Centrocytic
ML—Centroblastic-centrocytic (follicular
    and diffuse types)

HIGH GRADE
ML—Centroblastic
ML—Lymphoblastic,
    Burkitt
    Convoluted
ML—Immunoblastic

Working Formulation (North and South America)
LOW GRADE
ML—Diffuse, small lymphocytic type
    (with *CLL), plasmacytoid type
ML—Follicular, small cleaved cell
ML—Follicular, mixed small cleaved and
    large cell

INTERMEDIATE GRADE
ML—Follicular, large cell
ML—Diffuse, small cleaved cell
ML—Diffuse, small and large cell
ML—Diffuse, large cell

HIGH GRADE
ML—Large cell, immunoblastic
ML—Lymphoblastic
ML—Small noncleaved, Burkitt

ML, Malignant lymphoma.
*CLL, Lymphoma occurring in conjunction with chronic lymphocytic leukemia.

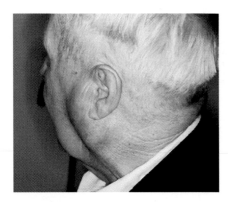

FIGURE 12-15

Lymphoma. A common head and neck clinical presentation of multiple, coalesced, persistently enlarged, firm, rubbery lymph nodes in the cervical area.

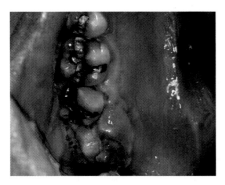

FIGURE 12-16

Lymphoma. HIV-associated lesion present on the gingiva and tuberosity.

CLINICAL

Non-Hodgkin lymphomas usually arise within lymph nodes; however, particularly within the oral cavity, extranodal disease is occasionally encountered. Indeed, those lymphomas associated with acquired immunodeficiency syndrome (AIDS) are frequently extranodal in location, being encountered in such tissues as the brain, oral mucosa, and the gut. Non-Hodgkin lymphomas are more frequently encountered in males than females and tend to occur in an older age group than those with Hodgkin lymphoma. Most patients are in the fourth or fifth decades of life. The earliest sign is a lymph node enlargement that persists or progressively enlarges. Low-grade fever and night sweats are common symptoms.

In the head and neck regions, non-Hodgkin lymphoma will manifest as a firm or rubbery cervical node enlargement that persists for over 1 month without any diminution in size (Figure 12-15). Inguinal and axillary nodes may also be involved as can the liver and spleen. In the later stages of disease multiple node groups may be affected along with hepatosplenomegaly.

Extranodal lymphomas arising within the oral cavity can occur centrally in the jawbones or arise in the oral soft tissue. In primary lymphoma of bone, patients may complain of pain and paresthesia or simply note osseous enlargements, usually in the mandible. Radiographs will disclose an irregular, poorly marginated radiolucency, and teeth in the affected area may show divergence or root resorption. Clinically, the teeth in an affected area often become loose. Soft tissue involvement may be seen anywhere in the oral mucosa, being more often identified as an enlargement or swelling on the gingiva or on the palate.

In human immunodeficieny virus (HIV) infections, malignant lymphoma is the second most commonly encountered malignancy after Kaposi sarcoma and extranodal localization in the oral cavity is frequently observed, generally identified on the palatal gingiva (Figure 12-16). Intraosseous lymphomas of the jaws in AIDS patients are extremely rare. The oral tumors are usually ulcerated, exhibit a rapid growth rate, and are frequently tumefactive or fungating.

A specific form of non-Hodgkin lymphoma occurs in the facial region and is referred to as **malignant** or **polymorphous reticulosis.** The tumor has an affinity for the midline structures of the face and will proliferate in the region of the nasal septum, causing osteolytic change with invasion into the ethmoids and through the nasal floor and palate. These lesions may occasionally perforate through the palate, yielding a large necrotic mass within the oral cavity. Similar clinical findings are encountered in Wegener granulomatosis or midline lethal granuloma, immunopathologic disorders characterized by vasculitis. They are biologically unrelated to polymorphous reticulosis, usually a form of T-cell lymphoma.

HISTOPATHOLOGY

In most forms of non-Hodgkin lymphoma the peripheral blood leukocyte count is normal. One form, diffuse lymphocytic lymphoma, is often associated with chronic lymphocytic leukemia, and therefore a leukocytosis with circulating leukemic blast cells will be encountered. Microscopically, the normal lymph node architecture is destroyed and malignant lymphocytes frequently invade the lymph node capsule. The affected node is significantly enlarged, and the growth pattern is divided into two major subcategories: diffuse, in which sheets of lymphoid cells prevail, and nodular, in which the malignant cells form confluent ovoid clusters that resemble markedly enlarged germinal centers (Figure 12-17). In nodular lymphomas there is little or no intervening medullary lymphoid tissue. As a group the lymphomas with a nodular pattern carry a better prognosis than those that are diffuse.

The histopathologic subtyping is based on the differentiation of the lym-

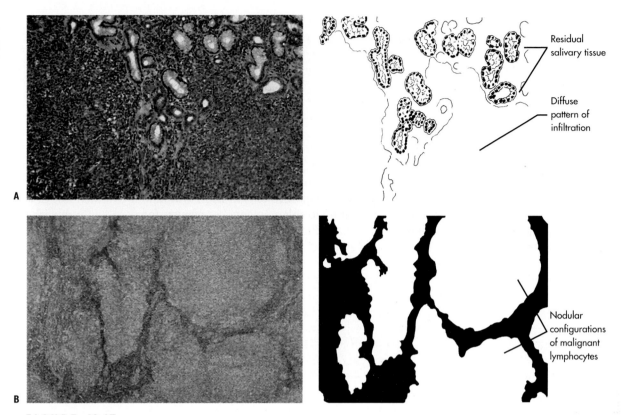

FIGURE 12-17

Lymphoma. A, Atypical lymphocytes infiltrating palatal salivary gland tissue in diffuse form of non-Hodgkin lymphoma. **B,** Nodular pattern of proliferation in non-Hodgkin lymphoma.

phoid precursor cells; the more primitive, anaplastic tumors are high grade, and the more differentiated tumors, which bear a greater resemblance to mature lymphocytes, are low grade. As mentioned previously, the two major classification systems are those proposed by the workshop on lymphoma classification in the United States and the Kiel classification that evolved in Europe (Box 12-1). There are a variety of cell surface markers, which are useful in these classification schemes, that identify lymphoid cells at varying stages of maturation. Both classifications take into account the resemblance of B-cell lymphoma populations to the B-cell region of the lymph node (centrocytes, centroblasts, or follicular center cells). The large-cell lymphomas emulate large follicular center cells or lymphoblasts. Intermediate-size cells with pale chromatin represent immunoblasts or lymphoblasts; and the well-differentiated cells are small and round, resembling mature lymphocytes. Box 12-1 compares the two major classification schemes. Most extranodal lymphomas occurring in AIDS are represented by intermediate-size lymphoblasts or large anaplastic blast cells. They are therefore high-grade lymphomas. The cells identified in malignant polymorphous reticulosis are pleomorphic-appearing lymphocytoid cells. They range from small lymphocytes to large blast-appearing cells. Mitotic figures and pleomorphism are common, and the cells tend to surround blood vessels (angiocentricity). There is frequently a significant amount of necrosis within the specimen, and the osseous trabeculas show osteoclastic resorption along the leading edge of the infiltrating tumor.

T-cell lymphomas associated with mycosis fungoides demonstrate characteristic histopathologic features on skin biopsy. The subcutaneous tissue is infiltrated diffusely with relatively monomorphic-appearing small lymphocytes, and clusters of lymphoid cells transmigrate into the overlying epithelium, referred to as **Pautrier microabscess;** the diagnosis can usually be confirmed by utilizing a monoclonal antibody to T-cell markers. The oral mucosa is rarely involved. Polyclonality refers to the ability of a population of lymphoid cells to synthesize a mixture of light and heavy chain immunoglobulins, whereas monoclonality is used for a population of cells that can only produce either a single type of light chain or a heavy chain immunoglobulin.

The pathologist is sometimes confronted with a lymphoctytic infiltrate or a proliferative lesion in a lymph node in which the histologic features are ambiguous. Tests for clonality are important because a monoclonal cell population occurs in malignancy, whereas polyclonal cells are most consistent with an inflammatory cell infiltrate. **Receptor gene rearrangement** assays will disclose clonality in lymphoid lesions. The B-cell receptor is the immunoglobulin molecule, whereas T-cells have a different type of receptor (Tcr). In diverse or polyclonal proliferations the B- and T-cell receptors normally evince a heterogeneous population of receptor gene rearrangements because each receptor molecule binds a different and unique antigen. Alternatively, only a single species of rearranged

FIGURE 12-18

Lymphoma. The immunoglobulin gene is intact in nonlymphoid tissue. When DNA from normal cells is cut with restriction enzymes, a germ line pattern is seen on electrophoresis *(column 2 bottom)*. In B-cell lymphomas, the immunoglobulin gene is rearranged identically in the malignant cells. This yields different length segments of DNA from the germ cell line bands derived from the normal cell population *(columns 3 and 4)*.

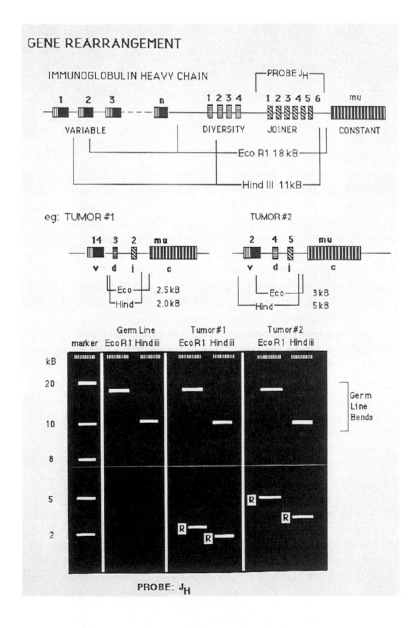

receptor genes will be identified in a monoclonal malignant proliferation (Figure 12-18).

TREATMENT

As with Hodgkin lymphoma the non-Hodgkin lymphomas are managed according to the stage of the disease and the histopathologic subtype. Multiregimented chemotherapy and radiation therapy are employed.

Burkitt Lymphoma

> ■ BURKITT LYMPHOMA: form of lymphoma first described in equatorial Africa that is associated with the Epstein-Barr virus and has a predilection for the jaws of children.

Burkitt lymphoma, first reported in the equatorial regions of Africa among young children, is associated with Epstein-Barr virus. The tumors typically involve extralymphoid sites, showing a predilection for the jaws and viscera, particulary the ovaries. Chromosomal abnormalities are a hallmark of this unique form of lymphoma. Translocation of a portion of chromosome 8 to chromosomes 2, 14, and 22 is regularly observed. The C-myc oncogene from chromosome 8 is then brought into proximity with the genes encoding immunoglobulin heavy (14), κ light (2), and λ light (22) chain genes. In these circumstances the immunoglobulin gene promoters are believed to cause overexpression of the C-myc oncogene, which is a DNA-binding transcription protein that is active in the initiation of cell cycling.

CLINICAL

Burkitt lymphoma is encountered in three distinct settings: (1) the classic endemic type found in equatorial Africa; (2) a non-African, nonendemic type that has been identified in Europe, the United States, and Asia; and (3) an AIDS-associated type. In African Burkitt lymphoma, children in the first decade of life are affected; however, some cases arise during teenage years. A 2:1 male/female ratio is encountered. Affected children usually present with massive tumors of the maxilla or mandible. The tumefactions are firm, and the oral mucosa overlying the masses is often hemorrhagic or ulcerated. Usually the masses are painless and no sensory deficits are noted. Radiographs disclose massive lesions undergoing osseous resorption with irregular margins and reactive bone occurring in the molar and premolar regions (Figure 12-19). Although most tumors are solitary, many can independently involve more than one jaw quadrant. Tooth displacement and root resorption are commonly encountered. Lymphomatous tissue is also present in the abdomen and may originate within the ovaries. In the nonendemic form, jaw tumors are only seen in 20% of the affected patients.

In AIDS patients, non-Hodgkin lymphoma is the second most prevalent neoplasm, with many of these lesions showing microscopic features in common with Burkitt lymphoma. The lymphomas resembling the Burkitt type tend to arise on the palate and gingiva. The CD4 count is invariably below 200 when the lymphoma first appears. Clinically the lesions appear as soft tissue nodular masses and many are hemorrhagic, thus resembling Kaposi sarcoma.

HISTOPATHOLOGY

The basic cell type is a medium round lymphoblast. A pathognomonic feature of the African form of Burkitt lymphoma is the presence of lacunae that contain macrophages with phagocytized cellular debris. These vacuolated lacunae are rather evenly dispersed among the malignant cell population and under low-power microscopy appear as a "starry sky" because the clear lacunae stand out

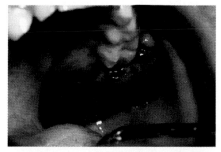
A

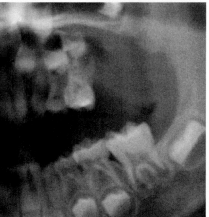
B

FIGURE 12-19

Burkitt lymphoma. A, Massive tumor of posterior maxilla of a young patient. **B,** Radiograph of same patient as **A** exhibiting a large ill-defined radiolucency.

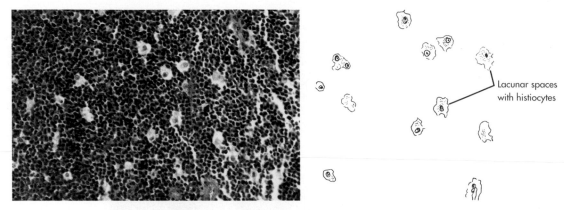

Lacunar spaces
with histiocytes

FIGURE 12-20

Burkitt lymphoma. Photomicrograph of "starry-sky" appearance that occurs when histiocytes residing within lacunae are scattered throughout diffuse sheets of malignant lymphocytes.

against the dark background of the densely packed lymphocytes (Figure 12-20). The malignant lymphocytes, which comprise the sheetlike proliferation, are characterized by large round nuclei with a prominent nuclear membrane, a stippled nucleoplasm, and prominent nucleoli that vary in number from 1 to 4. Each nucleus is surrounded by cytoplasm, which gives the sheets a syncytial appearance. Mitotic activity is often prominent. Tumor cells invade the periodontal ligament and may even extend into the pulps of developing teeth. Similar morphology is seen in the non-African, nonendemic form of Burkitt lymphoma and in HIV.

TREATMENT

Chemotherapy and radiation have been employed. Multidrug chemotherapy has dramatic effects on Burkitt lymphoma. Massive tumors may literally melt back to normal jaw dimensions within 2 weeks of initiation. Cyclophosphamide, vincristine sulfate, and methotrexate are commonly prescribed. The 5-year survival rate is less than 30%; and although response to chemotherapy is excellent, relapses and the appearance of new lesions tend to occur over time.

Multiple Myeloma

> ■ MULTIPLE MYELOMA: disseminated neoplasm of differentiated B lymphocytes or plasma cells located within bone.

> ■ SOLITARY PLASMACYTOMA: single tumor of plasma cells often located in the soft tissue of the upper air passages.

Multiple myeloma represents a third type of lymphoma that arises from bone marrow based B-cells, specifically, those that have undergone terminal differentiation into plasma cells. As with other lymphomas these tumors are believed to arise from a single cell type and therefore exhibit monoclonality. This clonality can be assessed in tissue sections or by biochemically evaluating the type of immunoglobulin secreted by the neoplastic cells. Multiple myeloma eventually becomes disseminated, involving multiple skeletal sites. This is probably accounted for by biochemical homing mechanisms for terminally differentiated B-cells invading other hematopoietic marrow sites.

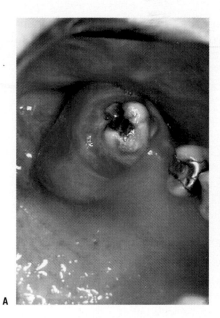

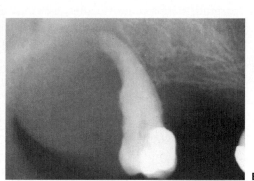

FIGURE 12-21

Multiple myeloma. A, Expansion of alveolar bone surrounding a maxillary molar. **B,** Radiograph of lesion depicted in **A** exhibiting a poorly defined radiolucency surrounding the molar.

The **solitary plasmacytoma** represents a clonal proliferation of plasma cells in an extramedullary site. Some patients have survived for many years with solitary extramedullary plasmacytoma, whereas others have eventually developed disseminated multiple myeloma.

CLINICAL

Multiple myeloma affects men and women equally and usually arises during the fourth, fifth, and sixth decades of life. Because the malignant cells occupy the marrow spaces without manifesting any specific signs or symptoms, the disease has often become widely disseminated by the time it is detected. A characteristic feature of multiple myeloma is deep bone pain. Osteolytic lesions are encountered in various bones and are usually quite prominent in the calvarium where they appear as coin-shaped, punched-out radiolucencies. Despite their malignant nature these radiolucent lesions are relatively well defined yet not corticated around their boundaries.

In the jaws the disease may simulate a toothache. Dental radiographs may also show coin-shaped, punched-out radiolucencies or widespread osseous destruction. The radiographic margins are moth eaten without cortication. Teeth within the area of malignancy may become loose (Figure 12-21).

The solitary plasmacytoma occurs as a pendulous mass, usually identified within the nasopharynx. Involvement of the oral mucosa is extremely rare. These plasma cell tumors are usually brought to the patient's attention by such symptoms as nasal speech or nasal stuffiness.

HISTOPATHOLOGY

Multiple myeloma and solitary plasmacytoma show the same microscopic features. Diffuse sheets of plasma cells are encountered with minimal fibrous stroma; rather, small capillary channels course among the plasma cells (Figure 12-22). The individual cells maintain both the nuclear eccentricity encountered in normal plasma cells and the peripheral chromatin beading. Importantly, binucleated forms are common, mitotic figures may be observed, and there is usually some degree of nuclear pleomorphism. Because plasmacytic infiltrates are quite common in the jaws, particularly in response to odontogenic infections, differentiation from myeloma is sometimes difficult. In most inflammatory conditions that are characterized by high plasma cell populations, other leukocytes

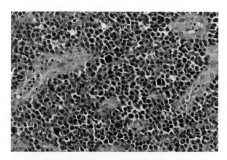

FIGURE 12-22

Multiple myeloma. Photomicrograph revealing diffuse sheets of atypical plasma cells with minimal fibrous connective tissue stroma.

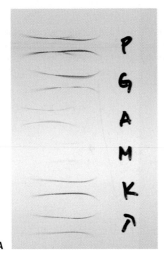

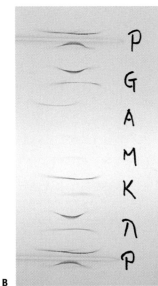

are also encountered and the stroma is collagenous. In myeloma, the cell population is usually homogeneous. Furthermore, the plasma cells of inflammation are polyclonal and will therefore express both κ and λ immunoglobulin light chains using immunohistochemistry. In multiple myeloma the plasma cell population is monoclonal and will express either λ or κ immunoglobulin light chains but not both.

Multiple myeloma, being a disseminated disease of immunoglobulin-secreting plasma cells, will affect a change in serum immunoglobulin levels (Figure 12-23). The total gamma globulins will be increased; and on serum immunoelectrophoresis, a monoclonal spike representing a single immunoglobulin class will account for the increased levels. Light chains from immunoglobulins are often excreted into the urine in myeloma and are referred to as Bence Jones protein.

TREATMENT

Multiple myeloma carries a poor prognosis despite intensive chemotherapy. Multidrug regimens are employed to arrest cell division in an attempt to eliminate the disease. Total body irradiation with bone marrow transplantation is another treatment option.

BLEEDING DISORDERS

Hemostasis is achieved by cooperative functions between blood thrombocytes and coagulation factors. During the primary stage of hemostasis, once a vessel wall is violated, platelet adhesion ensues. This adhesion phenomenon requires the presence of the von Willebrand factor and specific adhesion proteins on the thrombocyte plasma membrane. Platelet adhesion to the subintimal connective tissue then triggers biochemical changes within the thrombocytes with the release of proteins that facilitate aggregation between one platelet and its neighbor. These aggregated platelets then form the initial plug, which prevents bleeding (Figure 12-24). It is therefore axiomatic that individuals who have a deficiency in platelet numbers and individuals who have functional disturbances in platelet adhesion will suffer from bleeding episodes. In general, most platelet disorders are characterized by cutaneous and mucosal petechiae. The initial platelet plug is not stable but becomes a more adequate seal after the formation of a fibrin clot. Box 12-2 lists many of the causes of bleeding disorders (hemorrhagic diathesis) and easy bruising (purpura) encountered in patients.

FIGURE 12-23

Serum immunoelectrophoresis contrasting a polyclonal hypergammaglobulinemia of inflammation **(A)** with a monoclonal spike of a multiple myeloma **(B)**. *P,* Total immunoglobulins; *G,* IgG; *A,* IgA; *M,* IgM; *K,* kappa light chains; and λ, lambda light chains. Under *P,* the polyclonal increase in **A** is characterized by a broad curve, indicating a variety of immunoglobulin classes; whereas in **B** the monoclonal spike is small, indicating a single immunoglobulin class that is IgG with lambda clonality.

FIGURE 12-24

Thrombocyte function. When a vessel wall is damaged, platelets will adhere to the subintimal connective tissue aided by von Willebrand Factor VIII adhesion protein. Platelets aggregate with one another by virtue of other adhesion molecules, activated by ATP conversion to cyclic AMP.

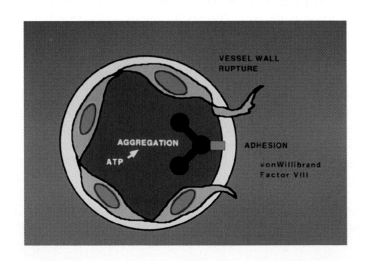

Platelet Disorders	*Vascular Wall Fragility*
Decreased number	Scurvy
Irradiation	Genetic
Chemotherapy	
Leukemia	*Coagulation Factor Deficiency*
Autoimmunity	Genetic
Defective adhesion	Primary liver disease
Genetic	Biliary obstruction
Defective aggregation	Steatorrhea
Genetic	Anticoagulant drugs
Prostaglandin inhibitors	

PLATELET DISORDERS

Thrombocytopenia

■ THROMBOCYTOPENIA: decrease in the number of circulating blood platelets that can be caused by a variety of factors.

Total circulating blood platelets are normally between 250,000 and 400,000 per cubic millimeter of blood. A decrease in number may occur due to a maturation arrest, a myelophthisic response in the marrow, or, after release into the circulation, immunologic events. Importantly, when the platelet count drops below 50,000 cells per cubic millimeter, severe catastrophic bleeding may occur subsequent to trauma or surgery. The most common underlying causes that result in thrombocytopenia include administration of cytotoxic chemotherapeutic drugs, leukemia, and autoimmune thrombocytopenic purpura, in which antiplatelet antibodies are observed. The autoimmune form occurs in HIV-infected patients as well and is often referred to as idiopathic thrombocytopenic purpura (ITP). The cause for the generation of antiplatelet antibodies is unknown.

CLINICAL
Petechial hemorrhages are the most common form of purpura encountered in thrombocytopenia and are characterized by pinpoint red or brown macules of the skin. Within the oral cavity, they may occur on any surface but are probably more frequently seen on the palate (Figure 12-25). In the differential diagnosis, however, it should be noted that palatal petechiae are more often caused by suction. Clicking the palate against the tongue is common when an individual suffers from an upper respiratory infection and has an "itchy throat." Palatal petechiae are also reported to occur from fellatio. Oral petechiae secondary to thrombocytopenia are usually accompanied by cutaneous petechiae as well. Additionally, patients may complain of spontaneous gingival hemorrhage.

LABORATORY
Thrombocytopenia is diagnosed by obtaining a platelet count. When leukemia is suspected, a complete blood count should be obtained because leukemia is frequently associated with a drop in the platelet count. The bleeding time is a clinical assessment of platelet numbers and adherence. This test is performed by placing a blood pressure cuff on the patient's arm and applying a pressure of 40

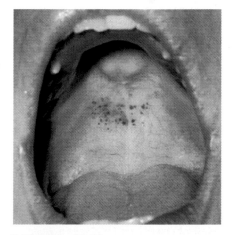

FIGURE 12-25

Palatal petechiae. Multiple small foci of superficial vessel bleeding occurs due to the fragility of the vessel wall or altered clotting factors when minor trauma to the area is encountered.

mm mercury. Below the cuff the forearm is penetrated with a 1 mm blood lancet. The small focus of hemorrhage is dabbed every 15 seconds with a piece of filter paper; when blood can no longer be identified on the paper, the bleeding time has been reached. In patients with normal functioning and adequate numbers of platelets, the bleeding time usually varies between 5 and 7 minutes.

TREATMENT

Before treatment can be planned, the underlying cause of a reduction in platelets must be determined. A platelet count below 50,000 can lead to a life-threatening hemorrhage after oral surgery. If surgery must be performed or if it is essential that an infected tooth be extracted, the patient will need to be hospitalized and platelet infusions must be administered.

Thrombasthenia

■ THROMBASTHENIA: functional group of diseases characterized by defective adherence or aggregation of platelets.

Although a hemorrhagic diathesis will occur when the number of platelets drops below critical levels, functional impairment can also result in purpura. Defects in platelet adhesion or aggregation culminate in inadequate plugging of ruptured vessels, and the disease is referred to as thrombasthenia. Aspirin toxicity with its effects on prostaglandin synthesis is one of the more clinically common defects in platelet adhesion and aggregation. There are also heritable diseases in which patients fail to synthesize functionally intact adhesion molecules on the platelet surface. One such disorder, which also affects the coagulation pathways, is von Willebrand disease in which an important adhesion molecule is defective. In addition, Factor VIII of the intrinsic pathway is also defective.

CLINICAL

In salicylate toxicity as well as von Willebrand disease and other rare forms of thrombasthenia, petechial hemorrhages are the hallmark. Therefore the clinical features simulate those seen in thrombocytopenia. Similarly, when petechiae occur within the oral cavity, the skin is usually also affected.

LABORATORY

The platelet count in thrombasthenia is normal. Whereas a functional assay for platelet aggregation can be performed in the clinical laboratory, the bleeding time is prolonged. In addition, assays are available to access levels of von Willebrand Factor VIII.

TREATMENT

Platelets that have become defective due to salicylate toxicity are impaired for the life of the platelet. Because new thrombocytes are constantly being synthesized, the defect is usually reversed within 1 week after withdrawal of aspirin. Dipyridamole is a platelet adhesion inhibitor prescribed to prevent thromboembolic disease. Prolonged bleeding can be a problem, and medical consultation should be sought before performing oral surgery. Currently, the heritable forms cannot be adequately treated; however, should a hemorrhagic crisis occur, platelet infusions will be necessary. von Willebrand disease is usually mild despite the fact that platelet adhesion and coagulation Factor VIII are defective. It is not uncommon for a diagnosis of von Willebrand disease to be made following prolonged bleeding subsequent to dental extraction, even in adult years.

CAPILLARY FRAGILITY

The fibrous coat or adventitia of small caliber vessels is defective or inadequate in ascorbic acid deficiency and in the heritable disease, hereditary hemorrhagic telangiectasia. Vitamin C is an important cofactor in collagen fibrillogenesis. When dietary intake is inadequate, collagen synthesis is impaired; and this is usually manifested in vessel walls. In hereditary hemorrhagic telangiectasia there is a structural deformity involving the integrity of the small vessel vascular wall.

Vitamin C Deficiency

■ SCURVY: systemic disease due to lack of vitamin C dietary intake in which vascular wall integrity and wound repair mechanisms are defective.

Vitamin C deficiency (scurvy) is rarely seen in the industrialized world because most individuals have sufficient vitamin C in their diets. Citrus fruits and tomatoes are the primary sources of this vitamin. Therefore scurvy is usually encountered in third world countries where adequate nutritional intake is not available.

CLINICAL

Purpura is one of the main manifestations of scurvy and occurs due to vascular wall fragility. The purpuric lesions may occur in the oral mucosa and on the skin and are represented by petechia and ecchymosis. Whereas the bruising usually occurs after traumatic provocation, in severe scurvy spontaneous purpura may be identified. Because the collagen fibers of the periodontal ligaments may also be defective, severe periodontal disease may be encountered and spontaneous tooth loss will occur. Scorbutic changes may also evolve in bone matrices, leading to pathologic fractures. Because vitamin C is important during healing, ulcerations or lacerations may persist and become secondarily infected. These ulcerations can involve the oral mucosa.

HISTOPATHOLOGY

Microscopically, vascular wall changes are not discernible in scurvy; although pathologic changes are identifiable with electron microscopy. Skin or mucosal biopsies show extravasation of erythrocytes, extravascular clot formation within tissue, and hemosiderin pigment deposition. The disease is diagnosed by assessing the patient's history, clinical findings, and serum ascorbic acid levels.

TREATMENT

Scurvy is reversed by adequate dietary intake of ascorbic acid. The vascular changes are reversible. Periodontal tissue breakdown, however, is permanent; lost alveolar bone will not regenerate after adequate vitamin intake.

Hereditary Hemorrhagic Telangiectasia

■ HEREDITARY HEMORRHAGIC TELANGIECTASIA: inherited disease in which vascular walls are defective and multiple vascular dilatations occur in the mucous membranes of the upper aerodigestive tract.

Inherited as an autosomal dominant trait, hereditary hemorrhagic telangiectasia **(Rendu-Osler-Weber syndrome)** affects the integrity of vascular walls. Lesions are most prominent in the head and neck areas, invariably involving the oral mucosa. The damaged vessels are dilatated, creating multiple reddish purple papules that are separated from one another by normal-appearing skin or mucosa. They typically occur on the dorsum of the tongue (Figure 12-26), on

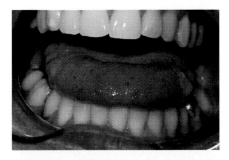

FIGURE 12-26

Hereditary hemorrhagic telangiectasia (Rendu-Osler-Weber syndrome). Multiple small raised reddish papules are present on the dorsum of the tongue. The patient also exhibited similar lesions on other mucosal surfaces and the skin.

the lips, and in the nasal mucosa. The affected vessels are larger than capillaries, and trauma may cause prolonged hemorrhaging. Epistaxis is common. The bleeding is usually stopped by direct compression.

HISTOPATHOLOGY

In hereditary hemorrhagic telangiectasia dilatated vascular channels engorged with erythrocytes are seen and erythrocyte extravasation is common, with the deposition of hemosiderin pigment in the perivascular connective tissue. The vessel wall defect is not appreciated with light microscopy; rather, electron microscopy is needed to demonstrate the tissue abnormality. There are no altered laboratory values regarding platelet numbers or aggregation in this disease. Clotting factors are normal.

TREATMENT

There is no treatment for this condition because it represents a structural defect. Hemorrhage can sometimes be problematic, and cases of severe epistaxis can occur. Compression with gauze or cotton packs will usually result in cessation of hemorrhage, and the affected vessel may be cauterized. For cosmetic reasons, particularly around the lip area, the cutaneous papules can be treated by laser therapy.

COAGULATION DISORDERS

The coagulopathies are diseases due to defective proteins that are components of the coagulation cascade (Figure 12-27). They may be **hereditary,** the result of mutations in the genes that encode a specific coagulation factor, or acquired, involving multiple coagulation factors. Most of the hereditary coagulopathies are quite rare, with the exception of hemophilia A. Acquired coagulation disorders occur primarily as a consequence of chronic liver disease and among patients taking antithrombotic medications such as Coumadin and Persantine. Because the majority of coagulation factors are synthesized within the liver, any disease that leads to the death of hepatocytes will result in a coagulopathic disorder. Therefore hepatitis, alcoholic cirrhosis, biliary atresia, and biliary cirrhosis can all be associated with prolonged bleeding times. Malabsorption syndromes, par-

FIGURE 12-27

Clotting factor pathways. The extent that the intrinsic pathway is able to function is assessed by the partial prothrombin time *(PTT),* whereas that of the extrinsic pathway is evaluated by a determination of the prothrombin time *(PT).* Both pathways converge into a common pathway culminating in the formation of a fibrin clot.

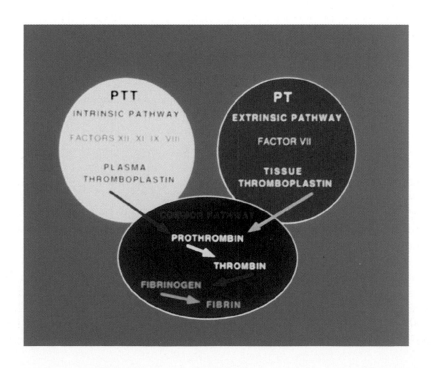

ticularly steatorrhea, involve defects in fat absorption. Inadequate absorption of fat results in a reduction of the fat-soluble vitamin K, an essential factor for the synthesis of five clotting factors, which predisposes to coagulopathies and a bleeding tendency.

Hemophilia

■ H E M O P H I L I A: group of bleeding diseases that evolve as a consequence of hereditary or acquired defects in the production of proteins necessary for normal blood coagulation.

The two major forms of hemophilia are hereditary; the defective proteins are components of the intrinsic pathway of the clotting that functions within blood vessels. Alternatively, the extrinsic pathway is activated extravascularly and is important in soft tissue clot formation and wound repair. Although a different group of clotting factors is required for the extrinsic pathway, the intrinsic and the extrinsic pathways culminate in the formation of thromboplastins. The two pathways then share a common route for the final synthesis of the fibrin protein network, the essence of normal clot formation. Genetic defects of the other clotting factors that occur are extremely rare.

CLINICAL

Purpura is the clinical sign common to all the coagulopathies. The purpuric lesions are characterized by diffuse purple, red, or brown macules commonly referred to as "bruises" or ecchymosis (Figure 12-28). These ecchymotic changes may be seen on the facial skin and the oral mucosa, typically occurring after minor trauma. Hemarthrosis (bleeding within the joints) is another common finding in coagulation disorders, being more prevalent in individuals with hereditary factor deficiency.

Hemophilia A, a hereditary deficiency of *Factor VIII,* and **hemophilia B,** a hereditary deficiency of *Factor IX,* are the most common of the genetic factor deficiencies. Hemophilia A is approximately ten times as prevalent as hemophilia B. **Afibrinogenemia,** a hereditary deficiency of *Factor I,* is even less commonly seen; deficiencies in the other specific factors are extremely rare. In all heritable coagulation disorders the disease becomes apparent in early childhood, often after the child engages in some physical activity that results in profound bruising or hemarthrosis. In addition, the eruption of deciduous teeth may trigger spontaneous gingival hemorrhage. Dental extraction or oral surgical procedures are contraindicated without taking appropriate precautions, which often necessitates hospitalization.

Acquired coagulopathy is commonly associated with liver cirrhosis and may be accompanied by a variety of other signs and symptoms depending on the severity of the liver parenchymal damage. The acquired coagulopathies encountered in liver disease and anticoagulant therapy share clinical features with those encountered in the three major forms of hemophilia (hemophilia A, hemophilia B, and afibrinogenemia). In addition to coagulation factors, the liver synthesizes a variety of other proteins including albumin. Albumin is the major protein component of blood and is largely responsible for maintaining the positive osmotic pressure in the vascular compartment. As albumin levels decrease and the total serum protein levels drop, intravascular osmotic pressure decreases, leading to loss of fluid from the vascular compartment to the surrounding tissues with resultant edema and ascitis. Because estrogens are metabolized in the liver thereby preventing their buildup in the blood, parenchymal necrosis of liver tissue will lead to increased estrogen levels that may predispose to breast enlargement (gynecomastia) in males. The conjugation of bilirubin by hepatocytes may also be impaired, leading to hyperbilirubinemia and jaundice. Last, chronic liver

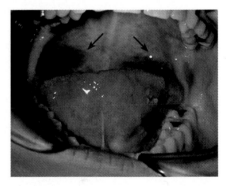

FIGURE 12-28

Ecchymosis. The areas of bilateral superficial interstitial bleeding of the posterior soft palate *(arrows)* present in this patient are commonly encountered after minor trauma in patients with hereditary or acquired coagulopathies.

failure with sclerosis induces a stasis in blood flow through the portal system with attending portal hypertension. This stasis culminates in the dilatation of veins that drain into the portal system, including the esophageal, hemorrhoidal, and umbilical veins. Esophageal varices, hemorrhoids, and abdominal *caput medusae* are signs of advanced liver disease and are attended by severe coagulation defects with ecchymosis.

Perhaps the most common cause of coaguloapathy is anticoagulant therapy. Coumadin, most commonly prescribed, interferes with the formation of many coagulation factors by inhibiting vitamin K, a coenzyme necessary for their synthesis of coagulation factors. Patients properly placed on anticoagulant therapy receive doses at levels that prevent spontaneous profound thrombosis yet do not place the patient in jeopardy of severe hemorrhaging. Nevertheless, the drug level cannot always be precisely monitored; and some of these patients will develop ecchymosis.

HISTOPATHOLOGY

Unlike platelet disorders in which petechial hemorrhages occur, coagulopathies are associated with more severe venous hemorrhage; and therefore the purpura is often large and more diffuse. Microscopically, diffuse zones of extravasated erythrocytes and deposits of hemosiderin pigment are present in the surrounding connective tissue. The diagnosis is best made by conducting assays that measure the intrinsic and extrinsic pathways of coagulation. The prothrombin time (PT) examines the extrinsic pathway, whereas the partial thromboplastin time (PTT) assesses the intrinsic pathway. Patients taking Coumadin or those with liver disease are usually monitored by the PT, whereas the PTT will be prolonged in hemophilia A and B.

TREATMENT

Oral surgical procedures in patients with a hemorrhagic diathesis can be life threatening if appropriate precautions are not observed. In general, a PT or PTT that is prolonged more than two times the laboratory control levels is an indication that oral or periodontal surgery should not be undertaken. If tooth extraction is required, the patient must be hospitalized and coagulation factor supplementation must be available.

ADDITIONAL READING

IRON DEFICIENCY ANEMIA

Dantas RO, Villanova MG. Esophageal motility impairment in Plummer-Vinson syndrome: correction by iron treatment. *Dig Dis Sci.* 1993; 38:968-71.

Geerlings SE, Statius van Eps LW. Pathogenesis and consequences of Plummer-Vinson syndrome. *Clin Investig.* 1992; 70:629-30.

Mohandas KM, Swaroop VS, Desai DC, Dhir V and others. Upper esophageal webs, iron deficiency anemia, and esophageal cancer. *Am J Gastroenterol.* 1991; 86:117-8.

Murphy PT, Hutchinson RM. Identification and treatment of anaemia in older patients. *Drugs Aging.* 1994; 4:113-27.

Seitz ML, Sabatino D. Plummer-Vinson syndrome in an adolescent. *J Adolesc Health.* 1991; 12:279-81.

Yip R. Iron deficiency: contemporary scientific issues and international programmatic approaches. *J Nutr.* 1994; 124:1479S-1490S.

PERNICIOUS ANEMIA

Greenberg, MS. Clinical and histologic changes of the oral mucosa in pernicious anemia. *Oral Surg Oral Med Oral Pathol.* 1981; 52:38-42.

Karnad AB, Krozser-Hamati A. Pernicious anemia: early identification to prevent permanent sequelae. *Postgrad Med.* 1992; 91:231-4.

Loffeld BC, van Spreeuwel JP. The gastrointestinal tract in pernicious anemia. *Dig Dis.* 1991; 9:70-7.

Pruthi RK, Tefferi A. Pernicious anemia revisited. *Mayo Clin Proc.* 1994; 69:144-50.

SICKLE CELL ANEMIA

Brown LD, Sebes JI: Sickle cell gnathopathy: radiologic assessment. *Oral Surg Oral Med Oral Pathol.* 1986; 61:653-6.

Mourshed F, Tuckson CR. A study of the radiographic features of the jaws in sickle-cell anemia. *Oral Surg Oral Med Oral Pathol.* 1974; 37:812-19.

Sanger RO, Greer RO, Auerbach RE. Differential diagnosis of some simple osseous lesions associated with sickle cell anemia. *Oral Surg Oral Med Oral Pathol.* 1977; 43:538.

Sears RS. The effects of sickle cell disease on dental and skeletal maturation. *ASDC J Dent Child.* 1981; 48:275.

THALASSEMIA

Cannell H. The development of oral and facial signs in beta-thalassaemia major. *Br Dent J.* 1988; 164:50.

Poyton HG, Davey KW. Thalassemia: changes visible in radiographs used in dentistry. *Oral Surg Oral Med Oral Pathol.* 1968; 25:564.

FETAL ERYTHROBLASTOSIS

Contreras M, de Silva M. The prevention and management of haemolytic disease of the newborn. *J R Soc Med.* 1994; 87:256-8.

Hadley AG, Kumpel BM. The role of Rh antibodies in haemolytic disease of the newborn. *Baillieres Clin Haematol.* 1993; 6:423-44.

AGRANULOCYTOSIS

Brna TG. Agranulocytosis from antiarrhythmic agents: what to watch for when a medication is first prescribed. *Postgrad Med.* 1991; 89:181-3, 187-8.

Lamster IB, Oshrain RL, Harper DS. Infantile agranulocytosis with survival into adolescence: periodontal manifestations and laboratory findings: a case report. *J Periodontol.* 1987; 8:34-9.

Mason RP, Fischer V. Possible role of free radical formation in drug-induced agranulocytosis. *Drug Saf.* 1992; (suppl 1): 45-50.

Meyer-Gessner M, Benker G, Lederbogen S, Olbricht T and others. Antithyroid drug-induced agranulocytosis: clinical experience with ten patients treated at one institution and review of the literature. *J Endocrinol Invest.* 1994; 17:29-36.

Ohishi M, Oobu K, Miyanoshita Y, Yamaguchi K. Acute gingival necrosis caused by drug-induced agranulocytosis. *Oral Surg Oral Med Oral Pathol.* 1988; 66:194-6.

Pisciotta AV, Konings SA, Ciesemier LL, Cronkite CE. On the possible mechanisms and predictability of clozapine-induced agranulocytosis. *Drug Saf.* 1992; 7(suppl 1):33-44.

Seger RA, Ezekowitz RA. Treatment of chronic granulomatous disease. *Immunodeficiency.* 1994; 5:113-30.

Strickland RD, Goldberg JS, Lazarus HM, Spetzler RF. Phenytoin-induced agranulocytosis after treatment for a gunshot wound to the face. *Oral Surg Oral Med Oral Pathol.* 1983; 56:500-1.

CYCLIC NEUTROPENIA

Bux J, Mueller-Eckhardt C. Autoimmune neutropenia. *Semin Hematol.* 1992; 29:45-53.

Dunkel IJ, Bussel JB. New developments in the treatment of neutropenia. *Am J Dis Child.* 1993; 147:994-1000.

Foucar K, Duncan MH, Smith KJ. Practical approach to the investigation of neutropenia. *Clin Lab Med.* 1993; 13:879-94.

Israel DS, Plaisance KI. Neutropenia in patients infected with human immunodeficiency virus. *Clin Pharm.* 1991; 10: 268-79.

Kaplan C, Morinet F, Cartron J. Virus-induced autoimmune thrombocytopenia and neutropenia. *Semin Hematol.* 1992; 29:34-44.

Little FM, Pais RC, Winton E, Ragab AH. Granulocyte colony-stimulating factor: a new approach in the treatment of childhood neutropenia. *J Med Assoc Ga.* 1992; 81:437-41.

Stroncek DF. Drug-induced immune neutropenia. *Transfus Med Rev.* 1993; 7:268-74.

Tsuda M, Urakami T, Watanabe S, Shimizu H and others. Recombinant human granulocyte colony-stimulating factor therapy for cyclic neutropenia associated with common variable immunodeficiency. *Acta Paediatr Jpn.* 1993; 35:124-6.

Welte K, Zeidler C, Reiter A, Riehm H. Effects of granulocyte colony-stimulating factor in children with severe neutropenia. *Acta Haematol Pol.* 1994; 25(2 suppl 1):155-62.

CHRONIC GRANULOMATOUS DISEASE

Allan D, Straton AG. Chronic granulomatous disease with associated oral lesions. *Br Dent J.* 1983; 154:110-2.

Cohen MS, Leong PA, Simpson DM. Phagocytic cells in periodontal defense: periodontal status of patients with chronic granulomatous disease of childhood. *J Periodontol.* 1985; 56:611-7.

Dinauer MC, Orkin SH. Chronic granulomatous disease. *Annu Rev Med.* 1992; 43:117-24.

Meyle J, Dopfer R. Chronic granulomatous disease: a special problem in dentistry. *Quintessence Int.* 1985; 16:221-3.

Scully C. Orofacial manifestations of chronic granulomatous disease of childhood. *Oral Surg Oral Med Oral Pathol.* 1981; 51:148-51.

Segal AW. Biochemistry and molecular biology of chronic granulomatous disease. *J Inherit Metab Dis.* 1992; 15:683-6.

Umeki S. Mechanisms for the activation/electron transfer of neutrophil NADPH oxidase complex and molecular pathology of chronic granulomatous disease. *Ann Hematol.* 1994; 68:267-77.

LEUKOCYTOSIS

Gin-Shaw S, Moore GP. Selected white cell disorders. *Emerg Med Clin North Am.* 1993; 11:495-516.

Warrell RP, de The H, Wang ZY, Degos L. Acute promyelocytic leukemia. *N Engl J Med.* 1993; 329:177-89; *N Engl J Med.* 1994; 330:141.

INFECTIOUS MONONUCLEOSIS

Bailey RE. Diagnosis and treatment of infectious mononucleosis. *Am Fam Physician.* 1994; 49:879-88.

Cassingham RJ. Infectious mononucleosis: a review of the literature, including recent findings on etiology. *Oral Surg Oral Med Oral Pathol.* 1971; 31:610.

Chetham MM, Roberts KB. Infectious mononucleosis in adolescents. *Pediatr Ann.* 1991; 20:206-13.

Holzel A. An early clinical sign in infectious mononucleosis. *Oral Surg Oral Med Oral Pathol.* 1959; 12:685.

Johnson PA, Avery C. Infectious mononucleosis presenting as a parotid mass with associated facial nerve palsy. *Int J Oral Maxillofac Surg.* 1991; 20:193-5.

Maddern BR, Werkhaven J, Wessel HB, Yunis E. Infectious mononucleosis with airway obstruction and multiple cranial nerve paresis. *Otolaryngol Head Neck Surg.* 1991; 104:529-32.

LEUKEMIA

Auerbach M. Acute myeloid leukemia in patients more than 50 years of age: special considerations in diagnosis, treatment, and prognosis. *Am J Med.* 1994; 96:180-5.

Bradstock KF. The diagnostic and prognostic value of immunophenotyping in acute leukemia. *Pathology.* 1993; 25:367-74.

Debru C. Preconceived ideas in the classification of leukemia. *Blood Cells.* 1993; 19:537-41; discussion 542-7.

Declerck D, Vinckier F. Oral complications of leukemia. *Quintessence Int.* 1988; 19:575-83.

Elbaz O, Mahmoud LA. Tumor necrosis factor and human acute leukemia. *Leuk Lymphoma.* 1994; 12:191-5.

Garfunkel AA, Glick M. Common oral findings in two different diseases: leukemia and AIDS: part 2. *Compendium.* 1992; 13:550, 552-3, 556.

Glick M, Garfunkel AA. Common oral findings in two different diseases: leukemia and AIDS: part 1. *Compendium.* 1992; 13:432, 434, 436.

Gulati SC, Nath B. Leukemia and bone marrow microenvironment. *Stem Cells (Dayt).* 1994; 12:225-6.

Hozumi M. Fundamentals of chemo-differentiation therapy of myeloid leukemia. *Anticancer Res.* 1994; 14:1177-92.

Lowenberg B. Leukemia and myelodysplasia. *Cancer Chemother Biol Response Modif.* 1993; 14:371-82.

Neame PB, Soamboonsrup P, Quigley JG, Pewarchuck W. The use of monoclonal antibodies and immune markers in the diagnosis, prognosis, and therapy of acute leukemia. *Transfus Med Rev.* 1994; 8:59-75.

Ratnam KV, Khor CJ, Su WP. Leukemia cutis. *Dermatol Clin.* 1994; 12:419-31.

Sachs L. The cellular and molecular environment in leukemia. *Blood Cells.* 1993; 19:709-26; discussion 727-30.

Sachs L. The molecular control of hemopoiesis and leukemia. *C R Acad Sci III.* 1993; 316:871-91.

Williams MC, Lee GT. Childhood leukemia and dental considerations. *J Clin Pediatr Dent.* 1991; 15:160-4.

Wingard JR. Viral infections in leukemia and bone marrow transplant patients. *Leuk Lymphoma.* 1993; 11(suppl 2): 115-25.

Yeager KA, Miaskowski C. Advances in understanding the mechanisms and management of acute myelogenous leukemia. *Oncol Nurs Forum.* 1994; 21:541-8.

HODGKIN LYMPHOMA

Dyer MJ. The new genetics and non-Hodgkin lymphoma. *Eur J Cancer.* 1990; 26:1099-102.

La Via MF, Self SE. Immunophenotypic analysis of non-Hodgkin's lymphomas. *Recenti Prog Med.* 1990; 81:629-34.

Leventhal BG, Kato GJ. Childhood Hodgkin and non-Hodgkin lymphomas. *Pediatr Rev.* 1990; 12:171-9.

McClain KL, Heise R, Day DL, Lee CK and others. Hodgkin's disease in children: correlation of clinical characteristics, staging procedures, and treatment at the University of Minnesota. *Am J Pediatr Hematol Oncol.* 1990; 12:147-54.

Mueller N. Epidemiologic studies assessing the role of the Epstein-Barr virus in Hodgkin's disease. *Yale J Biol Med.* 1987; 60:321-32.

Oza AM, Lister TA. Diagnosis and staging of Hodgkin's disease. *Curr Opin Oncol.* 1990; 2:832-7.

Pinkus GS, Lones M, Shintaku IP, Said JW. Immunohistochemical detection of Epstein-Barr virus-encoded latent membrane protein in Reed-Sternberg cells and variants of Hodgkin's disease. *Mod Pathol.* 1994; 7:454-61.

Rosenberg SA. The treatment of Hodgkin's disease. *Ann Oncol.* 1994; 2:17-21.

Tedeschi L, Romanelli A, Dallavalle G, Tavani E and others. Stages I and II non-Hodgkin's lymphoma of the gastrointestinal tract: retrospective analysis of 79 patients and review of the literature. *J Clin Gastroenterol.* 1994; 18:99-104.

NON-HODGKIN LYMPHOMA

Eisenbud L, Sciubba J, Mir R, Sachs SA. Oral presentations in non-Hodgkin's lymphoma: a review of thirty-one cases: part I: data analysis. *Oral Surg Oral Med Oral Pathol.* 1983; 56:151-156.

Green TL, Eversole LR. Oral lymphomas in HIV-infected patients: association with Epstein-Barr virus DNA. *Oral Surg Oral Med Oral Pathol.* 1989; 67:437-442.

Handlers JP, Howell RE, Abrams AM, Melrose RJ. Extranodal oral lymphoma: part I: a morphologic and immunoperoxidase study of 34 cases. *Oral Surg Oral Med Oral Pathol.* 1989; 61:362-367.

Hashimoto N, Kurihara K, Pathologic characteristics of oral lymphomas. *J Oral Pathol.* 1982; 11:214-227.

Ioachim HL, Dorsett B, Cronin W, Maya M and others. Acquired immunodeficiency syndrome-associated lymphomas: clinical, pathologic, immunologic, and viral characteristics of 111 cases. *Hum Pathol.* 1991; 22:659-673.

BURKITT LYMPHOMA

Kornblau SM, Goodacre A, Cabanillas F. Chromosomal abnormalities in adult nonepidemic Burkitt's lymphoma and leukemia: 22 new reports and review of 148 cases from the literature. *Hematol Oncol.* 1991; 9:63-78.

MULTIPLE MYELOMA

Bross DA, Perez-Atayde A, Mandell VS, Hyams JS and others. Hereditary hemorrhagic telangiectasia presenting in early childhood. *J Pediatr Gastroenterol Nutr.* 1994; 18:497-500.

Kikuchi K, Kowada M, Sasajima H. Vascular malformations of the brain in hereditary hemorrhagic telangiectasia (Rendu-Osler-Weber disease). *Surg Neurol.* 1994; 41:374-80.

Rhodus NL, Kuba R. Hereditary hemorrhagic telangiectasia with florid osseous dysplasia: report of a case with differential diagnostic considerations. *Oral Surg Oral Med Oral Pathol.* 1993; 75:48-53.

Siegel MB, Keane WM, Atkins JF, Rosen MR. Control of epistaxis in patients with hereditary hemorrhagic telangiectasia. *Otolaryngol Head Neck Surg.* 1991; 105:675-9.

Sureda A, Cesar J, Garcia Frade LJ, Garcia Avello A and others. Hereditary hemorrhagic telangiectasia: analysis of platelet aggregation and fibrinolytic system in seven patients. *Acta Haematol.* 1991; 85:119-23.

THROMBOCYTOPENIA

Blockmans D, Vermylen J. HIV-related thrombocytopenia. *Acta Clin Belg.* 1992; 47:117-23.

De masi R, Bode AP, Knupp C, Bogey W and others. Heparin-induced thrombocytopenia. *Am Surg.* 1994; 60:26-9.

Eisenberg MJ, Kaplan B. Cytomegalovirus-induced thrombocytopenia in an immunocompetent adult. *West J Med.* 1993; 158:525-6.

Fischereder M, Jaffe JP. Thrombocytopenia following acute acetaminophen overdose. *Am J Hematol.* 1994; 45:258-9.

Hohlfeld P, Forestier F, Kaplan C, Tissot JD and others. Diagnosis and management of foetal thrombocytopenia. *Nouv Rev Fr Hematol.* 1993; 35:413-8.

Kaplan C, Morel-Kopp MC, Clemenceau S, Daffos F. Fetal and neonatal alloimmune thrombocytopenia: current trends in diagnosis and therapy. *Transfus Med.* 1992; 2:265-71.

Phillips DE, Payne DK, Mills GM. Heparin-induced thrombotic thrombocytopenia. *Ann Pharmacother.* 1994; 28:43-6.

Rutherford CJ, Frenkel EP. Thrombocytopenia: issues in diagnosis and therapy. *Med Clin North Am.* 1994; 78:555-75.

THROMBASTHENIA

Clemetson KJ, Clemetson JM. Molecular pathology of the Bernard-Soulier syndrome, platelet-type von Willebrand's disease and Glanzmann's thrombasthenia. *Beitr Infusionther.* 1993; 31:168-73.

Perutelli P, Mori PG. Biochemical and molecular basis of Glanzmann's thrombasthenia. *Haematologica.* 1992; 77:421-6.

Tardio DJ, McFarland JA, Gonzalez MF. Immune thrombocytopenic purpura: current concepts. *J Gen Intern Med.* 1993; 8:160-3.

VITAMIN C DEFICIENCY

Fornstedt B, Carlsson A. Vitamin C deficiency facilitates 5-S-cysteinyldopamine formation in guinea pig striatum. *J Neurochem.* 1991; 56:407-14.

Mao X, Yao G. Effect of vitamin C supplementations on iron deficiency anemia in Chinese children. *Biomed Environ Sci.* 1992; 5:125-9.

Taniguchi M, Imamura H, Shirota T, Okamatsu H and others. Improvement in iron deficiency anemia through therapy with ferric ammonium citrate and vitamin C and the effects of aerobic exercise. *J Nutr Sci Vitaminol (Tokyo).* 1991; 37:161-71.

Wegger I, Palludan B. Vitamin C deficiency causes hematological and skeletal abnormalities during fetal development in swine. *J Nutr.* 1994; 124:241-8.

HEREDITARY HEMORRHAGIC TELANGIECTASIA

Bross DA, Perez-Atayde A, Mandell VS, Hyams JS and others. Hereditary hemorrhagic telangiectasia presenting in early childhood. *J Pediatr Gastroenterol Nutr.* 1994; 18:497-500.

Kikuchi K, Kowada M, Sasajima H. Vascular malformations of the brain in hereditary hemorrhagic telangiectasia (Rendu-Osler-Weber disease). *Surg Neurol.* 1994; 41:374-80.

Rhodus NL, Kuba R. Hereditary hemorrhagic telangiectasia with florid osseous dysplasia: report of a case with differential diagnostic considerations. *Oral Surg Oral Med Oral Pathol.* 1993; 75:48-53.

Siegel MB, Keane WM, Atkins JF, Rosen MR. Control of epistaxis in patients with hereditary hemorrhagic telangiectasia. *Otolaryngol Head Neck Surg.* 1991; 105:675-9.

Sureda A, Cesar J, Garcia Frade LJ, Garcia Avello A and others. Hereditary hemorrhagic telangiectasia: analysis of platelet aggregation and fibrinolytic system in seven patients. *Acta Haematol.* 1991; 85:119-23.

HEMOPHILIA

Blanchette V, Walker I, Gill P, Adams M and others. Hepatitis C infection in patients with hemophilia: results of a national survey. Canadian Hemophilia Clinic Directors Group. *Transfus Med Rev.* 1994; 8:210-7.

Furie B, Limentani SA, Rosenfield CG. A practical guide to the evaluation and treatment of hemophilia. *Blood.* 1994; 84:3-9.

Hoyer LW. Hemophilia A. *N Engl J Med.* 1994; 330:38-47.

Kazazian HH. The molecular basis of hemophilia A and the present status of carrier and antenatal diagnosis of the disease. *Thromb Haemost.* 1993; 70:60-2.

Lillicrap D. The molecular pathology of hemophilia A. *Transfus Med Rev.* 1991; 5:196-206.

Lozier JN, Santagostino E, Kasper CK, Teitel JM and others. Use of porcine factor VIII for surgical procedures in hemophilia A patients with inhibitors. *Semin Hematol.* 1993; 30(2 suppl 1):10-21.

Lusher JM, Warrier I. Hemophilia A. *Hematol Oncol Clin North Am.* 1992; 6:1021-33.

Mudad R, Kane WH. DDAVP in acquired hemophilia A: case report and review of the literature. *Am J Hematol.* 1993; 43:295-9.

Pfaff JA, Geninatti M. Hemophilia. *Emerg Med Clin North Am.* 1993; 11:337-63.

Roberts HR. Molecular biology of hemophilia B. *Thromb Haemost.* 1993; 70:1-9.

Roberts HR, Eberst ME. Current management of hemophilia B. *Hematol Oncol Clin North Am.* 1993; 7:1269-80.

Tozman EC. Sickle-cell disease, hemophilia, and hematology. *Curr Opin Rheumatol.* 1993; 5:95-8.

INDEX

Vascular tissue lesions, 305-12
  angiosarcomas, 310
  hamartomatous/benign neoplasms, *307*,
    307-9
  hemangiomas, *307*, 307-9, *308*, *309*
  hyperplasias, 305-7, *306*
  Kaposi sarcoma, *311*, 311-12, *312*
  lymphangiomas, *309*, 309-10, *310*
  pyogenic granulomas, 305-7, *306*
Vegetable allergies, 268
Venereal Disease Research Laboratory test
    (VDRL), for syphilis, 225
Venereal warts, from condyloma
    acuminatum, 213
Vermilionectomy, for cheilitis glandularis,
    271
Verruca vulgaris, *212*, 212-13
Verrucous carcinomas, *182*, 182-83, *183*
Verrucous hyperplasias, 168
Vertical impactions, 5, *5*
Vestigial tract cysts, *55*, 55-56
Vietnam, oral submucous fibrosis in, 169-
    70, *170*
Viral infections, *197*, 197-221
  acute lymphonodular pharyngitis, 209
  acute nonspecific ulcers, 219, *219*
  candidiasis, 218, *219*
  condyloma acuminatum, *213*, 213-14
  coxsackie viruses, 207-9
  cytomegalovirus, *207*, *207*
  deep invasive fungal infections, 219
  EBV, 206-7
  focal epithelial hyperplasias, 214
  gingivitis/periodontitis, 219, *219*
  hairy leukoplakia, 217-18, *218*
  hand, foot, mouth disease, 208, *208*
  herpangina, 208, *208*
  herpes simplex, *198*, 198-99, *199*
    secondary oral, *200*, 200-201, *201*
  herpes viruses, 198-208
  herpes zoster, 204-5, *205*
  herpetic whitlow, 201-4, *202*, *203*
  with HIV, 214-21, *215*, 221
  human papilloma viruses, 211-13
  infectious mononucleosis, *206*, 206-7
  Kaposi sarcoma, 219, *220*, 221
  measles, 13, 210-11
  mumps, 211, 331-32
  non-Hodgkin lymphoma, 221, *221*
  paramyxoviruses, 210-11
  retroviruses, 214-21, *215*
  rubella, 209-10
  squamous papillomas, 212
  togavirus, 209-10
  varicella, 204, *204*
  varicella-zoster virus, *204*, 204-5,
    205
  verruca vulgaris, *212*, 212-13
Viral parotitis, 331, *332*
Virus-associated leukocytosis, 392-93
Vitamin A deficiencies, 13
Vitamin B$_{12}$
  for aphthous minor, 247
  for pernicious anemia, 384

Vitamin C deficiencies, 13, 409
Vitamin D, for hyperparathyroidism, 103
Vitamin K, inhibition of, 412
von Willebrand Factor VIII, in
    thrombasthenia assessments, 408
VZV; *see* Varicella-zoster viruses (VZV)

W
Warthin tumors, 343
Warts
  in condyloma acuminatum, 213
  in verruca vulgaris, 212
Weight loss, in HIV pre-AIDS symptoms,
    216
Western countries, Paget's disease in, 99
White blood cell disorders, 387-90
  agranulocytosis, 388-89, *389*
  bacteria-associated leukocytosis, 392
  Burkitt lymphoma, 403-4, *404*
  cyclic neutropenia, 390
  Hodgkin lymphoma, 396t, 396-99, *399*
  infectious mononucleosis, 393-94
  leukemias, 394-96, *395*
  leukocytosis, *391*, 391-94
    virus-associated, 392-93
  leukopenia, 388-90
  multiple myelomas, 404-6, *405*, *406*
  neoplasms, 394-406
  neutrophil function disorders, 390
  non-Hodgkin lymphoma, 399-403, *400*,
    401, *402*
  pediatric chronic granulomatous disease,
    391
White sponge nevus, *24*, 24-25
WHO; *see* World Health Organization
    (WHO)
Wilms tumor, with hemifacial hypertrophy,
    26, *26*
Women; *see* Females
World Health Organization (WHO)
  on cementoblastomas, 144-45, *145*
  on central odontogenic fibromas, 141-
    42, *142*
  on leukoplakia, 164
  on odontogenic fibromas, 140
  on periapical cemento dysplasias, 90
Wormian bones, 31

X
Xerophthalmia, immune-mediated, 332
Xerostomia
  with AIDS, 217
  from *candida albicans*, 370
  from radiation injuries, 370
  with Sjögren syndrome, 333, 334

Z
Zone depths, in dental caries, *66*, 66-68, *67*
Zygomycosis, 237, *237*